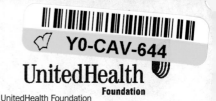
UnitedHealth

Foundation

UnitedHealth Foundation
P.O. Box 1459 Minneapolis, MN 55440-1459

July, 2002

Dear Colleague,

We at UnitedHealth Foundation are once again pleased to provide our nation's pediatricians with a complimentary copy of the BMJ Publishing Group's increasingly relevant publication, *Clinical Evidence*. This marks the fifth edition that we have been privileged to distribute. *Clinical Evidence* is an international resource that benefits from considerable input by clinical experts from the United States.

We are particularly excited to present you with this *new edition* of *Clinical Evidence* called *Clinical Evidence Pediatrics*. As the pace of clinical and evidence-based health research has intensified, the BMJ noted that both the content and size of *Clinical Evidence* was expanding. Given that the goal is to provide useful information in a convenient and easy to access format, the growing size of *Clinical Evidence* is becoming an issue. As such, we think the BMJ's decision to provide this pediatric version of *Clinical Evidence* was the right decision to support pediatricians in the practice of the best possible care to their patients. Of course, as a recipient of the UnitedHealth Foundation distribution you continue to have free access to *Clinical Evidence Online*. To make use of this feature, go to *www.clinicalevidence.com*. Once there, register as a recipient of UHF distribution.

We also want to bring to your attention the special role played in this pediatric edition by the American Academy of Pediatrics and their Section on Epidemiology. We are excited to work in collaboration with them and the BMJ Publishing Group to provide US pediatricians with this new edition. The American Academy of Pediatrics is to be commended for their leadership in advocating and supporting the best evidence-based health care for our nation's children.

We think that *Clinical Evidence Pediatrics* will support you in providing quality medicine that meets the high standards for which we all strive.

Sincerely,

Bill McGuire

William W. McGuire, M.D.
Chairman
UnitedHealth Foundation

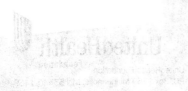

clinical
evidence

Pediatrics

The international source of the
best available evidence for
child health care

Reprinted from *Clinical Evidence*, Issue 7, 2002, published by the BMJ Publishing Group.

Editorial Office
BMJ Publishing Group, BMA House, Tavistock Square, London, WC1H 9JR, United Kingdom.
Tel: +44 (0)20 7387 4499 • Fax: +44 (0)20 7383 6242 • www.bmjpg.com

Subscription rates for the full *Clinical Evidence*
The complete edition of *Clinical Evidence* and *Clinical Evidence Concise* with companion CD-ROM are both published six monthly (June/December) by BMJ Publishing Group.The annual subscription rates for both publications (June, Issue 7, and December, Issue 8) are:

Personal: £75 • US$110 • Can$160
Institutional: £160 • US$240 • Can$345
Student/nurse: £35 • US$50 • Can$75

The above rates are for either the full print or the concise formats. The combined rates, for both formats, are:

Personal £110 • US$165 • Can$235
Institutional £220 • US$330 • Can$475
Student/nurse £60 • US$90 • Can$130

All individual subscriptions (personal, student, nurse) include online access at no additional cost. Institutional subscriptions are for full print/concise version only. Institutions may purchase online site licences separately. The Publishers offer discounts for any society or organisation buying bulk quantities for their members/specific groups. For further subscription information please visit the subscription pages of our website www.clinicalevidence.com or contact Miranda Lonsdale at mlonsdale@bmjgroup.com (outside the Americas) or Diane McCabe at ussales@bmjgroup.com (North and South Americas). You may also telephone us or fax us on the following numbers:

UK and ROW Tel: +44 (0)20 7383 6270 • Fax: +44 (0)20 7383 6402
Americas Tel: +1 800 373 2897/240 646 7000 • Fax: +1 240 646 7005

Contributors
If you are interested in becoming a contributor to *Clinical Evidence* please contact us at clinicalevidence@bmjgroup.com.

Rights
For information on translation rights, please contact Daniel Raymond-Barker at draymond-barker@bmjgroup.com.

British Library Cataloguing in Publication Data
A catalogue record for this book is available from the British Library:
ISBN 0-7279-1795-1

Permission to reproduce
Please contact Josephine Woodcock at jwoodcock@bmjgroup.com when requesting permission to reprint all or part of any contribution in *Clinical Evidence* or its specialty editions.

Legal Disclaimer
Care has been taken to confirm the accuracy of the information presented and to describe generally accepted practices. However, the authors, editors, and publishers are not responsible for errors or omissions or for any consequences from application of the information in this book and make no warranty, express or implied, with respect to the contents of the publication.

Categories presented in *Clinical Evidence* and other specialty editions indicate a judgement about the strength of the evidence available and the relative importance of benefits and harms. The categories do not indicate whether a particular treatment is generally appropriate or whether it is suitable for individuals.

Printed by Quebecor, Kingsport, Tennessee, USA.

Acknowledgements

For this pediatric edition of *Clinical Evidence*, the American Academy of Pediatrics (AAP) Section on Epidemiology would like to acknowledge the executive committee, especially Dan Neuspiel and Regina Rabinovich, present and past chairs of the AAP Section on Epidemiology, for enthusiastic support in getting this project under way, and also the members of the Section on Epidemiology for reviewing the content and selecting the topics to be included in this edition. We also thank the leadership of the American Academy of Pediatrics, especially Dr Joe Sanders, Dr Ed Zimmerman and Maureen DeRosa for support and assistance in completing the project. We also want to acknowledge the support of the UnitedHealth Foundation for underwriting the cost of printing and distributing this special edition.

The BMJ Publishing Group thanks the following people and organisations for their advice and support: The Cochrane Collaboration, and especially Iain Chalmers, Mike Clarke, Phil Alderson, Peter Langhorne and Carol Lefebvre; the NHS Centre for Reviews and Dissemination, and especially Jos Kleijnen and Julie Glanville; the NHS, and especially Tom Mann, Sir John Patteson, Ron Stamp, Veronica Fraser, Muir Gray and Ben Toth; the British National Formulary, and especially Dinesh Mehta, Eric Connor and John Martin; the Health Information Research Unit at McMaster University, and especially Brian Haynes and Ann McKibbon; the UnitedHealth Foundation, and especially Dr Reed Tuckson and Yvette Krantz; the clinicians, epidemiologists, and members of patient support groups who have acted as peer reviewers. The BMJ Publishing Group values the ongoing support it has received from the global medical community for *Clinical Evidence*. In addition to others, we wish to acknowledge the efforts of the UnitedHealth Foundation who have provided educational funding to support the wide dissemination of this valuable resource to many physicians and health professionals in the USA. It is hoped that the use of this material will continue to provide expert guidance for good patient outcome. We are grateful to the clinicians and patients who spare time to take part in focus groups, which are crucial to the development of *Clinical Evidence*. Finally, we would like to acknowledge the readers who have taken the time to send us their comments and suggestions.

Contents

Clinical Evidence Pediatrics

When the first issue of *Clinical Evidence* was published in 1999, the American Academy of Pediatrics' (AAP) Section on Epidemiology recognized that this was a valuable source of high quality information, but the topics relevant to pediatrics seemed lost among the many adult topics. We wondered then whether we might be able to team up with the BMJ Publishing Group to produce a specialty version of *Clinical Evidence* that was aimed just at clinicians who care for children. We felt that if we were able to make it comprehensive and widely applicable to primary care pediatricians, such a resource could be tremendously valuable to pediatricians in practice.

As *Clinical Evidence* developed, we worked closely with the BMJ Publishing Group towards this goal and this short volume is the first product of that effort. The full version of *Clinical Evidence* has plenty of information that is relevant to pediatric practice but, as might be expected in a publication originally aimed at general practitioners, includes lots of information not relevant to pediatrics; this made the book heavy and unwieldy as a quick reference for pediatricians.

Clinical Evidence Pediatrics contains all the child health topics published in *Clinical Evidence* in one easily accessible volume. Topics that apply to children alone, to both children and adults, and some topics that apply particularly to adolescents are included in this special pediatric edition. Members of the AAP Section on Epidemiology reviewed the list of topics and the content of each topic to be sure that these were of greatest value to US pediatricians. Time and cost restraints prevented us from changing the UK spellings and drug names, so conversion tables for measurements, terms and drug names are included at the front of the book to help with "translation". Members of the AAP, including committee and section leadership, were surveyed to determine what new topics would be of particular interest to US pediatricians; please use the response card in this book to add your own suggestions for potential future editions.

HOW TO USE CLINICAL EVIDENCE
Clinical Evidence is a book of evidence — no more and no less. Its purpose is to give you with the evidence you need to provide the best and most up-to-date care for your patients. Treatments are listed and categorized at the beginning of each topic according to what the best available evidence suggests (i.e. whether the treatment is *beneficial*, *likely to be beneficial*, has a *trade-off* between known benefits and harms, is of *unknown effectiveness*, or is *likely to be ineffective or harmful*).

The evidence is carefully and systematically collected (see How *Clinical Evidence* is put together, p xv), and is discussed and fully referenced in subsequent pages. This book makes no treatment recommendations, recognizing that the evidence, although absolutely necessary to good clinical decision making, must be considered in the context of the individual patient's clinical situation and personal preferences.

ACCESS
As a recipient of this book, you also have full access to the online version of *Clinical Evidence* — this is the full (adults and children) version. *Clinical Evidence* Online (www.clinicalevidence.com) is searchable and constantly updated. For information on PDA formats, please refer to the *Clinical Evidence* website homepage (www.clinicalevidence.com) for details and platform choices.

FEEDBACK

If US primary care pediatricians, many of whom are fellows of the AAP, find this volume useful, we would like to explore the development of an expanded version of *Clinical Evidence Pediatrics* that includes as many topics as US pediatricians require. Please let us know the benefits and limitations of this book and how it could be improved by pulling out the survey card at the end of the book and mailing or faxing us your comments. You may also complete the online feedback form at www.clinicalevidence.com to let us know what we can do to make this book as useful to you as possible.

Virginia A Moyer, MD, MPH, FAAP
Section Advisor on Child health
Professor of Pediatrics

About Clinical Evidence

The inspiration for *Clinical Evidence* came in a phone call in 1995. Tom Mann and his colleagues at the NHS Executive asked the BMJ Publishing Group to explore the possibility of developing an evidence "formulary" along the lines of the *British National Formulary*. They recognised that clinicians were under increasing pressure to keep up-to-date and to base their practice more firmly on evidence, but that few had the necessary time or skills to do this. Their idea was to provide a pocket book containing concise and regularly updated summaries of the best available evidence on clinical interventions. However, they didn't think that the NHS could develop such a formulary itself. "It would be marvellous", said Tom Mann, "if somebody would just do it". A small team at the BMJ set to work to produce a pilot version of what was then called the *Clinical Effectiveness Directory*.

Since that pilot, a great deal has changed. In collaboration with the American College of Physicians–American Society of Internal Medicine, we convened an international advisory board, held focus groups of clinicians, talked to patient support groups, and adopted countless good ideas from early drafts by our contributors. Throughout we have kept in mind an equation set out by Slawson et al.[1] This states that the usefulness of any source of information is equal to its relevance, multiplied by its validity, divided by the work required to extract the information. In order to be as useful as possible, we aimed for high relevance, high validity, and low work in terms of the reader's time and effort. We also kept in mind principles of transparency and explicitness. Readers needed to understand where our information came from and how it was assembled.

A UNIQUE RESOURCE
Clinical Evidence joins a growing number of sources of evidence-based information for clinicians. But it has several features that make it unique.

- Its contents are driven by questions rather than by the availability of research evidence. Rather than start with the evidence and summarise what is there, we have tried to identify important clinical questions, and then to search for and summarise the best available evidence to answer them.
- It identifies but does not try to fill important gaps in the evidence. In a phrase used by Jerry Osheroff, who has led much of the recent research on clinicians' information needs,[2] *Clinical Evidence* presents the dark as well as the light side of the moon. We feel that it will be helpful for clinicians to know when their uncertainty stems from gaps in the evidence rather than gaps in their own knowledge.
- It is updated every 6 months in print and monthly online. *Clinical Evidence* is also available in a concise format with companion CD-ROM.
- It specifically aims not to make recommendations. We feel that simply summarising the evidence will make it more widely useful. The experience of the clinical practice guideline movement has shown that it is nearly impossible to make recommendations that are appropriate in every situation. Differences in individual patients' baseline risks and preferences, and in the local availability of interventions, will always mean that the evidence must be individually interpreted rather than applied across the board. *Clinical Evidence* provides the raw material for developing locally applicable clinical practice guidelines, and for clinicians and patients to make up their own minds on the best course of action. We supply the evidence, you make the decisions.

COMPLEMENTARY BUT DIFFERENT
We are often asked how *Clinical Evidence* differs from two other high quality sources of evidence-based information: The *Cochrane Library*; and the evidence-based journals *ACP Journal Club*, *Evidence-Based Medicine*, *Evidence-Based Mental Health*, and *Evidence-Based Nursing*.

Clinical Evidence is complementary to but different from the work of the Cochrane Collaboration, which produces and publishes high quality systematic reviews of controlled trials.[3] *Clinical Evidence* has been called the friendly front end of the *Cochrane Library*, because it takes this and other, high quality information, and pulls it together in one place in a concise format. Many of our advisors and contributors are active members of the Cochrane Collaboration, and we are exploring closer ties between *Clinical Evidence* and the Collaboration in the way the evidence is searched for, summarised, and accessed by users.

Clinical Evidence is also complementary to but different from the evidence-based journals, which select and abstract the best and most clinically relevant articles as they appear in the world's medical literature. Together these journals form a growing archive of high quality abstracts of individual articles. *Clinical Evidence* takes a different approach. It begins not with the journals but with clinical questions. It is able to answer some. For others it simply reports that no good evidence was found.

DRUG NAMES

Clinical Evidence aims to present information on therapeutic drugs in a format that is relevant for an international audience. Only the generic or non-proprietary names of drugs rather than the brand names of drugs are used in *Clinical Evidence*, with a few exceptions where the brand name has become the commonly used name in clinical practice, for example EMLA cream (lidocaine-prilocaine). Difficulties arise when different names for the same drug are used in different parts of the world. The recommended International Name (rINN) or proposed International Name (pINN) is used where possible. Where an international name for a therapeutic drug is not available (e.g. aspirin), the most common name has been used. We have included a table of the drug names used in *Clinical Evidence* with the equivalent UK and US names (see p xxiii).

A WORK IN PROGRESS

Clinical Evidence is an evolving project. We knew before we started that we were undertaking an enormous task, but the more we worked the more we realised its enormity. We recognise that there is some mismatch between what we aim eventually to achieve and what we have achieved so far. Although we have made every effort to ensure that the searches are thorough and that the appraisals of studies are objective (see Searching and Appraising the literature p xv), we will inevitably have missed some important studies. In order not to make unjustified claims about the accuracy of the information, we use phrases such as "we found no systematic review"; rather than "there is no systematic review". In order to be as explicit as possible about the methods used for each contribution, we have asked each set of contributors to provide a brief methods section, describing the searches that were performed and how individual studies were selected.

UPDATING AND EXPANDING CLINICAL EVIDENCE

Our expectation is that *Clinical Evidence* will evolve rapidly in its early years. Indeed, it is already becoming a family of products, appearing in different formats and languages for different audiences. In particular, *Clinical Evidence* will evolve in response to the needs of clinicians. We have tried hard to anticipate those needs (not least by involving clinicians at every stage), but it is only when people begin to use *Clinical Evidence* in daily practice that we can know how best to develop it. That's why your feedback is so important to us, and we are arranging for various ways to evaluate the product.

REFERENCES

1. Slawson DC, Shaughnessy AF, Bennett JH. Becoming a medical information master: feeling good about not knowing everything. *J Fam Pract* 1994;38:505–513.
2. Ely JW, Osheroff JA, Ebell MJ, et al. Analysis of questions asked by family doctors regarding patient care. *BMJ* 1999; 319:358–361.
3. http://hiru.mcmaster.ca/cochrane/default.htm

A guide to the text

SUMMARY PAGE

The summary page for each topic presents the questions addressed, some key messages, and a list of the interventions covered, categorised according to whether they have been found to be effective or not. We have developed the categories of effectiveness from one of the Cochrane Collaboration's first and most popular products, *A guide to effective care in pregnancy and childbirth*.[1] The categories we now use are explained in the table below:

TABLE	Categorisation of treatment effects in *Clinical Evidence*
Beneficial	Interventions for which effectiveness has been demonstrated by clear evidence from RCTs, and for which expectation of harms is small compared with the benefits.
Likely to be beneficial	Interventions for which effectiveness is less well established than for those listed under "beneficial".
Trade off between benefits and harms	Interventions for which clinicians and patients should weigh up the beneficial and harmful effects according to individual circumstances and priorities.
Unknown effectiveness	Interventions for which there are currently insufficient data or data of inadequate quality.
Unlikely to be beneficial	Interventions for which lack of effectiveness is less well established than for those listed under "likely to be ineffective or harmful".
Likely to be ineffective or harmful	Interventions for which ineffectiveness or harmfulness has been demonstrated by clear evidence.

Fitting interventions into these categories is not always straightforward. For one thing, the categories represent a mix of several hierarchies: the level of benefit (or harm), the level of evidence (RCT or observational data), and the level of certainty around the finding (represented by the confidence interval). Another problem is that much of the evidence that is most relevant to clinical decisions relates to comparisons between different interventions rather than to comparison with placebo or no intervention. Where necessary, we have indicated the comparisons in brackets. A third problem is that interventions may have been tested, or found to be effective, in only one group of people, such as those at high risk of an outcome. Again, we have indicated this where possible. But perhaps most difficult of all has been trying to maintain consistency across different topics. We are working on refining the criteria for putting interventions under each category.

Interventions that cannot be tested in an RCT (perhaps because of ethical or practical reasons) are sometimes cited in the categorisation table, but they are always identified clearly with an asterix (for example, oxygen in severe acute asthma).

NEGATIVE FINDINGS

A surprisingly hard aspect to get right is the reporting of negative findings. As we have had to keep reminding ourselves, saying that there is no good evidence that a treatment works is not the same as saying that the treatment doesn't work. In trying to get this right, we may have erred too much on the side of caution; when in doubt we have changed summary phrases from, for example, "the review found no difference", to "the review found no evidence of a difference". We recognise that to get this right, we need a better handle on the power of individual systematic reviews and trials to demonstrate statistically significant differences between groups, and better information on what constitutes clinically important differences in the major outcomes for each intervention. In the meantime, we hope that the text makes a clear distinction between lack of benefit and lack of evidence of benefit.

OUTCOMES
Clinical Evidence focuses on outcomes that matter to patients, meaning those that patients themselves are aware of, such as symptom severity, quality of life, survival, disability, walking distance, and live birth rate. We are less interested in proxy outcomes such as blood lipid concentrations, blood pressure, or ovulation rates. Each topic includes a list of the main patient oriented outcomes, and where possible describes how these are measured. We have for the moment decided not to address the vexed question of what constitutes a clinically important change in an outcome, but we would welcome any suggestions.

EFFECTS, NOT EFFECTIVENESS
A key aim of *Clinical Evidence* is to emphasise the important trade offs between advantages and disadvantages of different treatment options. We therefore talk about the effects of interventions, both positive and negative, rather than the effectiveness, and for each question or intervention option we present data on benefits and harms under separate headings.

HARMS
"Harms" include adverse effects of treatment and inconvenience to the patient. Finding good evidence on harms of treatments is not easy. Ideally these would come from RCTs, but many trials are not sufficiently large or long term to capture rarer or more distant events, and many do not adequately report adverse effects. We have asked contributors to keep the negative effects of interventions in mind at all times. Where good evidence is available, we indicate the frequency of adverse effects. However, because RCTs are not reliable sources of evidence about harms, and because of the principle that a physician should strive to do no harm, we also include weaker forms of evidence about harms.

DRUG INFORMATION
We make no systematic attempt to provide information on drug dosages, formulations, indications, and contraindications. For this information, we refer readers to their national drug formularies. Drug dosages are included when a question explores the relative effects of different doses.

INFORMATION ON COST
We have decided not to include information on the cost or cost effectiveness of interventions. This is not because we believe cost to be unimportant, but because the question of what constitutes good evidence on cost is much disputed and because costs vary greatly both within and between countries. However, we believe that it will become increasingly untenable for clinicians to act without paying attention to resources. Future companion publications of *Clinical Evidence* may provide relevant information on costs.

NUMERICAL DATA
Whenever possible, data are presented in the same form as in the original studies. However, sometimes we have changed the units or type of information in an attempt to present the results in a systematic and easily interpretable form.

AN INTERNATIONAL APPROACH TO THE EVIDENCE
Clinical Evidence takes an international approach to the evidence. This means including drugs that are not licensed in some countries. It also means keeping in mind the practicalities of treating people in rich as well as poorer countries, by covering interventions even if they have been superseded (for example, single drug treatment for HIV infection as opposed to three drug treatment).

COMPETING INTERESTS

In line with the *BMJ*'s policy,[2] our aim is not to try to eliminate conflicts of interest but to make them explicit so that readers can judge for themselves what influence, if any, these may have had on the contributors' interpretation of the evidence. We therefore ask all contributors to let us know about any potential competing interests, and we append any that are declared to the end of the contribution. Where the contributor gives no competing interests, we record "none declared".

HOW TO USE THE INFORMATION IN CLINICAL EVIDENCE

The type of information contained in *Clinical Evidence* is necessary but not sufficient for the provision of effective, high quality health care. It is intended as an aid to clinical decision making, to be used in conjunction with other important sources of information. These other sources include estimates of people's baseline risk of a condition or outcome based on history, physical examination and clinical investigations; individual preferences; economic arguments; availability of treatments; and local expertise.

   Some guidance on how to apply research evidence in practice is available on our website (www.clinicalevidence.com) and in appendix 2.

REFERENCES

1. Enkin M, Keirse M, Renfrew M, et al. *A guide to effective care in pregnancy and childbirth*. Oxford: Oxford University Press, 1998.
2. Smith R. Beyond conflict of interest. *BMJ* 1998;317:219–292.

How Clinical Evidence is put together

The summaries in *Clinical Evidence* result from a rigorous process aimed at ensuring that the information they contain is both reliable and relevant to clinical practice.

SELECTING TOPICS
Clinical Evidence aims to cover common or important clinical conditions seen in primary and hospital care. To decide which conditions to cover in the first few issues, we reviewed national data on consultation rates, morbidity and mortality, and took advice from generalist clinicians and patient groups. Our website (www.clinicalevidence.com) provides a list of conditions that we are planning to cover in future issues. Further suggestions are welcome.

SELECTING THE QUESTIONS
The questions in *Clinical Evidence* concern the benefits and harms of preventative and therapeutic interventions, with emphasis on outcomes that matter to patients. Questions are selected for their relevance to clinical practice by section advisors and contributors, in collaboration with primary care clinicians and patient groups. Each new issue of *Clinical Evidence* will include new questions as well as updates of existing questions. Readers can suggest new clinical questions using the feedback slips to be found at the back of the book version and on the *Clinical Evidence* website (www.clinicalevidence.com), or by writing directly to *Clinical Evidence*.

SEARCHING AND APPRAISING THE LITERATURE
For each question, the literature is searched using the Cochrane Library, Medline, Embase and, occasionally, other electronic databases, looking first for good systematic reviews of RCTs; then for good RCTs published since the search date of the review. Where we find no good recent systematic reviews, we search for individual RCTs. The date of the search is recorded in the methods section for each topic. Of the studies that are identified in the search, we select and summarise only a small proportion. The selection is done by critically appraising the abstracts of the studies identified in the search, a task performed independently by information scientists using validated criteria similar to those of Sackett et al[1] and Jadad.[2,3] Where the search identifies more than one or two good reviews or trials, we select those we judge to be the most robust or relevant, using the full text of the article. Where we identify few or no good reviews or trials, we include other studies but highlight their limitations. Contributors, who are chosen for their expertise in the field and their skills in epidemiology, are asked to review our selection of studies, and to justify any additions or exclusions they wish to make.

Our search strategy and critical appraisal criteria are available on our website (www.clinicalevidence.com).

SUMMARISING THE EVIDENCE, PEER REVIEW, AND EDITING
The contributors summarise the evidence relating to each question. Each topic is then peer reviewed by the section advisors and by at least three external expert clinicians. The revised text is then extensively edited by editors with clinical and epidemiological training, and data are checked against the original study reports.

REFERENCES
1. Sackett DL, Haynes RB, Guyatt GH, Tugwell P. *Clinical Epidemiology: A basic science for clinical medicine*. 2nd ed. Boston: Little Brown, 1991.
2. Jadad A. Assessing the quality of RCTs: Why, what, how and by whom? In: Jadad A, ed. *Randomised Controlled Trials*. London: BMJ Books, 1998:45–60.
3. Jadad AR, Moore RA, Carroll D, Jenkinson C, et al. Assessing the quality of reports of randomized clinical trials: is blinding necessary? *Control Clin Trials* 1996;17:1–12.

Feedback and Error Correction

Despite the extensive peer review and quality checks, we expect that the text may contain some errors and/or inconsistencies. Please let us know if you find any errors, either by using the comment card at the back of the book or by emailing us at CEfeedback@bmjgroup.com.

Errors are graded as minor, moderate, and major based on an assessment of their potential impact. All errors are corrected in the next printed issue of *Clinical Evidence*. Anything other than a minor error is immediately corrected in the text displayed on our website (www.clinicalevidence.com) and a list of errors corrected is available. Any major errors are highlighted on the log-in page of the website.

If you wish to be notified automatically by e-mail of any corrections and updates, then register for the *Clinical Evidence* alerting service on our website. If you are using the information in *Clinical Evidence* to guide your clinical practice then it is essential to register so that you can remain as up-to-date as possible.

Absolute risk (AR) The probability that an individual will experience the specified outcome during a specified period. It lies in the range 0 to 1, or is expressed as a percentage. In contrast to common usage, the word "risk" may refer to adverse events (such as myocardial infarction) or desirable events (such as cure).

Absolute risk increase (ARI) The absolute difference in risk between the experimental and control groups in a trial. It is used when the risk in the experimental group exceeds the risk in the control group, and is calculated by subtracting the AR in the control group from the AR in the experimental group. This figure does not give any idea of the proportional increase between the two groups: for this, relative risk (RR) is needed (see below).

Absolute risk reduction (ARR) The absolute difference in risk between the experimental and control groups in a trial. It is used when the risk in the control group exceeds the risk in the experimental group, and is calculated by subtracting the AR in the experimental group from the AR in the control group. This figure does not give any idea of the proportional reduction between the two groups: for this, relative risk (RR) is needed (see below).

Allocation concealment A method used to prevent selection bias by concealing the allocation sequence from those assigning participants to intervention groups. Allocation concealment prevents researchers from (unconsciously or otherwise) influencing which intervention group each participant is assigned to.

Applicability The application of the results from clinical trials to individual people. A randomised trial only provides direct evidence of causality within that specific trial. It takes an additional logical step to apply this result to a specific individual. Individual characteristics will affect the outcome for this person.

Baseline risk The risk of the event occurring without the active treatment. Estimated by the baseline risk in the control group.

Bias Systematic deviation of study results from the true results, because of the way(s) in which the study is conducted.

Blinding/blinded A trial is fully blinded if all the people involved are unaware of the treatment group to which trial participants are allocated until after the interpretation of results. This includes trial participants and everyone involved in administering treatment or recording trial results.

Block randomisation Randomisation by a pattern to produce the required number of people in each group.

Case control study A study design that examines a group of people who have experienced an event (usually an adverse event) and a group of people who have not experienced the same event, and looks at how exposure to suspect (usually noxious) agents differed between the two groups. This type of study design is most useful for trying to ascertain the cause of rare events, such as rare cancers.

Case series Analysis of series of people with the disease (there is no comparison group in case series).

Clinically significant A finding that is clinically important. Here, "significant" takes its everyday meaning of "important" (compared with statistically significant; see below). Where the word "significant" or "significance" is used without qualification in the text, it is being used in its statistical sense.

Cluster randomisation A cluster randomised study is one in which a group of participants are randomised to the same intervention together. Examples of cluster randomisation include allocating together people in the same town, hospital, or school. If the results are then analysed by individuals rather than the group as a whole bias can occur.

Cohort study A non-experimental study design that follows a group of people (a cohort), and then looks at how events differ among people within the group. A study that examines a cohort, which differs in respect to exposure to some suspected risk factor (e.g. smoking), is useful for trying to ascertain whether exposure is likely to cause specified events (e.g. lung cancer). Prospective cohort studies (which track participants forward in time) are more reliable than retrospective cohort studies.

Completer analysis Analysis of data from only those participants who remained at the end of the study. Compare with intention to treat analysis, which uses data from all participants who enrolled (see below).

Confidence interval (CI) The 95% confidence interval (or 95% confidence limits) would include 95% of results from studies of the same size and design in the same population. This is close but not identical to saying that the true size of the effect (never exactly known) has a 95% chance of falling within the confidence interval. If the 95% confidence interval for a relative risk (RR) or an odds ratio (OR) crosses 1, then this is taken as no evidence of an effect. The practical advantages of a confidence interval (rather than a P value) is that they present the range of likely effects.

Controls In a randomised controlled trial (RCT), controls refer to the participants in its comparison group. They are allocated either to placebo, no treatment, or a standard treatment.

Crossover randomised trial A trial in which participants receive one treatment and have outcomes measured, and then receive an alternative treatment and have outcomes measured again. The order of treatments is randomly assigned. Sometimes a period of no treatment is used before the trial starts and in between the treatments (washout periods) to minimise interference between

the treatments (carry over effects). Interpretation of the results from crossover randomised controlled trials (RCTs) can be complex.

Cross sectional study A study design that involves surveying a population about an exposure, or condition, or both, at one point in time. It can be used for assessing prevalence of a condition in the population.

Effect size (standardised mean differences) In the medical literature, effect size is used to refer to a variety of measures of treatment effect. In *Clinical Evidence* it refers to a standardised mean difference: a statistic for combining continuous variables (such as pain scores or height), from different scales, by dividing the difference between two means by an estimate of the within group standard deviation.

Event The occurrence of a dichotomous outcome that is being sought in the study (such as myocardial infarction, death, or a four-point improvement in pain score).

Experimental study A study in which the investigator studies the effect of intentionally altering one or more factors under controlled conditions.

Factorial design A factorial design attempts to evaluate more than one intervention compared with control in a single trial, by means of multiple randomisations.

False negative A person with the target condition (defined by the gold standard) who has a negative test result.

False positive A person without the target condition (defined by the gold standard) who has a positive test result.

Fixed effects The "fixed effects" model of meta-analysis assumes, often unreasonably, that the variability between the studies is exclusively because of a random sampling variation around a fixed effect (see random effects below).

Hazard ratio (HR) Broadly equivalent to relative risk (RR); useful when the risk is not constant with respect to time. It uses information collected at different times. The term is typically used in the context of survival over time. If the HR is 0.5 then the relative risk of dying in one group is half the risk of dying in the other group.

Heterogeneity In the context of meta-analysis, heterogeneity means dissimilarity between studies. It can be because of the use of different statistical methods (statistical heterogeneity), or evaluation of people with different characteristics, treatments or outcomes (clinical heterogeneity). Heterogeneity may render pooling of data in meta-analysis unreliable or inappropriate.

Homogeneity Similarity (see heterogeneity above).

Incidence The number of new cases of a condition occurring in a population over a specified period of time.

Intention to treat analysis Analysis of data for all participants based on the group to which they were randomised and not based on the actual treatment they received.

Likelihood ratio The ratio of the probability that an individual with the target condition has a specified test result to the probability that an individual without the target condition has the same specified test result.

Meta-analysis A statistical technique that summarises the results of several studies in a single weighted estimate, in which more weight is given to results of studies with more events and sometimes to studies of higher quality.

Morbidity Rate of illness but not death.

Mortality Rate of death.

Negative likelihood ratio (NLR) The ratio of the probability that an individual with the target condition has a negative test result to the probability that an individual without the target condition has a negative test result. This is the same as the ratio (1-sensitivity/specificity).

Negative predictive value (NPV) The chance of not having a disease given a negative test result (not to be confused with specificity, which is the other way round; see below).

Not significant/non-significant (NS) In *Clinical Evidence*, not significant means that the observed difference, or a larger difference, could have arisen by chance with a probability of more than 1/20 (i.e. 5%), assuming that there is no underlying difference. This is not the same as saying there is no effect, just that this experiment does not provide convincing evidence of an effect. This could be because the trial was not powered to detect an effect that does exist, because there was no effect, or because of the play of chance.

Number needed to harm (NNH) One measure of treatment harm. It is the average number of people from a defined population you would need to treat with a specific intervention for a given period of time to cause one additional adverse outcome. NNH can be calculated as 1/ARI. In *Clinical Evidence*, these are usually rounded downwards.

Number needed to treat (NNT) One measure of treatment effectiveness. It is the number of people you would on average need to treat with a specific intervention for a given period of time to prevent one additional adverse outcome or achieve one additional beneficial outcome. NNT can be calculated as 1/ARR (see appendix 2). In *Clinical Evidence*, NNTs are usually rounded upwards.

NNT for a meta-analysis Absolute measures are useful at describing the effort required to obtain a benefit, but are limited because they are influenced by both the treatment and also by the baseline risk of the individual. If a meta-analysis includes individuals with a range of baseline risks, then no single NNT will be applicable to the people in that meta-analysis, but a single relative measure (odds ratio or relative risk) may be applicable if there is no heterogeneity. In *Clinical Evidence*, a NNT is provided for meta-analysis, based on a combination of the summary odds ratio (OR) and the mean baseline risk observed in average of the control groups.

Odds The odds of an event happening is defined as the probability that an event will occur, expressed as a proportion of the probability that the event will not occur.

Odds ratio (OR) One measure of treatment effectiveness. It is the odds of an event happening in the experimental group expressed as a proportion of the odds of an event happening in the control group. The closer the OR is to one, the smaller the difference in effect between the experimental intervention and the control intervention. If the OR is greater (or less) than one, then the effects of the treatment are more (or less) than those of the control treatment. Note that the effects being measured may be adverse (e.g. death or disability) or desirable (e.g. survival). When events are rare the OR is analagous to the relative risk (RR), but as event rates increase the OR and RR diverge.

Odds reduction The complement of odds ratio (1-OR), similar to the relative risk reduction (RRR) when events are rare.

Placebo A substance given in the control group of a clinical trial, which is ideally identical in appearance and taste or feel to the experimental treatment and believed to lack any disease specific effects. In the context of non-pharmacological interventions, placebo is usually referred to as sham treatments (see sham treatment below).

Positive likelihood ratio (LR+) The ratio of the probability that an individual with the target condition has a positive test result to the probability that an individual without the target condition has a positive test result. This is the same as the ratio (sensitivity/1-specificity).

Positive predictive value (PPV) The chance of having a disease given a positive test result (not to be confused with sensitivity, which is the other way round; see below).

Power A study has adequate power if it can reliably detect a clinically important difference (i.e. between two treatments) if one actually exists. The power of a study is increased when it includes more events or when its measurement of outcomes is more precise.

Pragmatic study An RCT designed to provide results that are directly applicable to normal practice (compared with explanatory trials that are intended to clarify efficacy under ideal conditions). Pragmatic RCTs recruit a population that is representative of those who are normally treated, allow normal compliance with instructions (by avoiding incentives and by using oral instructions with advice to follow manufacturers instructions), and analyse results by "intention to treat" rather than by "on treatment" methods.

Prevalence The proportion of people with a finding or disease in a given population at a given time.

Publication bias Occurs when the likelihood of a study being published varies with the results it finds. Usually, this occurs when studies that find a significant effect are more likely to be published than studies that do not find a significant effect, so making it appear from surveys of the published literature that treatments are more effective than is truly the case.

P value The probability that an observed or greater difference occurred by chance, if it is assumed that there is in fact no real difference between the effects of the interventions. If this probability is less than 1/20 (which is when the P value is less than 0.05), then the result is conventionally regarded as being "statistically significant".

Quasi randomised A trial using a method of allocating participants to different forms of care that is not truly random; for example, allocation by date of birth, day of the week, medical record number, month of the year, or the order in which participants are included in the study (e.g. alternation).

Random effects The "random effects" model assumes a different underlying effect for each study and takes this into consideration as an additional source of variation, which leads to somewhat wider confidence intervals than the fixed effects model. Effects are assumed to be randomly distributed, and the central point of this distribution is the focus of the combined effect estimate (see fixed effects above).

Randomised controlled trial (RCT) A trial in which participants are randomly assigned to two or more groups: at least one (the experimental group) receiving an intervention that is being tested and an other (the comparison or control group) receiving an alternative treatment or placebo. This design allows assessment of the relative effects of interventions.

Regression analysis Given data on a dependent variable and one or more independent variables, regression analysis involves finding the "best" mathematical model to describe or predict the dependent variable as a function of the independent variable(s). There are several regression models that suit different needs. Common forms are linear, logistic, and proportional hazards.

Relative risk (RR) The number of times more likely (RR > 1) or less likely (RR < 1) an event is to happen in one group compared with another. It is the ratio of the absolute risk (AR) for each group. It is analogous to the odds ratio (OR) when events are rare.

Relative risk increase (RRI) The proportional increase in risk between experimental and control participants in a trial.

Relative risk reduction (RRR) The proportional reduction in risk between experimental and control participants in a trial. It is the complement of the relative risk (1-RR).

Sensitivity The chance of having a positive test result given that you have a disease (not to be confused with positive predictive value [PPV], which is the other way around; see above).

Sensitivity analysis Analysis to test if results from meta-analysis are sensitive to restrictions on the data included. Common examples are large trials only, higher quality trials only, and more recent trials only. If results are consistent this provides stronger evidence of an effect and of generalisability.

Sham treatment An intervention given in the control group of a clinical trial, which is ideally identical in appearance and feel to the experimental treatment and believed to lack any disease specific effects (e.g. detuned ultrasound or random biofeedback).

Significant By convention, taken to mean statistically significant at the 5% level (see statistically significant below). This is the same as a 95% confidence interval not including the value corresponding to no effect.

Specificity The chance of having a negative test result given that you do not have a disease (not to be confused with negative predictive value [NPV], which is the other way around; see above).

Standardised mean difference (SMD) A measure of effect size used when outcomes are continuous (such as height, weight, or symptom scores) rather than dichotomous (such as death or myocardial infarction). The mean differences in outcome between the groups being studied are standardised to account for differences in scoring methods (such as pain scores). The measure is a ratio; therefore, it has no units.

Statistically significant Means that the findings of a study are unlikely to have arisen because of chance. Significance at the commonly cited 5% level ($P < 0.05$) means that the observed difference or greater difference would occur by chance in only 1/20 similar cases. Where the word "significant" or "significance" is used without qualification in the text, it is being used in this statistical sense.

Subgroup analysis Analysis of a part of the trial/meta-analysis population in which it is thought the effect may differ from the mean effect.

Systematic review A review in which specified and appropriate methods have been used to identify, appraise, and summarise studies addressing a defined question. It can, but need not, involve meta-analysis (see meta-analysis). In *Clinical Evidence*, the term systematic review refers to a systematic review of RCTs unless specified otherwise.

True negative A person without the target condition (defined by a gold standard) who has a negative test result.

True positive A person with the target condition (defined by a gold standard) who also has a positive test result.

Validity The soundness or rigour of a study. A study is internally valid if the way it is designed and carried out means that the results are unbiased and it gives you an accurate estimate of the effect that is being measured. A study is externally valid if its results are applicable to people encountered in regular clinical practice.

Weighted mean difference (WMD) A measure of effect size used when outcomes are continuous (such as symptom scores or height) rather than dichotomous (such as death or myocardial infarction). The mean differences in outcome between the groups being studied are weighted to account for different sample sizes and differing precision between studies. The WMD is an absolute figure and so takes the units of the original outcome measure.

Drug conversion list

The following information on drug nomenclature is provided by *Martindale: The Complete Drug Reference*, the foremost source for medicines information worldwide.[1]

Clinical Evidence name(s)*	International name†	UK name(s)‡	USA name(s)§
Acetaminophen see *Paracetamol*	Paracetamol	Paracetamol	Acetaminophen
Acetylcysteine	Acetylcysteine	Acetylcysteine	Acetylcysteine
Aciclovir	Aciclovir	Aciclovir	Acyclovir
Activated charcoal	—	Activated charcoal	Activated charcoal
Acyclovir see *Aciclovir*	Aciclovir	Aciclovir	Aciclovir
Adrenaline	Epinephrine	Adrenaline Epinephrine	Epinephrine
Albuterol see *Salbutamol*	Salbutamol	Salbutamol	Albuterol
Amethocaine see *Tetracaine*	Tetracaine	Amethocaine Tetracaine	Tetracaine
Aminophylline	Aminophylline	Aminophylline	Aminophylline
Amitriptyline	Amitriptyline	Amitriptyline	Amitriptyline
Amoxicillin	Amoxicillin	Amoxicillin	Amoxicillin
Arachis oil/chlorobutanol/ p-dichlorobenzene	—	Arachis oil p-Dichlorobenzene Chlorobutanol	Peanut oil p-Dichlorobenzene Chlorobutanol
Aspirin	—	Aspirin	Aspirin
Azithromycin	Azithromycin	Azithromycin	Azithromycin
Beclomethasone	Beclometasone	Beclometasone	Beclomethasone
Benzyl benzoate	—	Benzyl benzoate	Benzyl benzoate
Betamethasone	Betamethasone	Betamethasone	Betamethasone
Bichloroacetic acid	—	—	—
Bromhexine	Bromhexine	Bromhexine	None
Budesonide	Budesonide	Budesonide	Budesonide
Butenafine	Butenafine	Butenafine	Not available
Butoconazole	Butoconazole	Butoconazole	Butoconazole
Carbamazepine	Carbamazepine	Carbamazepine	Carbamazepine
Carbaryl	Carbaril	Carbaryl	Not available
S-Carboxymethylcysteine	Carbocisteine	Carbocisteine	Carbocysteine
Cefadroxil	Cefadroxil	Cefadroxil	Cefadroxil
Cefixime	Cefixime	Cefixime	Cefixime
Cefotaxime	Cefotaxime	Cefotaxime	Cefotaxime
Cefoxitin	Cefoxitin	Cefoxitin	Cefoxitin
Cefpodoxime-proxetil	Cefpodoxime proxetil	Cefpodoxime proxetil	Cefpodoxime proxetil
Ceftriaxone	Ceftriaxone	Ceftriaxone	Ceftriaxone

Clinical Evidence name(s)*	International name†	UK name(s)‡	USA name(s)§
Chloramphenicol	Chloramphenicol	Chloramphenicol	Chloramphenicol
Chlorhexidine/neomycin cream	Chlorhexidine Neomycin	Chlorhexidine Neomycin	Chlorhexidine Neomycin
Ciclopiroxolamine	Ciclopirox olamine	Ciclopirox olamine	Ciclopirox olamine
Cimetidine	Cimetidine	Cimetidine	Cimetidine
Ciprofloxacin	Ciprofloxacin	Ciprofloxacin	Ciprofloxacin
Cisapride	Cisapride	Cisapride	Cisapride
Clavulanic acid	Clavulanic acid	Clavulanic acid	Clavulanic acid
Clindamycin	Clindamycin	Clindamycin	Clindamycin
Clobetasol propionate	Clobetasol propionate	Clobetasol propionate	Clobetasol propionate
Clomipramine	Clomipramine	Clomipramine	Clomipramine
Clonidine	Clonidine	Clonidine	Clonidine
Clotrimazole	Clotrimazole	Clotrimazole	Clotrimazole
Co-proxamol	—	Co-proxamol	—
Cotrimoxazole	—	Co-trimoxazole	Co-trimoxazole
Crotamiton	Crotamiton	Crotamiton	Crotamiton
Cromolyn sodium see Sodium cromoglicate	Sodium cromoglicate	Sodium cromoglicate	Cromolyn sodium
Cyproheptadine	Cyproheptadine	Cyproheptadine	Cyproheptadine
Desipramine	Desipramine	Desipramine	Desipramine
Desmopressin	Desmopressin	Desmopressin	Desmopressin
Dexamethasone	Dexamethasone	Dexamethasone	Dexamethasone
Dexamfetamine	Dexamfetamine	Dexamfetamine	Dextroamphetamine
Dicyclomine see Dicycloverine	Dicycloverine	Dicyclomine Dicycloverine	Dicyclomine
Dicycloverine	Dicycloverine	Dicyclomine Dicycloverine	Dicyclomine
Dicloxacillin	Dicloxacillin	Dicloxacillin	Dicloxacillin
Doxycycline	Doxycycline	Doxycycline	Doxycycline
Econazole	Econazole	Econazole	Econazole
EMLA (lidocaine/prilocaine emulsion)	—	—	—
Epinephrine see Adrenaline	Epinephrine	Adrenaline Epinephrine	Epinephrine
Erythromycin	Erythromycin	Erythromycin	Erythromycin
Ethambutol	Ethambutol	Ethambutol	Ethambutol
Famciclovir	Famciclovir	Famciclovir	Famciclovir
Fenoterol	Fenoterol	Fenoterol	Fenoterol
Fenticonazole	Fenticonazole	Fenticonazole	Fenticonazole
Fluconazole	Fluconazole	Fluconazole	Fluconazole

Clinical Evidence name(s)*	International name†	UK name(s)‡	USA name(s)§
Flunisolide	Flunisolide	Flunisolide	Flunisolide
Fluorouracil	Fluorouracil	Fluorouracil	Fluorouracil
Fluoxetine	Fluoxetine	Fluoxetine	Fluoxetine
Fluticasone	Fluticasone	Fluticasone	Fluticasone
Fusidic acid	Fusidic acid	Fusidic acid	Fusidic acid
Gentamicin	Gentamicin	Gentamicin	Gentamicin
Griseofulvin	Griseofulvin	Griseofulvin	Griseofulvin
Hydrocortisone	Hydrocortisone	Hydrocortisone	Hydrocortisone
Ibuprofen	Ibuprofen	Ibuprofen	Ibuprofen
Idoxuridine	Idoxuridine	Idoxuridine	Idoxuridine
Imipramine	Imipramine	Imipramine	Imipramine
Imiquimod	Imiquimod	Imiquimod	Imiquimod
Indometacin	Indometacin	Indometacin	Indomethacin
Interferon alfa	Interferon alfa	Interferon alfa	Interferon alfa
Interferon beta	Interferon beta	Interferon beta	Interferon beta
Interferon gamma	Interferon gamma	Interferon gamma	Interferon gamma
Ipecacuanha	—	Ipecacuanha	Ipecac
Ipratropium bromide	Ipratropium bromide	Ipratropium bromide	Ipratropium bromide
Isoniazid	Isoniazid	Isoniazid	Isoniazid
Itraconazole	Itraconazole	Itraconazole	Itraconazole
Ivermectin	Ivermectin	Ivermectin	Ivermectin
Ketoconazole	Ketoconazole	Ketoconazole	Ketoconazole
Lactitol	Lactitol	Lactitol	Lactitol
Lactulose	Lactulose	Lactulose	Lactulose
Lamivudine	Lamivudine	Lamivudine	Lamivudine
Lidocaine	Lidocaine	Lignocaine Lidocaine	Lidocaine
Lignocaine see Lidocaine	Lidocaine	Lignocaine Lidocaine	Lidocaine
Lindane	Lindane	Lindane	Lindane
Lithium (carbonate or citrate)	—	Lithium carbonate Lithium citrate	Lithium carbonate Lithium citrate
Lomefloxacin	Lomefloxacin	Lomefloxacin	Lomefloxacin
Loperamide	Loperamide	Loperamide	Loperamide
Malathion	—	Malathion	Malathion
Mefenamic acid	Mefenamic acid	Mefenamic acid	Mefenamic acid
Metaproterenol see Orciprenaline	Orciprenaline	Orciprenaline	Metaproterenol
Methionine	Methionine	Methionine	Methionine

Clinical Evidence name(s)*	International name†	UK name(s)‡	USA name(s)§
Methylphenidate	Methylphenidate	Methylphenidate	Methylphenidate
Metronidazole	Metronidazole	Metronidazole	Metronidazole
Miconazole	Miconazole	Miconazole	Miconazole
Minocycline	Minocycline	Minocycline	Minocycline
Moclobemide	Moclobemide	Moclobemide	Moclobemide
Montelukast	Montelukast	Montelukast	Montelukast
Naftifine	Naftifine	Naftifine	Naftifine
Naproxen	Naproxen	Naproxen	Naproxen
Nedocromil	Nedocromil	Nedocromil	Nedocromil
Netilmicin	Netilmicin	Netilmicin	Netilmicin
Nevirapine	Nevirapine	Nevirapine	Nevirapine
Nitrofurantoin	Nitrofurantoin	Nitrofurantoin	Nitrofurantoin
Norfloxacin	Norfloxacin	Norfloxacin	Norfloxacin
Nystatin	Nystatin	Nystatin	Nystatin
Ofloxacin	Ofloxacin	Ofloxacin	Ofloxacin
Orciprenaline	Orciprenaline	Orciprenaline	Metaproterenol
Oxymetazoline	Oxymetazoline	Oxymetazoline	Oxymetazoline
Palivizumab	Palivizumab	Palivizumab	—
Paracetamol	Paracetamol	Paracetamol	Acetaminophen
Penicillin	Benzylpenicillin	Benzylpenicillin	Penicillin G
Permethrin	Permethrin	Permethrin	Permethrin
Phenoxymethylpenicillin	Phenoxymethylpenicillin	Phenoxymethylpenicillin	Penicillin V
Pidotimod	Pidotimod	—	—
Podophyllin	—	Podophyllum resin	Podophyllum resin
Podophyllotoxin	—	Podophyllotoxin	Podofilox
Polymyxin-bacitracin	Polymyxin Bacitracin	Polymyxin Bacitracin	Polymyxin Bacitracin
Prednisolone	Prednisolone	Prednisolone	Prednisolone
Prednisone	Prednisone	Prednisone	Prednisone
Probenecid	Probenecid	Probenecid	Probenecid
Pseudoephedrine	Pseudoephedrine	Pseudoephedrine	Pseudoephedrine
Pyrazinamide	Pyrazinamide	Pyrazinamide	Pyrazinamide
Ribavirin	Ribavirin	Tribavirin	Ribavirin
Rifampicin	Rifampicin	Rifampicin	Rifampin
Rifamycin	Rifamycin	Rifamycin	—
Rosaramicin	Rosaramicin	Rosaramicin	Rosaramicin
Salbutamol	Salbutamol	Salbutamol	Albuterol

Clinical Evidence name(s)*	International name†	UK name(s)‡	USA name(s)§
Salmeterol	Salmeterol	Salmeterol	Salmeterol
Senna	—	Senna	Senna
Sertaconazole	Sertaconazole	Sertaconazole	—
Simethicone	Simeticone	Simeticone	Simethicone
Sodium alginate	—	Sodium alginate	Sodium alginate
Sodium cromoglicate	Sodium cromoglicate	Sodium cromoglicate	Cromolyn sodium
Spectinomycin	Spectinomycin	Spectinomycin	Spectinomycin
Streptomycin	Streptomycin	Streptomycin	Streptomycin
Sulfacetamide	Sulfacetamide	Sulfacetamide	Sulfacetamide
Sulfadiazine	Sulfadiazine	Sulfadiazine	Sulfadiazine
Sulfamethoxazole	Sulfamethoxazole	Sulfamethoxazole	Sulfamethoxazole
Terbinafine	Terbinafine	Terbinafine	Terbinafine
Terbutaline	Terbutaline	Terbutaline	Terbutaline
Terconazole	Terconazole	Terconazole	Terconazole
Tetracaine	Tetracaine	Amethocaine Tetracaine	Tetracaine
Tioconazole	Tioconazole	Tioconazole	Tioconazole
Tobramycin	Tobramycin	Tobramycin	Tobramycin
Tolnaftate	Tolnaftate	Tolnaftate	Tolnaftate
Triamcinolone	Triamcinolone	Triamcinolone	Triamcinolone
Trichloroacetic acid	—	—	—
Trifluorothymidine see Trfluridine	Trifluridine	—	Trifluridine
Trifluridine	Trifluridine	—	Trifluridine
Trimethoprim-polymyxin	Trimethoprim Polymyxin	Trimethoprim Polymyxin	Trimethoprim Polymyxin
Trimethoprim-sulfamethoxazole see Cotrimoxazole	—	Co-trimoxazole	Co-trimoxazole
Undecenoic acid	—	Undecenoic acid	Undecenoic acid
Valaciclovir	Valaciclovir	Valaciclovir	Valacyclovir
Venlafaxine	Venlafaxine	Venlafaxine	Venlafaxine
Vidarabine	Vidarabine	Vidarabine	Vidarabine
Xylitol	—	Xylitol	Xylitol
Zafirlukast	Zafirlukast	Zafirlukast	Zafirlukast
Zidovudine	Zidovudine	Zidovudine	Zidovudine

*Clinical Evidence name: the name that appears in the Clinical Evidence index.
†International name: the recommended International Non-proprietary Name (rINN) or proposed International Non-proprietary Name (pINN).
‡UK name(s): the British Approved Name (BAN) or BP British Pharmacopoeia (BP) 2001 name.
§USA name: United States Formulary (USNF) 20th Edition, 2002 name or United States Pharmacopoeia (USP) 25th Edition, 2002 name.

1. Sweetman SC, editor. Martindale: The Complete Drug Reference. 33rd edition. London: Pharmaceutical Press, 2002. See http://www.pharmpress.com or contact martindale@rpsgb.org.uk

Metric equivalent for height and weight

Height		Weight	
Inches	**Cm**	**Lb**	**Kg**
18	45.7	5	2.3
19	48.3	6	2.7
20	50.8	7	3.2
21	53.3	8	3.6
22	55.9	9	4.1
23	58.4	10	4.5
24	61.0	15	6.8
25	63.5	20	9.1
26	66.0	25	11.4
27	68.6	30	13.6
28	71.1	35	15.9
29	73.7	40	18.2
30	76.2	50	22.7
31	78.7	60	27.2
32	81.3	70	31.8
33	83.8	80	36.3
34	86.4	90	40.9
35	88.9	100	45.4
36	91.4	110	49.9
37	94.0	120	54.5
38	96.5	130	59.0
39	99.1	140	63.6
40	101.6	150	68.1
45	114.3	160	72.6
50	127.0	170	77.2
55	139.7	180	81.7
60	152.4	190	86.3
65	165.1	200	90.8
70	177.8	210	95.3
75	190.5		

Centigrade-Fahrenheit equivalents

	Centigrade (C)	Fahrenheit (F)
Freezing	0.0	32.0
Body temperature range	36.0	96.8
	36.5	97.7
	37.0	98.6
	37.5	99.5
	38.0	100.4
	38.5	101.3
	39.0	102.2
	39.5	103.1
	40.0	104.0
	40.5	104.9
	41.0	105.8
	41.5	106.7
	42.0	107.6
Boiling	100.0	212.0

UK and US terms

UK / US

A
a tenth / one-tenth
acute glaucoma / acute narrow-angle glaucoma
adrenaline / epinephrine
aetiology / etiology
after effect / aftereffect
ageing / aging
allogenic / allogeneic
amenorrhoea / amenorrhea
amoebic, amoebiasis / amebic, amebiasis
anaesthesia / anesthesia
anaesthetic / anesthetic
analyse / analyze
antenatal / prenatal
antiacne / anti-acne
aortic incompetance / aortic regurgitation
apnoea / apnea
arrector / erector
artificial ventilation / artificial respiration or rescue breathing

B
bacteraemic / bacteremic
barrier cream / emollient cream
behaviour / behavior
blocked nose / stuffy nose
blueish / bluish
bow leg / bowleg
breast feed, breast feeding / breastfeed, breastfeeding
buphthalmos / congenital glaucoma
byproduct / by-product

C
caesarean section / cesarean section
callus (adj) / callous (adj) (noun is callus)
case series / case reports
casualty (first aid) / victim ("casualties", in US are usually dead)
casualty department / emergency room
channelled / channeled
chest drain / chest tube
chiropodist / podiatrist
coeliac disease / celiac disease
combined contraception pill / combination oral contraceptives
coronary heart disease / coronary artery disease
cot / crib
cotton bud / cotton swab
counselling / counseling
cranial diabetes / central diabetes
childminder / day care

D
desferrioxamine / deferoxamine
diarrhoea / diarrhea
diathermycoagulation / diathermocoagulation
disc / disk
diverticular disease / diverticulosis
Down's syndrome / Down syndrome
d-penicillamine / penicillamine
dummy / pacifier
dysaethesia / dysethesia
dysmenorrhoea / dysmenorrhea
dyspnoea / dyspnea

E
ear defenders / hearing protective devices
ear drops / eardrops
ear drum / eardrum
ear wax / earwax
end point / endpoint
energy / calories
exclude / rule out
extrinsic allergic alveolitis / hypersensitivity pneumonitis
eye drops / eyedrops

F
faeces / feces
false colour (x rays) / color-enhanced (X-rays)
feed, feeds (infant meal) / feeding, feedings
fibre / fiber
fibreoptic / fiberoptic
fibrosing alveolitis / interstitial fibrosis
fit / seizure
flexural psoriasis / inverse psoriasis
focusing errors / refractive errors

G
galactorrhoea / galactorrhea
gall stones / gallstones

gastro-oesophageal reflux disease (GORD) /
   gastroesophageal reflux disease (GERD)
giddiness / dizziness
gingivae / gingiva
glycaemic / glycemic
glyceryl trinitrate / nitroglycerin
gonadotrophin / gonadotropin
gonorrhoea / gonorrhea
greasy / oily
guaiphenesin / guaifenesin
gynaecomastin / gynecomastia

H

haemangiomata / hemangiomata
haemochromatosis / hemochromatosis
haemodialysis / hemodialysis
haemoglobin / hemoglobin
haemolysis / hemolysis
haemolytic / hemolytic
haemorrhage / hemorrhage
harms / risks
heat pad / heating pad
hot flushes / hot flashes
humour / humor
hyoscine hydrobromide / scopolamine
   hydrobromide
hypercholesterolaemia /
   hypercholesterolemia
hyperlipidaemia / hyperlipidemia
hypermetropia / hyperopia
hyperuricaemia / hyperuricemia
hypoglycaemia / hypoglycemia
hypoxaemia / hypoxemia
hysterosalpingogram / hydrosonography

I

indirect laryngoscopy / flexible fiberoptic
   laryngoscopy
information tag / emergency bracelet
interferon alpha / interferon alfa
ischaemic / ischemic

L

labour / labor
leukaemia / leukemia
localised / localized
long sight / farsightedness
looking after your back / taking care of
   your back
lymphoedema / lymphedema

M

menotrophin / menotropin
methohexitone / methohexital
mitozantrone / mitoxantrone
mitral incompetance / mitral
   regurgitation
moracizine / moricizine
mould / mold

N

naevus, nacvi / nevus, nevi
nail body / nail plate
nail root / nail matrix
named after / named for
nappy / diaper
nasendoscopy / nasal endoscopy
nasendoscope / nasal endoscope
nebuliser / nebulizer
nipple cream / moisturizing cream
non-opioid / nonopioid
non-perfumed / nonperfumed
non-smoker / nonsmoker
non-steroidal / nonsteridal
non-ulcer dyspepsia / nonulcer
   dyspepsia
noradrenaline / norepinephrine
norethisterone / norethindrone

O

odour / odor
oedema / edema
oesophagus / esophagus
oestrogen / estrogen
on prescription / by prescription
optician, optometrist / ophthalmologist
over sensitive / oversensitive
oxidisation / oxidation

P

painkiller / analgesic
paracetamol / acetaminophen
paralyse / paralyze
pass urine / urinate
pass wind / pass gas
pelvic floor exercises / Kegel exercises
per cent / percent
period / menstrual period, menstruation
persistent anxiety state / generalized
   anxiety disorder
physiotherapy / physical therapy
phlegm / sputum

pile(s) / hemorrhoid(s)
pilonidal sinus / pilonidal cyst
placenta praevia / placenta previa
plaster / adhesive bandage
polycythaemia / polycythemia
possetting / spitting up
premature labour / preterm labor
preventative / preventive
pre-eclampsia / preeclampsia

R

radio-opaque dye / radiopaque dye
radiotherapy / radiation therapy,
  treatment
realise / realize
re-attach / reattach
recognise / recognize
reducing diet / weight-loss diet
resolve (the disease resolves) / clears
  up, disappears, etc
ribbon gauze / nasal tampons, spongers
rifampicin / rifampin

S

sandpit / sandbox
sanitary towels / sanitary napkins
seborrhoea / seborrhea
seborrhoeic / seborrheic
semi-liquid / semiliquid
septicaemia / septicemia
severely / profoundly
short sight / nearsightedness
sickle cell anaemia / sickle-cell anemia
skin-tunnelled catheter / skin-tunneled
  venous catheter
sleep apnoea / sleep apnea
sodium cromoglycate / cromolyn sodium
sodium valproate / valproate sodium
soiling / defecation

solar keratosis / actinic keratosis
spectacles / glasses (or cycglasses)
sulphasalazine / sulfasalazine
sulphate / sulfate
sulphonamide / sulfonamide
sulphonylurca / sulfonylurca
sunbeds / sunlamps / tanning booths
suppleness / flexibility

T

tachypnoea / tachypnea
teat (bottle) / nipple (bottle as well as
  breast)
tendon hammer / reflex hammer
thalassaemia / thalassemia
threadworm(s) / pinworm(s)
though / although
thyroid tumours / thyroid nodules
tiredness / fatigue
tonometer / applantation tonometer
tonometry / applantation tonometry
trace / tracing
trainers / sneakers
tranquiliser / tranquilizer
tumour / tumor

V

venesection / phlebotomy
videocystometrogram / video
  urodynamics

W

wart paint / wart remover
waters (amniotic fluid) / water
weal / wheal
weep / ooze
wind / gas, burp

Acute gastroenteritis in children

Search date October 2001

Jacqueline Dalby-Payne and Elizabeth Elliott

INTERVENTIONS

Key Messages

- We found no systematic review or RCTs on "clear fluids" (water, carbonated drinks, and translucent fruit juices) versus oral rehydration solutions for treatment of mild to moderate dehydration caused by acute gastroenteritis.

- One systematic review in children with mild to moderate dehydration found no significant difference between oral versus intravenous fluids in duration of diarrhoea, time spent in hospital, or weight gain at discharge. One RCT in children with severe dehydration found that oral versus intravenous fluids significantly reduced the duration of diarrhoea and increased weight gain at discharge, and were associated with fewer adverse effects.

- Two RCTs found that, in children with mild to moderate dehydration, loperamide versus placebo significantly reduced the duration of diarrhoea. Another RCT found no significant difference between loperamide versus placebo in the duration of diarrhoea. We found insufficient evidence to assess the risk of adverse effects.

- One systematic review has found that lactose-free feeds versus lactose-containing feeds reduce the duration of diarrhoea in children with mild to severe dehydration. Subsequent RCTs found conflicting results.

DEFINITION   Acute gastroenteritis is characterised by rapid onset of diarrhoea with or without vomiting, nausea, fever, and abdominal pain.[1] In children, the symptoms and signs can be non-specific.[2] Diarrhoea is defined as the frequent passage of unformed liquid stools.[3]

INCIDENCE/ PREVALENCE   Worldwide, about 3–5 billion cases of acute gastroenteritis occur in children under 5 years of age each year.[4] In the UK, acute gastro-enteritis accounts for 204/1000 general practitioner consultations each year in children under 5 years of age.[5] Gastroenteritis leads to hospital admission in 7/1000 children under 5 years of age per year in the UK[5] and 13/1000 in the USA.[6] In Australia, gastroenteritis accounts for 6% of all hospital admissions in children under 15 years of age.[7]

AETIOLOGY/ RISK FACTORS   In developed countries, acute gastroenteritis is predominantly caused by viruses (87%), of which rotavirus is most common;[8–11] bacteria cause most of the remaining cases, predominantly *Campylobacter*, *Salmonella*, *Shigella*, and *Escherichia coli*. In developing countries bacterial pathogens are more frequent, although rotavirus is also a major cause of gastroenteritis.

PROGNOSIS   Acute gastroenteritis is usually self limiting but if untreated can result in morbidity and mortality secondary to water and electrolyte losses. Acute diarrhoea causes 4 million deaths per year in children under 5 years of age in Asia (excluding China), Africa, and Latin America, and over 80% of deaths occur in children under 2 years of age.[12] Although death is uncommon in developed countries, dehydration secondary to gastroenteritis is a significant cause of morbidity and need for hospital admission.[6,7,13]

AIMS   To reduce the duration of diarrhoea and quantity of stool output, and duration of hospital stay; to prevent and treat dehydration; to promote weight gain following rehydration; to prevent persistent diarrhoea associated with lactose intolerance (see glossary, p 5).

OUTCOMES   Total stool volume; duration of diarrhoea (time until permanent cessation); failure rate of oral rehydration treatment (as defined by individual RCTs); weight gain following rehydration; length of hospital stay; mortality.

METHODS   *Clinical Evidence* search and appraisal October 2001.

QUESTION   **What are the effects of treatments for acute gastroenteritis?**

OPTION   **CLEAR FLUIDS**

We found no systematic review or RCTs on "clear fluids" (water, carbonated drinks, and translucent fruit juices) versus oral rehydration solutions for treatment of mild to moderate dehydration caused by acute gastroenteritis.

Benefits: We found no systematic review or RCTs of "clear fluids" versus oral rehydration solutions.

Harms: We found no RCTs.

Comment: In this review, oral rehydration solutions are defined as glucose plus electrolyte or food (e.g. rice) based electrolyte solutions. Fruit juices and carbonated drinks are low in sodium and potassium, and usually have a high sugar content, which can exacerbate diarrhoea.

| OPTION | **ORAL VERSUS INTRAVENOUS FLUIDS** |

One systematic review in children with mild to moderate dehydration in developed countries found no significant difference between oral versus intravenous fluids in duration of diarrhoea, time spent in hospital, or weight gain at discharge. One RCT in children with severe dehydration in a developing country found that oral versus intravenous fluids significantly reduced the duration of diarrhoea and increased weight gain at discharge, and was associated with fewer adverse effects.

Benefits: **Mild to moderate dehydration:** We found one systematic review (search date 1993, 6 RCTs, 371 children in developed countries with acute gastroenteritis, most with mild to moderate dehydration and in hospital)[14] and two additional RCTs comparing oral versus intravenous rehydration (see table 1, p 7).[21,22] The review and the additional RCTs found no significant difference between oral versus intravenous fluids in the duration of diarrhoea, time spent in hospital, or weight gain at discharge. If children responded poorly to oral fluids they were given intravenous fluids, which was used as a measure of failure of oral fluids. However, the failure rate of intravenous treatment was not recorded. **Severe dehydration:** We found one RCT (470 children in Iran with acute gastroenteritis with severe dehydration) comparing oral versus intravenous fluids (see table 1, p 7).[23] It found no significant difference in the death rate with oral versus intravenous fluids (2/236 [1%] v 5/234 [2%]; RR 0.4, 95% CI 0.08 to 2.02). No cause of death was given. Oral versus intravenous treatment significantly reduced the duration of diarrhoea (4.8 days v 5.5 days; difference 0.7 days; P < 0.01), and increased weight gain at discharge (percentage increase in admission weight 9% v 7%; P < 0.001). Failure of oral treatment (defined as the need to move to intravenous treatment) occurred in 1/236 children (0.4%; 95% CI not provided).

Harms: **Mild to moderate dehydration:** The systematic review reported no adverse effects.[14] One additional RCT (100 children in Afghanistan) reported fever and rigors in 9/50 children (18%) receiving intravenous fluids versus none receiving oral fluids.[21] **Severe dehydration:** The RCT in children in Iran found that more children receiving intravenous treatment vomited during the first 6 hours of rehydration (70/234 [30%] v 47/236 [20%]; RR 0.64, 95% CI 0.46 to 0.89).[23] There was no significant difference in the risk of peri-orbital oedema (RR 0.99, 95% CI 0.25 to 3.92) or abdominal distention (RR 8.9, 95% CI 0.48 to 164). Phlebitis at the injection site requiring antibiotics occurred in 5/234 (2%) of children. In the same RCT, subgroup analysis of 58 children with hypernatraemia found that fewer children taking oral versus intravenous fluids developed seizures during rehydration, although the result did not quite reach significance (2/34 [6%] v 6/24 [25%]; RR 0.23, 95% CI 0.05 to 1.07).

Comment: The quality of the RCTs was difficult to assess because of poor reporting; only one reported the method of allocation concealment[17] and one reported the method of randomisation.[21] Blinding of outcomes was impossible owing to the nature of the intervention. Intention to treat analysis was used in all but one RCT.[17]

OPTION   LOPERAMIDE

Two RCTs found that, in children with mild to moderate dehydration, loperamide versus placebo significantly reduced the duration of diarrhoea. Another RCT found no significant difference between loperamide versus placebo in the duration of diarrhoea. We found insufficient evidence to assess the risk of adverse effects.

Benefits: We found no systematic review. We found five RCTs in children with acute diarrhoea (701 children, most with mild to moderate dehydration; (see table 2, p 8).[24–28] Of the three RCTs that assessed the duration of diarrhoea, two[24,26] found that loperamide versus placebo significantly reduced duration of diarrhoea (largest RCT, 315 children; risk of having diarrhoea at 24 h, 36/100 [36%] loperamide v 112/203 [55%] with placebo; RR 0.83, 95% CI 0.73 to 0.94).[24] Another RCT found no significant difference.[25] The results of other outcomes are included in table 2, p 8.

Harms: Four RCTs reported no adverse effects from loperamide.[24-26,28] One RCT reported mild abdominal distension, excessive sleep, and lethargy in children taking loperamide (3/16 [19%] with loperamide 0.8 mg/kg v 1/18 [6%] taking 0.4 mg/kg v 0/18 [0%] taking placebo; RR loperamide v placebo 4.9, 95% CI 0.28 to 86). Adverse effects caused one child to withdraw from the trial.[27] We found one evidence based guideline that identified case studies reporting lethargy, intestinal ileus, respiratory depression, and coma, especially in infants.[2]

Comment: We found insufficient evidence to estimate accurately the risk of adverse effects of loperamide in children.

OPTION   LACTOSE-FREE FEEDS

One systematic review has found that lactose-free feeds versus lactose-containing feeds reduce the duration of diarrhoea in children with mild to severe dehydration. Subsequent RCTs found conflicting results.

Benefits: We found one systematic review (search date not stated, 13 RCTs, 873 children with mild to severe dehydration)[29] and four subsequent RCTs[30–33] comparing lactose-containing versus lactose-free feeds. The review was limited by flaws in its methodology (see comment below). The review found that lactose-containing versus lactose-free feeds significantly increased "treatment failure" (89/399 [22%] v 56/474 [12%]; RR 2.1, 95% CI 1.6 to 2.7). The definition of treatment failure varied between trials and included increasing severity or persistence of diarrhoea or recurrence of dehydration. Lactose-free feeds versus lactose-containing feeds significantly reduced the duration of diarrhoea (9 RCTs; 826 children with mild or no dehydration receiving oral rehydration treatment; 92 h with lactose v 88 h with lactose-free; SMD 0.2 h after initiation of the study; P = 0.001). When the three RCTs that included children given additional solid food were excluded, lactose-free versus lactose-containing feeds also significantly reduced the duration of diarrhoea (6 RCTs; 604 children; 95 h with lactose v 82 h with lactose-free; SMD 0.3 h; P < 0.001). Children receiving lactose-free versus lactose-containing feeds had significantly reduced stool frequency (4 RCTs; 387 children; 4.0 stool movements/day with lactose v 3.5 with lactose-free; SMD 0.3; P < 0.004). Total stool volume was greater in children who received lactose-containing diets (4 RCTs; 209 children; SMD 0.4 g; P = 0.002). Differences in weight gain during treatment could not be assessed because of the use of solid food in two studies and considerable heterogeneity between studies. We found four subsequent RCTs (see table 3, p 9).[30–33] Two found that lactose-free versus lactose-containing feeds significantly reduced the duration of diarrhoea,[30,33] and the other two found no significant difference.[31,32] The results of other outcomes are summarised in table 3, p 9

Harms: The one RCT assessing adverse effects reported none in the treatment or control groups.[32]

Comment: Although the systematic review stated criteria for inclusion and exclusion of RCTs, only published studies were included and the method of determining RCT quality was not stated.[29] There was considerable heterogeneity between studies. Lactose-free feeds were superior to lactose-containing feeds for the duration of diarrhoea. Differences for other outcomes, although statistically significant, were not clinically important.

GLOSSARY

Lactose intolerance Malabsorption of lactose can occur for a short period after acute gastroenteritis because of mucosal damage and temporary lactase deficiency.

REFERENCES

1. Armon K, Elliott EJ. Acute gastroenteritis. In Moyer VA, Elliott EJ, Davis RL, eds. *Evidence Based Pediatrics and Child Health.* London: BMJ Books, 2000;273–286.

2. Practice parameter: the management of acute gastroenteritis in young children. American Academy of Pediatrics, Provisional Committee on Quality Improvement, Subcommittee on Acute Gastroenteritis. *Pediatrics* 1996;97:424–435.

3. Critchley M. *Butterworths Medical Dictionary Second Edition.* London: Butterworths & Co, 1986.

4. OPCS. *Mid-1993 population estimates for England and Wales.* London: HMSO, 1994.

5. OPCS. *Morbidity statistics from general practice. Fourth national study, 1991–1992.* London: HMSO, 1993.

6. Glass RI, Lew JF, Gangarosa RE, LeBaron CW, Ho MS. Estimates of morbidity and mortality rates for diarrheal diseases in American children. *J Pediatr* 1991;118:S27–S33.

7. Elliott EJ, Backhouse JA, Leach JW. Pre-admission management of acute gastroenteritis. *J Paediatr Child Health* 1996;32:18–21.

8. Conway SP, Phillips RR, Panday S. Admission to hospital with gastroenteritis. *Arch Dis Child* 1990; 65:579–584.

9. Finkelstein JA, Schwartz JS, Torrey S, Fleisher GR. Common clinical features as predictors of bacterial diarrhea in infants. *Am J Emerg Med* 1989;7: 469–473.

10. DeWitt TG, Humphrey KF, McCarthy P. Clinical predictors of acute bacterial diarrhea in young children. *Pediatrics* 1985;76:551–556.

11. Ferson MJ. Hospitalisations for rotavirus gastroenteritis among children under five years of age in New South Wales. *Med J Aust* 1996;164: 273–276.

12. Anonymous. *A manual for the treatment of diarrhoea. Programme for the control of diarrhoeal diseases.* Geneva: WHO, 1990.

13. Conway SP, Phillips RR, Panday S. Admission to hospital with gastroenteritis. *Arch Dis Child* 1990; 65:579–584.

14. Gavin N, Merrick N, Davidson B. Efficacy of glucose-based oral rehydration therapy. *Pediatrics* 1996;98:45–51. Search date 1993; primary sources Medline and experts and organisations involved in diarrhoea treatment contacted.

15. Santosham M, Daum RS, Dillman L, et al. Oral rehydration therapy of infantile diarrhea: a controlled study of well-nourished children hospitalized in the United States and Panama. *N Engl J Med* 1982;306:1070–1076.

16. Listernick R, Zieserl E, Davis AT. Outpatient oral rehydration in the United States. *Am J Dis Child* 1986;140:211–215.

17. Mackenzie A, Barnes G. Randomised controlled trial comparing oral and intravenous rehydration therapy in children with diarrhoea. *BMJ* 1991; 303:393–396.

18. Tamer AM, Friedman LB, Maxwell SR, Cynamon HA, Perez HN, Cleveland WW. Oral rehydration of infants in a large urban US medical center. *J Pediatr* 1985;107:14–19.

19. Vesikari T, Isolauri E, Baer M. A comparative trial of rapid oral and intravenous rehydration in acute diarrhoea. *Acta Paediatr Scand* 1987;76: 300–305.

20. Issenman RM, Leung AK. Oral and intravenous rehydration of children. *Can Fam Physician* 1993; 39:2129–2136.

21. Singh M, Mahmoodi A, Arya LS, Azamy S. Controlled trial of oral versus intravenous rehydration in the management of acute gastroenteritis. *Indian J Med Res* 1982;75: 691–693.

22. Oritiz A. Rehidratacion oral: Experiencia en el manejo de pacientes con gastroenteritis aguda en la sala de emergencia hospital pediatrico. *Bol Asoc Med P R* 1990;82:227–233.

23. Sharifi J, Ghavami F, Nowrouzi Z, et al. Oral versus intravenous rehydration therapy in severe gastroenteritis. *Arch Dis Child* 1985;60:856–860.

24. Diarrhoeal Diseases Study Group (UK). Loperamide in acute diarrhoea in childhood: results of a double blind, placebo controlled multicentre clinical trial. *BMJ Clin Res Ed* 1984; 289:1263–1267.

25. Owens JR, Broadhead R, Hendrickse RG, Jaswal OP, Gangal RN. Loperamide in the treatment of acute gastroenteritis in early childhood. Report of a two centre, double-blind, controlled clinical trial. *Ann Trop Paediatr* 1981;1:135–141.

26. Kassem AS, Madkour AA, Massoud BZ, Mehanna ZM. Loperamide in acute childhood diarrhoea: a double blind controlled trial. *J Diarrhoeal Dis Res* 1983;1:10–16.

27. Karrar ZA, Abdulla MA, Moody JB, Macfarlane SB, Al Bwardy M, Hendrickse RG. Loperamide in acute diarrhoea in childhood: results of a double blind, placebo controlled clinical trial. *Ann Trop Paediatr* 1987;7:122–127.

28. Bowie MD, Hill ID, Mann MD. Loperamide for treatment of acute diarrhoea in infants and young children. A double-blind placebo-controlled trial. *S Afr Med J* 1995;85:885–887.

29. Brown KH, Peerson JM, Fontaine O. Use of nonhuman milks in the dietary management of young children with acute diarrhea: a meta-analysis of clinical trials. *Pediatrics* 1994;93: 17–27. Search date not stated; primary sources Medline, hand searches of reference lists, and researchers contacted.

30. Allen UD, McLeod K, Wang EE. Cow's milk versus soy-based formula in mild and moderate diarrhea: a randomized, controlled trial. *Acta Paediatrica* 1994;83:183–187.

31. Clemente YF, Tapia CC, Comino AL, Lopez PL, Escriva TP, Gonzalez PJ. Lactose-free formula versus adapted formula in acute infantile diarrhea. *An Esp Paediatr* 1993;39:309–312.

32. Lozano JM, Cespedes JA. Lactose vs. lactose free regimen in children with acute diarrhoea: a randomized controlled trial. *Arch Latinoam Nutr* 1994;44:6–11.

33. Fayad IM, Hashem M, Husseine A, Zikri MA, Zikri MA, Santosham M. Comparison of soy-based formulas with lactose and with sucrose in the treatment of acute diarrhoea in infants. *Arch Pediatr Adolesc Med* 1999;153:675–680.

Jacqueline Dalby-Payne
Lecturer

Elizabeth Elliott
Associate Professor

Department of Paediatrics and Child Health
University of Sydney and The Children's Hospital at Westmead
Sydney
Australia

Competing interests: None declared.

TABLE 1 Oral versus intravenous fluids in mild to moderate[15–22] and severe dehydration[23] (see text, p 3).

Intervention (Na⁺ concentration)	Participants (age)	Duration of diarrhoea (d)	Stay in hospital (d)	Weight gain (%)	Stool output (ml/kg)	Failure of oral treatment (defined as the need to revert to iv treatment)*
Oral versus intravenous fluids in mild to moderate dehydration						
ORS (90, 50) v iv[15]	52 children from USA and 94 children in Panama with acute diarrhoea (3–24 months)	NS	NR	NS	USA: ORS (90) v iv (NS); ORS (50) v iv (193 v 112; P < 0.02). Panama: ORS (90) v iv (90 v 168; P < 0.001); ORS (50) v iv (NS)	1/98 (1%)
ORS (60) v iv[16]	29 children with acute diarrhoea (3–24 months)	NR	NR	NR	NR	2/15 (13%)
ORS (50) v iv[17]	111 children with acute diarrhoea (3–36 months)	NR	NS	NR	NR	2/52 (4%)
ORS (75, 50) v iv[18]	100 children with acute diarrhoea (3–33 months)	NR	NS	NS	NR	3/50 (6%)
ORS (60) v iv[19]	37 children with acute diarrhoea (< 5 y)	ORS < iv (1.0 ± 0.5 v 2.6 ±1.6; P < 0.001)	ORS < iv (2.7 ± 1.0 v 3.9 ± 1.7; P < 0.001)	ORS > iv ORS + 314 g v −16 g; P < 0.05	NS	2/20 (10%)
ORS (45, 74) v iv[20]	42 children with acute diarrhoea (6–31 months)	NR	NR	NS	NR	4/22 (18%)
ORS (3.5 g/L) v iv[21]	100 children with acute diarrhoea (mean age 11 y)	NS	NR	NS	NR	NR
ORS (75) v iv[22]	31 children with acute diarrhoea (mean age 4–5 y)	NS	NR	NS	NR	NR
Oral versus iv fluids in severe dehydration						
ORS (80,40) v iv[23]	470 children with acute diarrhoea (1–18 months)	ORS < iv (4.8 v 5.5; P < 0.01)	NR	ORS > iv (8.9% v 7.3%; P < 0.001)	NR	1/236 (0.4%)

d, day; iv, intravenous; NR, not reported; NS, non-significant; ORS, oral rehydration solution; y, year. *Although this outcome measures treatment failure of oral therapy it is not a comparative outcome as the number of children responding poorly to intravenous treatment was not recorded.

TABLE 2 Loperamide in mild to moderate dehydration: results of placebo controlled RCTs (see text, p 4).[24–28]

Intervention (loperamide dose mg/kg per day)	Participants	Duration of diarrhoea	Stay in hospital	Weight gain	Stool output
Loperamide (0.4, 0.8) v placebo[24]	315 children with acute diarrhoea and mild to moderate dehydration (3 months to 3 years)	L < P; risk of having diarrhoea at 24 hours; RR 0.83, 95% CI 0.73 to 0.94	NS	L > P; children with increased weight at 3 days: loperamide 0.8 mg v 0.4 mg v placebo: 58% v 51% v 36%	NR
Loperamide (0.2) v placebo[25]	50 children with acute diarrhoea (1–4 years)	NS	NS	NS	NR
Loperamide (0.2) v placebo[26]	100 children with acute diarrhoea and mild to moderate dehydration (< 2 years)	L < P; 59.1 hour v 81.1 hour; P < 0.05	NR	NS	NS
Loperamide (0.4, 0.8) v placebo[27]	53 children with acute diarrhoea (3 months to 3 years)	NR	NR	L > P; children with increased weight at 3 days: loperamide 0.8 mg v 0.4 mg v placebo: 88% v 50% v 39%; RR 0.53, 95% CI 0.29 to 0.97	NR
Loperamide (0.8) v placebo[28]	185 children with acute gastroenteritis and mild to moderate dehydration (3–18 months).	NR	NS	NR	NR

NR, not reported; NS, non-significant.

TABLE 3 Lactose-containing versus lactose-free feeds in children with mild to severe dehydration: results of subsequent RCTs (see text, p 5), [30–33].

Intervention	Participants	Duration of diarrhoea	Weight gain	Total stool output (ml/kg)	Treatment failure
Cow's milk v soy-based formula[30]	76 children with acute diarrhoea and mild to moderate dehydration (2–12 months)	L > LF; 6.6 v 4.5 days; P < 0.01	NS	NR	NS
Lactose v lactose-free formula[31]	60 children with acute diarrhoea (< 1 year)	NS	NS	NR	NR
Lactose v lactose-free formula[32]	52 children with acute diarrhoea and mild to moderate dehydration (1–24 months)	NS	NS	NR	NS
Soy-based formula with lactose v soy-based formula with sucrose[33]	200 boys with acute diarrhoea (3–18 months)	L > LF; 39 hours v 23 hours; P > 0.001	NS	L > LF; mean 164 (95% CI 131 to 208) v 89 (95% 55 to 87); P < 0.001	NS

NR, not recorded; NS, non-significant; L, lactose-containing; LF, lactose-free.

Acute otitis media

Search date June 2001

Paddy O'Neill

QUESTIONS

INTERVENTIONS

TREATMENT

Likely to be beneficial

Trade off between benefits and harms

PREVENTION

Likely to be beneficial

Trade off between benefits and harms

To be covered in future updates

Myringotomy, surgery

Covered elsewhere in *Clinical Evidence*

Key Messages

Treatment

- One RCT found that ibuprofen or paracetamol versus placebo reduced earache after 2 days in children receiving antibiotic treatment.
- Systematic reviews have found conflicting evidence about antibiotics versus placebo in acute otitis media. The most recent review found that antibiotics reduced the proportion of children still in pain at 2–7 days and reduced the risk of developing contralateral acute otitis media. We found no clear evidence favouring any particular antibiotic.
- One RCT found that immediate versus delayed antibiotic treatment reduced the number of days of earache, ear discharge, and amount of daily paracetamol used after the first 24 hours of illness but found no difference in daily pain scores. It also found an increase in diarrhoea with immediate versus delayed antibiotic treatment.
- One systematic review has found that 10 day courses of antibiotics versus 5 day courses reduce treatment failure, relapse, or re-infection in the short term (at 8–10 days), but found no significant difference in the long term (at 20–30 days). Two subsequent RCTs found similar results.

Prevention

- One systematic review has found that long term antibiotic prophylaxis versus placebo reduces recurrences of acute otitis media. However, one subsequent RCT found no significant difference between antibiotic prophylaxis and placebo.
- We found insufficient evidence on which antibiotic to use, for how long, and how many previous episodes of acute otitis media justify the starting of preventive treatment.

- One RCT found that xylitol syrup or chewing gum versus controls reduced the incidence of acute otitis media. It found no significant difference with xylitol lozenges versus control gum. More children taking xylitol versus control withdrew because of abdominal pain or other unspecified reasons.

DEFINITION   Otitis media is an inflammation in the middle ear. Subcategories include acute otitis media (AOM), recurrent AOM, and chronic suppurative otitis media. AOM presents with systemic and local signs, and has a rapid onset. The persistence of an effusion beyond 3 months without signs of infection defines otitis media with effusion (also known as "glue ear"). Chronic suppurative otitis media is characterised by continuing inflammation in the middle ear causing discharge (otorrhoea) through a perforated tympanic membrane.

INCIDENCE/   AOM is common and has a high morbidity and low mortality. In the
PREVALENCE   UK about 30% of children under 3 years old visit their general practitioner with AOM each year and 97% receive antimicrobial treatment.[1] By 3 months of age, 10% of children have had an episode of AOM. It is the most common reason for outpatient antimicrobial treatment in the USA.[2]

AETIOLOGY/   The most common bacterial causes for AOM in the USA and UK are
RISK FACTORS *Streptococcus pneumoniae, Haemophilus influenzae,* and *Moraxella catarrhalis.* Similar pathogens are found in Colombia.[3] The incidence of penicillin resistant *S pneumoniae* has risen, but rates differ between countries. The most important risk factors for AOM are young age and attendance at daycare centres such as nursery schools. Other risk factors include being white; male sex; and a history of enlarged adenoids, tonsillitis, or asthma; multiple previous episodes; bottle feeding; a history of ear infections in parents or siblings; and use of a soother or pacifier. The evidence for an effect of environmental tobacco smoke is controversial.[1]

PROGNOSIS   In about 80% of children the condition resolves in about 3 days without antibiotic treatment. Serious complications are rare but include hearing loss, mastoiditis, meningitis, and recurrent attacks.[1] The World Health Organization estimates that each year 51 000 children under the age of 5 years die from complications of otitis media in developing countries.[4]

AIMS   To reduce the severity and duration of pain and other symptoms, to prevent complications, and to minimise adverse effects of treatment.

OUTCOMES   Pain control (in infants this can be assessed by surrogate measures such as parental observation of distress/crying and analgesic use); incidence of complications such as deafness (usually divided into short and long term hearing loss), recurrent attacks of AOM, mastoiditis, and meningitis; resolution of otoscopic appearances; incidence of adverse effects of treatment.

METHODS   *Clinical Evidence* search and appraisal June 2001.

OPTION   ANALGESICS

One RCT found that ibuprofen or paracetamol versus placebo reduced earache after 2 days in children receiving antibiotic treatment.

Benefits: We found no systematic review but found one RCT (219 children aged 1–6 years with otoscopically diagnosed acute otitis media and receiving antibiotic treatment with cefaclor for 7 days) comparing the effect of three times daily treatment with ibuprofen or paracetamol versus placebo for 48 hours on earache (otalgia) and related outcomes.[5] It found that earache after 2 days was reduced with ibuprofen versus placebo (AR 5/71 [7%] with ibuprofen v 19/75 [25%] with placebo; RR 0.28, 95% CI 0.11 to 0.71; NNT 5, 95% CI 3 to 15) and with paracetamol versus placebo (AR 7/73 [10%] v 19/75 [25%] with placebo; RR 0.38, 95% CI 0.17 to 0.85; NNT 6, 95% CI 3 to 28). It found no difference between paracetamol and ibuprofen for reducing earache and no difference for ibuprofen or paracetamol versus placebo for other outcomes (appearance of the tympanic membrane; rectal temperature; and parental assessment of appetite, sleep, and playing activity).

Harms: The RCT found that 11 children experienced mild nausea, vomiting, and abdominal pain (5 [7%] taking ibuprofen, 3 [4%] taking paracetamol, and 3 [4%] taking placebo). None were withdrawn from treatment.[5]

Comment: The evidence from this RCT is limited because the assessment of the child's pain relief was based on parental observation using a scale of 0 or 1. The paracetamol versus placebo result has been recalculated by *Clinical Evidence* from data in the original publication, and corrects the stated conclusions of the RCT.

OPTION   ANTIBIOTICS

Systematic reviews have found conflicting evidence about antibiotics versus placebo in acute otitis media. The most recent review found that antibiotics reduced the proportion of children still in pain at 2–7 days and reduced the risk of developing contralateral acute otitis media. We found no clear evidence favouring any particular antibiotic. One RCT found that immediate versus delayed antibiotic treatment reduced the number of days of earache, ear discharge, and amount of daily paracetamol used after the first 24 hours of illness but found no difference in daily pain scores. It also found an increase in diarrhoea with immediate versus delayed antibiotic treatment.

Benefits: We found three systematic reviews and one subsequent RCT.[6–9]
Versus placebo or no treatment: One systematic review (search date 1992, 5400 children aged 4 months to 18 years, 33 RCTs) identified four RCTs (535 children receiving analgesics or other symptomatic relief).[6] It found a significant reduction in symptoms with a range of antibiotics (cephalosporins, erythromycin, penicillins, trimethoprim–sulfamethoxazole [co-trimoxazole]) versus placebo after 7–14 days' treatment (ARR 13.7%, 95% CI 8.2% to

19.2%; NNT 7).[6] The second systematic review (search date 1997, 741 children aged less than 2 years, 4 RCTs comparing antibiotics versus placebo alone or versus placebo with myringotomy) found no significant difference in clinical improvement between the two groups (OR 1.31, 95% CI 0.83 to 2.08).[7] A third systematic review (search date 2000, 2202 children aged 6 months to 15 years, 9 RCTs) compared early use of antibiotics versus placebo.[8] It found that antibiotics (e.g. erythromycin and penicillins) versus placebo reduced the proportion of children still in pain 2–7 days after presentation (175/1160 with antibiotics v 234/1128 with placebo; ARR 5.6%, 95% CI 2.5% to 8.7%; RR 0.72, 95% CI 0.62 to 0.85; NNT 17). In addition, fewer children experienced contralateral acute otitis media (35/329 with antibiotics v 56/337 with placebo; ARR 5.9%, 95% CI 1.0% to 10.8%; RR 0.65 95% CI 0.45 to 0.94).[8] The review found no difference in the rate of subsequent attacks of acute otitis media (187/864 with antibiotics v 175/804 with placebo; RR 1.00, 95% CI 0.83 to 1.19), abnormal tympanometry at 1 month (85/234 with antibiotic v 91/238 with placebo; RR 0.94, 95% CI 0.74 to 1.19), or abnormal tympanometry at 3 months (38/182 with antibiotic v 49/188 with placebo; RR 0.80, 95% CI 0.55 to 1.16). Four RCTs (717 children) reported pain outcomes 24 hours after presentation. All four found no difference in pain outcomes with antibiotics versus placebo (RR 1.02, 95% CI 0.85 to 1.22). Most RCTs did not state the time interval between onset of symptoms and starting treatment: the two RCTs that did stated 1–24 hours and about 30 hours. Only 1/2202 children developed mastoiditis (in a penicillin treated group).[8] **Choice of antibiotic regimen:** One systematic review (search date 1992, 5400 children aged 4 months to 18 years, 33 RCTs) found no differences between different antibiotics in rate of treatment success at 7–14 days or of middle ear effusion at 30 days.[6] **Immediate versus delayed antibiotic treatment:** We found one RCT (315 children aged 6 months to 10 years) comparing immediate versus delayed antibiotic (amoxycillin or erythromycin) use.[9] It found that after the first 24 hours of illness, immediate versus delayed antibiotic use reduced the duration of earache (mean difference –1.10 days, 95% CI –0.54 to –1.48), duration of ear discharge (mean difference –0.66 days, 95% CI –0.19 to –1.13), number of disturbed nights (mean difference –0.72 days, 95% CI –0.30 to –1.13), number of days crying (mean difference –0.69 days, 95% CI –0.31 to –1.08), and the number of teaspoons of paracetamol used (mean difference –0.52 teaspoons daily, 95% CI –0.26 to –0.79). The RCT found no significant difference in mean daily pain score (mean difference –0.16, 95% CI –0.42 to +0.11), number of daily episodes of distress (mean difference –0.12, 95% CI –0.34 to +0.11), or days absence from school (mean difference –0.18, 95% CI –0.76 to +0.41).

Harms: One systematic review gave no information on adverse events.[6] Another review found that antibiotics increased the risk of vomiting, diarrhoea, or rashes (AR 57/345 [17%] with antibiotics v 38/353 [11%] with control; RR 1.55, 95% CI 1.11 to 2.16; NNH 17, 95% CI 9 to 152).[8] The RCT comparing immediate versus delayed treatment with antibiotics found that immediate treatment increased diarrhoea (AR 25/135 [19%] with immediate v 14/150

[9%] with delayed; RR 1.9, 95% CI 1.08 to 3.66), but had no significant effect on rash (AR 6/133 [5%] with immediate v 8/149 [5%] with delayed; RR 0.84, 95% CI 0.30 to 2.36).[9]

Comment: The first systematic review[6] excluded two placebo controlled trials that were included in the second review[8] because they included myringotomy as part of the treatment. This may have biased the results in favour of antibiotic treatment and may explain the higher absolute risk reduction quoted in the first review.[6] We found inadequate evidence for the effectiveness of antibiotics in countries where the incidence of complicating mastoiditis is high.

| OPTION | SHORT VERSUS LONGER COURSES OF ANTIBIOTICS |

One systematic review has found that 10 day courses of antibiotics versus 5 day courses reduce treatment failure, relapse, or re-infection in the short term (at 8–19 days), but found no significant difference in the long term (at 20–30 days). Two subsequent RCTs found similar results.

Benefits: We found one systematic review[10] and two subsequent RCTs.[11,12] The systematic review (search date 1998, 30 RCTs in children aged 4 wks to 18 years with acute otitis media) found that treatment failure, relapse, or re-infection at an early evaluation (8–19 days) were more likely to occur with shorter courses of antibiotics (5 days) than with longer courses (8–10 days) (summary OR compared with longer courses 1.52, 95% CI 1.17 to 1.98). However, by 20–30 days, there were no differences between treatment groups (summary OR 1.22, 95% CI 0.98 to 1.54). The first subsequent RCT (385 younger children with newly diagnosed acute otitis media, mean age 13.3 months, range 4.0–30.0 months) compared amoxicillin/clavulanate in three divided doses for 10 days versus 5 days followed by 5 days of placebo.[11] Clinical success or failure was assessed at 12–14 days and again at 28–42 days after starting treatment. Intention to treat analysis found that the 10 day regimen increased clinical success on days 12–14 compared with the 5 day regimen (AR 158/186 [85%] for 10 days v 141/192 [73%] for 5 days; RR 1.16, 95% CI 1.04 to 1.28; NNT 8, 95% CI 5 to 30). However, by days 28–42, there was no significant difference in clinical success between the two groups (AR 108/185 [58%] for 10 days v 102/190 [54%] for 5 days; RR 1.09, 95% CI 0.91 to 1.30). The second subsequent RCT compared cefpodoxime–proxetil twice daily at 8 mg/kg daily for 10 days versus for 5 days followed by 5 days of placebo. It found that success rates were higher with the 10 days versus 5 days treatment group after 12–14 days (AR 199/222 [90%] for 10 days v 180/226 [80%] for 5 day treatment; RR 1.13, 95% CI 1.04 to 1.22; NNT 10, 95% CI 6 to 30), but no significance was found after 28–42 days (AR 149/222 [67%] for 10 days v 141/226 [62%] for 5 day treatment; RR 1.08, 95% CI 0.94 to 1.23).[12]

Harms: The systematic review (search date 1998)[10] and the two subsequent RCTs[11,12] found no difference with short versus long courses of antibiotics for diarrhoea and/or vomiting and rash.

Comment: None.

| OPTION | LONG TERM ANTIBIOTIC TREATMENT |

One systematic review has found that long term antibiotic prophylaxis versus placebo reduces recurrences of acute otitis media. However, one subsequent RCT found no significant difference between antibiotic prophylaxis and placebo. We found insufficient evidence on which antibiotic to use, for how long, and how many episodes of acute otitis media justify starting preventive treatment.

Benefits: **Versus placebo:** We found one systematic review and one subsequent RCT. The systematic review (search date 1993) identified 33 RCTs comparing antibiotics versus placebo to prevent recurrent acute otitis media (AOM) and otitis media with effusion.[13] Nine of the trials (945 people) looked at recurrent AOM only. It was not clear from the review which of the studies referred only to children; four either included the word "children" in the title or appeared in paediatric journals. Most studies defined recurrent AOM as at least three episodes of AOM in 6 months. The most commonly used antibiotics were amoxycillin, co-trimoxazole, and sulfamethoxazole, given for 3 months to 2 years. All nine studies showed a lower rate of recurrence with antibiotic treatment, although in seven the difference was not significant. Overall, the review found that antibiotics slightly reduced recurrence of AOM (AR of recurrence per person per month 0.08 with antibiotics v 0.19 with placebo; ARR 11%, 95% CI 3% to 19%; NNT per month to prevent 1 acute episode 9, 95% CI 5 to 33). The subsequent RCT (194 children aged 3 months to 6 years with 3 documented episodes of AOM within the preceding 6 months) compared amoxycillin 20 mg/kg daily either once or twice daily versus placebo.[14] The children were followed up monthly if asymptomatic or within 3–5 days if they had symptoms of upper respiratory tract infection for up to 90 days. The RCT found no significant difference between antibiotics versus placebo in preventing recurrent AOM (RR of remaining AOM free children diagnosed by otoscopy and tympanometry 1.00, 95% CI 0.66 to 1.52 using completer analysis, 36 children lost to follow up). Calculations including those children lost to follow up yielded similar results whether the outcomes were assumed in favour of placebo or in favour of antibiotics. **Choice and duration of antibiotic:** The systematic review found no significant difference in rate of recurrence between antibiotics. Greater treatment effect was seen with treatment lasting less than 6 months, but the confidence intervals overlapped (ARR for recurrence with courses < 6 months 21%, 95% CI 7% to 49%; ARR with courses > 6 months 4%, 95% CI 1% to 9%).[13]

Harms: The studies gave no information on harms.

Comment: None.

Acute otitis media

Child health

OPTION	XYLITOL CHEWING GUM OR SYRUP

One RCT found that xylitol syrup or chewing gum versus controls reduced the incidence of acute otitis media. It found no significant difference with xylitol lozenges versus control gum. More children taking xylitol versus control withdrew because of abdominal pain or other unspecified reasons.

Benefits: We found no systematic review but found one RCT (857 children, 54% boys) comparing xylitol (either as chewing gum, syrup, or lozenges) versus control (syrup or chewing gum).[15] The RCT randomised children into two groups according to ability to chew gum. Children who could chew gum received xylitol gum (8.4 g daily, 179 children), xylitol lozenges (10 g daily, 176 children), or control gum (xylitol 0.5 g daily, 178 children). Children who could not chew gum received xylitol syrup (10 g daily, 159 children) or control syrup (0.5 g daily, 165 children). Each time the child showed any signs of acute respiratory infection, acute otitis media (AOM) was excluded using tympanometry and otoscopy. Follow up was for 3 months. In the first group, xylitol gum versus control gum significantly reduced the number of children with at least one episode of AOM (AR 29/179 [16%] v 49/178 [28%]; RR 0.59, 95% CI 0.39 to 0.89; NNT 8, 95% CI 5 to 36) but no significant difference was found with xylitol lozenges versus control gum (AR 39/176 [22%] v 49/178 [28%]; RR 0.81, 95% CI 0.56 to 1.16). In the second group, xylitol syrup versus control syrup reduced the number of children with at least one episode of AOM (AR 46/159 [29%] v 68/165 [41%]; RR 0.70, 95% CI 0.52 to 0.95; NNT 8, 95% CI 4 to 53).

Harms: The RCT found that more children taking xylitol lozenges or syrup versus control treatment withdrew from the trial (xylitol lozenges v control gum, 26/176 [15%] v 8/178 [5%], P < 0.001; xylitol syrup v control syrup, 30/159 [19%] v 17/165 [10%], P < 0.03). Most withdrawals were because of either an unwillingness to take the intervention, having left the area, or because of abdominal discomfort.[15] We found no evidence about the long term effects of xylitol.

Comment: The children in this study received xylitol or the control intervention five times daily, a regimen that might be difficult to maintain long term. The incidence of AOM in those who withdrew from the trial was not described; therefore, the reported effect of xylitol may be under or overestimated.

REFERENCES

1. Froom J, Culpepper L, Jacobs M, et al. Antimicrobials for acute otitis media? A review from the International Primary Care Network. *BMJ* 1997;315:98–102.
2. Del Mar C, Glasziou P, Hayem M. Are antibiotics indicated as initial treatment for children with acute otitis media? A meta-analysis. *BMJ* 1997; 314:1526–1529. Search date 1994; primary sources Medline and Current Contents.
3. Berman S. Otitis media in developing countries. *Pediatrics* 1995;96:126–131.
4. World Health Organization. *World Development Report 1993: Investing in Health.* Oxford: Oxford University Press,1993:215–222.
5. Bertin L, Pons G, d'Athis P, et al. A randomized double blind multicentre controlled trial of ibuprofen versus acetaminophen and placebo for symptoms of acute otitis media in children. *Fundam Clin Pharmacol* 1996;10:387–392.
6. Rosenfeld RM, Vertrees JE, Carr J, et al. Clinical efficacy of antimicrobial drugs for acute otitis media: meta-analysis of 5400 children from thirty-three randomised trials. *J Pediatr* 1994;124: 355–367. Search date June 1992; primary sources Medline and Current Contents.
7. Damoiseaux RA, van Balen FAM, Hoes AW, de Melker RA. Antibiotic treatment of acute otitis

media in children under two years of age: evidence based? *Br J Gen Pract* 1998;48: 1861–1864. Search date January 1997; primary sources Medline, Embase, and hand searched references.

8. Glasziou PP, Del Mar CB, Sanders SL. Antibiotics for acute otitis media in children (Cochrane Review). In: The Cochrane Library, Issue 3, 2001. Oxford: Update Software. Search date April 2000; primary sources Medline, Current Contents, and reference lists.

9. Little P, Gould C, Williamson I, Moore M, Warner G, Dunleavey J. Pragmatic randomised controlled trial of two prescribing strategies for childhood acute otitis media. *BMJ* 2001;322:336–342.

10. Kozyrskj AL, Hildes-Ripstein GE, Longstaffe SEA, et al. Short course antibiotics for acute otitis media. In: The Cochrane Library, Issue 3, 2000. Oxford: Update Software. Search date 1998; primary sources Medline, Embase, Science Citation Index, Current Contents, hand searches of reference lists, and personal contacts.

11. Cohen R, Levy C, Boucherat M, Langue J, de la Rocque F. A multicenter randomized, double blind trial of 5 versus 10 days of antibiotic therapy for acute otitis media in young children. *J Pediatr* 1998;133:634–639.

12. Cohen R, Levy C, Boucherat M, et al. Five vs. ten days of antibiotic therapy for acute otitis media in young children. *Pediatr Infect Dis J* 2000;19: 458–463.

13. Williams RL, Chalmers TC, Stange KC, Chalmers FT, Bowin SJ. Use of antibiotics in preventing recurrent acute otitis media and in treating otitis media with effusion: a meta-analytic attempt to resolve the brouhaha. *JAMA* 1993;270: 1344–1351. (Published erratum appears in *JAMA* 1994;27:430.) Search date April 1993; primary sources Medline and Current Contents.

14. Roark R, Berman S. Continuous twice daily or once daily amoxicillin prophylaxis compared with placebo for children with recurrent acute otitis media. *Pediatr Infect Dis J* 1997;16:376–378.

15. Uhari M, Kontiokari T, Niemela MA. Novel use of xylitol sugar in preventing acute otitis media. *Pediatrics* 1998;102:879–884.

Paddy O'Neill
General Practitioner
Norton Medical Centre
Stockton on Tees
UK

Competing interests: None declared.

Asthma in children

Search date June 2001

Duncan Keeley

Key Messages

Treating acute asthma in children

■ One prospective cohort study and clinical experience support the need for oxygen in acute asthma.

- One systematic review has found that multiple doses of ipratropium bromide plus a β_2 agonist (fenoterol or salbutamol) versus β_2 agonist alone reduce hospital admission rates and improve lung function in children with severe asthma exacerbations. Combination treatment with single dose of ipratropium bromide plus a β_2 agonist (fenoterol, salbutamol or terbutaline) improves lung function but does not reduce hospital admission rates in children with mild to moderate asthma exacerbations.

- One systematic review, in children with acute but not life threatening asthma who were old enough to use a spacer, has found no significant difference in hospital admission rates with a metered dose inhaler plus a spacer versus nebulisation for delivery of β_2 agonists (fenoterol, salbutamol or terbutaline) or β agonist (orciprenaline). Children using a metered dose inhaler with a spacer may have shorter stays in emergency departments, less hypoxia, and lower pulse rates compared with children receiving β_2 agonist by nebulisation.

- One systematic review has found that early administration of oral corticosteroids (prednisone or prednisolone) versus placebo reduces hospital admission in children with acute asthma exacerbations.

- One systematic review found no consistent differences in hospital admission rates or forced expiratory volume in 1 second (FEV_1) between initial treatment with high dose inhaled corticosteroids versus oral corticosteroids in acute moderately severe asthma. Three RCTs found no significant difference; one RCT found that oral corticosteroids reduced hospital admission and improved lung function. One subsequent RCT found that inhaled corticosteroids improved lung function. These RCTs excluded children with the most severe attacks.

- We found conflicting evidence from one systematic review and one RCT on the effects of intravenous theophylline in acute asthma. Treatment was frequently stopped because of adverse effects.

Single agent prophylaxis in childhood asthma

- One systematic review has found that prophylactic inhaled corticosteroids (betamethasone, beclometasone budesonide, flunisolide, or fluticasone) versus placebo improve symptoms and lung function in children with asthma.

- RCTs have found that inhaled corticosteroids (beclometasone, budesonide, or fluticasone) versus inhaled long acting β_2 agonists (salmeterol) or inhaled nedocromil improve symptoms and lung function in children with asthma.

- One RCT found no significant difference in improving symptoms with inhaled beclometasone versus theophylline.

- Two systematic reviews of studies with long term follow up and a subsequent long term RCT have found no evidence of growth retardation in children with asthma treated with inhaled corticosteroids. Some shorter term studies found reduced growth velocity.

Additional treatments in childhood asthma inadequately controlled by standard dose inhaled corticosteroids

- One RCT, of the addition of a second dose of inhaled corticosteroid (beclometasone) found no significant differences in lung function, symptom scores, exacerbation rates or bronchial reactivity, but found significant reduction of growth velocity at 1 year.

- One RCT found that addition of a long acting β_2 agonist (salmeterol) increased peak expiratory flow rates in the first few months of treatment but found no increase after 1 year. A second short term RCT also found increased morning peak expiratory flow rates and more symptom free days at 3 months with addition of a long acting β_2 agonist (salmeterol).

- One small brief RCT found that addition of theophylline versus placebo to previous treatment significantly increased the number of symptom free days and significantly reduced the use of additional β agonist and additional corticosteroid medication. We found insufficient evidence to weigh these short term benefits and possible long term harms.

- One brief crossover RCT found small improvements in lung function and fewer asthma exacerbation days with addition of leukotriene receptor antagonist (montelukast) to inhaled corticosteroid (budesonide) in children with persistent asthma.

Treating acute wheeze in infants

- We found conflicting evidence from RCTs. Transient hypoxia may be caused by nebulised bronchodilators, particularly with air driven nebulisers, and seems less likely when using metered dose inhalers/spacers (see bronchiolitis, p 46).

- We found limited and conflicting evidence from one systematic review of small RCTs on the effects of inhaled ipratropium bromide for clinical outcomes in wheezing children.

- We found no evidence that oral corticosteroids improve outcomes in acute wheezing infants.

Prophylaxis in wheezing infants

- We found weak and conflicting evidence on the effects of prophylaxis with inhaled corticosteroids in wheezing infants.

DEFINITION   **Childhood asthma** is characterised by chronic or recurrent cough and wheeze. The diagnosis is confirmed by demonstrating reversible airway obstruction in children old enough to perform peak flow measurements or spirometry. Diagnosing asthma in children requires exclusion of other causes of recurrent respiratory symptoms. **Wheezing in infancy** may be caused by acute viral infection (see bronchiolitis, p 46), episodic viral associated wheeze, or asthma. These are not easy to distinguish clinically.

INCIDENCE/   Surveys have found increasing prevalence of wheeze and shortness
PREVALENCE   of breath, and diagnosed asthma in children. The increase is more than can be explained by an increased readiness to diagnose asthma. One questionnaire study from Aberdeen, Scotland, surveyed 2510 children aged 8–13 years in 1964 and 3403 children in 1989. Over the 25 years, prevalence of wheeze rose from 10% to 20%; episodes of shortness of breath from 5% to 10%; and diagnosis of asthma from 4% to 10%.[1] One prospective cohort study (826 neonates reviewed at 3 and 6 years of age) found that 34% had experienced at least one wheezing illness before age 3 years, 14% wheezed before age 3 years and were still wheezing at age 6, and 15% had a wheezing illness in the past year at age 6 but had not wheezed before age 3.[2]

AETIOLOGY/ RISK FACTORS	Asthma is more common in children with a personal or family history of atopy. Precipitating factors include infection, house dust mites, allergens from pet animals, exposure to tobacco smoke, and anxiety.
PROGNOSIS	A historical cohort study of wheezing in the first year of life found that 14% of children with one attack and 23% of children with four or more attacks (recalled at age 5 years) had experienced at least one wheezing illness in the past year at age 10.[3]
AIMS	To reduce or abolish cough and wheeze; to attain best possible lung function; to reduce the risk of severe attacks; to minimise sleep disturbance and absence from school; to minimise adverse effects of treatment; and to allow normal growth.
OUTCOMES	Wheeze; cough; nights disturbed by asthma; days lost from school or normal activities; hospital admission and duration of stay in hospital (subjective proxy outcome measures for severity of asthma exacerbations); lung function tests (peak expiratory flow rates and forced expiratory volume in 1 second); blood oxygen saturation in acute attacks; and airway hyperresponsiveness (measured using methacholine challenge tests).
METHODS	*Clinical Evidence* search and appraisal June 2001.

QUESTION What are the effects of treatments for acute asthma in children?

OPTION OXYGEN

One prospective cohort study and clinical experience support the need for oxygen in acute asthma.

Benefits:
We found no systematic review or RCTs. One double blind, prospective cohort study (280 children) found that decreased oxygen saturation upon entry to an emergency department was correlated with increased treatment with intravenous aminophylline (see glossary, p 33) and corticosteroids, and increased rates of hospital admission or subsequent readmission (arterial oxygen saturation ≤ 91% v arterial oxygen saturation ≥ 96%: OR 35, 95% CI 11 to 150; for arterial oxygen saturation 92–95% v ≥ 96%: OR 4.2, 95% CI 2.2 to 8.8).[4]

Harms:
We found no evidence about harms.

Comment:
A RCT of oxygen versus no oxygen treatment in acute severe asthma would be considered unethical. The cohort study does not address directly whether oxygen should be given therapeutically but it does suggest, along with clinical experience, that oxygen should continue to be given promptly to children with acute asthma.[4]

OPTION IPRATROPIUM BROMIDE ADDED TO β_2 AGONISTS

One systematic review has found that multiple doses of ipratropium bromide plus a β_2 agonist (fenoterol or salbutamol) versus the β_2 agonist alone reduce hospital admission rates and improve lung function in children with severe asthma exacerbations. Combination treatment with a

single dose of ipratropium bromide plus a β_2 agonist (fenoterol, salbutamol, or terbutaline) versus the β_2 agonist alone improves lung function but does not reduce hospital admission rates in children with mild to moderate asthma exacerbations.

Benefits: We found one systematic review (search date 2000, 13 RCTs, children aged 18 months to 17 years with acute asthma) comparing effects of combined inhaled anticholinergics plus β_2 agonists versus β_2 agonists alone on hospital admission rate.[5] **Single dose:** The systematic review found that in children with mild to moderate exacerbations, adding a single dose of ipratropium bromide to β_2 agonists (fenoterol, salbutamol [see glossary, p 33] or terbutaline) versus the β_2 agonist alone significantly improved forced expiratory volume in 1 second (FEV_1) at 1 hour (3 RCTs: SMD 0.57, 95% CI 0.21 to 0.93) and at 2 hours (3 RCTs: SMD 0.53, 95% CI 0.17 to 0.90), but found no significant reduction in hospital admission (3 RCTs: RR 0.93, 95% CI 0.65 to 1.32).[5] **Multiple doses:** The systematic review found that in children with mild, moderate, or severe exacerbations, adding multiple doses of ipratropium bromide to a β_2 agonist (fenoterol or salbutamol) improved FEV_1 (4 RCTs: WMD 9.7 of predicted FEV_1, 95% CI 5.7 to 13.7, 1 h after last ipratropium bromide inhalation) and reduced hospital admissions (6 RCTs: RR 0.75, 95% CI 0.62 to 0.89; NNT 13, 95% CI 8 to 32). Subgroup analysis found significant reduction only in children with severe exacerbations (baseline FEV_1 < 50% of predicted or change of 7 to 9 in baseline clinical score after last combined inhalation, RR 0.71, 95% CI 0.58 to 0.89; NNT 7, 95% CI 5 to 20).[5]

Harms: The systematic review found no significant increase in risk of nausea (3 RCTs: RR 0.59, 95% CI 0.30 to 1.14), vomiting (3 RCTs: RR 1.03, 95% CI 0.37 to 2.87), or tremor (4 RCTs: RR 1.01, 95% CI 0.63 to 1.63) in children treated with multiple doses of ipratropium bromide.[5]

Comment: None.

OPTION	METERED DOSE INHALER PLUS SPACER DEVICES VERSUS NEBULISERS FOR DELIVERING β_2 AGONISTS

One systematic review, in children with acute but not life threatening asthma who were old enough to use a spacer, has found no significant difference in hospital admission rates with a metered dose inhaler plus a spacer versus nebulisation for delivery of β_2 agonists (fenoterol, salbutamol or terbutaline) or β agonist (orciprenaline). Children using a metered dose inhaler with a spacer may have shorter stays in emergency departments, less hypoxia, and lower pulse rates compared with children receiving β_2 agonist by nebulisation.

Benefits: We found one systematic review (search date 1999, 16 RCTs, 686 children with acute asthma but excluding life threatening asthma) comparing spacer/holding chamber attached to a metered dose inhaler versus single or multiple treatment with nebuliser for delivery of β_2 agonists (fenoterol, salbutamol [see glossary, p 33] or terbutaline) or β agonist (orciprenaline [see glossary, p 33]).[6] The review found no significant difference between spacer and multiple treatments with nebulisers in hospital admission rates (OR 0.91,

95% CI 0.4 to 2.1). It found a significant increase in pulse rate with nebulisers (WMD 8.3% from baseline, 95% CI 5.0% to 11.5%). One RCT (152 children $\geq$ 2 years) found that the time spent in the emergency department was shorter in children using metered dose inhaler plus spacer (WMD –37 min, 95% CI –50 to –24 min).[7] Two small RCTs included in the review comparing delivery of β_2 agonists (salbutamol or terbutaline) via spacer versus single treatment with nebuliser found less deterioration in blood gases with the spacer.[6]

Harms: The systematic review found no significant deterioration in any of the outcome measures with delivery of β_2 agonists using metered dose inhaler plus a spacer versus nebulisation.[6]

Comment: These findings suggest that, in children old enough to use a spacer, metered dose inhaler with spacer could be substituted for nebulisation in the treatment of acute asthma in emergency departments and hospital wards.

OPTION   ORAL CORTICOSTEROIDS

One systematic review has found that early oral corticosteroids (prednisone or prednisolone) versus placebo reduce hospital admission in children with acute asthma exacerbations.

Benefits: We found one systematic review (search date 1999, 3 RCTs comparing corticosteroid v placebo within 45 min of arrival at the emergency department).[8] It found that oral corticosteroid (1–2 mg/kg prednisone or prednisolone) versus placebo significantly reduced admission rates in children with acute asthma exacerbations (OR 0.24, 95% CI 0.11 to 0.53).[8]

Harms: The systematic review included RCTs in adults and did not report separately on adverse reactions in children given oral corticosteroids; overall it found no significant difference with oral corticosteroids versus placebo.[8] We found few reports of adverse effects with short courses of systemic corticosteroids. Several case reports have associated systemic corticosteroid treatment with severe varicella infection. One case control study (167 cases, 134 controls) in otherwise immunocompetent children with complicated and uncomplicated varicella infection did not find significant risk attributable to corticosteroid exposure (OR 1.6, 95% CI 0.2 to 17), but it was too small to exclude a clinically important risk.[9]

Comment: None.

OPTION   HIGH DOSE INHALED CORTICOSTEROIDS

One systematic review has found no consistent differences in hospital admission rates or increase in flow expiratory volume in 1 second between initial treatment with high dose inhaled corticosteroids versus oral corticosteroids in acute moderately severe asthma. Three RCTs found no significant difference; one RCT in children with severe attacks found that oral corticosteroids reduced hospital admission and improved lung function. One subsequent RCT found that inhaled corticosteroids improved lung function. These RCTs excluded children with the most severe attacks.

Benefits: **High dose inhaled versus oral:** We found one systematic review (search date not stated, 4 RCTs),[10] one subsequent RCT,[11] and one additional RCT.[12] The systematic review compared effects of initial treatment with high dose inhaled corticosteroids versus oral corticosteroids in hospital emergency departments on admission rates.[10] The results from the four RCTs were not pooled because of marked heterogeneity between studies. One RCT (100 children with acute asthma ≥ 5 years, mean initial flow expiratory volume in 1 second [FEV_1] 45%) compared fluticasone (2 mg through metered dose inhaler with spacer) versus prednisone (2 mg/kg orally).[13] It found that prednisone reduced hospital admission (10% prednisone v 31% fluticasone; P = 0.01) and increased mean FEV_1 at 4 hours (9% fluticasone v 19% prednisone; P ≤ 0.001).[13] The second RCT (111 children aged 1–17 years) compared dexamethasone (1.5 mg/kg via nebuliser) versus prednisone (2 mg orally).[14] It found no significant difference between nebulised dexmethasone versus oral prednisone in hospital admission (12/56 [21%] with dexamethasone v 44/55 [31%] with prednisone; ARR 9.5%, 95% CI −8% to 21%; RR 0.69, 95% CI 0.36 to 1.27), but found fewer relapses with nebulised dexamethasone within 48 hours after discharge (0/44 [0%] v 6/38 [16%]; ARR −16%, 95% CI −27% to −4.5%); however, all children in the RCT received a 5 day course of prednisone (2 mg/kg daily) on discharge.[14] Two other RCTs compared budesonide (800 μg via nebuliser at 1, 30, and 60 mins; 1600 μg via turbohaler) versus prednisolone (2 mg/kg orally).[15,16] Overall, no significant differences were found between the groups in admission rates (OR for inhaled corticosteroids v oral corticosteroids 0.49, 95% CI 0.22 to 1.07).[15,16] The subsequent RCT (321 children aged 4–16 years, peak expiratory flow rate 40–75% predicted) compared nebulised fluticasone (1 mg twice daily for 7 days) versus oral prednisolone (2 mg/kg for 4 days then 1 mg/kg for 3 days). It found that nebulised fluticasone versus oral prednisolone improved mean morning peak expiratory flow rate over 7 days (difference 9.5 L/min, 95% CI 2 L/min to 17 L/min). No significant differences were found in symptom scores, withdrawals, or adverse events.[11] The additional RCT (46 children, aged 15–16 years, admitted to hospital with severe exacerbations of asthma) compared nebulised budesonide 2 mg hourly with oral prednisolone 2 mg/kg at admission and after 24 hours.[12] It found no significant difference between groups in FEV_1 at 24 hours or at 3 and 24 days after admission. All children in this trial were treated with 800 μg budesonide daily following discharge from hospital.

Harms: The systematic review found no significant adverse effects with inhaled corticosteroids.[10]

Comment: These RCTs suggest that high dose inhaled corticosteroids may be substituted for oral corticosteroids in the initial phase of treatment of moderately severe acute asthma. This may be useful for children who vomit oral corticosteroids or for children with frequent exacerbations where there is concern about the cumulative dose of oral steroids. One RCT was funded by the manufacturers of fluticasone.[11]

OPTION INTRAVENOUS THEOPHYLLINE

We found conflicting evidence from one systematic review and one RCT on the effects of intravenous theophylline in acute asthma. Treatment was frequently stopped because of adverse effects.

Benefits:
We found one systematic review (search date 1994, 6 small RCTs, 164 children aged 1.5–18 years)[17] and one subsequent RCT.[18] The review found no significant difference with intravenous theophylline versus placebo added to routine treatment (mean difference in forced expiratory volume in 1 second [FEV_1] +39% of predicted; P = 0.25).[17] The subsequent RCT (163 children aged 1–19 years with acute asthma, 43% admitted to intensive care) compared intravenous aminophylline (see glossary, p 33) versus placebo. It found significantly greater improvement in FEV_1 at 6 hours (mean increase in FEV_1 10%, 95% CI 4% to 17%), less additional oxygen needed in the first 30 hours (median 6 h with additional intravenous v 18 h with placebo; P = 0.015) and significantly reduced likelihood of intubation (absolute risk 0% with aminophylline v 6% with placebo; P = 0.03).[18]

Harms:
The systematic review (search date 1994) did not specifically look for information on adverse effects but concluded that theophylline may have slight detrimental effect as children receiving theophylline versus placebo had slightly longer hospital stays (mean difference 0.31 days; P = 0.03) and received more β_2 agonist (salbutamol) treatments (mean difference 2.1; P = 0.02).[17] The subsequent RCT found that more children had their infusions stopped with aminophylline versus placebo because of adverse effects (mainly nausea and vomiting) (32% v 5%; OR 8.7, 95% CI 2.9 to 28.4; P < 0.0001).[18] Theophylline can cause serious adverse effects (cardiac arrhythmia or convulsion) if therapeutic blood concentrations are exceeded.

Comment:
The trials in the review were too small to exclude a clinically important effect.

QUESTION What are the effects of single agent prophylaxis in childhood asthma?

OPTION INHALED CORTICOSTEROIDS

One systematic review has found that prophylactic inhaled corticosteroids (betamethasone, beclometasone, budesonide, flunisolide, or fluticasone) versus placebo improve symptoms and lung function in children with asthma. RCTs have found that inhaled corticosteroids (beclometasone, budesonide, or fluticasone) versus inhaled long acting β_2 agonists (salmeterol) or inhaled nedocromil improve symptoms and lung function in children with asthma. One RCT found no significant difference in improving symptoms with inhaled beclometasone versus theophylline. Two systematic reviews of studies with long term follow up and a subsequent long term RCT have found no evidence of growth retardation in children with asthma treated with inhaled corticosteroids. Some shorter term studies found reduced growth velocity.

Benefits: **Versus placebo:** We found one systematic review (search date 1996, 24 RCTs, 1087 children, 10/24 RCTs in preschool children, duration 4–88 wks) comparing effects of regular inhaled corticosteroids (betamethasone, beclometasone, budesonide, flunisolide, or fluticasone) versus placebo on asthma symptoms (see comment below), concomitant drug use, and peak expiratory flow rate (PEFR).[19] It found that corticosteroids significantly improved symptom score (overall weighted relative improvement in symptom score 50%, 95% CI 49% to 51%), reduced β_2 agonist use (RR 0.37, 95% CI 0.36 to 0.38), reduced oral corticosteroid use (RR 0.68, 95% CI 0.66 to 0.70), and improved peak flow rate (weighted mean improvement in PEFR 11% predicted, 95% CI 9.5% to 12.5%). **Versus theophylline:** We found no systematic review. We found one RCT (195 children aged 6–16 years, followed for 12 months) comparing inhaled beclometasone (360 µg daily) versus oral theophylline.[20] It found no significant difference with inhaled beclometasone versus oral theophylline in the mean asthma symptom score (0 = no symptoms, 6 = incapacitating symptoms: mean score 0.5 to 0.8 for beclometasone v 0.6 to 0.9 for theophylline) with less use of bronchodilators and oral corticosteroids with inhaled beclometasone. **Versus sodium cromoglicate:** We found no systematic review. Several small comparative RCTs have found sodium cromoglicate to be less effective than inhaled corticosteroids in improving symptoms and lung function. **Versus nedocromil:** We found one RCT (1041 children aged 5–12 years, forced expiratory volume in 1 second [FEV_1] 94% predicted) that compared inhaled budesonide (200 µg twice daily) and inhaled nedocromil (8 mg twice daily) versus placebo for 4–6 years.[21] It found that budesonide was superior to nedocromil, and that nedocromil was superior to placebo in several measures of asthma symptoms and morbidity (see table 1, p 35). The mean change in post-bronchodilator FEV_1 over the study period was not significantly different among the three groups. **Versus inhaled long acting β_2 agonists:** We found no systematic review but found two RCTs of beclometasone (200 µg twice daily) versus salmeterol (50 µg twice daily) for 1 year. The first RCT (67 children aged 6–16 years) found that beclometasone was more effective than salmeterol in improving FEV_1 (mean change of FEV_1 −4.5% of predicted with salmeterol, 95% CI −9.0% to +0.1% v 10% with beclometasone, 95% CI not provided; mean difference beclometasone v salmeterol 14.2%, 95% CI 8.3% to 20%), reducing use of rescue salbutamol (see glossary, p 33) (0.44 uses/day with salmeterol v 0.07 uses/day with beclometasone; P ≤ 0.001).[22] Both treatments improved symptom scores (3% of children asymptomatic before the trial with salmeterol v 6% with beclometasone; 36% at 1 year with salmeterol v 55% with beclometasone) and PEFR (improvement in morning PEFR 49 L/min with salmeterol v 61 L/min with beclometasone), but there was no significant difference between treatments at 1 year. There were two exacerbations in the beclometasone group compared with 17 in the salmeterol group. The second RCT (241 children aged 6–14 years) compared beclometasone (81 children) versus salmeterol (80 children) versus placebo (80 children).[23] It found that beclometasone reduced airway hyperresponsiveness more than salmeterol (P = 0.003). Beclometasone versus placebo reduced rescue bronchodilator use (P ≤ 0.001) and treatment withdrawals because of exacerbations (P = 0.03). Salmeterol versus placebo did not significantly reduce the use of a rescue bronchodilator (P = 0.09) or treatment withdrawals because of exacerbations (P = 0.55). Both salmeterol and beclometasone improved FEV_1 compared with placebo, but the difference between beclometasone and salmeterol was not significant. **Versus oral leukotriene receptor antagonists:** We found one systematic review (search date 1999, 10 RCTs).[24] All studies were brief (6–12 wks), although some had longer unblinded extensions. Only two studies included children. One of these (involving montelukast) remains unpublished. Another study (451 people aged 12 years and older) compared zafirlukast and low dose fluticasone. It found that fluticasone caused greater improvement in lung function (increase in mean morning PEFR 50 L/min v 12 L/min) and symptoms (change in percentage of symptom free days 28% v 16%).[25] The systematic review, mainly of results for adults, found similar exacerbation rates but inhaled corticosteroids resulted in better improvements in lung function and symptoms when compared with leukotriene receptor antagonists. We found 1 RCT (336 children, 6–14 years; 8 wk duration) comparing oral montelukast versus placebo in children with asthma (FEV_1 50% to 85% of predicted value). It found improvement with montelukast versus placebo (increase from baseline FEV_1 8.23%, 95% CI 6.3% to 10.1% v 3.6%, 95% CI 1.3 to 5.9%; P < 0.001).[26]

Harms: **Inhaled corticosteroids versus placebo:** One systematic review (search date 1996) found no significant difference with inhaled corticosteroids (betamethasone, budesonide, flunisolide, or fluticasone) versus placebo in adrenal function (12 RCTs) and found clinical cases of oral candidiasis (four RCTs).[19] Observational studies have found little or no biochemical evidence of change in bone metabolism with inhaled corticosteroids.[27,28] Two cross sectional studies using a slit lamp to screen for lenticular changes in children taking long term inhaled corticosteroids (beclometasone, budesonide) found no posterior subcapsular cataracts.[29,30] The systematic review identified eight RCTs reporting growth velocity and found no significant difference with inhaled corticosteroids versus placebo.[19] One systematic review (search date 1993, 21 studies) reported height for age in 810 children with asthma treated with oral or inhaled corticosteroids. It found no evidence of growth impairment with inhaled beclometasone (12 studies, 331 children).[31] A second systematic review (search date 1999, 3 RCTs) identified one RCT (94 children, 7–9 years) comparing effect of inhaled beclometasone 400 μg daily versus placebo on growth as a primary outcome measure in children with recurrent viral induced wheeze.[32] It found a significant decrease in growth with beclometasone versus placebo (mean growth at end of 7 month treatment period, 2.7 cm v 3.7 cm; 95% CI –1.4 to –0.6; P < 0.0001) and found no significant catch up growth during a follow up 4 month washout period.[33] A large RCT (1041 children with mild to moderate asthma) compared budesonide (400 μg daily) versus nedocromil versus placebo with 4–6 years' follow up.[21] The mean increase in height in the budesonide group was 1.1 cm less than in the placebo group (22.7 cm v 23.8 cm; P = 0.005); the difference occurred mainly within the first year of treatment.[21] Two RCTs comparing beclometasone with salmeterol found slowing in linear growth with beclometasone (growth over year of treatment 5.4 cm[22] and 6.1 cm in the salmeterol groups, 4.0 cm[22] and 4.7 cm[23] in the beclometasone groups; P = 0.004;[22] P = 0.007).[23] **Theophylline:** One RCT found that continuous oral theophylline was associated with a higher frequency of headache, gastric irritation, and tremor than beclometasone (360 μg daily).[20] One systematic review (search date not stated, 12 studies, 340 children) of the behavioural and cognitive effects of theophylline found no evidence of significant adverse effects.[34] Another RCT compared inhaled beclometasone (360 μg daily) versus oral theophylline for 1 year.[20] It found a significantly higher rate of growth (more notable in boys) with the theophylline group (mean rate of growth in prepubescent boys 4.3 cm/year v 6.2 cm/year). This effect was not sufficient to be noticed by the children or by their parents, and no child was withdrawn from the study on this account.[20] **Sodium cromoglicate:** Sodium cromoglicate may cause cough, throat irritation, and bronchoconstriction, but no long term adverse effects have been reported. **Versus theophylline or sodium cromoglicate:** One controlled, prospective study compared 216 children treated with budesonide (400–600 μg daily) with 62 children treated with theophylline or sodium cromoglicate over 3–5 years' follow up.[35] No significant changes in growth velocity were found at doses up to 400 μg (5.5 cm/year with budesonide v 5.6 cm/year with controls). The adult height of 142 of these budesonide treated children (mean treatment period 9.2 years, mean daily dosage 412 μg) was compared with 18 controls never treated with inhaled corticosteroids and 51 healthy siblings. There were no significant differences. Children in all groups attained their target adult height (mean difference between measured and target adult height: +0.3 cm, 95% CI –0.6 to +1.2 for budesonide treated children; –0.2 cm, 95% CI –2.4 to +2.1 for control children with asthma; +0.9 cm, 95% CI –0.4 to +2.2 for healthy siblings).[36] **Inhaled long acting β_2 agonists:** These agents occasionally cause tremor or tachycardia. Three large RCTs found no evidence of important adverse effects from salmeterol over 1 year.[22,23,37] **Oral leukotriene receptor antagonists:** One placebo controlled RCT found similar incidence of adverse effects with leukotriene receptor antagonists and with placebo.[26] A systematic review (search date 1994) found that leukotriene receptor antagonists compared with corticosteroids were associated with increased risk of withdrawal because of adverse effects (3 RCTs; RR 1.9, 95% CI 1.1 to 3.3).[24] Gastrointestinal symptoms and headaches have been reported with both montelukast and zafirlukast. Allergic granulomatosis (Churg Strauss syndrome) has been reported in people taking either drug, possibly because of reduction in steroid treatment unmasking a pre-existing condition.

Comment: None.

QUESTION **What are the effects of additional treatments in childhood asthma inadequately controlled by standard dose inhaled corticosteroids?**

OPTION INCREASED DOSE OF INHALED CORTICOSTEROID

One RCT, of the addition of a second dose of inhaled corticosteroid (beclometasone) to previous treatment, found no significant differences in lung function, symptom scores, exacerbation rates, or bronchial reactivity and found an adverse effect on growth velocity at 1 year.

Benefits: We found no systematic review but found one RCT (177 children, age 6–16 years, 1 year of follow up, mean pre-bronchodilator flow expiratory volume in 1 second [FEV_1] 86% predicted) comparing beclometasone (200 µg twice daily), salmeterol (50 µg twice daily), and placebo in children already taking beclometasone (200 µg twice daily).[38] No significant differences were found at 1 year in lung function (mean change in FEV_1: 5.8% of predicted, 95% CI 2.9% to 8.7% with double dose beclometasone v 4.3%, 95% CI 2.1 to 6.5 with placebo), symptom scores, exacerbation rates, bronchial reactivity, or changes in airway responsiveness (1.30 units of methacholine, 95% CI 0.73 to 1.87 with salmeterol v 0.80, 95% CI 0.33 to 1.27 with placebo). No benefit of either adding salmeterol or a second dose of beclometasone was found in this group of children whose compliance with pre-existing medication was good.

Harms: Growth was significantly slower in children receiving higher dose inhaled corticosteroids (3.6 cm, 95% CI 3.0 to 4.2 with double dose beclometasone v 5.1 cm, 95% CI 4.5 to 5.7 with salmeterol v 4.5 cm, 95% CI 3.8 to 5.2 with placebo).

Comment: Higher dose inhaled corticosteroids are frequently used despite lack of evidence of benefit. In some children, higher prescribed doses may compensate for poor compliance or incorrect inhaler technique.

OPTION ADDITION OF REGULAR LONG ACTING β_2 AGONIST

One RCT found that addition of a long acting β_2 agonist (salmeterol) versus placebo significantly increased peak expiratory flow rates in the first few months of treatment, but found no significant increase after 1 year. A second short term RCT also found increased morning peak expiratory flow rates and more symptom free days at 3 months with addition of a long acting β_2 agonist (salmeterol).

Benefits: We found no systematic review but found two RCTs.[38,39] One RCT (177 children) found that at 1 year the addition of salmeterol did not improve lung function, airway responsiveness, symptom scores, exacerbation rates, or bronchial reactivity.[38] Salmeterol versus placebo increased mean morning peak expiratory flow rates (PEFRs) slightly after 3 months (difference: +12 L/min). There were no significant differences in symptom scores at any time. The second RCT (210 children, 4–16 years, 12 weeks' follow up, mean morning PFER 79% predicted) compared salmeterol (50 µg twice daily) versus placebo in children inadequately controlled on inhaled corticosteroids (average dose 750 µg daily).[39] At 12 weeks, mean morning PEFR (relative to the predicted PEFR) was 4% higher in the salmeterol group. Mean evening PEFR was not significantly different. The median proportion of symptom free days improved more with salmeterol than with placebo (60% v 30% for the third month of treatment).

Harms: The RCTs found no significant adverse effects associated with salmeterol.[38,39]

Comment: The second RCT was organised and funded by the manufacturer of salmeterol. Studies of adults with poor control on low dose inhaled corticosteroids have found greater benefit with additional long-acting β_2 agonists than with higher doses of inhaled steroid.

OPTION	ADDITION OF ORAL THEOPHYLLINE

One small brief RCT found that addition of theophylline versus placebo to previous treatment significantly increased the number of symptom free days and significantly reduced the use of additional β agonist and additional corticosteroid medication. We found insufficient evidence to weigh these short term benefits and possible long term harms.

Benefits: We found no systematic review but found one RCT (double blind crossover trial, 33 children, age 6–19 years, recruited from a hospital asthma clinic, 22 children used inhaled beclometasone [mean 533 µg/day], 11 used oral prednisolone [mean 30 mg alternate days]).[40] It found that the addition for 4 weeks of oral theophylline (serum concentration 10–20 µg/mL) versus placebo increased the mean number of symptom free days (63% with theophylline v 42% with placebo; $P \leq 0.01$). Inhaled β agonist (orciprenaline [see glossary, p 33]) was needed twice as often with placebo (0.5 doses/day with theophylline v 1.0 with placebo; $P \leq 0.01$). Additional daily prednisolone was needed by fewer children while on theophylline than while on placebo (3/32 with theophylline v 10/32 with placebo; $P = 0.02$).

Harms: In the RCT, short term adverse effects included mild transient headache and nausea in six children after the crossover from placebo to the theophylline dose that they had previously tolerated.[40]

Comment: One child was excluded from the analysis because of poor compliance. The RCT was too brief to assess long term harms.

OPTION	ADDITION OF ORAL LEUKOTRIENE RECEPTOR ANTAGONISTS

One short duration crossover RCT in children with persistent asthma found small improvements in lung function and fewer asthma exacerbation days with addition of a leukotriene receptor antagonist (montelukast) to inhaled corticosteroid (budesonide).

Benefits: We found no systematic review but found one crossover RCT (279 children aged 6–14 years previously treated with inhaled corticosteroid for at least 6 wks, with mean flow expiratory volume in 1 second (FEV_1) 78% predicted after 1 month run-in with budesonide 200 µg) comparing adding oral montelukast 5 mg versus placebo to inhaled budesonide over 4 weeks.[41] It found a slight increase in

FEV_1 with montelukast versus placebo (primary efficacy analysis of 251 children, relative change of FEV_1, relative to baseline: 4.6% v 3.3%, 95% CI −0.1 to 2.7%, P = 0.06; per-protocol analysis of 205 children, 6.0% v 4.1%, 95% CI 0.5 to 3.4%; P = 0.01). It found fewer asthma exacerbation days (decrease from baseline peak flow of > 20%, or increase from baseline of β_2 agonist use of > 70%) with montelukast versus placebo (12.2% v 15.9%; P = 0.01). No significant differences were found in quality of life measurements, global evaluations or asthma attacks requiring unscheduled medical intervention or treatment with oral corticosteroid.

Harms: The RCT found no significant difference with montelukast versus placebo in asthma exacerbation, upper respiratory tract infection, headache, cough, pharyngitis, and fever.[41]

Comment: The RCT in children was brief (4 wks treatment).[41] We found one large RCT of montelukast added to beclometasone in adults with inadequately controlled asthma that found benefit over a 16 week period.[42] Both RCTs were funded by the manufacturers of montelukast.

QUESTION **What are the effects of treatments for acute wheezing in infancy?**

OPTION β_2 AGONISTS DELIVERED BY NEBULISER OR METERED DOSE INHALER/SPACER

We found conflicting evidence from RCTs. Transient hypoxia may be caused by nebulised bronchodilators, particularly with air driven nebulisers, and seems less likely with metered dose inhalers plus spacers (see bronchiolitis, p 46).

Benefits: We found no systematic review but found many hospital based RCTs of nebulised β_2 agonists versus normal saline in infants and young children with acute wheezing. Some, but not all, have found short term improvements in clinical respiratory distress scores with β_2 agonists.[43] We found no large RCTs with clinical outcomes. Small RCTs with physiological rather than clinical end points found that giving β_2 agonists by metered dose inhaler with spacer to wheezy infants was effective, with less likelihood than nebulisation to show transient reduction of lung function.[44,45] A large single blind RCT (123 children aged 1–24 months with moderate to severe wheezing, city hospital emergency department in Santiago, Chile) compared nebulised salbutamol (see glossary, p 33) (0.25 mg/kg 3 times in 1 h) with salbutamol by metered dose inhaler plus spacer (2 puffs 5 times in 1 h). In children assessed as non-responders after the first hour, treatment was repeated for a second hour together with intramuscular betamethasone. Withholding of β_2 agonists from a control group was considered unethical. Reduction in clinical severity score (≤ 5) was significantly better with metered dose inhaler plus spacer versus nebulisation after 1 hour (clinical severity score ≤ 5: 56/62 [90%] v 43/61 [71%]; OR 3.9, 95%

CI 1.5 to 10.4; P = 0.01) but not after 2 hours (100% v 94%; P > 0.05). Only one child (in the nebuliser group) was hospitalised because of treatment failure.[46]

Harms: Some infants have transiently decreased oxygen saturation after nebulisation, especially with air driven nebulisers.[43] Nebulised β_2 agonists are known to cause tachycardia, tremor, and hypokalaemia, but serious adverse effects are rare.

Comment: None.

OPTION INHALED IPRATROPIUM BROMIDE

We found limited and conflicting evidence from one systematic review on the effects of inhaled ipratropium bromide for clinical outcomes in wheezing children.

Benefits: We found one systematic review (search date 1998, 321 children, six RCTs) of ipratropium bromide for wheeze in children under 2 years.[47] One included RCT found that adding ipratropium bromide to β_2 agonists resulted in fewer children receiving further treatment 45 minutes after initial treatment in the emergency room (OR 0.22, 95% CI 0.08 to 0.61), but a second similar study found no additional benefit. A third included RCT (31 hospitalised children) comparing ipratropium bromide versus placebo found no significant difference in the duration of hospitalisation (WMD –0.4 days, 95% CI –1.4 to +0.61). Adding ipratropium bromide to β_2 agonist had no effect on duration of hospitalisation compared with β_2 agonist alone (WMD –0.4 days, 95% CI –1.41 to +0.61). In one home based, 2 month crossover trial, parents preferred regular nebulised ipratropium bromide to nebulised water, but there was no significant reduction in the frequency of reported symptoms during treatment.[47]

Harms: No evidence of harm specific to the use of ipratropium bromide was found in these studies.

Comment: The studies were too small to exclude a clinically important effect of ipratropium bromide.

OPTION ORAL CORTICOSTEROIDS

We found no evidence that oral corticosteroids improve outcomes in acute wheezing infants.

Benefits: We found no systematic review. One outpatient study compared oral prednisolone versus placebo (38 acutely wheezing children aged 3–17 months, including 30 children previously admitted with wheeze). It found no significant differences in outcome between the two groups in the 56 episodes studied.[48]

Harms: No important adverse effects were identified.[48]

Comment: Acute infantile wheezing may be because of bronchiolitis. This is often difficult to separate from other acute wheezing, and is dealt with elsewhere (see bronchiolitis, p 46).

We found weak and conflicting evidence on the effects of prophylaxis with inhaled corticosteroids in wheezing infants.

Benefits: We found no systematic review. We found inconsistent results of placebo controlled trials on inhaled corticosteroids in recurrent or persistent infant wheezing. Some found improvements in symptom scores and reduced administration of additional treatments. Other studies did not find beneficial effect. We found a greater tendency for positive findings in studies of older children and in studies involving administration by metered dose inhaler and spacer rather than nebuliser. We found no RCTs of continuous oral theophylline in infants, and the small numbers of trials with inhaled sodium cromoglicate were mainly negative.

Harms: We found no good evidence on the long term safety of treatment with continuous inhaled corticosteroids in infancy. Known effects of using nebuliser and facemasks include oral candidiasis and thinning of facial skin.

Comment: Administering inhaled treatments to infants is difficult. RCTs of treatment for infant wheezing used a variety of drugs, dosages, and devices, and were sometimes conducted in populations with differing proportions of children with asthma rather than other types of infant wheeze. These factors may explain the inconsistent results.

GLOSSARY

Aminophylline A stable combination of theophylline and ethylenediamine; the ethylenediamine is added to increase the solubility of theophylline in water.

Orciprenaline is known as metaproterenol in USA; it is a non-selective β agonist.

Salbutamol is known as albuterol in USA; it is a short acting selective β_2 agonist.

REFERENCES

1. Russell G, Ninan TK. Respiratory symptoms and atopy in Aberdeen school children: evidence from two surveys 25 years apart. *BMJ* 1992;304: 873–875.

2. Martinez FD, Wright AL, Taussig L, et al. Asthma and wheezing in the first six years of life. *N Engl J Med* 1995;333:132–138.

3. Park ES, Golding J, Carswell F, et al. Pre-school wheezing and prognosis at 10. Arch Dis Child 1986;61:642–646.

4. Geelhoed GC, Landau LI, Le Souef PN. Evaluation of SaO2 as a predictor of outcome in 280 children presenting with acute asthma. *Ann Emerg Med* 1994;23:1236–1241.

5. Plotnick LH, Ducharme FM. Combined inhaled anticholinergics and β_2 agonists in the initial management of acute paediatric asthma. In: The Cochrane Library, Issue 2, 2001. Oxford: Update Software. Search date 2000; primary sources Medline, Embase, Cinahl, hand searches of bibliographies of references, and contact with pharmaceutical companies for details of unpublished trials and personal contacts.

6. Cates CJ. Holding chambers versus nebulisers for β-agonist treatment of acute asthma. In: The Cochrane Library, Issue 2, 2001. Oxford: Update Software. Search date 1999; primary sources Medline and Cochrane Airways Review Group Register.

7. Chou KJ, Cunningham SJ, Crain EF. Metered-dose inhalers with spacers vs nebulizers for pediatric asthma. *Arch Pediatr Adolesc Med* 1995;149: 201–205.

8. Rowe BH, Spooner C, Ducharme FM, Bretzlaff JA, Bota GW. Early emergency department treatment of acute asthma with systemic corticosteroids (Cochrane Review) In: The Cochrane Library, Issue 2, 2001 Oxford: Update Software. Last amended November 2000. Search date 1999; primary sources cochrane Airways Review Group Register, Embase, Medline, Cinahl, and hand searches.

9. Patel H, Macarthur C, Johnson D. Recent corticosteroids use and the risk of complicated varicella in otherwise immunocompetent children. *Arch Pediatr Adolesc Med* 1996;150:409–414.

10. Edmonds ML, Camargo CA Jr, Pollack CV Jr, Rowe BH. Early use of inhaled corticosteroids in the emergency department treatment of acute asthma. In: The Cochrane Library, Issue 2, 2002. Oxford: Update Software. Search date not stated; primary sources Cochrane Airways Group Register, and hand searches of bibliographies.

11. Manjra AI, Price J, Lenney W et al. Efficacy of nebulised fluticasone propionate compared with oral prednisolone in children with an acute exacerbation of asthma. *Respir Med* 2000;94: 1206–1214

12. Matthews EE, Curtis PD, McLain B, Morris L, Turbitt M. Nebulized budesonide versus oral

steroid in severe exacerbations of childhood asthma. *Acta Paediatr* 1999;88:841–843.

13. Schuh S, Resiman J, Alshehri M, et al. A compariosn of inhaled fluticasone and oral prednisone for children with severe acute asthma. *N Engl J Med* 2000;343:689–694.

14. Scarfone RJ, Loiselle JM, Wiley JF II, et al. Nebulized dexamethasone versus oral prednisone in the emergency treatment of asthmatic children. *Ann Emerg Med* 1995;26:480–486.

15. Volowitz B, Bentur L, Finkelstein Y, et al. Effectiveness and safety of inhaled corticosteroids in controlling acute asthma attacks in children who were treated in the emergency department: a controlled comparative study with oral prednisolone. *J Allergy Clin Immunol* 1998;102: 1605–1609.

16. Devidayal S, Singhi S, Kumar L, Jayshree M. Efficacy of nebulized budesonide compared to oral prednisolone in acute bronchial asthma. *Acta Paediatr* 1999;88:835–840.

17. Goodman DC, Littenberg B, O'Connor GT, et al. Theophylline in acute childhood asthma: a meta-analysis of its efficacy. Pediatr Pulmonol 1996;21: 211–218. Search date 1994; primary source Medline.

18. Yung M, South M. Randomised controlled trial of aminophylline for severe acute asthma. *Arch Dis Child* 1998;79:405–410.

19. Calpin C, Macarthur C, Stephens D, et al. Effectiveness of prophylactic inhaled steroids in childhood asthma: a systematic review of the literature. *J Allergy Clin Immunol* 1997;100: 452–457. Search date 1996; primary source Medline.

20. Tinkelman DG, Reed C, Nelson H, et al. Aerosol beclomethasone dipropionate compared with theophylline as primary treatment of chronic, mild to moderately severe asthma in children. *Pediatrics* 1993;92:64–77.

21. The Childhood Asthma Management Program Research Group. Long-term effects of budesonide or nedocromil in children with asthma. *N Engl J Med* 2000;343:1054–1063.

22. Verberne A, Frost C, Roorda R, et al. One year treatment with salmeterol compared with beclomethasone in children with asthma. *Am J Respir Crit Care Med* 1997;156:688–695.

23. Simons FER and the Canadian Beclomethasone Dipropionate – Salmeterol Xinafoate Study Group. A comparison of beclomethasone, salmeterol and placebo in children with asthma. *N Engl J Med* 1997;337:1659–1665.

24. Ducharme FM, Hicks GC. Anti-leukotriene agents compared to inhaled corticosteroids in the management of recurrent and/or acute asthma. In: The Cochrane Library, Issue 3, 2000. Search date 1999; primary sources Medline, Embase, Cinahl, hand searches of reference lists, and personal contact with colleagues and internal headquarters of leukotriene producers.

25. Bleecker ER, Welch MJ, Weinstein SF, et al. Low dose inhaled fluticasone proprionate versus oral zafirlukast in the treatment of persistent asthma. *J Allergy Clin Immunol* 2000;105(6 Pt 1):1123–1129.

26. Knorr B, Matz J, Bernstein JA, et al. Montelukast for chronic asthma in 6–14 year old children. *JAMA* 1998;279:1181–1186.

27. Wolthers OD, Riis BJ, Pedersen S. Bone turnover in asthmatic children treated with oral prednisolone or inhaled budesonide. *Pediatr Pulmonol* 1993;16:341–346.

28. Reilly SM, Hambleton G, Adams JE, Mughaal MZ. Bone density in asthmatic children treated with inhaled corticosteroids. *Arch Dis Child* 2001; 84(2):183–184.

29. Simons FE, Persaud MP, Gillespie CA, et al. Absence of posterior subcapsular cataracts in young patients treated with inhaled corticosteroids. *Lancet* 1993;342:776–778.

30. Abuektish F, Kirkpatrick JN, Russell G. Posterior subcapsular cataract and inhaled steroid therapy. *Thorax* 1995;50:674–676.

31. Allen DB, Mullen M, Mullen B. A meta-analysis of the effect of oral and inhaled steroids on growth. *J Allergy Clin Immunol* 1994;93:967–976. Search date 1993; primary sources literature search of leading medical journals 1956–1993.

32. Sharek PJ, Bergman DA. Beclomethasone for asthma in children: effects on linear growth. In: The Cochrane Library, Issue 2, 2001. Oxford: Update Software. Search date 1999; primary source Cochrane Airways Group Asthma Trials Register.

33. Doull 1995, Freezer NJ, Holgate ST. Growth of prepubertal children with mild asthma treated with inhaled beclometasone dipropionate. *Am J Resp Crit Care Med* 1995;151:1715–1719.

34. Stein MA, Krasowski M, Leventhal BL, et al. Behavioural and cognitive effects of theophylline and caffeine. *Arch Pediatr Adolesc Med* 1996;50: 284–288. Search date not stated; primary sources Medline, Psychlit, Dissertation Abstracts, and hand searched references.

35. Agertoft L, Pedersen S. Effects of long-term treatment with an inhaled corticosteroid on growth and pulmonary function in asthmatic children. *Respir Med* 1994;88:373–381.

36. Agertoft L, Pedersen S. Effect of long-term treatment with inhaled budesonide on adult height in children with asthma. *N Engl J Med* 2000;343: 1064–1069.

37. Lenney W, Pedersen S, Boner AL, Ebbutt A, Jenkins M, on behalf of an international study group. Efficacy and safety of salmeterol in childhood asthma. *Eur J Pediatr* 1995;154: 983–990.

38. Verberne A, Frost C, Duiverman E, Grol M, Kerrebijn K. Addition of salmeterol versus doubling the dose of beclomethasone in children with asthma. *Am J Respir Crit Care Med* 1998;158: 213–219.

39. Russell G, Williams DAJ, Weller P, Price J. Salmeterol xinafoate in children on high dose inhaled steroids. *Ann Allergy Asthma Immunol* 1995;75:423–428.

40. Nassif EG, Weinberger M, Thompson R, Huntley W. The value of maintenance theophylline in steroid dependent asthma. *N Engl J Med* 1981;304: 71–75.

41. Simons FER, Villa JR, Lee BW, et al. Montelukast added to budesonide in children with persistent asthma: a randomized double blind crossover study. *J Pediatr* 2001;138(5):694–698.

42. Laviolette M, Malmstrom K, Lu S, et al. Montelukast added to inhaled beclomethasone in treatment of asthma. *Am J Respir Crit Care Med* 1999;160:1862–1868.

43. Alario AJ, Lewander W, Dennehy P, et al. The efficacy of nebulised metaproterenol in wheezing infants and young children. *Am J Dis Child* 1992; 146:412–418.

44. Kraemer R, Frey U, Sommer CW, et al. Short-term effect of albuterol, delivered via a new auxiliary device, in wheezy infants. *Am Rev Respir Dis* 1991;144:347–351.

45. Yuksel B, Greenough A. Comparison of the effects on lung function of different methods of bronchodilator administration. *Respir Med* 1994;88:22.

46. Rubilar L, Castro-Rodrguez JA, Girardi G. Randomized controlled trial of salbutamol via metered-dose inhaler with spacer verus nebuliser

for acute wheezing in children less than 2 years of age. *Pediatr Pulmonol* 2000;29:264–269.

47. Everard M, Kurian M. Anticholinergic drugs for wheeze in children under the age of two years. In: The Cochrane Library, Issue 2, 2001. Oxford: Update Software. Search date 1998; primary sources Cochrane Airways Group Register and hand search of respiratory care and paediatric journals.

48. Webb M, Henry R, Milner AD. Oral corticosteroids for wheezing attacks under 18 months. *Arch Dis Child* 1986;61:15–19.

Duncan Keeley
General Practitioner
Thame
Oxfordshire
UK

Competing interests: The author has received occasional consultancy fees or assistance with organisation of, or travel to, meetings from companies including Allen and Hanburys, Astra, MSD, Zeneca, 3M, and Boots.

TABLE 1 Comparison of inhaled budesonide, nedocromil, and placebo over 4–6 years on several measures of asthma symptoms and morbidity (see text, p 25).[21]

Intervention	Budesonide (311 children)	Nedocromil (312 children)	Placebo (418 children)
Prednisone courses per 100 person years	70	102	122
Urgent care visits due to asthma per 100 person years	12	16	22
Hospitalisations due to asthma per 100 person years	2.5	4.3	4.4
Beclomethasone or other asthma medications added	6.6%	17.1%	18.7%

Attention deficit hyperactivity disorder in children

Search date June 2001

Paul Ramchandani, Carol Joughin and Morris Zwi

QUESTIONS

INTERVENTIONS

Likely to be beneficial

Unknown effectiveness

See glossary, p 43

Key Messages

- One systematic review has found that methylphenidate versus placebo reduces core symptoms of attention deficit hyperactivity disorder in the short term but may disturb sleep and appetite. The review could not draw firm conclusions about the effects of methylphenidate versus dexamfetamine or tricyclic anti-depressants. The review also found that methylphenidate versus psychological/behavioural treatment improves symptoms in the medium term, but the clinical importance of these findings is unclear.

- Limited evidence from two systematic reviews suggests that dexamfetamine versus placebo improves some behavioural outcomes but the clinical importance of these findings is unclear.

- Limited evidence from one systematic review suggests that clonidine versus placebo reduces core attention deficit hyperactivity disorder symptoms, but the clinical importance of these findings is unclear.

- One systematic review of two small RCTs found insufficient evidence about psychological or behavioural treatments; one subsequent RCT found no significant difference between psychological/behavioural treatment versus standard care in behavioural rating scales.

- One systematic review found inconsistent results for combination treatments (medication plus psychological/behavioural treatment) versus placebo in attention deficit hyperactivity disorder. A second systematic review has found that combination treatments versus psychological/behavioural treatments alone significantly improve attention deficit hyperactivity disorder symptoms.

DEFINITION	Attention deficit hyperactivity disorder is "a persistent pattern of inattention and/or hyperactivity and impulsivity that is more frequent and severe than is typically observed in individuals at a comparable level of development" (DSM-IV).[1] Inattention, hyperactivity, and impulsivity are commonly known as the core symptoms of attention deficit hyperactivity disorder. Symptoms must be present for at least 6 months, observed before the age of 7 years, and "clinically significant impairment in social, academic, or occupational functioning" must be evident in more than one setting. The symptoms must not be better explained by another disorder such as an anxiety disorder (see glossary, p 43), mood disorder, psychosis, or autistic disorder.[1] The World Health Organization's International Statistical Classification of Diseases and Related Health Problems (ICD-10)[2] uses the term "hyperkinetic disorder" for a more restricted diagnosis. It differs from the DSM-IV classification[3] as all three problems of attention, hyperactivity, and impulsiveness must be present, more stringent criteria for "pervasiveness" across situations must be met, and the presence of another disorder is an exclusion criterion.
INCIDENCE/ PREVALENCE	Prevalence estimates of attention deficit hyperactivity disorder vary according to the diagnostic criteria used and the population sampled. DSM-IV prevalence estimates among school children range from 3–5%,[1] but other estimates vary from 1.7–16%.[4,5] No objective test exists to confirm the diagnosis of attention deficit hyperactivity disorder, which remains a clinical diagnosis. Other conditions frequently coexist with attention deficit hyperactivity disorder. Oppositional defiant disorder (see glossary, p 43) is present in 35% (95% CI 27% to 44%) of children with attention deficit hyperactivity disorder, conduct disorder (see glossary, p 43) in 26% (95% CI 13% to 41%), anxiety disorder in 26% (95% CI 18% to 35%), and depressive disorder (see glossary, p 43) in 18% (95% CI 11% to 27%).[6]
AETIOLOGY/ RISK FACTORS	The underlying causes of attention deficit hyperactivity disorder are not known.[6] There is limited evidence that it has a genetic component.[7–9] Risk factors also include psychosocial factors.[10] There is increased risk in boys compared to girls, with ratios varying from 3:1[6] to 4:1.[3]
PROGNOSIS	More than 70% of hyperactive children may continue to meet criteria for attention deficit hyperactivity disorder in adolescence, and up to 65% of adolescents may continue to meet criteria for attention deficit hyperactivity disorder in adulthood.[5] Changes in diagnostic criteria cause difficulty with interpretation of the few outcome studies. One cohort of boys followed up for an average of 16 years found a ninefold increase in antisocial personality disorder and a fourfold increase in substance misuse disorder.[7]
AIMS	To reduce inattention, hyperactivity and impulsivity, and to improve psychosocial and educational functioning in affected children and adolescents, with minimal adverse effects of treatment.
OUTCOMES	Children's behaviour, such as Conners Teacher's Rating Scales (see glossary, p 43); school performance, such as School Situations Questionnaire (see glossary, p 43); adverse effects.
METHODS	*Clinical Evidence* search and appraisal June 2001.

OPTION   METHYLPHENIDATE

One systematic review has found that methylphenidate versus placebo
reduces core symptoms of attention deficit hyperactivity disorder in the
short term but may disturb sleep and appetite. The review could not draw
firm conclusions about the effects of methylphenidate versus
dexamfetamine or tricyclic antidepressants. The review also found that
methylphenidate versus psychological/behavioural treatment improves
symptoms in the medium term, but the clinical importance of these
findings is unclear.

Benefits: We found one systematic review (search date 2000).[11] Most
studies were conducted in the USA, used a diagnosis of attention
deficit disorder (DSM-III) or attention deficit hyperactivity disorder
(DSM-IIIR or DSM-IV), and included children aged between 5–18
years, mostly recruited from psychiatric and other hospital outpatient clinics. **Versus placebo:** The systematic review included,
but did not pool results from, 13 rigorously selected short term RCTs
(1177 children, aged 5–18 years).[11] Three RCTs (99 children)
found no significant difference in core symptoms between methylphenidate versus placebo. The other 10 RCTs found that methylphenidate (dose range 0.56–0.72 mg/kg daily or 5–35 mg daily for
trials reporting in those units) versus placebo significantly improved
the Conners Teacher's Rating Scale (see glossary, p 43) hyperactivity index (see comment below). The same systematic review
found similar results in 17 other RCTs (643 children), which were
less stringent in terms of homogeneity of participants, outcome
measures, and methodological quality. **Versus dexamfetamine:**
The systematic review[11] identified four poorly reported crossover
RCTs (224 children, aged 5–18 years) comparing methylphenidate
(dose range 0.6 mg–4.5 mg/kg daily or 20 mg daily for trials
reporting in those units) versus dexamfetamine (dose
0.39–2.6 mg/kg daily or 10 mg daily for trials reporting in those
units) but, because of heterogeneity, could not pool their results.
Three RCTs (99 children, aged 5–12 years) found no significant
difference with methylphenidate versus dexamfetamine in the outcomes of interest. The other RCT found improvement with methylphenidate versus dexamfetamine for some, but not all outcome
measures. No firm conclusions can be drawn. **Versus tricyclic
antidepressants:** The systematic review[11] identified, but could not
pool, the results of two poorly reported crossover RCTs (105
children) comparing methylphenidate (dose 0.4 mg/kg daily or
mean 20 mg daily for trials reporting in those units) versus imipramine (dose 1–2 mg/kg daily or mean 65 mg daily for trials
reporting in those units). One RCT (75 children) found no significant
differences in clinical outcomes after 1 year, and the other RCT (30
children) found that imipramine versus methylphenidate improved
some but not all outcomes in the short term. No firm conclusions
can be drawn. **Versus psychological/behavioural treatment:** We
found one systematic review (search date 2000) that identified four
RCTs comparing methylphenidate versus psychological/behavioural

treatment (see glossary, p 43).[11] Three of the RCTs (192 children, aged 5–12 years) were poorly reported and compared a variety of psychological/behavioural treatments (individual cognitive training [see glossary, p 43] over 12 wks; parent and teacher training; behaviour treatment for 8 wks) versus methylphenidate (5–60 mg daily). Overall, these three RCTs found limited evidence that, in the medium term, methylphenidate versus psychological/behavioural treatment improved symptoms. The fourth RCT (579 children, aged 7–10 years) compared medication treatment (144 children, double blind titration of methylphenidate dose, switched to alternative medication after 28 days if response unsatisfactory, mean initial dose 30.5 mg daily) versus intensive behavioural management versus combined medication and intensive behavioural management versus standard community care.[12] A total of 74% of the children in the medication group were taking methylphenidate at the end of the study. Initial results were not presented as the number of children who improved, but only as P values. Methylphenidate versus psychological/behaviour treatment improved some, but not all, of the symptoms of attention deficit disorder. Subsequent secondary analysis has developed these findings (see comment below).

Harms: The systematic review (search date 2000)[11] did not combine results on harms because of heterogeneity and incomplete data reporting. It presented the number of RCTs that had found significant results (see comment below). **Versus placebo:** The following symptoms were found by at least one RCT to be significantly more common in children receiving methylphenidate: sleep disorders; anorexia or appetite disturbance; headache; motor tics; irritability; and abdominal pain (see table 1, p 45). We found no good evidence of effects of methylphenidate on growth rates in children. **Versus dexamfetamine:** Out of the four RCTs identified by the systematic review, two RCTs reported no significant difference with methylphenidate versus dexamfetamine for anorexia or appetite disturbance and one RCT reported no significant difference in motor tics, abdominal pain, and irritability. **Versus psychological/ behavioural treatment:** The one large RCT comparing medication with intensive behavioural treatment (see glossary, p 43)[12] found that, of the children receiving either medication management or combined medication and intensive behavioural treatment, 50% reported mild adverse effects, 11% had moderate adverse effects, and 3% experienced severe adverse effects.

Comment: The RCT comparing medication versus intensive behavioural treatment is the largest and most rigorous currently available RCT of attention deficit hyperactivity disorder treatments.[12] Subsequent secondary analysis suggests that 56% of the children taking medication improved compared to 34% of these in the behavioural treatment group.[13] There is also a suggestion that children with comorbid behaviour problems (oppositional defiant disorder/ conduct disorder) demonstrated a stronger response to medication than those without comorbid behaviour problems, and that children with attention deficit hyperactivity disorder and anxiety disorders were likely to respond equally well to behavioural or medication treatments.[14] There are some concerns about the methods used in the RCT and caution should be exercised when using the results of secondary analysis, as they are more susceptible to bias than the primary outcome analyses.[15] It should also be noted that the principal outcome measures were rating scales based on impressions of parents and teachers; they did not include the child's view or direct measures of their response to treatment. Long term effects on psychosocial adjustment, educational success, or behavioural improvement are unclear. We found no evidence about methylphenidate for pre-school children.[16] The abbreviated Conners Teacher's Rating Scale has been used widely in treatment studies and has been researched, validated, and standardised to measure treatment effects in attention deficit hyperactivity disorder.[17] However, the clinical importance of the effect of methylphenidate versus placebo on the abbreviated Conners Teacher's Rating Scale remains unclear.

OPTION   DEXAMFETAMINE SULPHATE

Limited evidence from two systematic reviews suggests that dexamfetamine versus placebo improved some behavioural outcomes but the clinical importance of these findings is unclear.

Benefits: **Versus placebo:** We found two systematic reviews.[5,16] The first systematic review (search date 1997, 4 RCTs, 61 children aged 6–12 years, dexamfetamine 0.46–0.75 mg/kg daily) found that dexamfetamine versus placebo improved the change in the abbreviated Conners Teacher's Rating Scale (see glossary, p 43) (WMD –4.8, 95% CI –6.4 to –2.9).[16] The second later systematic review (search date 1997, 3 RCTs, 150 children aged 6–16 years, dexamfetamine 5–20 mg daily) only evaluated longer term studies (> 12 wks).[5] It found some evidence of positive outcomes (including improved concentration and hyperactivity) with dexamfetamine versus placebo. However, some methodological problems were identified with the studies in this review.[5] The clinical importance of these findings is unclear. **Versus methylphenidate:** See benefits of methylphenidate, p 38.

Harms: **Versus placebo:** The second systematic review found that dexamfetamine significantly increased anorexia and appetite disturbance in three RCTs.[5] **Versus methylphenidate:** See harms of methylphenidate, p 39.

Comment: See comment of methylphenidate for the principal outcome measures, p 39.

OPTION   CLONIDINE

Limited evidence from one systematic review suggests that clonidine versus placebo reduced core attention deficit hyperactivity disorder symptoms, but the clinical importance of these findings is unclear.

Benefits: **Versus placebo:** We found one systematic review (search date 1999, 6 RCTs, 143 children, mean age 11 years, dose of clonidine 0.1–0.24 mg daily for 4–12 wks).[18] One of the six RCTs was a comparison of clonidine versus methylphenidate, rather than versus placebo,[19] and the rating scales of the clinical features of attention deficit hyperactivity disorder completed by parents, teachers, and clinicians were combined in the systematic review. A meta-analysis of the six RCTs found that clonidine versus placebo improved this combined rating scale (effect size 0.58, 95% CI 0.27 to 0.89). The clinical importance of this result is unclear (see comment below), and the results should be treated with caution. **Versus methylphenidate or combined treatment:** We found no systematic review but found one small RCT (3 groups of 8 boys aged 6–16 years with attention deficit hyperactivity disorder and either comorbid oppositional defiant disorder [see glossary, p 43] or conduct disorder [see glossary, p 43]) comparing clonidine (mean dose 0.17 mg daily) versus methylphenidate (mean dose 35 mg daily) versus clonidine plus methylphenidate.[19] Most outcomes were not significantly different between the three groups. However, methylphenidate versus clonidine significantly improved the teacher reported School Situations Questionnaire (see glossary, p 43) (P < 0.009). The clinical importance of this isolated result from a single small RCT is unclear.

Harms: **Versus placebo:** The systematic review[18] included information from 10 studies of harms. Not all were high quality RCTs, and their results are difficult to interpret. In children taking clonidine, nine of 10 studies found sedation in children; six studies found increased irritability. Electrocardiographs were recorded in two placebo controlled RCTs, which found no abnormalities. **Versus methylphenidate or combined treatment:** One small RCT (24 boys)[19] found that two of eight children on clonidine developed new onset bradycardia. Four of eight children on a combination of clonidine and methylphenidate developed bradycardia.

Comment: The systematic review[18] noted larger effect sizes in smaller and lower quality studies. Inclusion of the RCT of clonidine versus methylphenidate[19] in the systematic review creates difficulties in using that review to indicate the effects of clonidine versus placebo. The RCT[19] had a larger effect size than most other included studies, and it is likely to have inflated the final result of the meta-analysis. The results used by the systematic review for that RCT were not described in the original RCT report, and may have been a less reliable comparison of baseline and end of the study measures rather than a rigorous comparison of randomly allocated groups. Harms were reported as the number of studies that recorded a specific adverse effect or not rather then the number of children experiencing adverse effects.

| OPTION | PSYCHOLOGICAL/BEHAVIOURAL TREATMENT |

One systematic review of two small RCTs found insufficient evidence; one subsequent RCT found no significant difference with psychological/behavioural treatment versus standard care in behavioural rating scales.

Benefits: **Versus standard care:** We found one systematic review (search date 1997, 2 RCTs, 50 children aged 6–13 years),[16] and a subsequent RCT.[12] The systematic review found no significant difference between psychological/behavioural treatment (see glossary, p 43) versus standard care in teacher rating scales (SMD –0.40, 95% CI –1.28 to +0.48) or parent ratings (1 RCT, 26 children, WMD –3.8, CI –9.6 to +2.0). The RCTs identified by the systematic review were small and the clinical importance of these results is unclear. The subsequent RCT (290 children)[12] found no significant difference between intensive behavioural treatments versus standard community care. In children with comorbid anxiety disorders (see glossary, p 43), the RCT found that intensive behavioural treatment resulted in better clinical outcomes. **Versus methylphenidate:** See benefits of methylphenidate, p 38.

Harms: Harms were not reported.

Comment: Children in the trials had different diagnoses, presentations, and clinical needs. Secondary analysis of one RCT[12] suggests small benefit with intensive behavioural treatment versus standard community care (34% of children improved with intensive behavioural treatment v 25% with standard community care group).[13] However, caution should be exercised in interpreting the results of secondary analysis as they are more susceptible to bias than the primary outcome analyses.[15]

OPTION	MEDICATION PLUS PSYCHOLOGICAL/BEHAVIOURAL TREATMENT

One systematic review found inconsistent results for combination treatments (medication plus psychological/behavioural treatment) versus placebo in attention deficit hyperactivity disorder. A second systematic review has found that combination treatments versus psychological/behavioural treatments alone significantly improve attention deficit hyperactivity disorder symptoms.

Benefits: **Versus control/placebo:** We found one systematic review (search date 1997, 3 RCTs, 35 children aged 5–13 years).[16] It found that combination of medication with psychological/behavioural treatments versus control/placebo improved parent ratings of attention deficit hyperactivity disorder (Conners Parent's Rating Scale WMD −7.3, 95% CI −12.3 to −2.4), but not teacher ratings of attention deficit hyperactivity disorder (Conners Teacher's Rating Scale [see glossary, p 43] WMD 1.3, 95% CI −0.7 to +3.2). The clinical importance of these findings is unclear.[16] **Versus stimulant drugs alone:** See benefits of methylphenidate, p 38. **Versus psychological/behavioural treatments alone:** We found one systematic review (search date 2000, 11 RCTs, 428 children aged 5–18 years).[11] It found that methylphenidate plus behavioural treatments versus behavioural treatments alone significantly improved attention deficit hyperactivity disorder behaviours, symptoms, and measures of academic achievement. No significant difference was found in social skills or in measures of the relationship between parents and children.[11] The review separately assessed one RCT,[12] which found that combined drug and intensive behavioural treatment versus intensive behavioural treatment alone significantly improved three of five measures of attention deficit hyperactivity disorder core symptoms (see glossary, p 43), one of three measures of aggression/oppositional behaviour, one of three measures of anxiety depression, and one of three measures of academic achievement.[12]

Harms: The RCTs found no evidence of adverse effects. See harms of methylphenidate, p 39.

Comment: The RCT[12] is the largest and most methodologically rigorous study of attention deficit hyperactivity disorder treatments with high standards for reporting and follow up of nearly all children (see comment under methylphenidate, p 39).[15] The results of a secondary analysis of this RCT[12] suggest that children with attention deficit hyperactivity disorder and comorbid anxiety respond equally well to medication management or intensive behavioural treatment (see comment of methylphenidate about secondary analysis, p 39);[14] however, secondary analysis indicated that combined medication management plus intensive behavioural treatment was better than medication management alone.[14]

GLOSSARY

Anxiety disorder A range of conditions with features including apprehension, motor tension, and autonomic overactivity.

Behavioural treatment Treatment using insights from learning theory to achieve specific changes in behaviour. It is usually highly structured. It can be used with either children with attention deficit hyperactivity disorder or their parents/carers.

Cognitive training Brief structured treatment aimed at changing dysfunctional beliefs.

Conduct disorder Conduct disorders include a repetitive pattern of antisocial, aggressive, or defiant conduct, which violate age appropriate social expectations.[2]

Conners Teacher's Rating Scales Widely used rating scales for assessment of symptoms of attention deficit hyperactivity disorder used extensively in both clinical work and epidemiological studies. There are 10 item parent and teacher questionnaires which can be used for children aged 3–17 years.

Core symptoms Inattention, hyperactivity, and impulsivity are commonly known as the core symptoms of attention deficit hyperactivity disorder.[5]

Depressive disorder Characterised by persistent low mood, loss of interest and enjoyment, and reduced energy.

Oppositional defiant disorder The presence of markedly defiant, disobedient, provocative behaviour, but without the severely dissocial or aggressive acts seen in conduct disorder.[2]

Psychological/behavioural treatments Includes any of the following methods: contingency management methods (e.g. behaviour modification); cognitive–behavioural therapy; individual psychotherapy; parent training or education; teacher training and education; parent and family counselling/therapy; social skills training; and electroencephalogram, biofeedback, or relaxation treatment.

School Situations Questionnaire A teacher completed questionnaire, which measures the pervasiveness of child behaviour problems across 12 school situations.[20]

REFERENCES

1. American Psychiatric Association. *Diagnostic and Statistical Manual of Mental Disorders, 4th Edition (DSM-IV)*. American Psychiatric Association, Washington DC, 1994.

2. World Health Organization. *International Statistical Classification of Diseases and Related Health Problems, Tenth Revision, Vol 3*. Geneva; World Health Organization, 1994.

3. Taylor E, Sergeant J, Doepfner M, et al. Clinical guidelines for hyperkinetic disorder. European Society for Child and Adolescent Psychiatry. *Eur Child Adolesc Psychiatry* 1998;7:184–200.

4. Goldman LS, Genel M, Bezman RJ, Slanetz PJ. Diagnosis and treatment of attention-deficit/hyperactivity disorder in children and adolescents.

Council on Scientific Affairs, American Medical Association. *JAMA* 1998;279:1100–1107.

5. Jadad AR, Boyle M, Cunningham C, Kim M, Schachar R. *Treatment of attention-deficit/hyperactivity disorder*. Evidence report/technology assessment: No 11 (Prepared by McMaster University under Contract No. 290–97-0017). Rockville MD, 1999. Agency for Health Care Policy and Research and Quality. Search date 1997; primary sources Medline, Cinahl, HealthStar, PsychInfo, Embase, Cochrane Library, hand searched reference lists, and organisations funding research on attention deficit hyperactivity disorder and researchers contacted. http://hstat.nlm.nih.gov/hq.Hquest/screen/DirectAccess/db/3143.

6. Green M, Wong M, Atkins D, et al. *Diagnosis and treatment of attention-deficit/hyperactivity disorder in children and adolescents.* Council on Scientific Affairs, American Medical Association. Technical Review No.3 (Prepared by Technical Resources International, Inc. under Contract No. 290-94-2024.). Agency for Health Care Policy and Research, AHCPR Publication No. 99-0050. Rockville MD, 1999.

7. Finkel MF. The diagnosis and treatment of the adult attention deficit hyperactivity disorders. *Neurologist* 1997;3:31-44.

8. Hertzig MEE, Farber EAE. *Annual progress in child psychiatry and child development, 1996.* New York: Brunner/Mazel Inc, 1997:602.

9. Kaminester DD. Attention deficit hyperactivity disorder and methylphenidate: When society misunderstands medicine. *McGill J Med* 1997;3: 105-114.

10. Taylor E, Sandberg S, Thorley G, Giles S. *The epidemiology of childhood hyperactivity.* London, Institute of Psychiatry. Maudsley Monographs 1991;33.

11. Lord J, Paisley S. *The clinical effectiveness and cost-effectiveness of methylphenidate for hyperactivity in childhood.* London: National Institute for Clinical Excellence, Version 2, August 2000. Search date 2000; primary sources Jadad et al. (reference 5 above), Medline, Cinahl, Healthstar, PsychInfo, and Embase.

12. Jensen PS, Arnold LE, Richters JE, et al. A 14-month randomized clinical trial of treatment strategies for attention-deficit/hyperactivity disorder. The MTA Cooperative Group. Multimodal Treatment Study of Children with ADHD. *Arch Gen Psychiatry* 1999;56:1073-1086.

13. Swanson JM, Kraemer HC, Hinshaw SP, et al. Clinical relevance of the primary findings of the MTA; success rates based on severity of ADHD and ODD symptoms at the end of treatment. *J Am Acad Child Adolesc Psychiatry* 2001;40:168-179.

14. Jensen PS, Hinshaw SP, Kraemer HP, Lenora N, et al. ADHD comorbidity findings from MTA study: comparing comorbid subgroups. *J Am Acad Child Adolesc Psychiatry* 2001;40:147-158.

15. Boyle MH, Jadad AR. Lessons from large trials: the MTA study as a model for evaluating the treatment of childhood psychiatric disorder. *Can J Psychiatry* 1999;44:991-998.

16. Miller A, Lee SK, Raina P, Klassen A, Zupanic J, Olsen L. A review of therapies for attention-deficit/ hyperactivity disorder. 1998. Canadian Coordinating Office for Health Technology Assessment. Search date 1997; primary sources Medline, Current Contents, hand search of review articles, textbooks, British Columbia Methylphenidate Survey, and Intercontinental Medical Statistics for information on drug prescription and utilization in Canada.

17. Goyette CH, Conners CK, Ulrich RF. Normative data on revised Conners parent and teacher rating scales. *J Abnorm Child Psychol* 1978;6:221-236.

18. Connor DF, Fletcher KE, Swanson JM. A meta-analysis of clonidine for symptoms of attention-deficit hyperactivity disorder. *J Am Acad Child Adolesc Psychiatry* 1999;38:1551-1559. Search date 1999; primary sources Medline, PsychInfo, Current Contents, Social and Behavioral Sciences, and Current Contents Clinical Medicine, and hand searches of non-peer reviewed research reports, book chapters, chapter bibliographies, and individual report references.

19. Connor DF, Barkley RA, Davis HT. A pilot study of methylphenidate, clonidine, or the combination in ADHD comorbid with aggressive oppositional defiant or conduct disorder. *Clin Pediatr (Phila)* 2000;39:15-25.

20. Barkley RA. *Attention-Deficit Hyperactivity Disorder: A handbook for diagnosis and treatment.* New York: Guilford Press, 1990.

Paul Ramchandani
MRC Research Training Fellow
University of Oxford
Department of Psychiatry
Warneford Hospital
Oxford
UK

Carol Joughin
Project Manager
FOCUS Royal College of Psychiatrists Research Unit
London
UK

Morris Zwi
Consultant Child and Adolescent Psychiatrist
Child and Family Consultation Centre
Richmond
Surrey
UK

Competing interests: None declared. The opinions expressed are those of the authors and do not necessarily reflect those of the Royal College of Psychiatrists.

Child health

TABLE 1	The number of RCTs reporting significant adverse effects with methylphenidate versus placebo (see text, p 39).[11]

Adverse effect	Number of trials
Anorexia or appetite disturbance	7/12 (58%)
Motor tics	1/2 (50%)
Irritability	2/9 (22%)
Sleep disorder	4/20 (20%)
Abdominal pain	2/10 (20%)
Headache	2/10 (20%)

Search date October 2001

Juan M Lozano and Elaine Wang

Key Messages

Treatment

- Two good quality systematic reviews have found that inhaled bronchodilators improve overall clinical scores in children with bronchiolitis in the short term, but found no evidence that bronchodilators reduce admission rates or produce a clinically important improvement in oxygen saturation.
- One systematic review and eight additional RCTs found limited and conflicting evidence on the effects of corticosteroids in children with bronchiolitis.
- One RCT found no evidence that routine use of antibiotics improved clinical scores in children with bronchiolitis.
- One systematic review found no good evidence that ribavirin (tribavirin) reduced mortality, the risk of respiratory deterioration, or length of hospital stay in children admitted to hospital with respiratory syncytial virus bronchiolitis. It found some evidence that ribavirin reduced the duration of ventilation. One small subsequent RCT found no significant differences in hospital stay, oxygen needs, recurrence of disease, or admission rates.
- We found insufficient evidence to determine the effect of immunoglobulin treatment on clinical outcomes for children with bronchiolitis.

Preventing transmission in hospital

- We found no evidence that cohort segregation, handwashing, or the wearing of gowns, masks, or eye-nose goggles by carers reduced transmission rates between children in hospital.

Prevention in high risk children

- One systematic review has found that, in children born prematurely, in children with bronchopulmonary dysplasia, and in children with a combination of risk factors, prophylactic respiratory syncytial virus immunoglobulin or palivizumab (monoclonal antibody) reduces admission rates to hospital and intensive care units.

DEFINITION Bronchiolitis is a virally induced acute bronchiolar inflammation that is associated with signs and symptoms of airway obstruction. Diagnosis is based on clinical findings. Clinical manifestations include fever, rhinitis (inflammation of the nasal mucosa), tachypnoea, expiratory wheezing, cough, rales, use of accessory muscles, apnoea (absence of breathing), dyspnoea (difficulty in breathing), alar flaring (flaring of the nostrils), and retractions (indrawing of the intercostal soft tissues on inspiration). The disease severity (see glossary, p 54) of bronchiolitis may be classified clinically as mild, moderate, or severe.

INCIDENCE/ PREVALENCE Bronchiolitis is the most common lower respiratory tract infection in infants, occurring in a seasonal pattern with highest incidence in the winter in temperate climates,[1] and in the rainy season in warmer countries. Each year in the USA, about 21% of infants have lower respiratory tract disease and 6–10/1000 infants are admitted to hospital for bronchiolitis (1–2% of children under 12 months of age).[2] The peak rate of admission occurs in infants aged between 2–6 months.[3]

AETIOLOGY/ RISK FACTORS Respiratory syncytial virus is responsible for bronchiolitis in 70% of cases. This figure reaches 80–100% in the winter months. However, in early spring parainfluenza virus type 3 is often responsible.[1]

PROGNOSIS **Morbidity and mortality:** Disease severity is related to the size of the infant, and to the proximity and frequency of contact with infective infants. Children at increased risk of morbidity and mortality are those with congenital heart disease, chronic lung disease, history of premature birth, hypoxia, and age less than 6 weeks.[4] Other factors associated with a prolonged or complicated hospital stay include a history of apnoea or respiratory arrest, pulmonary consolidation seen on a chest radiograph, and (in North America) native American or Inuit race.[5] The risk of death within 2 weeks is high for children with congenital heart disease (3.4%) or chronic lung disease (3.5%) compared with other groups combined (0.1%).[4] Rates of admission to intensive care units (range 31–36%) and need for mechanical ventilation (range 11–19%) are similar among all high risk groups.[4] The percentage of these children needing oxygen supplementation is also high (range 63–80%).[4] In contrast, mortality in children with bronchiolitis but without these risk factors is less than 1%, and rates of intensive care units admission and ventilation in such children are markedly lower (15% and 8%).[6] **Long term prognosis:** Information on long term prognosis varies among studies. One small prospective study of two matched cohorts (25 children with bronchiolitis; 25 children without) found no evidence that bronchiolitis requiring outpatient treatment is associated with an increased risk of asthma in the long term.[7] Possible confounding factors include variation in illness severity, smoke exposure, and crowding.[8] We found one prospective study in 50 randomly selected infants admitted with bronchiolitis, followed up by questionnaire for 5 years and a visit in the fifth year. It found a doubling of asthma incidence compared with the general population, although there was large (30%) loss to follow up and no matched control group.[9]

AIMS To decrease morbidity and mortality, shorten hospital stay, and prevent transmission of infection, with minimum adverse effects.

OUTCOMES Death rate; rates of hospital admission; rate of intubation or admission to intensive care units clinical score (clinical score is a subjective, unvalidated measure that is based on judgements made by the clinician); rates of clinical and serological infection. Oxygen saturation is a proxy outcome, but the clinical significance and sensitivity of this outcome are unclear.

METHODS *Clinical Evidence* search and appraisal October 2001. Studies were appraised independently by the two authors and then reviewed again together to resolve differences by consensus. Titles were scanned and, if the article seemed relevant, the abstract was obtained and appraised to determine if the complete article was to be reviewed.

QUESTION **What are the effects of treatment for children with bronchiolitis?**

OPTION **BRONCHODILATORS (INHALED SALBUTAMOL, INHALED ADRENALINE [EPINEPHRINE])**

Two good quality systematic reviews have found that inhaled bronchodilators achieve short term improvement in overall clinical scores in children treated in hospitals, emergency departments, and outpatient clinics, although they found no evidence that bronchodilators reduce admission rates or produce a clinically important improvement in oxygen saturation.

Benefits: We found two systematic reviews. The first review (search date 1998, 8 RCTs, 485 children) evaluated children in outpatient clinics or the emergency department and after admission to hospital.[10] The second review (search date 1995, 5 RCTs, 251 children) considered children treated in outpatient clinics.[11] Four RCTs were common to both reviews. The first review found that, in the short term, bronchodilators improved clinical scores in children with mild and moderately severe bronchiolitis (lack of improvement in clinical score, bronchodilator v placebo, RR 0.76, 95% CI 0.60 to 0.95).[10] Both reviews[10,11] found no evidence that bronchodilators improved oxygen saturation by a clinically important amount (mean difference in oxygen saturation +1.2%, 95% CI +0.8% to +1.6%[11]). Both reviews 10,11 found no evidence that bronchodilators versus placebo reduced admission rates in children treated in outpatient clinics or the emergency department (RR 0.85, 95% CI 0.47 to 1.53;[10] 23/97 [24%] children treated with bronchodilator admitted v 21/90 [23%] with placebo; RR 1.0, 95% CI 0.6 to 1.7[11]).

Harms:	One systematic review reported tachycardia, increased blood pressure, decreased oxygen saturation, flushing, hyperactivity, prolonged cough, and tremor following use of bronchodilators. The review did not report frequency of adverse events.[10] The second review did not report harms.[11]
Comment:	None of the RCTs used respiratory failure as an outcome. One systematic review found significant heterogeneity among RCTs in the effects of bronchodilators on oxygen saturation.[10] Discrepancies in primary studies included differences in study populations such as inclusion of sedated children, short duration of follow up, and validity of clinical scores. Bronchodilators may improve the clinical appearance of a child through a general stimulatory effect rather than by improving respiratory function.[12]

OPTION	CORTICOSTEROIDS

One systematic review and eight additional RCTs found limited and conflicting evidence on the effects of corticosteroids in children with bronchiolitis.

Benefits:	We found one systematic review (search date 1999, 6 RCTs, 347 children in hospital)[13] and eight additional RCTs (858 children) of corticosteroids versus placebo in children with bronchiolitis.[14–21] Three of the additional RCTs had been mentioned in the systematic review but excluded because of data inconsistency,[18] treatment outside hospital,[19] or failure to report the outcome markers sought by the systematic review.[20] The systematic review found no significant difference in the mean length of stay in all the RCTs that reported length of stay (5 RCTs: WMD −0.43 days, 95% CI −1.05 to +0.18 days), in the four RCTs with clearly identified randomisation methods (WMD −0.35 days, 95% CI −0.84 to +0.14 days), and after exclusion of RCTs that included children with previous wheezing (4 RCTs: WMD −0.29 days, 95% CI −0.71 to +0.13 days).[13] Interpretation of the effect of corticosteroids versus placebo on clinical symptoms found by the systematic review is difficult (see comment below). The RCTs in the systematic review reported different clinical scales at varying times after starting treatment. The scales usually included measurements of oxygen saturation, wheezing, accessory muscle use, and respiratory rate. Results reported 72 hours after starting treatment were too heterogeneous for analysis. Only three RCTs (197 children) provided results for 24 hours after starting treatment. The systematic review pooled the standardised effect size for clinical scores from these three RCTs and found that corticosteroids versus placebo produced a significant improvement. Although statistically significant, the clinical importance of such an improvement is not clear as different scales are combined across studies. Seven of the eight additional RCTs that compared the clinical score found no significant benefit from corticosteroids (see table 1, p 56).[14-17,19-21] One RCT found a statistically significant transient improvement in a "bronchiolitis score" with oral prednisolone for 2 days. This is of doubtful clinical importance.[21] Three small long term follow up RCTs (3 years,[22] 3–5 years,[23] and 2 years[24]) used telephone questionnaires to examine the effect of corticosteroids during the acute episode on subsequent wheezing. Two of the three RCTs did not observe any benefit

Bronchiolitis

from corticosteroids. The third was an unblinded RCT in which 117 hospitalised infants (mean age 2.6 months, requiring hospital treatment because of respiratory syncytial virus bronchiolitis) were allocated to be in a control group (41 infants), and received inhaled budesonide for 7 days (40 infants), or inhaled budesonide for 2 months (36 infants).[24] However, this RCT had several problems that compromised its validity (see comment below).

Harms: The acute adverse effects of oral corticosteroids are well documented, and include hyperglycaemia and immunosuppression. The RCTs did not give information on these.

Comment: The evidence presented in the published systematic review[13] is difficult to interpret because some of the RCTs did not exclude children with a history of wheezing who may have asthma, a condition likely to respond to corticosteroids. The clinical scales used in the RCTs included oxygen saturation, but the clinical relevance of changes in this item are unclear. Even if the results are accepted at face value, the clinical significance of an effect size is unclear. Furthermore, eight RCTs with more than double the number of people were not included in the meta-analysis. All of these RCTs, except one, did not find a benefit of corticosteroids and the single RCT that did only observed a transient improvement in clinical score at one timepoint. Another systematic review is under way (E Wang, personal communication, 2001). We found inadequate evidence to evaluate the effects of systemic versus inhaled corticosteroids. The unblinded RCT comparing two different regimens of inhaled budesonide in hospitalised children[24] had several problems that further compromised its validity. Diagnosis of asthma was based only on a telephone survey; the children were not assessed to establish if they had received additional interventions or exposures that could explain the results.

OPTION	ROUTINE ANTIBIOTICS

One unblinded RCT found no evidence that routine antibiotics are of clinical benefit in children admitted to hospital with bronchiolitis and uncomplicated respiratory syncytial virus pneumonia, although the study was not powerful enough to rule out a clinically important effect.

Benefits: We found no systematic review. We found one unblinded RCT (138 children admitted to hospital with clinically apparent pneumonia, 45% of whom were diagnosed with respiratory syncytial virus [RSV] infection) comparing the routine use of antibiotics versus no antibiotics (no placebo). It found no significant difference between treatment groups in the proportion infected with RSV. It found no evidence that antibiotics reduced duration of hospital stay or respiratory rate, or improved clinical symptoms, clinical signs, or radiographic assessment scores for pulmonary disease.[25]

Harms: The RCT did not report harms, although potential risks include superinfection with resistant bacteria and drug reactions.

Comment: The RCT was unblinded and used block randomisation (children randomised in groups of 20). This reduces confidence in the results. Two children initially treated without antibiotics were switched to antibiotics because of complicating purulent infections. Analysis was by intention to treat.

| OPTION | RIBAVIRIN |

One systematic review found no good evidence that ribavirin (tribavirin) reduced mortality, the risk of respiratory deterioration, or length of hospital stay in children admitted to hospital with respiratory syncytial virus bronchiolitis. It found some evidence that ribavirin reduced the duration of ventilation. One subsequent RCT found no evidence that ribavirin reduced duration of hospital stay or admission rate due to lower respiratory tract symptoms during the first year after the acute episode.

Benefits: We found one systematic review (search date 1999, 10 small RCTs).[26] The review found that, in children and infants hospitalised with respiratory syncytial virus bronchiolitis, ribavirin compared with placebo did not significantly reduce mortality (5/86 [6%] with ribavirin v 7/72 [10%] with placebo, RR 0.61, 95% CI 0.21 to 1.75), respiratory deterioration (4/56 [7%] with ribavirin v 11/60 [18%] with placebo; RR 0.42, 95% CI 0.15 to 1.17), or length of hospital stay (1.9 days less with ribavirin v placebo, 95% CI –0.9 to +4.6 days), but duration of ventilation was significantly reduced (1.2 days, 95% CI 0.2 to 3.4 days).[26] The high mortality in both groups may have been because of severe disease at baseline. One subsequent RCT (40 hospitalised infants who received ribavirin or placebo within 12 h of admission) found no differences in outcomes measured during the acute episode, such as the duration of oxygen supplementation need (ribavirin 2.72 days v placebo 1.92 days; mean difference 0.80 days, 95% CI –0.73 to +2.32 days) or hospital stay (ribavirin 4.94 days v placebo 3.36 days; mean difference 1.58 days, 95% CI –0.18 to +3.35 days).[27] This RCT also followed the infants for 1 year after the initial episode. It found no significant differences in admission rates associated with recurrent lower respiratory illness (2/16 [13%] with ribavirin v 3/19 [16%] with placebo; RR 0.79, 95% CI 0.15 to 4.17) or the use of bronchodilators (5/16 [31%] with ribavirin v 8/19 [42%] with placebo; RR 0.74, 95% CI 0.30 to 1.82). However, the sample size may have been too small to rule out a clinically important difference.

Harms: We found no results from prospective studies. The review did not report harms. We found case reports of headaches and contact lens dysfunction in carers. Ribavirin has been reported to be associated with acute bronchospasm in treated children. The standard aerosol is sticky, and clogging of ventilatory equipment has been reported.[28]

Comment: We found one small prospective study comparing pulmonary function tests in 54 children previously randomised to inpatient treatment with ribavirin or placebo.[29] It found no evidence of long term differences in outcome, although the study was not powerful enough to rule out a clinically important difference.

Bronchiolitis

OPTION   IMMUNOGLOBULINS (POOLED IMMUNOGLOBULINS, RSV IG)

We found insufficient evidence from small, low powered RCTs that immunoglobulins improved clinical outcomes in children admitted to hospital with bronchiolitis.

Benefits: We found no systematic review but found five RCTs (4 using albumin solution as control, 1 using saline, 335 children in total).[30-34] Two RCTs used pooled immunoglobulins, two RCTs used respiratory syncytial virus (RSV) Ig, and one RCT used palivizumab (synthetic monoclonal antibody). Neither RCT using RSV Ig found evidence that RSV Ig shortened hospital stay compared with albumin (in high risk children [see glossary, p 54]: mean duration of hospital stay 8.41 days with RSV Ig v 8.89 days with albumin; P = NS; in non-high risk children: mean stay 4.58 days with RSV Ig v 5.52 days with albumin; P = NS).[30,31] The third RCT (35 children) found no evidence that palivizumab reduced hospital stay (mean 14.5 days, 95% CI 12.4 to 16.6 days with RSV Ig v 11.5 days, 95% CI 10.0 to 13.0 with placebo; P = 0.25), duration of ventilation (mean 8.8 days, 95% CI 6.5 to 11.1 days with palivizumab v 6.2 days, 95% CI 4.7 to 7.7 days with placebo; P = 0.45), or duration of treatment with supplemental oxygen (mean 12.3 days, 95% CI 10.0 to 14.6 days with palivizumab v 9.5 days, 95% CI 7.9 to 11.1 days with placebo; P = 0.47).[34] Neither of the remaining RCTs found any evidence that pooled immunoglobulins improved outcome in children with bronchiolitis.

Harms: The RCTs found that RSV Ig was associated with elevation of liver enzymes and anoxic spells (no frequencies given).[30] One unblinded RCT (249 children) of prophylactic RSV Ig found that adverse effects occurred in about 3% of treated children.[35] This RCT and a subsequent analysis of the data found that effects included increased respiratory rate, mild fluid overload during the first infusion, urticarial reaction at the infusion site, mild decreases in oxygen saturation, and fever (no frequencies given).[35,36]

Comment: Four RCTs used albumin as control. The effects of albumin in bronchiolitis are not known.

QUESTION   What are the effects of measures to prevent transmission in hospital?

OPTION   NURSING INTERVENTIONS (COHORT SEGREGATION, HANDWASHING, GOWNS, MASKS, GLOVES, AND GOGGLES)

We found no direct evidence from RCTs that cohort segregation, handwashing, use of gowns, masks, gloves, or goggles reduced nosocomial transmission of respiratory syncytial virus to other children. Handwashing is a well established technique for reducing cross-infection in other contexts, so RCTs may not be ethically feasible.

Benefits: We found no systematic review and no good quality RCTs examining effects of cohort segregation (see glossary, p 54), handwashing, gowns, masks, gloves, or goggles, used either singly or in combination on nosocomial transmission of bronchiolitis in children.

Harms: **Cohort segregation:** Potential risks of cohort segregation include misdiagnosing respiratory syncytial virus infection and putting non-infected patients at risk by subsequent placement into the wrong cohort. **Handwashing:** Dermatitis is an adverse effect of repeated handwashing. **Other interventions:** No harms reported.

Comment: **Single nursing interventions:** We found four observational studies comparing nosocomial infection rates in separate series of children before and after introduction of cohort segregation, handwashing, gowns and masks, and goggles. No study adjusted results for variations in baseline incidence. Three studies found a lower incidence of transmission after introduction of cohort segregation alone, handwashing alone, and eye-nose goggles alone.[37–39] The fourth study found no significant difference in transmission after introducing gowns and masks.[40] **Combinations of nursing interventions:** We found one RCT (58 medical personnel caring for children admitted with bronchiolitis), which found no significant difference in nosocomial infection rate in staff when they used gowns and masks in addition to handwashing (5/28 [18%] of those using gowns, masks, and handwashing v 4/30 [13%] in the control group; RR 1.3, 95% CI 0.4 to 3.6).[41] The RCT did not report transmission rates in the children. One non-randomised prospective trial (233 children at risk of severe nosocomial infection) compared transmission rates in wards adopting different nursing policies. It found that a combination of cohort segregation, gowns, and gloves reduced nosocomial transmission rates compared with all other policies (cohort segregation alone, gown and gloves alone, no special precautions) taken together. However, the control interventions did not remain constant throughout the trial, the results were based on an interim analysis, and the definition of "at risk" children was not clearly stated.[42]

QUESTION What are the effects of prophylactic measures in high risk children?

OPTION IMMUNOGLOBULINS

One systematic review has found that, in children born prematurely or children with bronchopulmonary dysplasia, prophylactic respiratory syncytial virus Ig or palivizumab (monoclonal antibody) given monthly reduces hospital admission and admission to intensive care.

Benefits: We found one systematic review (search date 1999, 4 RCTs, 2598 children) comparing monthly RSV Ig or palivizumab (monoclonal antibody) versus placebo or no prophylaxis.[35] Three of the RCTs used intravenous respiratory syncytial virus (RSV) Ig and one used intramuscular palivizumab. Two of the RCTs using RSV Ig were unblinded and both of these used no prophylaxis as the control intervention. The review found that RSV Ig versus placebo reduced admission to hospital (OR 0.48, 95% CI 0.37 to 0.64) and intensive care unit (OR 0.47, 95% CI 0.29 to 0.77), but did not reduce the incidence of mechanical ventilation (OR 0.99, 95% CI 0.48 to 2.07).[35]

Harms: See harms of immunoglobulins, p 52.

Child health

Bronchiolitis

Comment: Premature infants included in the RCTs were children under 6 months old, with gestational age at birth less than either 32 or 35 weeks. Children with bronchopulmonary dysplasia were under 2 years old and still undergoing treatment for this anomaly. Planned subgroup analysis in the review found that prophylaxis reduced hospital admission in children whose only risk factor was prematurity (OR 0.27, 95% CI 0.15 to 0.49) and in children with bronchopulmonary dysplasia alone (OR 0.54, 95% CI 0.37 to 0.80), but not in children with cardiac comorbidity alone (OR 0.64, 95% CI 0.37 to 1.10).

GLOSSARY

Cohort segregation Children infected with different viral strains are segregated from each other and treated separately, with the aim of preventing cross-infection.
Disease severity Mild: not requiring hospitalisation. Moderate: requiring hospitalisation but not intubation. Severe: requiring intubation or artificial ventilation.
High risk children Premature infants with or without bronchopulmonary dysplasia, or infants and children with congenital heart disease.

REFERENCES

1. Phelan P, Olinsky A, Robertson C. *Respiratory illness in children.* 4th ed. London: Blackwell Scientific Publications, 1994.
2. Gruber W. Bronchiolitis. In: Long S, Pickering L, Prober C, eds. *Principles and practice of pediatric infectious diseases.* 1st ed. New York: Churchill Livingstone, 1997:1821.
3. Glezen WP, Taber LH, Frank AL, Kessel JA. Risk of primary infection and reinfection with respiratory syncytial virus. *Am J Dis Child* 1986;140: 543–546.
4. Navas L, Wang E, de Carvalho V, Robinson J, PICNIC. Improved outcome of respiratory syncytial virus infections in a high-risk hospitalized population of Canadian children. *J Pediatr* 1992; 121:348–354.
5. Wang EEL, Law BJ, Stephens D, PICNIC. Pediatric Investigators Collaborative Network on Infections in Canada (PICNIC) study of morbidity and risk factors with RSV disease. *J Pediatr* 1995;126: 212–219.
6. Wang EEL, Law BJ, Boucher F, et al. Pediatric Investigators Collaborative Network on Infections in Canada (PICNIC) study of admission and management variation in patients hospitalized with respiratory syncytial viral lower respiratory infection. *J Pediatr* 1996;129:390–395.
7. McConnochie KM, Mark JD, McBride JT, et al. Normal pulmonary function measurements and airway reactivity in childhood after mild bronchiolitis. *J Pediatr* 1985;107:54–58.
8. McConnochie KM, Roghmann KJ. Parental smoking, presence of older siblings and family history of asthma increase risk of bronchiolitis. *Am J Dis Child* 1986;140:806–812.
9. Sly PD, Hibbert ME. Childhood asthma following hospitalization with acute viral bronchiolitis in infancy. *Pediatr Pulmonol* 1989;7:153–158.
10. Kellner JD, Ohlsson A, Gadomski AM, Wang EEL. Bronchodilators for bronchiolitis. In: The Cochrane Library, Issue 3, 2001. Oxford: Update Software. Search date 1998; primary sources Medline, Embase, Reference Update, reference lists of articles, and files of the authors.
11. Flores G, Horwitz RI. Efficacy of beta 2-agonists in bronchiolitis: a reappraisal and meta-analysis. *Pediatrics* 1997;100:233–239. Search date 1995; primary sources Medline and hand searched references and selected journals.
12. Gadomski AM, Lichenstein R, Horton L, King J, Keane V, Permutt T. Efficacy of albuterol in the management of bronchiolitis. *Pediatrics* 1994;93: 907–912.
13. Garrison MM, Christakis DA, Harvey E, Cummings P, Davis RL. Systemic corticosteroids in infant bronchiolitis: a meta-analysis. *Pediatrics* 2000; 105:e44. Search date 1999; primary sources Medline, Embase, and Cochrane Clinical Trials Registry.
14. Richter H, Seddon P. Early nebulized budesonide in the treatment of bronchiolitis and the prevention of postbronchiolitic wheezing. *J Pediatr* 1998;132: 849–853.
15. Bulow SM, Nir M, Levin E. Prednisolone treatment for respiratory syncytial virus infection: a randomized controlled trial of 147 infants. *Pediatrics* 1999;104:77.
16. Tal A, Bavilski C, Yohai D, Bearman JE, Gorodischer R, Moses SW. Dexamethasone and salbutamol in the treatment of acute wheezing in infants. *Pediatrics* 1983;71:13–18.
17. Cade A, Brownlee KG, Conway, SP. Randomised placebo-controlled trial of nebulised corticosteroids in acute respiratory syncytial viral bronchiolitis. *Arch Dis Child* 2000;82:126–130.
18. Connolly JH, Field CM, Glasgow JF, Slattery CM, MacLynn DM. A double blind trial of prednisolone in epidemic bronchiolitis due to respiratory syncytial virus. *Acta Paediat Scand* 1969;58: 116–120.
19. Berger I, Argaman Z, Schwartz SB. Efficacy of corticosteroids in acute bronchiolitis: short-term and long-term follow-up. *Pediatr Pulmonol* 1998; 26:162–166.
20. Leer JA, Green JL, Heimlich EM, et al. Corticosteroid treatment in bronchiolitis. A controlled collaborative study in 297 infants and children. *Am J Dis Child* 1969;117:495–503.
21. Goebel J, Estrada B, Quinonez J, et al. Prednisolone plus albuterol versus albuterol alone in mild to moderate bronchiolitis. *Clin Pediatr* 2000;39:213–220.
22. Reijonen TM, Kotaniemi-Syrjanen A, Korhonen K, Korppi M. Predictors of asthma three years after hospital admission for wheezing in infancy. *Pediatrics* 2000;106:1406–1412.
23. Van Woensel JBM, Kimpen JLL, Sprikkelman AB, Ouwehand A, Van Aalderan WMC. Long-term

effects of prednisolone in the acute phase of bronchiolitis caused by respiratory syncytial virus. *Pediatr Pulmonol* 2000;30:92–96.

24. Kajosaari M, Syvanen P, Forars M, Juntunen-Backman K. Inhaled corticosteroids during and after respiratory syncytial virus-bronchiolitis may decrease subsequent asthma. *Pediatr Allergy Immunol* 2000;11:198–202.

25. Fris B, Andersen P, Brenoe E, et al. Antibiotic treatment of pneumonia and bronchiolitis: a prospective randomised study. *Arch Dis Child* 1984;59:1038–1045.

26. Randolph AG, Wang EEL. Ribavirin for respiratory syncytial virus lower respiratory tract infection. In: The Cochrane Library, Issue 3, 2001. Oxford: Update Software. Search date 1999; primary sources Medline, hand searched references, and noted experts contacted.

27. Everard ML, Swarbrick A, Rigby AS, Milner AD. The effect of ribavirin to treat previously healthy infants admitted with acute bronchiolitis on acute and chronic respiratory morbidity. *Respir Med* 2001; 95:275–280.

28. Johnson EM. Developmental toxicity and safety evaluations of ribavirin. *Pediatr Infect Dis J* 1997; 9(suppl):85–87.

29. Long CE, Voter KZ, Barker WH, Hall CB. Long term follow-up of children hospitalized with respiratory syncytial virus lower respiratory tract infection and randomly treated with ribavirin or placebo. *Pediatr Infect Dis J* 1997;16:1023–1028.

30. Rodriguez WJ, Gruber WC, Welliver RC, et al. Respiratory syncytial virus (RSV) immune globulin intravenous therapy for RSV lower respiratory tract infection in infants and young children at high risk for severe RSV infections. *Pediatrics* 1997;99: 454–461.

31. Rodriguez WJ, Gruber WC, Groothuis JR, et al. Respiratory syncytial virus immune globulin treatment of RSV lower respiratory tract infection in previously healthy children. *Pediatrics* 1997; 100:937–942.

32. Hemming VG, Rodriguez W, Kim HW, et al. Intravenous immunoglobulin treatment of respiratory syncytial virus infections in infants and young children. *Antimicrob Agents Chemother* 1987;31:1882–1886.

33. Rimensberger PC, Burek-Kozlowska A, Morell A, et al. Aerosolized immunoglobulin treatment of respiratory syncytial virus infection in infants. *Pediatr Infect Dis J* 1996;15:209–216.

34. Malley R, DeVincenzo J, Ramilo O, et al. Reduction of respiratory syncytial virus (RSV) in tracheal aspirates in intubated infants by use of humanized monoclonal antibody to RSV F protein. *J Infect Dis* 1998;178:1555–1561.

35. Wang EEL, Tang NK. Immunoglobulin for preventing respiratory syncytial virus infection. In: The Cochrane Library, Issue 3, 2001. Oxford: Update Software. Search date 1999; primary sources Cochrane Acute Respiratory Infections Trials Register, Medline, abstracts from the Pediatric Academy Meetings and the Intersciences Conference on Antimicrobial Agents and Chemotherapy from 1994 to 1997.

36. Groothuis JR, Levin MJ, Rodriguez W, et al. Use of intravenous gamma globulin to passively immunize high-risk children against respiratory syncytial virus: safety and pharmacokinetics. *Antimicrob Agents Chemother* 1991;35:1469–1473.

37. Krasinski K, LaCouture R, Holzman R, Waithe E, Bonk S, Hanna B. Screening for respiratory syncytial virus and assignment to a cohort at admission to reduce nosocomial transmission. *J Pediatr* 1990;116:894–898.

38. Isaacs D, Dickson H, O'Callaghan C, Sheaves R, Winter A, Moxon ER. Handwashing and cohorting in prevention of hospital acquired infections with respiratory syncytial virus. *Arch Dis Child* 1991;66: 227–231.

39. Gala CL, Hall CB, Schnabel KC, et al. The use of eye-nose goggles to control nosocomial respiratory syncytial virus infection. *JAMA* 1986;256: 2706–2708.

40. Hall CB, Douglas RG. Nosocomial respiratory syncytial virus infections: should gowns and masks be used? *Am J Dis Child* 1981;135:512–515.

41. Murphy D, Todd JK, Chao RK, Orr I, McIntosh K. The use of gowns and masks to control respiratory illness in pediatric hospital personnel. *J Pediatr* 1981;99:746–750.

42. Madge P, Paton JY, McColl JH, Mackie PLK. Prospective controlled study of four infection-control procedures to prevent nosocomial infection with respiratory syncytial virus. *Lancet* 1992;340: 1079–1083.

Juan M Lozano
Associate Professor
Department of Paediatrics and Clinical Epidemiology Unit
School of Medicine
Javeriana University
Bogotá DC
Colombia

Elaine Wang
Associate Professor
Hospital for Sick Children
University of Toronto and Aventis Pasteur
Toronto
Canada

Competing interests: EW has received reimbursement from ICN Pharmaceuticals, the manufacturer of ribavirin, for attending a symposium. She has also been paid for speaking by Abbott Canada (the distributor of a RSV monoclonal antibody) as well as for participating at a clinical trials site by Medimmune (the manufacturer of a RSV monoclonal antibody).

TABLE 1 Studies of corticosteroids versus placebo in bronchiolitis: results of RCTs (see text, p 49).

Study	Allocation/blinding	Intervention	Number of children	Outcome	Results
Richter et al[14]	Random/blinded	Nebulised budesonide	40	Clinical score and condition at 6 months	No benefit
Bulow et al[15]	Random/blinded	Prednisolone/methylprednisolone	147	Hospital stay; supportive measures in hospital; condition at 1 month and 1 year after discharge	No benefit
Tal et al[16]	Random/blinded, factorial design	Dexamethasone/placebo salbutamol/placebo	32	Clinical score and hospital stay	No benefit
Cade et al[17]	Random/blinded	Budesonide	161	Hospital stay; time taken to be symptom free; readmission rates; GP consultation	No benefit
Connolly et al[18]	Random/blinded	Prednisolone	95	Duration of illness after hospitalisation	No benefit
Berger et al[19]	Random/blinded	All had salbutamol; prednisone	38	Clinical score; oxygen saturation; condition at 7 days and 2 years later	No benefit
Leer et al[20]	Random/blinded	Betamethasone	297	Nine respiratory tract signs; fever and complications after admission	No benefit
Goebel et al[21]	Random/blinded	All children received salbutamol (oral or inhaled) prednisolone	48	Bronchiolitis score at day 2	Transient effect only on day 2

Search date February 2002

Kate Ackerman and David Creery

INTERVENTIONS

*Although we found no direct
evidence to support their use,
widespread consensus holds that
(on the basis of indirect evidence
and extrapolation from adult
data) these interventions should
be universally applied to children
who have arrested. Placebo
controlled trials would be
considered unethical.

See glossary, p 63

Key Messages

- Outcome following out of hospital cardiorespiratory arrest in children is poor, and it is unclear at what stage intervention becomes futile.

- Prospective and retrospective observational studies have consistently found that out of hospital cardiorespiratory arrest in children, where the cause is uncertain (such as in fatal and near miss sudden infant death syndrome), has a far worse prognosis than arrest from any other cause.

- It is widely accepted that cardiopulmonary resuscitation and ventilation should be undertaken in children who have arrested. Placebo controlled trials would be considered unethical. We found no prospective evidence on the effects of training parents to perform cardiopulmonary resuscitation.

- One RCT found no evidence that endotracheal intubation improves survival or neurological outcome compared with bag-mask ventilation in children who have arrested in the community.

- We found no prospective evidence on the effects of bicarbonate, calcium, different doses of adrenaline (epinephrine), or direct current cardiac shock to improve the outcome of non-submersion out of hospital cardiorespiratory arrest in children.

Cardiorespiratory arrest

DEFINITION Non-submersion out of hospital cardiorespiratory arrest in children is a state of pulselessness and apnoea occurring outside of a medical facility and not caused by submersion in water.[1]

INCIDENCE/ PREVALENCE We found 12 studies (3 prospective, 9 retrospective) reporting the incidence of non-submersion out of hospital cardiorespiratory arrest in children (see table 1, p 64).[2–13] Eleven studies reported the incidence in both adults and children, and eight reported the incidence in children.[2–9,11–13] Incidence of arrests in the general population ranged from 2.2–5.7/100 000 people a year (mean 3.1, 95% CI 2.1 to 4.1). Incidence of arrests in children ranged from 6.9–18.0/100 000 children a year (mean 10.6, 95% CI 7.1 to 14.1).[8] One prospective study (300 children) found that about 50% of out of hospital cardiorespiratory arrests occurred in children under 12 months, and about two thirds occurred in children under 18 months.[11]

AETIOLOGY/ RISK FACTORS We found 26 studies reporting the causes of non-submersion pulseless arrests (see glossary, p 63) in a total of 1574 children. The commonest causes of arrest were undetermined causes as in sudden infant death syndrome (see glossary, p 63) (39%), trauma (18%), chronic disease (7%), and pneumonia (4%) (see table 2, p 65).[1,3–12,14–28]

PROGNOSIS We found no systematic review that investigated non-submersion arrests alone. We found 27 studies (5 prospective, 22 retrospective; total of 1754 children) that reported only on out of hospital arrest.[1–12,14–28] The overall survival rate following out of hospital arrest was 5% (87 children). Nineteen of these studies (1140 children) found that of the 48 surviving children, 12 (25%) had no or mild neurological disability and 36 (75%) had moderate or severe neurological disability. We found one systematic review (search date 1997), which reported outcomes after cardiopulmonary resuscitation for both in hospital and out of hospital arrests of any cause, including submersion in children.[29] Studies were excluded if they did not report survival. The review found evidence from prospective and retrospective observational studies that out of hospital arrest of any cause in children carries a poorer prognosis than arrest within hospital (132/1568 children [8%] survived to hospital discharge after out of hospital arrest v 129/544 children [24%] after in hospital arrests). About half of the survivors were involved in studies that reported neurological outcome. Of these, survival with "good neurological outcome" (i.e. normal or mild neurological deficit) was higher in children who arrested in hospital compared with those who arrested elsewhere (60/77 surviving children [78%] in hospital v 28/68 [41%] elsewhere).[29]

AIMS To improve survival and minimise neurological sequelae in children suffering non-submersion out of hospital cardiorespiratory arrest.

OUTCOMES Out of hospital death rate; rate of death in hospital without return of spontaneous circulation; return of spontaneous circulation with subsequent death in hospital; and return of spontaneous circulation with successful hospital discharge with mild, moderate, severe, or no neurological sequelae; adverse effects of treatment.

METHODS
Clinical Evidence search and appraisal February 2002. In addition, we searched citation lists of retrieved articles and relevant review articles. Studies reporting out of hospital arrest in adults that listed "adolescent" as a MeSH heading were also reviewed. Both authors reviewed the retrieved studies independently and differences were resolved by discussion. We selected studies reporting out of hospital cardiorespiratory arrests in children. Studies were excluded if data relating to submersion could not be differentiated from non-submersion data (except where we found no data relating exclusively to non-submersion arrest; in such cases we have included studies that did not differentiate these types of arrest, and have made it clear that such evidence is limited by this fact). Some features of cardiorespiratory arrest in adults appear to be different from arrest in children, so studies were excluded if data for adults could not be differentiated from data for children.

| QUESTION | What are the effects of treatments for non-submersion out of hospital cardiorespiratory arrest? |

| OPTION | AIRWAY MANAGEMENT AND VENTILATION |

It is widely accepted that good airway management and rapid ventilation should be undertaken in a child who has arrested, and it would be considered unethical to test its role in a placebo controlled trial.

Benefits:
We found no studies comparing airway management and ventilation versus no intervention.

Harms:
We found insufficient information.

Comment:
It would be considered unethical to test the role of airway management and ventilation in a placebo controlled trial.

| OPTION | INTUBATION VERSUS BAG-MASK VENTILATION |

One controlled trial found no evidence of a difference in survival or neurological outcome between bag-mask ventilation and endotracheal intubation in children requiring airway management in the community.

Benefits:
We found no systematic review. We found one high quality controlled trial (830 children requiring airway management in the community, including 98 children who had arrested after submersion) comparing (using alternate day allocation) bag-mask ventilation versus endotracheal intubation (given by paramedic staff trained in these techniques).[30] Treatments were not randomised; each was allocated on alternate days. Analysis was by intention to treat (see comment below). The trial found no significant difference in rates of survival or good neurological outcome (normal, mild deficit, or no change from baseline function) between the two treatment groups (105/349 [30%] survived after bag-mask ventilation v 90/373 [24%] after intubation; OR 1.36, 95% CI 0.97 to 1.89; good neurological outcome achieved in 80/349 [23%] of children after bag-mask ventilation v 70/373 [19%] after intubation; OR 1.27, 95% CI 0.89 to 1.83; OR for non-submersion cardiorespiratory arrest calculated by author).

Harms: The trial found that time spent at the scene of the arrest was longer when intubation was intended, and this was the only significant determinant of a longer total time from dispatch of paramedic team to arrival at hospital (mean time at scene 9 min with bag-mask v 11 min with intubation; P < 0.001; mean total time 20 min with bag-mask v 23 min with intubation; P < 0.001).[30] However, the trial found no significant difference between bag-mask ventilation and intubation for complications common to both treatments (complications in 727 children for whom data were available, bag-mask v intubation: gastric distension 31% v 7%; P = 0.20; vomiting 14% v 14%; P = 0.82; aspiration 14% v 15%; P = 0.84; oral or airway trauma 1% v 2%; P = 0.24). A total of 186 children across both treatment groups were thought by paramedical staff to be successfully intubated. Of these, oesophageal intubation occurred in three children (2%); the tube became dislodged in 27 children (14%; unrecognised in 12 children, recognised in 15); right main bronchus intubation occurred in 33 children (18%); and an incorrect size of tube was used in 44 children (24%). Death occurred in all but one of the children with oesophageal intubation or unrecognised dislodging of the tube.[30]

Comment: **Population characteristics:** The baseline characteristics of children did not differ significantly between groups in age, sex, ethnicity, or cause of arrest. The trial did not report the frequency of pulseless arrest (see glossary, p 63) versus respiratory arrest (see glossary, p 63). **Intention to treat:** Intubation and bag-mask ventilation are not mutually exclusive. The study protocol allowed bag-mask ventilation before intubation and after unsuccessful intubation. Of 420 children allocated to intubation, 115 received bag-mask ventilation before intubation, 128 received bag-mask ventilation after attempted intubation, four were lost to follow up, and the remainder received intubation that was believed to be successful. Of 410 children allocated to bag-mask ventilation, 10 children were intubated successfully (although in violation of study protocol), nine received bag-mask ventilation after attempted intubation, six were lost to follow up, and the remainder received bag-mask ventilation in accordance with study protocol.[30]

OPTION	INTRAVENOUS ADRENALINE (EPINEPHRINE)

Intravenous adrenaline (epinephrine) at "standard dose" (0.01 mg/kg) is a widely accepted treatment for establishing return of spontaneous circulation. We found no prospective evidence comparing adrenaline (epinephrine) versus placebo, or comparing standard or single doses versus high or multiple doses of adrenaline (epinephrine), in children who have arrested in the community.

Benefits: We found no systematic review, no RCTs, and no prospective observational studies.

Harms: We found no prospective data in this context.

Comment: **Versus placebo:** Standard dose adrenaline (epinephrine) is a widely accepted treatment for arrests in children. Placebo controlled trials would be considered unethical. **High versus low dose:** Two small retrospective studies (128 people) found no evidence of a difference in survival to hospital discharge between low or single dose and high or multiple dose adrenaline (epinephrine), although the studies were too small to rule out an effect.[8,12]

OPTION   INTRAVENOUS BICARBONATE

We found no RCTs on the effects of intravenous bicarbonate in out of hospital cardiorespiratory arrest in children.

Benefits: We found no RCTs.

Harms: We found insufficient evidence.

Comment: Bicarbonate is widely believed to be effective in arrest associated with hyperkalaemic ventricular tachycardia or fibrillation, but we found no prospective evidence supporting this.

OPTION   INTRAVENOUS CALCIUM

We found no RCTs on the effects of intravenous calcium in out of hospital cardiorespiratory arrest in children.

Benefits: We found no RCTs.

Harms: We found insufficient evidence.

Comment: Calcium is widely believed to be effective in arrest associated with hyperkalaemic ventricular tachycardia or fibrillation, but we found no prospective evidence supporting this.

OPTION   BYSTANDER CARDIOPULMONARY RESUSCITATION

It is widely accepted that cardiopulmonary resuscitation and ventilation should be undertaken in children who have arrested. Placebo controlled trials would be considered unethical. We found no RCTs on the effects of training parents to perform cardiopulmonary resuscitation. One systematic review of observational studies has found that children who were witnessed having an arrest and who received bystander cardiopulmonary resuscitation were more likely to survive to hospital discharge.

Benefits: We found no RCTs. We found one systematic review (search date 1997) of prospective and retrospective studies.[29] This concluded that survival was improved in children who were witnessed to arrest and received cardiopulmonary resuscitation from a bystander. Of 150 witnessed arrests outside hospital, 28/150 (19%) survived to hospital discharge. Of those children who received bystander cardiopulmonary resuscitation, 20/76 (26%) survived to discharge.[29] The review did not report survival rates in children whose arrests were not witnessed, but the overall survival rate for out of hospital cardiac arrest was 8%. **Training parents to perform cardiopulmonary resuscitation:** We found no systematic review and no RCTs examining the effects of training parents to perform cardiopulmonary resuscitation in children who have arrested outside hospital.

Harms: Potential harms include those resulting from unnecessary chest compression after respiratory arrest with intact circulation.

Cardiorespiratory arrest

Comment: The review of observational studies found that children who received bystander cardiopulmonary resuscitation had a hospital discharge rate of 20/76 (26%) versus 8/74 (11%) for children who also had their arrests witnessed but had not received cardiopulmonary resuscitation. Cardiopulmonary resuscitation was not randomly allocated and children resuscitated may be systematically different from those who did not receive resuscitation. The apparent survival rates for witnessed arrests and arrests with bystander initiated cardiopulmonary resuscitation may be artificially high because of inappropriate evaluation of true arrest. However, assuming confounding variables were evenly distributed between groups, then the best estimate of the benefit of cardiopulmonary resuscitation is a 15% absolute increase in the probability that children will be discharged alive from hospital.

OPTION   DIRECT CURRENT CARDIAC SHOCK

It is widely accepted that children who arrest outside hospital and are found to have ventricular fibrillation or pulseless ventricular tachycardia should receive direct current cardiac shock treatment. Placebo controlled trials would be considered unethical. We found no RCTs on the effects of direct current cardiac shock in children who have arrested in the community, regardless of the heart rhythm.

Benefits: We found no systematic review and no RCTs.

Harms: We found insufficient evidence.

Comment: **In children with ventricular fibrillation:** One retrospective study (29 children with ventricular fibrillation who had arrested out of hospital from a variety of causes, including submersion) found that of 27 children who were defibrillated, 11 survived (5 with no sequelae, 6 with severe disability). The five children with good outcome all received defibrillation within 10 minutes of arrest (time to defibrillation not given for those who died). Data on the two children who were not defibrillated were not presented.[31] **In children with asystole:** One retrospective study in 90 children with asystole (see glossary, p 63) (including those who had arrested after submersion) found that 49 (54%) had received direct current cardiac shock treatment. None of the children survived to hospital discharge, regardless of whether or not direct current cardiac shock was given.[32] We found one systematic review (search date 1997) of observational studies (1420 children who had arrested outside hospital) that recorded electrocardiogram rhythm.[29] Bradyasystole or pulseless electrical activity (see glossary, p 63) were found in 73%, whereas ventricular fibrillation or pulseless ventricular tachycardia (see glossary, p 63) were found in 10%.[29] The review found that survival after ventricular fibrillation or ventricular tachycardia arrest was higher than after asystolic arrest in children. Survival to discharge reported in the systematic review was 39/802 (5%) for children with initial rhythm asystole (see glossary, p 63) and 30% (29/97) with initial rhythm ventricular fibrillation (see glossary, p 63) or ventricular tachycardia.[29]

GLOSSARY

Asystole The absence of cardiac electrical activity

Bradyasystole Bradycardia clinically indistinguishable from asystole

Initial rhythm asystole The absence of cardiac electrical activity at initial determination

Initial rhythm ventricular fibrillation Electrical rhythm is ventricular fibrillation at initial determination

Pulseless arrest Absence of palpable pulse

Pulseless electrical activity The presence of cardiac electrical activity in absence of a palpable pulse

Pulseless ventricular tachycardia Electrical rhythm of ventricular tachycardia in absence of a palpable pulse

Respiratory arrest Absence of respiratory activity

Sudden infant death syndrome The sudden unexpected death of a child, usually between the ages of 1 month and 1 year, for which a thorough postmortem examination does not define an adequate cause of death. Near miss sudden infant death syndrome refers to survival of a child after an unexpected arrest of unknown cause

REFERENCES

1. Schindler MB, Bohn D, Cox PN, et al. Outcome of out of hospital cardiac or respiratory arrest in children. N Engl J Med 1996;335:1473–1479.

2. Broides A, Sofer S, Press J. Outcome of out of hospital cardiopulmonary arrest in children admitted to the emergency room. Isr Med Assoc J 2000;2:672–674.

3. Eisenberg M, Bergner L, Hallstrom A. Epidemiology of cardiac arrest and resuscitation in children. Ann Emerg Med 1983;12:672–674.

4. Applebaum D, Slater PE. Should the Mobile Intensive Care Unit respond to pediatric emergencies? Clin Pediatr (Phila) 1986;25:620–623.

5. Tsai A, Kallsen G. Epidemiology of pediatric prehospital care. Ann Emerg Med 1987;16:284–292.

6. Thompson JE, Bonner B, Lower GM. Pediatric cardiopulmonary arrests in rural populations. Pediatrics 1990;86:302–306.

7. Safranek DJ, Eisenberg MS, Larsen MP. The epidemiology of cardiac arrest in young adults. Ann Emerg Med 1992;21:1102–1106.

8. Dieckmann RA, Vardis R. High-dose epinephrine in pediatric out of hospital cardiopulmonary arrest. Pediatrics 1995;95:901–913.

9. Kuisma M, Suominen P, Korpela R. Paediatric out of hospital cardiac arrests — epidemiology and outcome. Resuscitation 1995;30:141–150.

10. Ronco R, King W, Donley DK, Tilden SJ. Outcome and cost at a children's hospital following resuscitation for out of hospital cardiopulmonary arrest. Arch Pediatr Adolesc Med 1995;149:210–214.

11. Sirbaugh PE, Pepe PE, Shook JE, et al. A prospective, population-based study of the demographics, epidemiology, management, and outcome of out of hospital pediatric cardiopulmonary arrest. Ann Emerg Med 1999;33:174–184.

12. Friesen RM, Duncan P, Tweed WA, Bristow G. Appraisal of pediatric cardiopulmonary resuscitation. Can Med Assoc J 1982;126:1055–1058.

13. Hu SC. Out of hospital cardiac arrest in an Oriental metropolitan city. Am J Emerg Med 1994;12:491–494.

14. Barzilay Z, Somekh E, Sagy M, Boichis H. Pediatric cardiopulmonary resuscitation outcome. J Med 1988;19:229–241.

15. Bhende MS, Thompson AE. Evaluation of an end-tidal CO$_2$ detector during pediatric cardiopulmonary resuscitation. Pediatrics 1995;95:395–399.

16. Brunette DD, Fischer R. Intravascular access in pediatric cardiac arrest. Am J Emerg Med 1988;6:577–579.

17. Clinton JE, McGill J, Irwin G, Peterson G, Lilja GP, Ruiz E. Cardiac arrest under age 40: etiology and prognosis. Ann Emerg Med 1984;13:1011–1015.

18. Hazinski MF, Chahine AA, Holcomb GW, Morris JA. Outcome of cardiovascular collapse in pediatric blunt trauma. Ann Emerg Med 1994;23:1229–1235.

19. Losek JD, Hennes H, Glaeser P, Hendley G, Nelson DB. Prehospital care of the pulseless, nonbreathing pediatric patient. Am J Emerg Med 1987;5:370–374.

20. Ludwig S, Kettrick RG, Parker M. Pediatric cardiopulmonary resuscitation. A review of 130 cases. Clin Pediatr (Phila) 1984;23:71–75.

21. Nichols DG, Kettrick RG, Swedlow DB, Lee S, Passman R, Ludwig S. Factors influencing outcome of cardiopulmonary resuscitation in children. Pediatr Emerg Care 1986;2:1–5.

22. O'Rourke PP. Outcome of children who are apneic and pulseless in the emergency room. Crit Care Med 1986;14:466–468.

23. Rosenberg NM. Pediatric cardiopulmonary arrest in the emergency department. Am J Emerg Med 1984;2:497–499.

24. Sheikh A, Brogan T. Outcome and cost of open- and closed-chest cardiopulmonary resuscitation in pediatric cardiac arrests. Pediatrics 1994;93:392–398.

25. Suominen P, Rasanen J, Kivioja A. Efficacy of cardiopulmonary resuscitation in pulseless paediatric trauma patients. Resuscitation 1998;36:9–13.

26. Suominen P, Korpela R, Kuisma M, Silfvast T, Olkkola KT. Paediatric cardiac arrest and resuscitation provided by physician-staffed emergency care units. Acta Anaesthesiol Scand 1997;41:260–265.

27. Torphy DE, Minter MG, Thompson BM. Cardiorespiratory arrest and resuscitation of children. *Am J Dis Child* 1984;138:1099–1102.
28. Walsh R. Outcome of pre-hospital CPR in the pediatric trauma patient [abstract]. *Crit Care Med* 1994;22:A162.
29. Young KD, Seidel JS. Pediatric cardiopulmonary resuscitation: a collective review. *Ann Emerg Med* 1999;33:195–205. Search date 1997; primary sources Medline and bibliographic search.
30. Gausche M, Lewis RJ, Stratton SJ, et al. Effect of out of hospital pediatric endotracheal intubation on survival and neurological outcome. *JAMA* 2000;283:783–790.
31. Mogayzel C, Quan L, Graves JR, Tiedeman D, Fahrenbruch C, Herndon P. Out of hospital ventricular fibrillation in children and adolescents: causes and outcomes. *Ann Emerg Med* 1995;25:484–491.
32. Losek JD, Hennes H, Glaeser PW, Smith DS, Hendley G. Prehospital countershock treatment of pediatric asystole. *Am J Emerg Med* 1989;7:571–575.

Kate Ackerman
The Children's Hospital
Boston
USA

David Creery
Children's Hospital of Eastern Ontario
Ottawa
Canada

Competing interests: None declared.

TABLE 1	Incidence of non-submersion out of hospital cardiorespiratory arrest in children* (see text p 58).		
Reference	Location	Year	Incidence per 100 000 people in total population	Incidence per 100 000 children
12	Manitoba, Canada	1982	2.9	ND
3	King County, USA	1983	2.4	9.9
4	Jerusalem, Israel	1986	2.5	6.9
5	Fresno, USA	1987	5.7	ND
6	Midwestern USA	1990	4.7	ND
7	King County, USA	1992	2.4	10.1
13	Taipei, Taiwan	1994	1.3	ND
8	San Francisco, USA	1995	2.2	16.1
9	Helsinki, Finland	1995	1.4	9.1
10	Birmingham, USA	1995	ND	6.9
11	Houston, USA	1999	4.9	18.0
2	Southern Israel	2000	3.5	7.8

* Incidence represents arrests per 100 000 population per year. ND, no data.

TABLE 2	Causes of non-submersion out of hospital cardiorespiratory arrest in children* (see text p 58).			
Cause	Number of arrests (%)		Number of survivors (%)	
Undetermined	691	(43.9)	1	(0.1)
Trauma	311	(19.8)	10	(3.2)
Chronic disease	126	(8.0)	9	(7.1)
Pneumonia	75	(4.8)	6	(8.0)
Non-accidental injury	23	(1.5)	2	(8.7)
Aspiration	20	(1.3)	0	(0)
Overdose	19	(1.2)	3	(15.8)
Other	309	(19.6)	28	(9.1)
Total	1574 (100)		59	(3.7)

*Figures represent the numbers of arrests/survivors in children with each diagnosis.

Constipation

Search date August 2001

Gregory Rubin

INTERVENTIONS

Key Messages

- We found no RCTs on effects of increasing dietary fibre in children.

- Two RCTs found improvement in stool frequency and symptoms of constipation with cisapride versus placebo after 8–12 weeks of treatment in an outpatient setting. We found no evidence from primary care settings. Cisapride has been withdrawn in several countries because of suspected adverse cardiac effects.

- We found limited evidence that osmotic laxatives may increase stool frequency and soften stools in infants. One small RCT found short term benefit from the addition of toilet training or biofeedback.

- We found no RCTs of the effects of stimulant laxatives in children.

- RCTs found short term benefit from adding biofeedback training to conventional treatment in childhood constipation. Two of the RCTs found no significant difference after 1 year.

DEFINITION	Constipation is characterised by infrequent bowel evacuations, hard, small faeces, or difficult or painful defecation. The frequency of bowel evacuation varies from person to person.[1] Encopresis is defined as involuntary bowel movements in inappropriate places at least once a month for 3 months or more, in children aged 4 years and older.[2]
INCIDENCE/ PREVALENCE	Constipation with or without encopresis is common in children. It accounts for 3% of consultations to paediatric outpatient clinics and 25% of paediatric gastroenterology consultations in the USA.[3] Encopresis has been reported in 1.5% of children at school entry. The peak incidence is at 2–4 years of age.
AETIOLOGY/ RISK FACTORS	No cause is discovered in 90–95% of children with constipation. Low fibre intake and a family history of constipation may be associated factors.[4] Psychosocial factors are often suspected, although most children with constipation are developmentally normal.[3] Chronic constipation can lead to progressive faecal retention, distension of the rectum, and loss of sensory and motor function. Organic causes for constipation are uncommon, but include Hirschsprung's disease (1/5000 births; male : female 4 : 1: constipation invariably present from birth), cystic fibrosis, anorectal physiological abnormalities, anal fissures, constipating drugs, dehydrating metabolic conditions, and other forms of malabsorption.[3]
PROGNOSIS	Childhood constipation can be difficult to treat and often requires prolonged support, explanation, and medical treatment. In one long term follow up study of children presenting under the age of 5 years, 50% recovered within 1 year and 65–70% recovered within 2 years; the remainder required laxatives for daily bowel movements or continued to soil for years.[3] It is not known what proportion continue to have problems into adult life, although adults presenting with megarectum or megacolon often have a history of bowel problems from childhood.
AIMS	To remove faecal impaction and to restore a bowel habit in which stools are soft and passed without discomfort.
OUTCOMES	Number of defaecations per week; number of episodes of soiling per month; gut transit time; use of laxatives.
METHODS	*Clinical Evidence* search and appraisal August 2001. Keywords: constipation, diet therapy, diagnosis, therapy, psychology, stimulant laxatives, dietary fibre, lactulose. The search was limited to infants and children. Trials were selected for inclusion if they focused on the management of constipation or encopresis, or both; if they were relevant to primary health care; and if they included children without an organic cause for constipation.

QUESTION What are the effects of treatments?

OPTION INCREASED DIETARY FIBRE

We found no RCTs on the effects of increasing dietary fibre in children.

Benefits: We found no RCTs on the effects of increasing dietary fibre on constipation in children.

Harms: We found insufficient data.

Comment: None.

OPTION | CISAPRIDE

Two RCTs found improvement in stool frequency and symptoms of constipation with cisapride versus placebo after 8–12 weeks of treatment in an outpatient setting. We found no evidence from primary care settings. Cisapride has been withdrawn in several countries because of suspected adverse cardiac effects.

Benefits: We found no systematic review but found two RCTs. One RCT (69 children, aged 4–18 years, with idiopathic constipation) compared cisapride (0.3 mg/kg/day as a syrup) versus placebo following clearance of accumulated stool. It found that after 8 weeks cisapride significantly increased stool frequency (mean stool frequency/wk 6.75 v 1.31) and decreased gut transit time.[5] The second RCT (40 children, aged 2–16 years), analysed by intention to treat, found significant benefit for cisapride over placebo at 12 weeks, measured by a composite of improved stool frequency, absence of faecal soiling, and no use of other laxatives (improvement in composite index 14/20 [70%] with cisapride v 7/20 [35%] with placebo; RR 2.0, CI 1.03 to 3.88; NNT 3, 95% CI 1 to 24).[6]

Harms: The RCTs did not report harms; see comment below.

Comment: Cisapride is licensed for use in children in the Republic of Ireland. Its license has been suspended in the UK and Germany, and its marketing stopped in the USA, because of its association with heart rhythm abnormalities in adults. See comments on cisapride under gastro-oesophageal reflux in children, p 85.

OPTION | OSMOTIC LAXATIVES

We found limited evidence that osmotic laxatives may increase stool frequency and soften stools in infants. One small RCT found short term benefit from the addition of toilet training or biofeedback.

Benefits: We found no systematic review and no placebo controlled trials of osmotic laxatives in children. We found two small RCTs comparing the effects of lactitol versus lactulose on stool frequency and consistency in 51 and 39 children with constipation.[7,8] Both preparations resulted in a significant increase in stool frequency at 4 weeks and normal consistency of stools at 2 weeks compared with baseline.[7,8] A third RCT (220 non-breastfed, constipated infants aged 0–6 months) compared 2% versus 4% lactulose mixed with an artificial milk preparation.[9] At 14 days, over 90% of parents in both groups reported easy passage of normal or thin consistency stools (P < 0.05 compared with baseline). **With toilet training or biofeedback:** One RCT (87 children with encopresis) compared medical treatment (enemas and osmotic or stimulant laxatives) with and without toilet training.[10] A third arm of the trial evaluated biofeedback. Children receiving toilet training used significantly fewer laxatives and required fewer treatment sessions than those in the other two groups. Toilet training and biofeedback produced similar reductions in rates of soiling, which were greater than those achieved by medical treatment alone (P < 0.04).

Harms: One study found that children taking lactulose experienced significantly more abdominal pain and flatus than those taking lactitol (English abstract only; detailed results will be reported following translation).[7]

Comment: The benefits shown in these studies are comparisons of outcomes before and after treatment, and were not necessarily due to the treatments.[7,8] Toilet training consisted of reinforcement and scheduling to promote response to the urge to defecate, and instruction and modelling to promote appropriate straining.[10]

OPTION   STIMULANT LAXATIVES

We found no placebo controlled RCTs of the effects of stimulant laxatives in children.

Benefits: We found one systematic review (search date not stated), which found no RCTs of adequate methodological rigour comparing stimulant laxatives versus either placebo or alternative treatment in children.[11] We found no placebo controlled RCTs of the effects of stimulant laxatives in children. **With toilet training or biofeedback:** See osmotic laxatives, p 68.

Harms: None identified.

Comment: The studies we found were all comparative, used multiple interventions, had small sample sizes, or both. One quasi-randomised study (using last hospital number digit to allocate patients) compared senna versus mineral oil concentrate in 37 children aged 3–12 years with chronic constipation.[12] The study found that senna versus mineral oil after 6 months was less effective in reducing involuntary faecal soiling (8/18 [44%] with senna v 1/19 [5%] with mineral oil; RR 8.44, 95% CI 1.52 to 16.7). No significant differences were found in the number of children with relapses of constipation symptoms during the treatment period (12/19 [63%] with senna v 16/18 [89%] with mineral oil; RR 0.71, 95% CI 0.48 to 1.04).[12]

OPTION   BIOFEEDBACK TRAINING

RCTs found that biofeedback plus conventional treatment (laxatives alone or laxatives plus dietary advice and toilet training) versus conventional treatment alone significantly improved defaecation dynamics and reduced rates of soiling after 3–7 months. Two of the RCTs found no significant difference in soilin g stool frequency or laxative use after 1 year.

Benefits: We found no systematic review. Four RCTs compared conventional treatment (laxatives alone or laxatives plus dietary advice and toilet training) with or without biofeedback in 87,[10] 192,[13] 129,[14] and 41[15] children with constipation, encopresis, or both. The biofeedback compared 2–6 weeks of training[15] or seminars.[13] Three RCTs found that biofeedback significantly improved defaecation dynamics,[13,15] and rates of soiling,[10] after 3–7 months but none of the RCTs found significant improvement in soiling, stool frequency, or laxative use at 1 year or more.

Harms: None identified.

Comment: None.

REFERENCES

1. Nelson R, Wagget J, Lennard-Jones JE, Barnes PRH. Constipation and megacolon in children and adults. In: Misiewicz JJ, Pounder RE, Venables CW, eds. *Diseases of the gut and pancreas*. 2nd ed. Oxford: Blackwell Science, 1994.

2. American Psychiatric Association. *Diagnostic and statistical manual of mental disorders*. 4th ed. Washington, DC: American Psychiatric Association, 1994.

3. Loening-Baucke V. Chronic constipation in children. *Gastroenterology* 1993;105:557–1563.

4. Roma E, Adamidis D, Nikolara R, Constantopoulos A, Messaritakis J. Diet and chronic constipation in children: the role of fiber. *J Pediatr Gastroenterol Nutr* 1999;28:169–174.

5. Halibi IM. Cisapride in the management of chronic pediatric constipation. *J Pediatr Gastroenterol Nutr* 1999;28:199–202.

6. Nurko MD, Garcia-Aranda JA, Worona LB, Zlochisty O. Cisapride for the treatment of constipation in children: a double blind study. *J Pediatr* 2000;136:35–40.

7. Pitzalis G, Mariani P, Chiarini-Testa MR, et al. Lactitol in chronic idiopathic constipation of childhood. *Pediatr Med Chir* 1995;17:223–226.

8. Martino AM, Pesce F, Rosati U. The effects of lactitol in the treatment of intestinal stasis in childhood. *Minerva Pediatr* 1992;44:319–323.

9. Hejlp M, Kamper J, Ebbesen F, Hansted C. Infantile constipation and allomin-lactulose. Treatment of infantile constipation in infants fed with breast milk substitutes: a controlled trial of 2% and 4% allomin-lactulose. *Ugeskr Laeger* 1990;152:1819–1822.

10. Cox DJ, Sutphen J, Borowitz S, et al. Contribution of behaviour therapy and biofeedback to laxative therapy in the treatment of pediatric encopresis. *Ann Behav Med* 1998;20:70–76.

11. Price KJ, Elliott TM. What is the role of stimulant laxatives in the management of childhood constipation and soiling? (Cochrane Review). In: The Cochrane Library, Issue 3, 2001. Oxford: Update Software. Search date not stated.

12. Sondheimer JM, Gervaise EP. Lubricant versus laxative in the treatment of chronic functional constipation of children: a comparative study. *J Pediatr Gastroenterol Nutr* 1982;1:223–226.

13. Van der Plas RN, Benninga MA, Büller HA, et al. Biofeedback training in treatment of childhood constipation: a randomised controlled study. *Lancet* 1996;348:776–780.

14. Loening-Baucke V. Biofeedback treatment for chronic constipation and encopresis in childhood: long term outcome. *Pediatrics* 1995;96: 105–111.

15. Loening-Baucke V. Modulation of abnormal defecation dynamics by biofeedback treatment in chronically constipated children with encopresis. *J Pediatr* 1990;116:214–222.

Gregory Rubin
Professor of Primary Care
University of Sunderland
Sunderland
UK

Competing interests: None declared.

Search date May 2001

Martin Osmond

INTERVENTIONS

Key Messages

- We found that treatment of croup in primary care settings has not yet been evaluated adequately in RCTs.
- RCTs in primary paediatric assessment units (PAUs) have found that systemic steroids, nebulised steroids, and nebulised adrenaline (epinephrine) all improve symptoms. Systemic and nebulised steroids have also been found to reduce hospital admissions.
- RCTs found no evidence of a difference between systemic and nebulised steroids, but the trials were too limited to rule out a clinically important difference.
- RCTs have found that systemic steroids, nebulised steroids in PAUs, and nebulised adrenaline all improve symptoms in children admitted to hospital. Systemic and nebulised steroids have also been found to reduce hospital stay and re-attendance.
- We found no good evidence to compare the effectiveness of systemic and nebulised steroids in hospitals.
- We found no good evidence to compare the effectiveness of nebulised adrenaline and steroids in hospitals.
- The effectiveness of inhaling humidified air/oxygen in hospitals has not been evaluated adequately.
- None of the RCTs we reviewed, in over 1000 infants with childhood croup, described any deaths related either to croup itself or to any associated treatment.

DEFINITION Croup is an acute clinical syndrome characterised by a harsh, barking cough, inspiratory stridor, and hoarse voice, caused by laryngeal or tracheal obstruction. Mild fever and rhinorrhoea may also be present. The most important differential diagnoses are acute epiglottitis, inhalation of a foreign body, and bacterial tracheitis. The RCTs in this review excluded children with previous upper airway abnormalities, previous prolonged intubation, severe croup (cyanosis with impaired consciousness), and recent treatment with steroids. The conclusions of the review should not be applied to children with these clinical features.

INCIDENCE/ Croup occurs in about 3% of children aged under 6 years per year,[1]
PREVALENCE and causes 2–3% of hospital admissions in young children in the UK.[2] One retrospective Belgian study of 5–8 year olds found that 16% of children had suffered from croup, and 5% had experienced recurrent croup (3 or more episodes).[3]

AETIOLOGY/ Croup is believed to be mainly viral in origin, but atopy plays a part
RISK FACTORS in some children. The most common virus isolated is parainfluenza types 1, 2, or 3. Other viruses include influenza, adenovirus, respiratory syncytial virus, and rhinovirus.

PROGNOSIS Fewer than 2% of children with croup are admitted to hospital in the UK.[1] Of those admitted, only 1–2% require intubation. Mortality is low: of 208 children who were given artificial airways over a 10 year period, two died.[4] Symptoms of upper airway obstruction can be extremely distressing to the child and to the family.

AIMS To reduce suffering and distress, need for hospital admission, duration of hospital stay, rates of intubation, and mortality, without undue adverse effects.

OUTCOMES Severity of symptoms and signs of upper airway obstruction, rates of hospital admission, visits to a medical practitioner or re-attendance to an accident and emergency department, intubation rates, mortality, and adverse effects of treatment. A commonly used definition of a clinically significant improvement is 2 points or more of the validated Westley croup score (maximum score, or most severe, 17)[5] within a predefined timescale. The Westley score comprises the sum of five clinical parameters: conscious level, cyanosis, stridor, air entry, and chest wall retractions. Intubation and death are rare in children with croup, so trials recruiting large numbers of children would be needed to exclude a difference in rates between interventions.

METHODS *Clinical Evidence* search and appraisal May 2001. Data were extracted from trials that used randomisation (not quasi-randomisation) and intention to treat analysis. Most children in the studies were cared for in institutions with excellent staffing and monitoring facilities. RCTs performed in hospital settings studied children with more severe croup than those performed in assessment units.

What are the effects of treatment in primary care settings?

We found insufficient evidence about the treatment of croup in primary care settings.

Benefits: We found no systematic review or RCTs evaluating interventions versus placebo in acute childhood croup in primary care settings.

Harms: Insufficient data.

Comment: It is surprising that there is no evidence relating to children with croup in the primary care setting as this is where the great majority of children with croup are treated.

QUESTION **What are the effects of treatment in primary paediatric assessment units?**

OPTION **SYSTEMIC STEROIDS VERSUS PLACEBO IN PAEDIATRIC ASSESSMENT UNITS**

Three RCTs have found that a single dose of oral or intramuscular steroids significantly improves symptoms within 5 hours, reduces the likelihood of admission to hospital by 75%, and reduces the need for further treatment after discharge by 70%.

Benefits: We found two systematic reviews (both search dates 1997), which included three relevant trials of systemic steroids versus placebo for children with croup in PAUs (see glossary, p 79).[6,7] However, they did not analyse these three trials[8–10] separately from other included studies. The three RCTs included 230 children seen at primary PAUs in Australia, Canada, and the USA. One RCT compared a single intramuscular dose of 0.6 mg/kg dexamethasone, given shortly after arrival in the assessment unit, versus placebo.[8] The other RCTs compared 0.15 mg/kg oral dexamethasone[9] and 0.6 mg/kg intramuscular dexamethasone[10] versus placebo in children ready for discharge from the assessment unit. **Symptom improvement:** Intramuscular dexamethasone (0.6 mg/kg) significantly improved the croup score within 5 hours (96 children; change in croup score: dexamethasone v placebo, -2.9 v -1.3).[8] **Admission to hospital:** Intramuscular dexamethasone given shortly after arrival in the assessment unit reduced admissions to hospital (RR of admission compared with placebo 0.25, 95% CI 0.13 to 0.49; NNT to prevent 1 additional admission 2, 95% CI 1 to 3).[8] **Re-attendance:** For the week after discharge, all three RCTs reported lower rates of re-attendance to any medical practitioner or institution in children given steroids (RR for re-attendance compared with placebo 0.33, 95% CI 0.19 to 0.56; NNT to prevent 1 additional child re-attending 12, 95% CI 6 to 60).[8–10]

Harms: None reported.

Comment: The children were observed for up to 5 hours in a PAU before discharge was decided. Some children were treated with nebulised adrenaline.[10]

**RCTs have found that nebulised steroids versus placebo reduce the
likelihood of a poor response within 2–5 hours by more than 50%, and
halve the risk of hospital admission.**

Benefits: We found three systematic reviews (search dates 1997,[6] 1997,[7]
and not stated[11]), which included four RCTs comparing nebulised
steroids versus placebo for children with croup in PAUs (see glossary, p 79).[8,12-14] However, the reviews combined the results with
RCTs of hospital based treatment. **Symptom improvement:** The
four relevant RCTs (250 children) evaluated treatment in assessment units. They compared a single dose of inhaled steroids versus
placebo, given after humidified oxygen.[8,12-14] Combined data from
the three RCTs, which dichotomised outcomes into either good
(improvement in croup score of 2 or more) or poor response,
showed a significantly reduced likelihood of a poor response within
2–5 hours after treatment (RR 0.44, 95% CI 0.29 to 0.67).[12-14]
Admission to hospital: Rate of admission was halved (RR 0.55,
95% CI 0.38 to 0.81; NNT to prevent 1 additional admission 4,
95% CI 3 to 8).[8,12-14] **Re-attendance:** The four RCTs found no
evidence of a significant difference in rates of further admission
(RR 0.74, 95% CI 0.26 to 2.08), or consultations with other health
practitioners (RR 0.86, 95% CI 0.34 to 2.19) in the week after
discharge from the assessment unit.[8,12-14]

Harms: Nebulised steroids seem to be well tolerated. In one of these four
RCTs, two neutropenic children suffered bacterial tracheitis after
treatment with nebulised dexamethasone.[14]

Comment: We found insufficient evidence to compare regimens of nebulised
steroids. In the RCTs, children were observed for up to 5 hours in the
assessment unit and all received humidified air or oxygen; in one
RCT, both groups also received oral dexamethasone 0.6 mg/kg.[13]
One pilot RCT (17 children in hospital) compared inhaled steroid
(fluticasone propionate 1000 µg, 2 doses) versus placebo delivered by a metered dose inhaler and spacing device, as a potential
treatment that could be given at home. It found no evidence of
benefit, but was too small to rule out a clinically significant effect.[15]
We found another systematic review (search date 1997) that did
not analyse separately data from trials of nebulised steroids versus
placebo.[6]

**RCTs have found that systemic dexamethasone and nebulised
budesonide are equally effective in reducing symptoms. One RCT has
found that oral dexamethasone reduces the rate of admission compared
with nebulised budesonide.**

Benefits: We found one systematic review (search date 1997),[7] which
included a single RCT,[16] and we found two additional RCTs.[8,17] The
RCTs (280 children with acute croup attending an assessment unit)
compared oral dexamethasone 0.6 mg/kg versus nebulised

budesonide 2 mg,[16,17] and intramuscular dexamethasone 0.6 mg/kg versus nebulised budesonide 4 mg.[8] The RCTs found no significant difference between nebulised budesonide and systemic dexamethasone in rates of symptom resolution or re-attendance after discharge, although fewer children on oral dexamethasone were admitted (RR oral v nebulised steroids 0.53, 95% CI 0.34 to 0.81).[8]

Harms: None reported.

Comment: None.

OPTION   **NEBULISED ADRENALINE (EPINEPHRINE) IN PAEDIATRIC ASSESSMENT UNITS**

One small RCT has found that nebulised adrenaline (epinephrine) versus placebo, given in the assessment unit to children suffering from croup, significantly improves symptoms within 30 minutes. Symptoms returned to pre-intervention severity in a third of children within 2 hours.

Benefits: We found no systematic review. **Adrenaline versus placebo:** We found one RCT (54 children with stridor at rest seen in an assessment unit) comparing nebulised racemic adrenaline (0.5 mg/kg diluted to 2 ml with 0.9% sodium chloride) versus saline placebo.[18] It found a significant improvement in croup scores 30 minutes after treatment with adrenaline (mean scores 2.0 v 3.6 on placebo; P < 0.01).[18] The trial found no significant reduction in duration of stay in the assessment unit (mean stay [range]: 11.5 h [5–21] v 13.3 h [6–24]). **Adrenaline combined with steroids:** We found no RCTs. Two prospective cohort studies assessed 115 children treated with nebulised adrenaline and dexamethasone 0.6 mg/kg in an assessment unit. Of the 55–66% who responded satisfactorily, all were discharged after 3–4 hours' observation, and none re-attended for further medical care within 24–48 hours.[19,20]

Harms: We found no evidence of a significant difference in adverse effects after treatment with adrenaline or placebo. Of the children who had improved by 30 minutes, a considerable proportion relapsed, although there was no significant difference in the rate of relapse (return of croup scores to the pretreatment value) between the two groups (35% with adrenaline v 25% with placebo; RR adrenaline v placebo 1.41, 95% CI 0.36 to 5.51). This raises the question of whether children given nebulised adrenaline and then discharged may come to harm when symptoms recur. No children discharged in the RCT re-attended for further treatment.[18] Children were observed for a minimum of 5 hours (up to 24 h). During this time, 40% of treated children and 48% of controls were given a further dose of adrenaline whereas 52% of treated children and 58% of controls received oral betamethasone (6 mg) before final discharge. These differences were not significant.

Comment: None.

QUESTION   What are the effects of treatment in hospital?

OPTION   INHALATION OF HUMIDIFIED AIR/OXYGEN IN HOSPITAL

The effectiveness of inhaling humidified air/oxygen has not been evaluated adequately.

Benefits: We found no systematic review. We found one RCT (16 children), which compared up to 12 hours' care in a humidified atmosphere (air with relative humidity 87–95%) versus normal care.[21] It found no significant difference in recovery rates (mean croup scores at 6 h were 3.1 v 3.8).

Harms: None reported.

Comment: The study was not blinded and selection, performance, and detection biases remain possible. A systematic review of the effects of humidified air is in preparation.[22]

OPTION   SYSTEMIC STEROIDS IN HOSPITAL

RCTs have found that giving systemic corticosteroids to children admitted with croup significantly improves symptoms by 12 hours and reduces hospital stay. Limited evidence suggests that a single dose of oral dexamethasone 0.3 mg/kg is as effective as 0.6 mg/kg in children admitted with croup.

Benefits: We found two systematic reviews (search dates 1999[23] and not stated[11]), which combined data from 11 relevant RCTs (904 children), and we found one additional RCT not included in either review (41 children).[24] The most common regimen was intramuscular or oral dexamethasone 0.3–0.6 mg/kg as a single dose on admission or repeated over 24–48 hours. **Symptom improvement:** RCTs that evaluated symptomatic improvement at 12–24 hours found that significantly more children responded to steroids than to placebo (response defined as ≥ 2 points improvement of croup score; RR of response 1.23, 95% CI 1.13 to 1.33; NNT to achieve response in 1 additional child 7, 95% CI 5 to 10). **Hospital stay:** Four RCTs evaluated duration of hospital stay. Three found a significant reduction in hospital stay on dexamethasone compared with placebo (median stay 20 v 13 h,[17] mean stay 91 v 49 h,[25] and 9 v 3 days[24]). The fourth RCT found no significant difference.[26] **Intubation rates:** Seven RCTs in the systematic review and two subsequent RCTs gave data on intubation rates.[17,23,24] Children given systemic steroids were less at risk of intubation than children taking placebo (RR 0.21, 95% CI 0.06 to 0.69). This combined estimate is dominated by one small study with a much higher than average rate of intubation (5/32 children).[24]

Harms: Systemic steroids seem to be well tolerated. We found three RCTs (130 children) reporting rates of secondary bacterial infection.[24,26,27] These reported nine cases of pneumonia, one of septicaemia, one of bacterial tracheitis, one of otitis media, and one of sinusitis. Six cases were in treated children and seven in controls (RR for infection compared with placebo 0.94, 95% CI 0.33 to 2.69).

Comment: A significant reduction in time to symptom resolution may not reduce hospital stay, which is influenced by hospital policies and referral patterns, availability of treatment in the community, parental access to transportation and communications, and the tendency to discharge children at a certain time each day.[28]

OPTION **HIGH VERSUS LOW DOSE SYSTEMIC STEROID REGIMENS IN HOSPITAL**

Limited evidence suggests that a single dose of oral dexamethasone 0.3 mg/kg is as effective as 0.6 mg/kg in children admitted with croup.

Benefits: We found one systematic review (search date 1997),[7] which included one RCT (120 children admitted with croup) comparing different single doses of oral dexamethasone (0.6 v 0.3 mg/kg and 0.3 v 0.15 mg/kg).[25] It found no significant differences in rate of improvement in croup score, duration of hospital stay, or intubation rates. However, children given the lower dose of dexamethasone were more likely to be given nebulised adrenaline than those given the higher dose (RR 2.32, 95% CI 1.02 to 5.28). We found no studies comparing other systemic regimens.

Harms: None reported.

Comment: None.

OPTION **NEBULISED STEROIDS IN HOSPITAL**

RCTs have found that children admitted with croup given corticosteroids versus placebo improve more rapidly, leave hospital sooner, and are less likely to re-attend. We found insufficient evidence on the effect of nebulised steroids on intubation rates.

Benefits: We found one systematic review (search date not stated,[11] 4 RCTs,[17,29-31] 252 children admitted to hospital with croup) comparing nebulised steroids with placebo. However, this review combined the results with RCTs conducted in PAUs (see glossary, p 79). **Symptom improvement:** One RCT evaluated budesonide 1 mg, two doses, 30 minutes apart.[29] The risk of an inadequate response by 2 hours was significantly reduced (RR 0.40, 95% CI 0.19 to 0.83; NNT to prevent 1 additional inadequate response 2, 95% CI 1 to 8). **Hospital stay:** Another RCT compared nebulised budesonide 2 mg initially, followed by 1 mg every 12 hours, versus placebo, and found a significant reduction in hospital stay (mean stay 36 v 55 h).[30] The third RCT compared budesonide 2 mg single dose versus placebo and reported a significant reduction in the number of children staying in hospital for more than 24 hours (RR 0.37, 95% CI 0.16 to 0.88; NNT 3, 95% CI 2 to 14).[17] **Intubation rates:** Data from the three RCTs found that there was no significant effect on intubation rates (RR of intubation 0.18, 95% CI 0.01 to 3.67).[17,29,30] **Relapse rate:** The fourth RCT compared nebulised budesonide 2 mg versus placebo given every 12 hours while in hospital.[31] It found that budesonide accelerated clinical improvement (decrease in croup score by 2 points or more) compared with placebo (P = 0.013), and reduced the rate of further medical attendance in the 3 days after discharge (re-attendance rate 1/34 with budesonide *v* 7/32 with placebo; P = 0.02).

Harms: Nebulised steroids seem to be well tolerated. Two RCTs reported adverse effects. One RCT reported one episode of nausea and one episode of distress caused by firm application of the face mask for 10 minutes.[30] The other RCT reported emotional distress in six of 42 children treated with budesonide nebulisers and nine of 40 children treated with placebo.[31] In four children with severe croup (1 treated with budesonide and 3 with placebo), this led to interventional treatment outside of the protocol (nebulised adrenaline).

Comment: The optimal regimen of nebulised steroids has not yet been established.

OPTION   SYSTEMIC VERSUS NEBULISED STEROIDS IN HOSPITAL

We found no RCTs undertaken outside of PAUs of oral versus nebulised steroids for croup.

Benefits: We found no systematic review and no RCTs investigating the effects of oral versus nebulised steroids in hospital.

Harms: We found no evidence.

Comment: None.

OPTION   NEBULISED ADRENALINE (EPINEPHRINE) IN HOSPITAL

One small RCT has found that nebulised adrenaline (epinephrine) versus placebo given in the assessment unit to children suffering from croup significantly improves symptoms within 30 minutes. Symptoms returned to pre-intervention severity in a third of children within 2 hours.

Benefits: We found no systematic review. **Versus placebo:** We found three RCTs (53 children admitted to hospital with croup) comparing nebulised adrenaline versus placebo. Two RCTs did not show improvement with adrenaline, but were too small to exclude a clinically significant difference.[32,33] The other small RCT compared aerosolised racemic adrenaline versus 0.9% saline, both delivered by intermittent positive pressure breathing.[5] Children given adrenaline experienced greater reductions in croup score. The reduction was greatest within 30 minutes of treatment and was not apparent at 2 hours (mean croup scores at 30 min 1.7 *v* 3.1). **Nebuliser versus intermittent positive pressure breathing:** We found one RCT (14 children) comparing nebulised adrenaline delivered by intermittent positive pressure breathing versus nebulised adrenaline alone.[34] It found no significant difference in resolution of symptoms (mean croup scores at 30 min 3.1 *v* 2.4). **L-adrenaline versus racemic adrenaline:** We found one RCT (31 children) comparing racemic adrenaline versus L-adrenaline.[35] It found no significant difference in croup scores (mean scores at 30 min, 3.8 *v* 4.8).

Harms: There was no significant difference in the risk of cardiovascular adverse effects with L-adrenaline or racemic adrenaline. Three children receiving racemic adrenaline were intubated (RR of intubation with racemic v L-adrenaline 6.59, 95% CI 0.37 to 118).[35] Children given nebulised adrenaline need medical observation because symptoms may return to pretreatment severity (see harms of nebulised adrenaline in PAUs, p 75).

Comment: Racemic adrenaline comprises equal amounts of D- and L-isomers and was historically chosen in favour of the more readily available L-form in the belief that it caused fewer adverse cardiovascular effects.

OPTION	NEBULISED ADRENALINE VERSUS STEROIDS IN HOSPITAL

We found no good evidence to compare the effectiveness of nebulised adrenaline (epinephrine) and steroids.

Benefits: We found one systematic review (search date 1997),[7] which identified one RCT (66 children admitted to hospital with croup) comparing nebulised adrenaline 4 mg versus nebulised budesonide 2 mg.[36] This trial found no significant difference in duration of hospital stay (mean difference in hospital stay, adrenaline v budesonide, −5.8 h, 95% CI −22.8 h to +11.2 h) or in croup scores (mean change −2.9 v −1.7; P = 0.08). We found no RCTs comparing nebulised adrenaline versus oral steroids.

Harms: None reported.

Comment: Nebulised adrenaline and steroids may have an additive effect through different modes of action, although whether this leads to improved outcomes is unknown.

GLOSSARY

Primary paediatric assessment unit (PAU) An emergency room or accident and emergency department with the facilities to monitor closely the clinical condition of a child with acute onset of inspiratory stridor.

REFERENCES

1. Denny FW, Murphy TF, Clyde WA Jr, Collier AM, Henderson FW. Croup: an 11-year study in a pediatric practice. *Pediatrics* 1983;71:871–876.

2. Phelan PD, Landau LI, Olinsily A. *Respiratory illness in children*. 2nd ed. Oxford: Blackwell Science,1982:32–33.

3. Van Bever HP, Wieringa MH, Weyler JJ, et al. Croup and recurrent croup: their association with asthma and allergy. *Eur J Pediatr* 1999;158:253–257.

4. McEniery J, Gillis J, Kilham H, Benjamin B. Review of intubation in severe laryngotracheobronchitis. *Pediatrics* 1991;87:847–853.

5. Westley CR, Cotton EK, Brooks JG. Nebulized racemic epinephrine by IPPB for the treatment of croup: a double-blind study. *Am J Dis Child* 1978; 132:484–487.

6. Ausejo M, Saenz A, Pham B, et al. The effectiveness of glucocorticoids in treating croup: meta-analysis. *BMJ* 1999;319:595–600. Search date 1997; primary sources Cochrane Controlled Trials Register, Embase, Medline, and letters to authors.

7. Ausejo M, Saenz A, Pham B, et al. Glucocorticoids for Croup. In: The Cochrane Library, Issue 1, 2001. Oxford: Update Software. Search date 1997; primary sources Cochrane Controlled Trials Register, Embase, Medline, and letters to authors. Substantially amended June 1999.

8. Johnson DW, Jacobson S, Edney PC, et al. A comparison of nebulised budesonide, intramuscular dexamethasone, and placebo for moderately severe croup. *N Engl J Med* 1998; 339:498–503.

9. Geelhoed GC, Turner J, Macdonald WBG. Efficacy of a small single dose of oral dexamethasone for outpatient croup: a double blind placebo controlled clinical trial. *BMJ* 1996;313:140–142.

10. Cruz MN, Stewart G, Rosenberg N. Use of dexamethasone in the outpatient management of acute laryngotracheitis. *Pediatrics* 1995;96: 220–223.

11. Griffin S, Ellis S, Fitzgerald-Barron A, Rose J, Egger M. Nebulised steroid in the treatment of croup: a systematic review of randomised controlled trials. *Br J Gen Pract* 2000;50:135–141. Search date

not stated; primary sources Cinahl, Cochrane Controlled Trials Register, Embase, Medline, hand searching of article bibliographies, pharmaceutical industry database.

12. Klassen TP, Feldman ME, Watters LK, Sutcliffe T, Rowe PC. Nebulized budesonide for children with mild-to-moderate croup. N Engl J Med 1994;331: 285–289.

13. Klassen TP, Watters LK, Feldman ME, Sutcliffe T, Rowe PC. The efficacy of nebulized budesonide in dexamethasone-treated outpatients with croup. Pediatrics 1996;97:463–466.

14. Johnson DW, Schuh S, Koren G, Jaffe DM. Outpatient treatment of croup with nebulized dexamethasone. Arch Pediatr Adolesc Med 1996; 150:349–355.

15. Jan Roorda R, Walhof CM. Effects of inhaled fluticasone propionate administered with metered dose inhaler and spacer in mild to moderate croup: A negative preliminary report. Pediatr Pulmonol 1998;25:114–117.

16. Klassen TP, Craig WR, Moher D, et al. Nebulized budesonide and oral dexamethasone for the treatment of croup: a randomized controlled trial. JAMA 1998;279:1629–1632.

17. Geelhoed GC, Macdonald WB. Oral and inhaled steroids in croup: a randomized, placebo-controlled trial. Pediatr Pulmonol 1995;20: 355–361.

18. Kristjansson S, Berg-Kelly K, Winso E. Inhalation of racemic adrenaline in the treatment of mild and moderately severe croup. Clinical symptom score and oxygen saturation measurements for evaluation of treatment effects. Acta Paediatr 1994;83:1156–1160.

19. Ledwith CA, Shea LM, Mauro RD. Safety and efficacy of nebulized racemic epinephrine in conjunction with oral dexamethasone and mist in the outpatient treatment of croup. Ann Emerg Med 1995;25:331–337.

20. Kunkel NC, Baker MD. Use of racemic epinephrine, dexamethasone, and mist in the outpatient management of croup. Pediatr Emerg Care 1996;12:156–159.

21. Bourchier D, Dawson KP, Fergusson DM. Humidification in viral croup: a controlled trial. Aust Paediatr J 1984;20:289–291.

22. Moore M, Little P. Humidified air inhalation for treating croup (Protocol for a Cochrane Review). In: The Cochrane Library, Issue 1, 2001. Oxford: Update Software. Date of most recent substantive amendment: 25 October 1999. Review expected to be published in Issue 1, 2002.

23. Kairys SW, Olmstead EM, O'Connor GT. Steroid treatment of laryngotracheitis: a meta-analysis of the evidence from randomized trials. Pediatrics 1989;83:683–693. Search date June 1999; primary sources Medline, Embase, and Cochrane Library.

24. Sumboonnanonda A, Suwanjutha S, Sirinavin S. Randomized controlled trial of dexamethasone in infectious croup. J Med Assoc Thai 1997;80: 262–265.

25. Geelhoed GC, Macdonald WBG. Oral dexamethasone in the treatment of croup: 0.15 mg/kg versus 0.3 mg/kg versus 0.6 mg/kg. Pediatr Pulmonol 1995;20:362–368.

26. Super DM, Cartelli NA, Broosks LJ, Lembo RM, Kumar ML. A prospective randomized double-blind study to evaluate the effect of dexamethasone in acute laryngotracheitis. J Pediatr 1989;115: 323–329.

27. Kuusela AL, Vesikari T. A randomized double-blind, placebo-controlled trial of dexamethasone and racemic epinephrine in the treatment of croup. Acta Paediatr Scand 1988;77:99–104.

28. Kemper KJ. Medically inappropriate hospital use in a pediatric population. N Engl J Med 1988;318: 1033–1037.

29. Husby S, Agertoft L, Mortensen S, Pedersen S. Treatment of croup with nebulised steroid (budesonide): a double blind, placebo controlled study. Arch Dis Child 1993;68:352–355.

30. Godden CW, Campbell MJ, Hussey M, Cogswell JJ. Double blind placebo controlled trial of nebulised budesonide for croup. Arch Dis Child 1997;76: 155–158.

31. Roberts GW, Master VV, Staugas RE, et al. Repeated dose inhaled budesonide versus placebo in the treatment of croup. J Paediatr Child Health 1999;35:170–174.

32. Gardner HG, Powell KR, Roden VJ, Cherry JD. The evaluation of racemic epinephrine in the treatment of infectious croup. Pediatrics 1973;52:52–55.

33. Taussig LM, Castro O, Beaudry PH, Fox WW, Bureau M. Treatment of laryngotracheobronchitis (croup). Am J Dis Child 1975;129:790–793.

34. Fogel JM, Berg IJ, Gerber MA, Sherter CB. Racemic epinephrine in the treatment of croup: nebulization alone versus nebulization with intermittent positive pressure breathing. J Pediatr 1982;101:1028–1031.

35. Waisman Y, Klein BL, Boenning DA, et al. Prospective randomized double-blind study comparing L-epinephrine and racemic epinephrine aerosols in the treatment of laryngotracheitis (croup). Pediatrics 1992;89:302–306.

36. Fitzgerald D, Mellis C, Johnson M, et al. Nebulized budesonide is as effective as nebulized adrenaline in moderately severe croup. Pediatrics 1996;97: 722–725.

Martin Osmond
Associate Professor of Pediatrics
University of Ottawa
Ottawa
Canada

Competing interests: None declared.

Search date September 2001

Yadlapalli Kumar and Rajini Sarvananthan

INTERVENTIONS

*Not widely licensed for use in children. Clinical use in adults has been restricted because of heart rhythm abnormalities.

Key Messages

- Small RCTs found that prone or left lateral positioning versus supine positioning improved oesophageal pH variables, but both positions are associated with sudden infant death syndrome.

- We found no clear evidence about the effects of feed thickeners. One small RCT found no significant difference between carob flour thickened feeds and placebo thickened feeds in regurgitation as reported by parents. Another small RCT found that carob flour versus traditional formula thickened with rice flour significantly reduced gastro-oesophageal reflux symptoms and episodes of vomiting.

- One small RCT found that sodium alginate versus placebo significantly reduced episodes of regurgitation as reported by parents.

- One systematic review of cisapride versus placebo found no significant improvement in clinical symptoms of gastro-oesophageal reflux. Cisapride has been withdrawn or its use restricted in several countries because of an association with heart rhythm abnormalities.

- One small RCT found that cimetidine (an H$_2$ antagonist) versus placebo significantly improved gastro-oesophageal reflux complicated by oesophagitis in children.

- We found no RCTs on the effects of proton pump inhibitors on gastro-oesophageal reflux in children.

- We found no RCTs on the effects of surgery on gastro-oesophageal reflux in children.

Gastro-oesophageal reflux in children

DEFINITION Gastro-oesophageal reflux disease is the passive transfer of gastric contents into the oesophagus due to transient or chronic relaxation of the lower oesophageal sphincter.[1] A survey of 69 children (median age 16 months) with gastro-oesophageal reflux disease attending a tertiary referral centre found that presenting symptoms were recurrent vomiting (72%), epigastric and abdominal pain (36%), feeding difficulties (29%), failure to thrive (28%), and irritability (19%).[2] Over 90% of children with gastro-oesophageal reflux disease have vomiting before 6 weeks of age.[1] Rare complications of the condition include oesophagitis with haematemesis and anaemia, respiratory problems (such as cough, apnoea, and recurrent wheeze), and failure to thrive.[1] A small comparative study (40 children) suggested that, when compared with healthy children, infants with gastro-oesophageal reflux disease had slower development of feeding skills and had problems affecting behaviour, swallowing, food intake, and mother–child interaction.[3]

INCIDENCE/ PREVALENCE Gastro-oesophageal regurgitation is considered a problem if it is frequent and persistent.[1] Regurgitation occurs in 18% of the general infant population.[4] In a study comparing the prevalence of gastro-oesophageal reflux disease in children with respiratory dysfunction (62 children) to a control group (387 children), the prevalence of excessive gastro-oesophageal reflux, diagnosed by pH metric criteria, was 42% and 8%, respectively.[5]

AETIOLOGY/ RISK FACTORS Risk factors for gastro-oesophageal reflux disease include immaturity of the lower oesophageal sphincter, chronic relaxation of the sphincter, increased abdominal pressure, gastric distension, hiatus hernia, and oesophageal dysmotility.[1] Premature infants and children with severe neurodevelopmental problems or congenital oesophageal anomalies are particularly at risk.

PROGNOSIS Regurgitation is considered benign, and most cases resolve spontaneously by 12–18 months of age.[6] However, with gastro-oesophageal reflux disease caused by hiatus hernia, 30% of cases persist until the age of 4 years.[7]

AIMS To relieve symptoms, maintain normal growth, prevent complications such as oesophagitis, and minimise adverse effects of treatment.

OUTCOMES Clinical condition (in terms of symptoms and growth); parental distress; incidence of complications (e.g. oesophagitis). Reflux Index, a measure of the percentage of time with a low oesophageal pH (frequently < 4), is an intermediate outcome often used in RCTs. Clinical interpretation of the resulting data is problematic.

METHODS *Clinical Evidence* search and appraisal September 2001. We also searched Cinahl.

QUESTION	What are the effects of treatment for symptomatic gastro-oesophageal reflux?

OPTION	DIFFERENT POSTURES

Small RCTs found that prone or left lateral positioning versus supine positioning improved oesophageal pH variables, but both positions are associated with sudden infant death syndrome.

Benefits: We found no systematic review or RCTs on the effect of posture on clinical symptoms, but found three small RCTs on effect of posture on oesophageal pH variables such as the reflux index. One RCT (crossover, 24 children, age < 5 months) found that the prone and left lateral positions versus the supine and right lateral positions significantly reduced the reflux index (P < 0.001); it found no significant effect with head elevation.[8] A second RCT (crossover, 15 children, age < 6 months) also found that the prone position (head elevated in a harness) versus supine positioning (in an infant seat where the head and trunk were elevated to 60°) significantly reduced the reflux index (P < 0.001).[9] The third RCT (crossover, 18 children, < 37 wks gestation but > 7 days old) compared prone versus left lateral versus right lateral positions over 24 hours. It found that prone and left lateral positions versus right lateral position significantly reduced reflux index (P < 0.001), the number of reflux episodes (P < 0.001), and duration of longest reflux episode (P < 0.001).[10]

Harms: The RCTs gave no information on adverse effects (see comment below).

Comment: All three RCTs measured the reflux index as a surrogate outcome, but it is difficult to interpret the clinical importance of the observed changes in the reflux index. One large, prospective cohort study found that prone sleeping position compared with supine position was associated with an increased risk of sudden infant death syndrome (OR 4.5, 95% CI 1.3 to 15.4).[11] The side sleeping position compared with the supine position also increased the risk of sudden infant death syndrome (at 2 months, adjusted OR 6.6, 95% CI 1.7 to 25.2).[12]

OPTION	FEED THICKENERS

We found no clear evidence. One small RCT found no significant difference between carob flour thickened feeds and placebo thickened feeds in regurgitation reported by parents. Another small RCT found that carob flour versus traditional formula thickened with rice flour significantly reduced gastro-oesophageal reflux symptoms and episodes of vomiting.

Benefits: We found no systematic review. **Versus placebo:** We found two RCTs. The first RCT (20 children, aged 1–16 wks with regurgitation > 5 times daily) found that feeds thickened with carob flour versus placebo thickener (Saint John's bread, which is free of fibre and polysaccharides) decreased regurgitation documented by parents after 1 week of treatment, but the difference was not significant (mean regurgitation score 2.2 v 3.3; P = 0.14).[13] The second RCT compared dry rice cereal versus isocaloric unthickened feeds but did not seek to report benefits (see harms below).[14] **Versus each other:** We found one RCT (24 children, age 5–11 months), which found that, after 2 weeks, carob flour versus traditional formula with rice significantly reduced a symptom score (mean relative reduction 70% v 49%; P < 0.01) and the frequency of vomiting recorded by parents (P < 0.05).[15]

Harms: The second RCT (24 children, age 0–6 months) found that feeds thickened with dry rice cereal versus isocaloric unthickened feeds significantly increased coughing after feeding (means: 3.1 cough salvos/h, 95% CI 1.5 to 4.7 with thickened feeds v 2.0, 95% CI 1.2 to 2.8 with unthickened feeds; P = 0.034).[15]

Comment: The clinical significance of changes in regurgitation scores is unclear.

OPTION SODIUM ALGINATE

One small RCT found that sodium alginate versus placebo significantly reduced the frequency of episodes of regurgitation reported by parents.

Benefits: We found no systematic review but found one RCT.[16] The RCT (20 children, mean age 28 months) found that sodium alginate versus lactose powder placebo for 8 days significantly reduced the frequency of regurgitation episodes reported by parents (frequency relative to untreated level 25–33% with sodium alginate v 0% with placebo). Sodium alginate versus placebo also significantly improved oesophageal pH variables (Euler-Byrne index and reflux time, P< 0.05).

Harms: The RCT found no adverse effects.[16]

Comment: The high sodium content of sodium alginate might be inappropriate in preterm babies.[17]

OPTION CISAPRIDE

One systematic review comparing cisapride versus placebo found no significant improvement in clinical symptoms of gastro-oesophageal reflux. Cisapride has been withdrawn or its use restricted in several countries because of an association with heart rhythm abnormalities.

Benefits: We found one good quality systematic review (8 RCTs, search date not stated).[18] It found no significant difference between cisapride versus placebo in clinical improvement (for symptoms at the end of treatment being "same or worse" v "improved": 7 RCTs, 236 children; OR 0.34, 95% CI 0.10 to 1.19) but a significant reduction of the reflux index (5 RCTs, 176 children; WMD –6.49, 95% CI –10.13 to –2.85). Confidence in these results is reduced by three potential biases: (i) the "same or worse" category included the subcategory of "slight improvement" and significant heterogeneity was found between studies on pooling results for this outcome; (ii) the review found evidence suggesting publication bias favouring

RCTs with positive outcomes; (iii) the reflux index is poorly correlated with clinical symptoms and the clinical importance of changes in reflux index are unclear.

Harms: The systematic review found a non-significant increase in adverse events with cisapride versus placebo (4 RCTs, 190 children; OR 1.8, 95% CI 0.87 to 3.7), but did not describe specific adverse effects.[18] See comment below.

Comment: Cisapride has been withdrawn or its use restricted in several countries because of an increased frequency of heart rhythm abnormalities that are associated with sudden death.[19] One case control study (201 children, age 1–12 months) found that cisapride significantly prolonged the QTc interval on electrocardiogram in a subgroup of infants younger than 3 months, but in older infants the difference was not significant.[20] A second case control study (252 infants) found similar results.[21] A third case control study (120 children) found prolonged QT interval in some normal children with or without cisapride.[22] Gastrointestinal adverse effects (borborygmi, cramps, and diarrhoea) occured in 2% of infants.[20] Rash, pruritus, urticaria, bronchospasm, extrapyramidal effects, headache, dose-related increases in urinary frequency, hyperprolactinaemia, and reversible liver function abnormalities were extremely rare.[20] Most macrolide antibiotics and cimetidine elevate plasma cisapride levels and may increase the clinical risk.[20]

OPTION   H$_2$ ANTAGONISTS

One small RCT found that cimetidine versus placebo significantly improved gastro-oesophageal reflux complicated by oesophagitis in children.

Benefits: We found no systematic review but found two small RCTs. The first RCT (double blind, 37 children with gastro-oesophageal reflux disease complicated by oesophagitis, age 1 month to 14 years) found that cimetidine (30–40 mg/kg daily) versus placebo significantly reduced the number of children with gastro-oesophageal reflux over 12 weeks (ARR 51%, 95% CI 21% to 81%; NNT 2, 95% CI 2 to 5). Improvement was defined in terms of either clinical or endoscopic findings.[23] A second crossover RCT (27 children with gastro-oesophageal reflux disease) compared different doses of cimetidine but reported only physiological outcomes (gastric pH, gastric acid suppression).[24] We found no RCTs of ranitidine in children.

Harms: The RCTs found no adverse effects.[23,24]

Comment: Cimetidine has been reported to cause bradycardia in a small subgroup of people and may increase cisapride plasma levels.[20] Uncontrolled studies of ranitidine have reported bronchospasm, acute dystonic reactions, sinus node dysfunction, bradycardia, and vasovagal reactions.[20]

OPTION   PROTON PUMP INHIBITORS

We found no RCTs about proton pump inhibitors for gastro-oesophageal reflux in children.

Gastro-oesophageal reflux in children

Benefits: We found no systematic review or RCT on proton pump inhibitors for gastro-oesophageal reflux in children. One small case series did not report clinical outcomes.[25]

Harms: We found no systematic review or RCTs.

Comment: Proton pump inhibitors have been reported to cause hepatitis, and omeprazole chronically elevates serum gastrin.[25]

OPTION	SURGERY

We found no RCTs about surgery for gastro-oesophageal reflux in children.

Benefits: We found no systematic review or RCT comparing surgery versus medical interventions, or one surgical procedure versus another.

Harms: A retrospective review (106 children) of modified Nissen's fundoplication found a failure rate of 8% and, when neurologically impaired children were included, a long term mortality of 8%.[26] If only neurologically normal children were considered, the mortality was 2% in the immediate postoperative period and 3% on long term follow up (3 deaths in 62 children; all deaths were in children with congenital abnormalities).

Comment: We found a cohort study of 22 children who had undergone anterior gastric fundoplication.[27] Twenty children (91%) remained asymptomatic at 2 years. Complications of surgical treatment include dumping, retching, intestinal obstruction, "gas bloat", and recurrence of gastro-oesophageal reflux disease.[17]

REFERENCES

1. Herbst JJ. *Textbook of Gastroenterology and Nutrition in Infancy*. 2nd ed. New York: Raven Press, 1989:803–813.
2. Lee WS, Beattie RM, Meadows N, et al. Gastro-oesophageal reflux: Clinical profiles and outcome. *J Paediatr Child Health* 1999;35:568–571.
3. Mathisen B, Worrall L, Masel J, et al. Feeding problems in infants with gastro-oesophageal reflux disease: a controlled study. *J Paediatr Child Health* 1999;35:163–169.
4. Boulton TJ, Rowley MP. Nutritional studies during early childhood. III. Incidental observations of temperament, habits, and experiences of ill-health. *Aust Paediatr J* 1979;15:87–90.
5. Sacré L, Vandenplas Y. Gastroesophageal reflux associated with respiratory abnormalities during sleep. *J Pediatr Gastroenterol Nutr* 1989;9:28–33.
6. Vandenplas Y, Belli D, Benhamou P, et al. A critical appraisal of current management practices for infant regurgitation – recommendations of a working party. *Eur J Pediatr* 1997;156:343–357.
7. Carre IJ. Natural history of partial thoracic stomach ("hiatus hernia") in children. *Arch Dis Child* 1959;34:344–353.
8. Tobin JM, McCloud P, Cameron DJS. Posture and gastro-oesophageal reflux: a case for left lateral positioning. *Arch Dis Child* 1997;76:254–258.
9. Orenstein SR, Whitington PF. Positioning for prevention of infant gastroesophageal reflux. *J Pediatr* 1983;103:534–537.
10. Ewer AK, James ME, Tobin JM. Prone and left lateral positioning reduce gastro-oesophageal reflux in preterm infants. *Arch Dis Child Fetal Neonatal Ed* 1999;81:F201–205.
11. Dwyer T, Ponsonby AB, Newman NM, et al. Prospective cohort study of prone sleeping position and sudden infant death syndrome. *Lancet* 1991;337:1244–1247.
12. Mitchell EA, Tuohy PG, Brunt JM, et al. Risk factors for sudden infant death syndrome following the prevention campaign in New Zealand. *Pediatrics* 1997;100:835–840.
13. Vandenplas Y, Hachimi-Idrissi S, Casteels A, et al. A clinical trial with an "anti-regurgitation" formula. *Eur J Pediatr* 1994;153:419–423.
14. Orenstein SR, Shalaby TM, Putnam PE. Thickening feedings as a cause of increased coughing when used as therapy for gastroesophageal reflux in infants. *J Pediatr* 1992;121:913–915.
15. Borrelli O, Salvia G, Campanozzi A, et al. Use of a new thickened formula for treatment of symptomatic gastroesophageal reflux in infants. *Ital J Gastroenterol Hepatol* 1997;29:237–242.
16. Buts JP, Barudi C, Otte JB. Double-blind controlled study on the efficacy of sodium alginate (Gaviscon) in reducing gastroesophageal reflux assessed by 24 hour continuous pH monitoring in infants and children. *Eur J Pediatr* 1987;146:156–158.
17. Davies AEM, Sandhu BK. Diagnosis and treatment of gastro-oesophageal reflux. *Arch Dis Child* 1995;73:82–86.
18. Augood C, MacLennan S, Gilbert R, Logan S. Cisapride treatment for gastro-oesophageal reflux in children (Cochrane Review). In: The Cochrane Library, Issue 3, 2001. Oxford: Update Software. Search date 2000; primary sources Cochrane Central Trials Register, Cochrane Specialised Trials register of the Cochrane Upper Gastrointestinal

and Pancreatic Diseases Group, Medline, Embase, Science Citation Index, and hand searched reference lists.

19. WHO Pharmaceuticals Newsletter, No.3, 2000. http://www.who.int/medicines/library/pnewslet/pn32000.html (accessed November 2001).
20. Vandenplas Y, Belli DC, Benatar A, et al. The role of cisapride in the treatment of pediatric gastroesophageal reflux. *J Pediatr Gastroenterol Nutr* 1999;28:518–528.
21. Benatar A, Feenstra A, Decraene T, Vandenplas Y. Effects of cisapride on corrected QT interval, heart rate, and rhythm in infants undergoing polysomnography. *Pediatrics* 2000;106(6):E85.
22. Ramirez-Mayans J, Garrido-Garcia LM, Huerta-Tecanhuey A, et al. Cisapride and QTc interval in children. *Pediatrics* 2000;106:1028–1030.
23. Cucchiara S, Gobio-Casali L, Balli F, et al. Cimetidine treatment of reflux esophagitis in children: An Italian multicentre study. *J Pediatr Gastroenterol Nutr* 1989;8:150–156.
24. Lambert J, Mobassaleh M, Grand RJ. Efficacy of cimetidine for gastric acid suppression in pediatric patients. *J Pediatr* 1992;120:474–478.
25. Gunasekaran TS, Hassall EG. Efficacy and safety of omeprazole for severe gastroesophageal reflux in children. *J Pediatr* 1993;123:148–154.
26. Spillane AJ, Currie B, Shi E. Fundoplication in children: Experience with 106 cases. *Aust NZ J Surg* 1996;66:753–756.
27. Bliss D, Hirschl R, Oldham K, et al. Efficacy of anterior gastric fundoplication in the treatment of gastroesophageal reflux in infants and children. *J Paediatr Surg* 1994;29:1071–1075.

Yadlapalli Kumar
Consultant Paediatrician Royal Cornwall Hospital
Treliske Truro Cornwall
UK

Rajini Sarvananthan
Lecturer in Paediatrics
Universiti Kebangsaan Malaysia
Malaysia

Competing interests: None declared.

Infantile colic

Search date September 2001

Teresa Kilgour and Sally Wade

Key Messages

- One systematic review has found that dicycloverine (dicyclomine) versus placebo reduces crying in infants with colic. One RCT found that dicycloverine versus placebo reduced colic in infants. Dicycloverine is associated with serious adverse effects.

- One RCT found no significant difference with simethicone (activated dimeticone) versus placebo for presence of colic when rated by carers. Another RCT found no significant difference with simethicone versus placebo in improvement as rated by parental interview, 24 hour diary, or behavioural observation. Another poor quality RCT found that simethicone versus placebo significantly reduced the number of crying attacks on days 4–7 of treatment.

- One small RCT found that soya based infant feeds versus cow's milk reduced the duration of crying in infants with colic.

- We found insufficient evidence from two RCTs to compare casein hydrolysate hypoallergenic formula versus cow's milk formula in infants with colic.

- One RCT found limited evidence that replacing cow's milk formula with whey hydrolysate formula reduced infant colic.

- Three RCTs found no significant difference in effects of low lactose (lactase treated) milk versus untreated milk in infants with colic.

- One small crossover RCT found that sucrose solution versus placebo increased parent rated improvement in symptoms of infantile colic.

- One small RCT found that herbal tea (containing extracts of chamomile, vervain, licorice, fennel, and balm mint in a sucrose solution) versus sucrose solution alone reduced parent rated symptoms of infantile colic.

- Two systematic reviews found conflicting evidence from four small RCTs on the effects of behavioural modification of parents' response to crying in infants with colic.

- We found no RCTs on the effects of cranial osteopathy in infants with colic.
- One RCT found no significant difference with massage versus a crib vibrator in colic related crying or in parental rating of symptoms of infantile colic.
- Two RCTs found inconclusive results about the effects of spinal manipulation in infants with colic

DEFINITION   Infantile colic is defined as excessive crying in an otherwise healthy baby. The crying typically starts in the first few weeks of life and ends by 4–5 months. Excessive crying is defined as crying that lasts at least 3 hours a day, for 3 days a week, for at least 3 weeks.[1]

INCIDENCE/   Infantile colic causes one in six families to consult a health profes-
PREVALENCE sional. One systematic review of fifteen community based studies found a wide variation in prevalence, which depended on study design and method of recording.[2] The two best prospective studies identified by the review yielded prevalence rates of 5% and 19%.[2] One RCT (89 breast and formula fed infants) found that, at 2 weeks of age, the prevalence of crying more than 3 hours a day was 43% among formula fed infants and 16% among breast fed infants. The prevalence at 6 weeks was 12% (formula fed) and 31% (breast fed).[3]

AETIOLOGY/   The cause of infantile colic is unclear and, despite its name, might
RISK FACTORS not have an abdominal cause. It may reflect part of the normal distribution of infantile crying. Other possible explanations are painful gut contractions, lactose intolerance, gas, or parental mis-interpretation of normal crying.[1]

PROGNOSIS   Infantile colic improves with time. One study found that 29% of infants aged 1–3 months cried for more than 3 hours a day, but by 4–6 months of age the prevalence had fallen to 7–11%.[4]

AIMS   To reduce infant crying and distress, and the anxiety of the family, with minimal side effects of treatment.

OUTCOMES   Duration of crying or colic, as measured on dichotomous, ordinal, or continuous scales; parents' perceptions of severity (recorded in a diary).

METHODS   *Clinical Evidence* search and appraisal September 2001. We searched Cinahl, the Cochrane Library, Embase, and Medline for publications using reduction in crying or colic as the main outcome. Trials were excluded for the following reasons: infants studied had normal crying patterns, infants were older than 6 months, interventions lasted less than 3 days, trials had no control groups or had low Jadad quality scores (see glossary, p 96).[5] Sometimes we pooled results from RCTs with different but comparable outcomes; effect sizes were calculated using a random effects model.

Child health

Infantile colic

OPTION   DICYCLOVERINE

One systematic review has found that dicycloverine (dicyclomine) versus placebo reduces crying in infants with colic. One RCT found that dicycloverine versus placebo reduced colic in infants.

Benefits: We found two systematic reviews.[1,6] The first systematic review (search date 1996)[1] identified five RCTs (134 infants) comparing the effect of dicycloverine (see glossary, p 96) versus placebo on crying or the presence of colic. It found that dicycloverine (most frequently 5 mg 4 times daily) versus placebo significantly reduced crying (SMD 0.46, 95% CI 0.33 to 0.60). The clinical importance of this result is unclear (see comment below). The second systematic review (search date 1999)[6] identified three RCTs included in the first systematic review,[1] but did not pool the results. One RCT found that dicycloverine versus placebo (cherry syrup) significantly reduced colic (elimination of colic: 63% with dicycloverine v 25% with placebo; RR 0.5, 95% CI 0.28 to 0.88; NNT 3, CI not provided).[7] The other two RCTs used definitions of colic that included symptoms but not duration and frequency, and reported results in terms of clinical scores. Both RCTs found significantly better mean clinical scores with dicycloverine versus placebo.[6]

Harms: Two of five RCTs[8,9] in the systematic reviews[1,6] compared harms of dicycloverine versus placebo. The first RCT (crossover design, 30 infants) found more drowsiness with dicycloverine versus placebo (4/30 [13%] v 1/30 [3%]; ARI +10%, 95% CI −4% to +24%).[8] The second RCT (crossover design, 25 infants) found more loose stools or constipation in infants on dicycloverine versus placebo (3/25 [12%] v 1/25 [4%]; ARI +8%, 95% CI −7% to +23%).[9] Case reports of harms in infants have included breathing difficulties, seizures, syncope, asphyxia, muscular hypotonia, and coma.[10]

Comment: Only one RCT stated measures to make the control syrup taste the same as the drug syrup.[8] The first review is limited because it pooled different outcome measures from RCTs and included crossover studies.[1] The crossover design is unlikely to provide valid evidence because infantile colic has a naturally variable course, and the effects of dicycloverine may continue even after a washout period.[11]

OPTION   SIMETHICONE (ACTIVATED DIMETICONE)

One RCT found no significant difference with simethicone (activated dimeticone) versus placebo in the presence of colic when rated by carers. Another RCT found no significant difference with simethicone versus placebo in improvement as rated by parental interview, 24 hour diary, or behavioural observation. Another, poor quality RCT found that simethicone versus placebo significantly reduced the number of crying attacks on days 4–7 of treatment.

Benefits: We found two systematic reviews (search dates 1996[1] and 1999,[6] same 3 RCTs in each review, 136 infants with infantile colic) comparing the effect of simethicone (see glossary, p 96) versus placebo on the duration of crying or the presence of colic. The first RCT (double blind, crossover, 83 infants aged 2–8 wks) compared 0.3 mL of simethicone versus placebo before feeds.[12] It found no significant difference in colic when rated by carers (28% improved with simethicone v 37% with placebo v 20% with both; effect size for simethicone versus placebo: –0.10, 95% CI –0.27 to +0.08). The second RCT (double blind, crossover trial, 27 infants aged 2–8 wks) found no significant difference with simethicone versus placebo in improvement as rated by parental interview, 24 hour diary, or behavioural observation (effect size +0.06, 95% CI –0.17 to +0.28).[13] The third RCT (26 infants aged 1–12 wks) was of unsatisfactory quality; it reported no details on how cases of colic were defined.[14] It found that simethicone versus placebo significantly reduced the number of crying attacks on days 4 to 7 of treatment (effect size +0.54, 95% CI +0.21 to +0.87).[14]

Harms: None of the RCTs reported adverse effects with either simethicone or placebo.

Comment: The crossover design of both RCTs limits their validity and clinical utility.

OPTION **REPLACEMENT OF COW'S MILK WITH SOYA BASED INFANT FEEDS**

One small RCT found that soya based infant feeds versus cow's milk reduced the duration of crying in infants with colic.

Benefits: We found two systematic reviews (search dates 1996[1] and 1999,[6] 2 RCTs). One RCT (19 infants) found that soya based infant feeds (see glossary, p 96) versus standard cow's milk formula reduced the duration of crying (4.3–12.7 h with soya based infant feeds v 17.3–20.1 h with cow's milk; mean difference –10.3 h, 95% CI –16 to –4 h).[15] The other RCT only considered infants admitted to hospital for colic and used weak methods (Jadad score 1).[16]

Harms: None reported.

Comment: Mothers were not told which milk the babies received, but differences between the milks may have been detected from smell and texture. No firm conclusions can be drawn about the effect of soya based infant feeds versus standard cow's milk formula because of the small size of the RCT.[15]

OPTION **REPLACEMENT OF COW'S MILK WITH CASEIN HYDROLYSATE MILK**

We found insufficient evidence from two RCTs to compare casein hydrolysate milk versus cow's milk formula in infants with colic.

Benefits: We found two systematic reviews (search dates 1996[1] and 1999[6]), which identified the same two RCTs. The first RCT (double blind, crossover, 17 infants) studied the effect of each of three changes of infant diet over 4 days.[17] Bottle fed infants received casein hydrolysate milk (see glossary, p 96) and cow's milk alternately. By the third change there was no notable difference in the incidence of colic between groups. A total of 8/17 (47%) infants left the study before completion. The second RCT (122 infants) compared bottle fed infants given casein hydrolysate milk versus cow's milk formula. It also compared breast fed infants with mothers on a hypoallergenic diet (see glossary, p 96) versus controls on an unmodified diet.[18] Thirty eight infants were bottle fed, but the RCT did not report how many of these babies received the active diet. This RCT pooled the results of breast and bottle fed babies and found that the active diet reduced infant distress as measured by parents on a validated chart. The number of bottle fed infants was too small to establish or exclude important effects in the bottle fed subgroup.

Harms: None reported.

Comment: The available evidence is insufficient to define the effects of casein hydrolysate milk on infantile colic.

| OPTION | REPLACEMENT OF COW'S MILK FORMULA BY WHEY HYDROLYSATE FORMULA |

One RCT found limited evidence that replacing cow's milk formula with whey hydrolysate formula reduced infant colic.

Benefits: We found two systematic reviews (search dates 1996[1] and 1999[6]) and one subsequent RCT.[19] The systematic reviews found no RCTs of adequate quality. The subsequent, double blind RCT (43 infants) found that whey hydrolysate formula (see glossary, p 96) (23 infants) versus standard cow's milk formula reduced the time that babies cried each day, measured by a validated parental diary (crying reduced by 63 min/day, 95% CI 1 to 127 min/day).[19]

Harms: None identified in the RCT.

Comment: Parents may not have been blind to the intervention. When asked, six indicated that they were aware of allocation, but two of these falsely identified the formula. When these infants' results were removed from the analysis, the crying time with whey hydrolysate formula versus standard cow's milk formula was significantly reduced by 58 minutes daily (P = 0.03).[18]

| OPTION | LOW LACTOSE (LACTASE TREATED) MILK |

Three RCTs found no significant difference in the effects of low lactose (lactase treated) milk versus untreated milk in infants with colic.

Benefits: We found two systematic reviews (search dates 1996[1] and 1999,[6] 2 RCTs) and one additional small RCT.[20] The first RCT in the systematic reviews (double blind, crossover, 10 weaned infants) compared bottle feeding using pooled breast milk versus low lactose (lactase treated) breast milk versus cow's milk versus low lactose (lactase treated) cow's milk.[21] It found no evidence that low lactose milk reduced the timing, severity, or duration of colic recorded by parents. The second RCT (12 breast fed infants) compared lactase versus placebo drops given within 5 minutes of feeding and found no differences for time spent feeding, sleeping, or crying. The additional small crossover RCT (13 infants) compared lactase treated milk versus placebo treated milk.[20] It found a non-significant reduction in crying time with lactase treated milk (1.1 h/day, 95% CI 0.2 to 2.1 h/day).

Harms: None reported.

Comment: The RCTs are too small to make firm conclusions. The babies were not selected on the basis of confirmed lactose intolerance.

OPTION SUCROSE SOLUTION

One small crossover RCT found that sucrose solution versus placebo increased parent rated improvement in symptoms of infantile colic.

Benefits: We found one systematic review (search date 1999, 1 RCT).[6] The small crossover RCT (19 infants) compared 2 mL of 12% sucrose solution versus placebo given to babies when they continued to cry despite comforting.[22] Parents, blind to the intervention, scored the effect of the treatment on a scale of 1–5. Treatments were crossed over after 3–4 days and again after 6–8 days. The RCT found that sucrose versus placebo significantly increased parent rated improvement (12/19 [63%] with sucrose v 1/19 [5%] with placebo; ARI 58%, 95% CI 10% to 89%; NNT 2, 95% CI 1 to 10; RR 12, 95% CI 3.0 to 19).

Harms: None reported.

Comment: No firm conclusion can be drawn about the effect of sucrose solution versus placebo because of the small size of the RCT.[22]

OPTION HERBAL TEA

One small RCT found that herbal tea (containing extracts of chamomile, vervain, licorice, fennel, and balm mint in a sucrose solution) versus sucrose solution alone reduced parent rated symptoms of infantile colic.

Benefits: We found two systematic reviews (search dates 1996[1] and 1999,[6] 1 RCT[23]). The RCT compared herbal tea (containing extracts of chamomile, vervain, licorice, fennel, and balm mint in a sucrose solution) (33 infants) versus sucrose solution alone (35 infants) given by parents up to three times daily in response to episodes of colic. Coding was only known to the pharmacist and the taste and smell of the tea and placebo were similar. Parents rated the response using a symptom diary. The RCT found that, at 7 days, herbal tea eliminated colic more frequently than sucrose solution (number of infants colic free: 19/33 [58%] with herbal tea v 9/35 [26%] with sucrose; ARI 32%, 95% CI 7% to 53%; RR 2.2, 95% CI 1.3 to 3.1; NNT 3, 95% CI 2 to 14).

Harms: None reported.

Comment: No firm conclusion can be drawn about the effect of herbal tea versus sucrose solution. The RCT did not state the exact proportion of the herbs used in the preparation.

Infantile colic

| OPTION | BEHAVIOURAL MODIFICATION |

Two systematic reviews found conflicting evidence from four small RCTs on the effects of behavioural modification of parents' response to crying in infants with colic.

Benefits: We found two systematic reviews (search dates 1996[1] and 1999,[6] 4 RCTs). **Focused counselling versus non-specific reassurance:** One RCT (22 infants) assessed maternal anxiety and the hours of crying each day by questionnaire. It found no evidence that counselling mothers about specific management techniques (responding to crying with gentle soothing motion, avoidance of over stimulation, using a pacifier, and prophylactic carrying) was any better than reassurance (see glossary, p 96) and support.[24] **Focused counselling versus car ride simulation:** The same RCT also allocated 16 infants (mean age 6.8 wks) to car ride simulation for up to 1 hour. There were no important differences between this group and the control group (11 infants) for crying times or maternal anxiety.[24] **Focused counselling versus elimination of cow's milk protein:** One RCT (20 infants) found that counselling parents to respond to their baby's cries by feeding, holding, offering a pacifier, stimulating, or putting the baby down to sleep, decreased duration and extent of crying more quickly than substitution of soya or cow's milk with hydrolysed casein formula (mean decrease in crying, recorded by parent diary, 2.1 h/day with counselling v 1.2 h/d with dietary change).[25] **Increased carrying versus general advice:** The third RCT (66 infants) randomised mothers of babies with colic to carry their infant, even when not crying, for at least an additional 3 hours a day or to a general advice group (to carry, check baby's nappy, feed, offer pacifier, place baby near mother, or use background stimulation such as music). The "advice to carry" group carried their babies for 4.5 hours daily compared with 2.6 hours daily in the general advice group. There was no effect on daily crying time (mean difference 3 min less, 95% CI 37 min less to 32 min more).[26] **Reducing stimulation versus non-specific interview:** The fourth RCT (42 infants, median age 10 wks) allocated mothers of infants to advice to reduce stimulation (mothers were advised to reduce stimulation by not patting, lifting, or jiggling the baby, or reducing auditory stimulation) versus an empathetic interview. For infants under 12 weeks, advice to reduce stimulation versus no advice improved a change rating scale for more infants (after 7 days: 14/15 [95%] improved with advice v 6/12 [50%] with control; ARI 43%, 95% CI 8% to 49%; RR 1.9, 95% CI 1.2 to 2.0; NNT 2, 95% CI 2 to 13).[27] Improvement in the change rating scale was defined as a score of +2 or better on a scale from −5 to +5 that was meant to indicate perceived change in crying since the start of the trial. It is unclear whether this scale has been validated (see comment below).

Harms: None reported.

Comment: Mothers given advice to reduce stimulation were also given permission to leave their infants if they felt they could no longer tolerate the crying. It is unclear whether the improved change score represents a true change in the hours that the baby cried, or altered maternal perception.

| OPTION | CRANIAL OSTEOPATHY |

We found no RCTs on the effects of cranial osteopathy in infants with colic.

Benefits: We found no systematic review and no RCTs on the effects of cranial osteopathy (see glossary, p 96) in infants with colic.

Harms: We found no RCTs.

Comment: None.

| OPTION | INFANT MASSAGE |

One RCT found no significant difference with massage versus a crib vibrator for colic related crying or parental rating of symptoms of infantile colic.

Benefits: We found no systematic review. **Versus usual care:** We found no RCTs. **Versus other care:** We found one RCT (58 infants, 47% with colic; see comment below) comparing massage versus a crib vibrator over a 4 week period.[28] Infant massage (performed 3 times daily) included gentle stroking of the skin over different parts of the head, body, and limbs, using olive oil and while maintaining eye contact. The crib vibrator was used for 25 minute periods at least 3 times daily (see comment below). Colic symptom ratings were obtained from parental diaries of crying. The RCT found no significant difference with massage versus a crib vibrator for colic related crying or parental rating of symptoms (AR for less crying: 64% v 52%; P = 0.24, CI not provided).[28]

Harms: None reported.

Comment: Only 47% of infants in the trial were specified to have colic, so the results may not apply to infants with colic.[28] The use of a crib vibrator as a control intervention is based on an earlier study in which a similar device was as effective as parental reassurance and support. It is unclear whether reduced crying in this RCT reflects the natural course of infantile colic or the specific effect of interventions. The RCT may have lacked power to detect clinically important effects. The available evidence is insufficient to define the effectiveness of infant massage in infantile colic.

| OPTION | SPINAL MANIPULATION |

Two RCTs found inconclusive results about the effects of spinal manipulation in infants with colic.

Benefits: We found no systematic review. We found two RCTs that considered the effects of spinal manipulation (see glossary, p 96).[29,30] **Versus simethicone (activated dimeticone):** One RCT (41 infants) compared 2 weeks of spinal manipulation versus 2 weeks of daily treatment with simethicone; parents recorded length of crying in a colic diary.[29] It found that spinal manipulation versus simethicone significantly reduced crying (mean reduction in crying for days 4–7: 2.4 h with spinal manipulation v 1.0 h with simethicone; P = 0.04; CI not provided).[29] Parents were not blinded to treatment. **Versus holding:** One RCT (86 infants) compared spinal palpation by a chiropractor versus holding of the infant by a nurse (3 times over 8 days).[29] The parents, who were blind to the intervention, rated symptom severity on a five point scale and recorded crying in a diary. The RCT found no significant difference with spinal palpation versus holding for crying reduction (by day 8, mean reduction 3.1 h for both groups; P = 0.98, CI not provided).[29]

Harms: None reported.

Comment: It is unclear whether reduced crying reflected effects of interventions or spontaneous improvement.

GLOSSARY

Behavioural modification Changing the way in which parents respond to their babies crying from colic.

Casein hydrolysate milk contains casein protein; it is used in the same way as soya based infant feeds.

Cranial osteopathy involves gentle manipulation of the tissues of the head by an osteopath.

Dicycloverine (dicyclomine) has direct antispasmodic action on the gastrointestinal tract and anticholinergic effects, which are similar to atropine.

Hypoallergenic diet In bottle fed infants, a hypoallergenic diet uses a casein hydrolysate formula. In breast fed infants, a hypoallergenic diet involves a maternal diet, free of artificial colourings, preservatives, and additives, and low in common allergens (e.g. milk, egg, wheat, nuts).

Jadad Scale This measures factors that impact on trial quality. Poor description of the factors, rated by low figures, are associated with greater estimates of effect. The scale includes three items: was the study described as randomised? (0–2); was the study described as double blind? (0–2); was there a description of withdrawals and drop outs? (0–1).[5]

Reassurance Informing the parent that infantile colic is a self limiting condition resolving by 3–4 months of age, and is not caused by disease or any fault in parental care.

Simethicone (activated dimeticone) has defoaming properties, which can aid dispersion of gas in the gastrointestinal tract.

Soya based infant feeds contain proteins from soya beans; the feeds are used as lactose free vegetable milks for those with lactose or cow's milk protein intolerance.

Spinal manipulation Chiropractic manual treatment of the infant's vertebral column.

Whey hydrolysate milk contains whey protein; it is used in the same way as soya based infant feeds.

REFERENCES

1. Lucassen PLB, Assendelf WJJ, Gubbels JW, Van Eijk JTM, Van Geldrop WJ, Knuistingh Neven A. Effectiveness of treatments for infantile colic: a systematic review. BMJ 1998;316:1563–1569. Search date 1996: primary sources Cochrane Controlled Trials Register, Embase, Medline, and reference searching.

2. Lucassen PLBJ, Assendelft WJJ, Van Eijk JTHM, Gubbels JW, Douwes AC, Van Geldrop WJ. Systematic review of the occurrence of infantile colic in the community. Arch Dis Child 2001; 84:398–403. Search date 1998; primary sources Embase and Medline.

3. Lucas A, St James-Roberts I. Crying, fussing and colic behaviour in breast and bottle-fed infants. Early Human Development 1998;53:9–19.

4. St James Roberts I, Halil A. Infant crying patterns in the first year: Normal community and clinical findings. J Child Psychol Psychiatry 1991;32:951–968.

5. Jadad AR, Moore RA, Carroll D, et al. Assessing the quality of reports of randomized clinical trials: is blinding necessary? Control Clin Trials 1996;17: 1–12.

6. Garrison MM, Christakis DA. A systematic review of treatments for infant colic. Pediatrics 2000; 106:184–190. Search date 1999; primary sources Medline, Cochrane Clinical Trials Registry, hand searches of reference lists, and authors.

7. Weissbluth M, Christoffel KK, Davis AT. Treatment of infantile colic with dicyclomine hydrochloride. J Pediatr 1984:104:951–955.

8. Hwang CP, Danielsson B. Dicyclomine hydrochloride in infantile colic. BMJ 1985;291:1014.

9. Gruinseit F. Evaluation of the efficacy of dicyclomine hydrochloride ("Merbentyl") syrup in the treatment of infantile colic. Curr Med Res Opin 1977;5:258–261.

10. Williams J, Watkin Jones R. Dicyclomine: worrying symptoms associated with its use in some small babies. *BMJ* 1984;288:901.

11. Fleiss JL. The crossover study. In: Fleiss JL, ed. *The design and analysis of clinical experiments.* New York: John Wiley and Sons, 1986.

12. Metcalf TJ, Irons TG, Sher LD, Young PC. Simethicone in the treatment of infantile colic: a randomized, placebo-controlled, multicenter trial. *Pediatrics* 1994;94:29–34.

13. Danielsson B, Hwang CP. Treatment of infantile colic with surface active substance (simethicone). *Acta Paediatr Scand* 1985;74:446–450.

14. Sethi KS, Sethi JK. Simethicone in the management of infant colic. *Practitioner* 1988; 232:508

15. Campbell JPM. Dietary treatment of infantile colic: a double-blind study. *J R Coll Gen Pract* 1989;39: 11–14.

16. Lothe L, Lindbert T, Jakobsson I. Cow's milk formula as a cause of infantile colic: a double-blind study. *Pediatrics* 1982;70:7–10.

17. Forsythe BWC. Colic and the effect of changing formulas: a double blind, multiple-crossover study. *J Pediatr* 1989;115:521–526.

18. Hill DJ, Hudson IL, Sheffield LJ, Shelton MJ, Menahem S, Hosking CS. A low allergen diet is a significant intervention in infantile colic: Results of a community based study. *J Allergy Clin Immunol* 1995;96:886–892.

19. Lucassen LB, Assendelft WJ, Gubbels LW, Van Eijk, Douwes AC. Infantile colic: crying time reduction with a whey hydrolysate; a double blind, randomized placebo-controlled trial. *Pediatrics* 2000;106:1349–1354.

20. Kearney PJ, Malone AJ, Hayes T, Cole M, Hyland M. A trial of lactase in the management of infant colic. *J Hum Nutrition Dietetics* 1998;11:281–285.

21. Stahlberg MR, Savilahti E. Infantile colic and feeding. *Arch Dis Child* 1986;61:1232–1233.

22. Markestad T. Use of sucrose as a treatment for infant colic. *Arch Dis Child* 1997;77:356–357.

23. Weizman Z, Alkrinawi S, Goldfarb D, Bitran C. Herbal teas for infantile colic. *J Pediatr* 1993;123: 670–671.

24. Parkin PC, Schwartz CJ, Manuel BA. Randomised controlled trial of three interventions in the management of persistent crying of infancy. *Pediatrics* 1993;92;197–201.

25. Taubman B. Parental counselling compared with elimination of cow's milk or soy milk protein for the treatment of infant colic syndrome: a randomized trial. *Pediatrics* 1988; 81:756–761.

26. Barr RG, McMullen SJ, Spiess H, Leduc DG, Yaremko J, Barfield R, et al. Carrying as a colic "therapy": a randomized controlled trial. *Pediatrics* 1991;87:623–630.

27. McKenzie S. Troublesome crying in infants: effect of advice to reduce stimulation. *Arch Dis Child* 1991;66:1461–1420.

28. Huhtala V, Lehtonen L, Heinonen R, Korvenranta H. Infant massage compared with crib vibrator in the treatment of colicky infants. *Pediatrics* 2000; 105:e84.

29. Wiberg JMM, Nordsteen J, Nilsson N. The short term effect of spinal manipulation in the treatment of infant colic: A randomized controlled clinical trial with a blinded observer. *J Manip Physiol Therap* 1999;22:517–522.

30. Olafsdottir E, Forshei S, Fluge G, Markestad T. Randomised controlled trial of infant colic treated with chiropractic spinal manipulation. *Arch Dis Child* 2001;84:138–141.

Teresa Kilgour
Staff Grade Community Paediatrician
City Hospitals Sunderland
Sunderland
UK

Sally Wade
Staff Grade Community Paediatrician
Archer Street Clinic
Darlington
UK

Competing interests: None declared.

Nocturnal enuresis

Search date October 2001

Sara Bosson and Natalie Lyth

INTERVENTIONS

Key Messages

- One systematic review has found that intranasal desmopressin versus placebo significantly reduces bedwetting by at least one night per week, and increases the chance of attaining 14 consecutive dry nights.

- One systematic review has found that tricyclic drugs (imipramine, desipramine) versus placebo significantly increase the chance of attaining 14 consecutive dry nights. It found no significant difference with imipramine versus an alarm during the treatment period, but found that children using an enuresis alarm had fewer wet nights per week after the treatment had stopped.

- One small RCT found that indometacin (indomethacin) versus placebo significantly increased the number of dry nights in children aged over 6 years with primary nocturnal enuresis.

- One small RCT found that carbamazepine versus placebo significantly increased the number of dry nights in children aged over 7 years with nocturnal enuresis caused by detrusor instability.

- One systematic review has found that significantly more children achieved 14 consecutive dry nights with enuresis alarms versus no treatment. It found insufficient evidence on the effects of dry bed training plus alarm versus alarm alone.

- One RCT found that significantly more children achieved 14 consecutive dry nights with a standard home alarm clock to wake the child immediately before their usual time of enuresis versus waking after 3 hours' sleep.

- One RCT found that significantly more children achieved 4 weeks of dryness with an alarm plus intranasal desmopressin (40 μg) versus an alarm alone.

- One systematic review has found that significantly more children achieve 14 consecutive dry nights with dry bed training and dry bed training plus alarm versus no treatment.
- We found no RCTs of ultrasound in children with primary nocturnal enuresis. We found one small controlled trial which found that ultrasound versus control reduced the number of wet nights.
- One RCT found no significant difference with laser acupuncture versus intra-nasal desmopressin in reduction of wet nights in children aged over 5 years with primary nocturnal enuresis.
- We found no RCTs on the best age to start treatment in children with nocturnal enuresis. Anecdotal experience suggests that reassurance is sufficient below the age of 7 years.

DEFINITION Nocturnal enuresis is the involuntary discharge of urine at night in the absence of congenital or acquired defects of the central nervous system or urinary tract in a child aged 5 years or older.[1] Disorders that have bedwetting as a symptom (termed "nocturnal inconti-nence") can be excluded by a thorough history, examination, and urinalysis. "Monosymptomatic" nocturnal enuresis is characterised by night time symptoms only and accounts for 85% of cases. Nocturnal enuresis is defined as primary if the child has never been dry for a period of more than 6 months, and secondary if such a period of dryness preceded the onset of wetting.

INCIDENCE/ Between 15% and 20% of 5 year olds, 7% of 7 year olds, 5% of
PREVALENCE 10 year olds, 2–3% of 12–14 year olds, and 1–2% of people aged 15 years and over wet the bed twice a week on average.[2]

AETIOLOGY/ Nocturnal enuresis is associated with several factors, including
RISK FACTORS small functional bladder capacity, nocturnal polyuria, and arousal dysfunction. Linkage studies have identified associated genetic loci on chromosomes 8q, 12q, 13q, and 22q11.[3–6]

PROGNOSIS Nocturnal enuresis has widely differing outcomes, from spontane-ous resolution to complete resistance to all current treatments. About 1% of adults remain enuretic. Without treatment, about 15% of children with enuresis become dry each year.[7]

AIMS To stay dry on particular occasions (e.g. when visiting friends); to reduce the number of wet nights; to reduce the impact of the enuresis on the child's lifestyle; to initiate successful continence; to avoid relapse, with minimal adverse effects.

OUTCOMES Rate of initial success (defined as 14 consecutive dry nights); average number of wet nights per week; number of relapses after initial success; average number of wet nights after treatment has ceased.

METHODS *Clinical Evidence* search and appraisal October 2001.

| QUESTION | What are the effects of treatments for short term relief of symptoms? |

| OPTION | DESMOPRESSIN |

One systematic review has found that intranasal desmopressin versus placebo significantly reduces bedwetting by at least one night per week and increases the chance of attaining 14 consecutive dry nights.

Benefits:
We found one systematic review (search date 1997).[8] **Versus placebo:** The review identified 16 RCTs comparing the effect of intranasal desmopressin (10–40 µg) versus placebo on mean number of wet nights per week. It found that each dose of desmopressin versus placebo significantly reduced bedwetting by at least one night per week (desmopressin 20 µg; RR −1.56, 95% CI −1.94 to −1.19). Three RCTs found that desmopressin versus placebo significantly increased the chance of attaining 14 consecutive dry nights (overall RR with desmopressin v placebo 4.6, 95% CI 1.4 to 15.0) (see table 1, p 105). **Other comparisons:** The review found insufficient evidence on lower versus higher doses of desmopressin and oral versus nasal administration of desmopressin.[8]

Harms:
The systematic review reported nasal discomfort, headache, nosebleeds, bad taste, rash, sight disturbance, and anorexia.[8] Rarely, water intoxication has been reported.

Comment:
The systematic review included only studies of interventions used to remedy either primary or secondary nocturnal enuresis (incontinence was excluded by medical examination or explicitly mentioned in the inclusion/exclusion criteria of included RCTs), and included a systematic measurement of baseline wetting and outcomes. Many of the included RCTs were of poor quality.

| OPTION | TRICYCLIC DRUGS |

One systematic review has found that tricyclic drugs (imipramine, desipramine) versus placebo significantly increase the chance of attaining 14 consecutive dry nights. It found no significant difference with imipramine versus an alarm during the treatment period, but found that children using an enuresis alarm have one fewer wet night per week after the treatment had stopped.

Benefits:
We found one systematic review (search date 1997, 22 RCTs, 1100 children).[9] Many of the trials were of poor quality. **Versus placebo:** The review identified 10 RCTs comparing effect of imipramine versus placebo on mean number of wet nights per week. It found that imipramine versus placebo reduced bedwetting by one night per week (WMD −0.84 nights, 95% CI −1.21 to −0.47 nights). It also found that tricyclic drugs (imipramine, desipramine) versus placebo significantly increased the chance of attaining 14 consecutive dry nights (imipramine, 4 RCTs: RR 5.0, 95% CI 2.4 to 10.4; desipramine, 1 RCT: RR 3.6, 95% CI 1.07 to 11.81) (see table 1, p 105). **Versus alarms:** The review (3 small RCTs, 103 children) found no significant difference in mean number of wet nights per week with imipramine versus an alarm during the treatment period.[9]

However, two of the three RCTs found that when the treatment had stopped, children using an enuresis alarm had one fewer wet night per week (WMD 1.03 nights, 95% CI 0.19 to 1.87 nights).[9]

Harms: The systematic review reported more adverse effects with tricyclic drugs versus placebo. These included anorexia, anxiety reaction, burning sensation, constipation, depression, diarrhoea, dizziness, drowsiness, dry mouth, headache, irritability, lethargy, sleep distur-bance, upset stomach, and vomiting.[9] The review also found that, when reported, tricyclic drugs were associated with more adverse effects than desmopressin (tricyclic drugs 83/480 [17.3%] v desmopressin 41/579 [7.1%]). Tricyclic drugs have been reported as fatal in overdose.

Comment: We found no good studies directly comparing tricyclic drugs versus desmopressin.

OPTION   INDOMETACIN

One small RCT found that indometacin (indomethacin) versus placebo significantly increased the number of dry nights in children aged over 6 years with primary nocturnal enuresis.

Benefits: We found no systematic review but found one RCT.[13] The RCT (85 children aged over 6 years with primary nocturnal enuresis) com-pared desmopressin versus indometacin (indomethacin) versus placebo. It found that indometacin suppository versus placebo significantly increased the number of dry nights over 3 weeks (mean number of dry nights 8.9 with indometacin v 3.8 with placebo; P < 0.005).[13]

Harms: The RCT did not report any adverse effects.

Comment: None.

OPTION   CARBAMAZEPINE

One small RCT found that carbamazepine versus placebo significantly increased the number of dry nights in nocturnal enuresis caused by detrusor instability in children aged over 7 years.

Benefits: We found no systematic review but found one RCT.[14] The RCT (double blind crossover study, 26 children aged 7–15 years with detrusor instability on videocystourethrography) found that car-bamazepine versus placebo significantly increased the number of dry nights over 30 days (mean number of dry nights 18.8 with carbamazepine v 3.9 with placebo; P < 0.001).

Harms: The RCT did not report any adverse effects.[14]

Comment: The study population had proven detrusor instability. It may not be possible to generalise these results to all children with nocturnal enuresis.

Nocturnal enuresis

QUESTION   What are the effects of long term treatments?

OPTION   ALARMS AND DRY BED TRAINING

One systematic review has found that significantly more children achieve 14 consecutive dry nights with enuresis alarms versus no treatment. It found insufficient evidence on the effect of dry bed training plus alarm versus alarm alone. One RCT found that significantly more children achieved 14 consecutive dry nights with a standard home alarm clock to wake the child immediately before their usual time of enuresis versus waking after 3 hours' sleep. One RCT found that significantly more children achieved 4 weeks of dryness with an alarm plus intranasal desmopressin (40 µg) versus an alarm alone. Another systematic review has found that significantly more children achieve 14 consecutive dry nights with dry bed training plus an alarm versus no treatment.

Benefits: **Alarm versus no treatment:** We found one systematic review (search date 1997).[10] It found that significantly more children achieved 14 consecutive dry nights with alarm versus no treatment (4 RCTs; RR 3.7, 95% CI 2.6 to 5.3) (see table 1, p 105). **Standard home alarm clock versus waking:** We found one RCT.[11] It found that significantly more children achieved 14 consecutive dry nights with a standard home alarm clock to wake the child immediately before their usual time of enuresis versus waking after 3 hours' sleep (RR 1.3, 95% CI not stated; P = 0.03) (see table 1, p 105). **Alarm plus desmopressin versus alarm alone:** We found one RCT.[15] It found that significantly more children achieved 4 weeks of dryness with alarm plus intranasal desmopressin (40 µg) versus alarm alone (27/36 [75%] with an alarm plus desmopressin v 16/35 [46%] with an alarm alone; P < 0.005). **Dry bed training versus no treatment:** We found one systematic review (search date 1996).[12] It found that significantly more children achieved 14 consecutive dry nights with dry bed training versus no treatment (1 RCT; RR 2.5, 95% CI 0.55 to 11.4) (see table 1, p 105). **Dry bed training plus alarm versus no treatment:** We found one systematic review (search date 1996).[12] It found that significantly more children achieved 14 consecutive dry nights with dry bed training plus an alarm versus no treatment (1 RCT; RR 10, 95% CI 2.69 to 37.24) (see table 1, p 105). **Dry bed training plus alarm versus alarm alone:** We found one systematic review (search date 1997).[10] It found that children using an alarm alone were as likely as those using an alarm plus dry bed training to achieve 14 consecutive dry nights, but the confidence intervals were wide.

Harms: One systematic review found that adverse effects of alarms were limited to minor inconvenience because of malfunction or disturbance.[12] No adverse effects were reported in the two RCTs.[11,15]

Comment: None.

OPTION   ULTRASOUND

We found no RCTs of ultrasound in children with primary nocturnal enuresis. We found one small controlled trial, which found that ultrasound versus control significantly reduced the number of wet nights.

Benefits: We found no RCTs of ultrasound in children with primary nocturnal enuresis.

Harms: We found no RCTs.

Comment: We found one controlled trial (35 children with primary nocturnal enuresis, aged 6–14 years) comparing ultrasound (27 children) versus control (8 children treated without the apparatus being switched on).[16] Ultrasound treatment was applied daily to lumbosacral skin for 10 sessions. The controlled trial found that ultrasound versus control significantly reduced the number of wet nights per week at 1 week, 3 months, 6 months, and 12 months after treatment ($P < 0.05$ at all times). The study did not find any adverse effects. It is not clear why this prospective study has such a difference in population size between ultrasound and control groups.[16]

OPTION   LASER ACUPUNCTURE

One RCT found no significant difference with laser acupuncture versus intranasal desmopressin in reduction of wet nights in children aged over 5 years with primary nocturnal enuresis.

Benefits: We found no systematic review. **Versus no treatment:** We found no RCTs. **Versus intranasal desmopressin:** We found one RCT (40 children aged > 5 years with primary nocturnal enuresis) comparing laser acupuncture versus intranasal desmopressin (20–40 µg for 3 months).[17] Laser acupuncture was applied to seven pre-defined acupuncture areas for 30 seconds per session for 10–15 sessions. Complete response was defined as a reduction in the number of wet nights of at least 90%. At 6 months, the RCT found no significant difference with laser acupuncture versus intranasal desmopressin in the reduction of wet nights (complete responders: 65% with laser acupuncture v 75% with desmopressin).

Harms: The RCT did not find any adverse effects with either laser acupuncture or intranasal desmopressin.[17]

Comment: Laser acupuncture treatment may not be widely available.

QUESTION   What is the best age to start treatment?

We found no RCTs on the best age to start treatment in children with nocturnal enuresis. Anecdotal experience suggests that reassurance is sufficient below the age of 7 years.

Benefits: We found no RCTs on the best age to start treatment in children with nocturnal enuresis (see comment below).

Harms: We found no RCTs.

Comment: Anecdotal experience suggests that reassurance is sufficient below the age of 7 years. Behavioural treatments, such as alarms, require motivation and commitment from the child and a parent. Anecdotal experience suggests that children under the age of 7 years may not exhibit the commitment needed. Minimum ages for which drugs are licensed vary among countries.

REFERENCES

1. Forsythe WI, Butler R. 50 years of enuretic alarms; a review of the literature. *Arch Dis Child* 1991;64: 879–885.
2. Blackwell C. *A guide to enuresis: a guide to treatment of enuresis for professionals.* Bristol: Eric, 1989.
3. Eiberg H. Total genome scan analysis in a single extended family for primary nocturnal enuresis: evidence for a new locus (ENUR 3) for primary nocturnal enuresis on chromosome 22q11. *Eur Urol* 1998;33:34–36.
4. Eiberg H. Nocturnal enuresis is linked to a specific gene. *Scand J Urol Nephrol* 1995;173(suppl): 15–17.
5. Arnell H, Hjalmas M, Jagervall G, et al. The genetics of primary nocturnal enuresis: inheritance and suggestion of a second major gene on chromosome 12q. *J Med Genet* 1997;34: 360–365.
6. Eiberg H, Berendt I, Mohr J. Assignment of dominant inherited nocturnal enuresis (ENUR 1) to chromosome 13q. *Nat Genet* 1995;10:354–356.
7. Forsythe WI, Redmond A. Enuresis and spontaneous cure rate of 1129 enuretics. *Arch Dis Child* 1974;49:259–263.
8. Glazener CMA, Evans JHC. Desmopressin for nocturnal enuresis in children. In: The Cochrane Library, Issue 3, 2001. Oxford: Update Software. Search date 1997; primary sources Medline, Embase, Amed, Assia, Bids, Cinahl, Psychlit, Sigle, and DHSS data.
9. Glazener CMA, Evans JHC. Tricyclic and related drugs for nocturnal enuresis in children. In: The Cochrane Library, Issue 3, 2001. Oxford: Update Software. Search date 1997; primary sources Medline, Embase, Amed, Assia, Bids, Cinahl, Psychlit, Sigle, and DHSS data.
10. Glazener CMA, Evans JHC. Alarm interventions for nocturnal enuresis in children (Cochrane Review). In: The Cochrane Library, Issue 3, 2001. Oxford: Update Software. Search date 1997; primary sources Medline, Embase, Amed, Assia, Bids, Cinahl, Psychlit, Sigle, and DHSS data.
11. El-Anany FG, Maghraby HA, Shaker SED, Abdel-Moneim AM. Primary nocturnal enuresis: a new approach to conditioning treatment. *Urology* 1999;53:405–409.
12. Lister-Sharp D, O'Meara S, Bradley M, Sheldon TA. University of York. NHS Centre for Reviews and Dissemination. August 1997. *A systematic review of the effectiveness of interventions for managing childhood nocturnal enuresis.* CRD Report 11. Search date 1996; primary sources Cochrane Library, Medline, Embase, and Psychlit.
13. Sener F, Hasanoglu E, Soylemezoglu O. Desmopressin versus indomethacin treatment in primary nocturnal enuresis and the role of prostaglandins. *Urology* 1998:52:878–881.
14. Al Waili NS. Carbamazepine to treat primary nocturnal enuresis: double-blind study. *Eur J Med Res* 2000;5:40–44.
15. Bradbury M. Combination therapy for nocturnal enuresis with desmopressin and an alarm device. *Scand J Urol Nephrol Suppl* 1997;183:61–63.
16. Kosar A, Akkus S, Savas S, *et al.* Effect of ultrasound in the treatment of primary nocturnal enuresis. *Scand J Urol Nephrol* 2000;34: 361–365.
17. Radmayr C, Schlager A, Studen M, Bartsch G. Prospective Randomised trial using laser acupuncture versus desmopressin in the treatment of nocturnal enuresis. *Eur Urol* 2001; 40:201–205.

Sara Bosson
Staff Grade Community Paediatrician
Weston Area Health Trust
Weston-Super-Mare
UK

Natalie Lyth
Associate Specialist Child Health
Northallerton Health Service Trust
Northallerton
UK

Competing interests: SB, none declared. NL has been reimbursed for attending a symposium by Ferring Pharmaceuticals, the manufacturer of desmotabs.

TABLE 1 Treatments for enuresis: advantages and disadvantages (see text, pp 100, 102).

	Initial success (14 consecutive dry nights)	Long term success	Evidence	Advantages	Disadvantages
Desmopressin[8]	RR v placebo 4.6, 95% CI 1.4 to 15.0	No better than placebo	Meta-analysis of 3 RCTs	Effective within days, few adverse effects with appropriate pretreatment advice	Case reports of water intoxication
Tricyclic drugs[9]	RR v placebo 5.0, 95% CI 2.4 to 10.4	No better than placebo (RR 1.1)	Meta-analysis of 4 RCTs	Effective within days	Risk of lethal overdose, frequent significant adverse effects
Alarm[10]	RR v no treatment 3.7, 95% CI 2.6 to 5.3	31–61% still dry at 3 months. Nine times less likely relapse than with desmopressin	Meta-analysis of 4 RCTs	Safe	Takes longer to become dry, needs good cooperation from child and family
Standard home alarm clock[11]	77.1% v 61.8% with waking after 3 hours' sleep (RR 1.3; P = 0.03)	No better at 3 months than waking after 3 hours' sleep (66% dry v 56%; P = 0.19)	1 RCT, 125 people	Safe, does not require bed wetting to initiate alarm	None reported
Dry bed training[12]	RR v no treatment 2.5, 95% CI 0.55 to 11.4	No better than no treatment (RR 0.4, 95% CI 0.14 to 1.13)	1 good quality RCT, 45 people	Safe	Requires high degree of motivation
Dry bed training plus alarm[12]	RR v no treatment 10, 95% CI 2.69 to 37.24	No better than alarm alone (RR 1.0, 95% CI 0.7 to 1.5)	1 RCT, 45 people	Safe	Requires an even greater input from the family than either treatment alone

Otitis media with effusion

Search date July 2001

Ian Williamson

INTERVENTIONS

Key Messages

- We found insufficient evidence on the effects of strategies for preventing otitis media with effusion (OME).
- One systematic review has found that antimicrobial drugs speed the resolution of OME, but are not effective in the long term. Adverse effects were frequently reported.
- We found little evidence of clinically significant benefit with oral steroids, but some evidence of adverse effects.
- RCTs have found short term benefit from autoinflation with a nasal balloon.
- We found insufficient evidence regarding sustained benefits from mechanical and surgical treatments.

DEFINITION   OME, or "glue ear", is serous or mucoid but not mucopurulent fluid in the middle ear. Children usually present with hearing loss and speech problems. In contrast to those with acute otitis media (see topic, p 10), children with OME do not suffer from acute ear pain, fever, or malaise. Hearing loss is usually mild and often identified when parents express concern regarding their child's behaviour, school performance, or language development.

INCIDENCE/   At any time, 5% of children aged 2–4 years have persistent (at least
PREVALENCE 3 months) bilateral hearing loss associated with OME. The prevalence declines considerably beyond age 6 years.[1] About 80% of children aged 10 years have been affected by OME at some time in the past. OME is the most common reason for referral for surgery in children in the UK. Middle ear effusions also occur infrequently in adults after upper respiratory tract infection or after air travel.

AETIOLOGY/   Contributory factors include upper respiratory tract infection and
RISK FACTORS narrow upper respiratory airways. Prospective case control studies have identified risk factors, including age 6 years or younger at first onset, daycare centre attendance, high number of siblings, low socioeconomic group, frequent upper respiratory tract infection, bottle feeding, and household smoking.[2,3] Most factors are associated with about twice the risk of developing OME.[4]

PROGNOSIS   In 5% of preschool children, OME (identified by tympanometric screening) persists for at least 1 year.[5,6] One large cohort study (534 children) found that middle ear disease increased reported hearing difficulty at age 5 years (OR 1.44, 95% CI 1.18 to 1.76) and was associated with delayed language development in children up to age 10 years.[7]

AIMS   To improve hearing and wellbeing; to avoid poor behavioural, speech, and educational development; and to prevent recurrent earache and otitis media.

OUTCOMES   Resolution of effusion (both speed and completeness) assessed by otoscopy, tympanometry, or global clinical assessment; hearing impairment, assessed by audiometry or tympanometry (although the positive predictive value of these tests has been reported as low as 49%);[8] developmental and behavioural tests; language and speech development; adverse effects of treatment. Patient centred outcomes in children with OME (e.g. disability or quality of life) need further development and evaluation.

METHODS   *Clinical Evidence* search and appraisal July 2001.

QUESTION   What are the effects of preventive interventions?

OPTION   AVOIDANCE OF MODIFIABLE RISK FACTORS

We found no RCTs that evaluated interventions to modify risk factors for OME, such as passive smoking and bottle feeding.

Benefits: We found no systematic review or RCTs of interventions aimed at modifying risk factors for OME.

Harms: We found insufficient data.

Otitis media with effusion

Comment: There is good epidemiological evidence that the risk of OME is increased by passive smoking,[2] bottle feeding,[3] low socioeconomic group, and exposure to a large number of other children.[8] Feasible preventive interventions may include strategies to reduce household smoking and encourage breast feeding.

QUESTION **What are the effects of treatments?**

OPTION **ANTIMICROBIAL DRUGS**

Two systematic reviews and one subsequent non-systematic review have found that resolution of OME occurred faster with antibiotics than with placebo or no treatment. They found no significant effect on longer term outcomes. Adverse effects with antibiotics were frequent.

Benefits: We found two systematic reviews[8,9] and one subsequent non-systematic review.[10] Both systematic reviews found that OME resolves faster with antimicrobial drugs. **Short term outcomes:** The first systematic review (search date 1992, 10 blinded RCTs, 1041 children with OME) compared antimicrobial drugs (amoxicillin with or without clavulanic acid, cefaclor, erythromycin, sulphisoxazole, sulfamethoxazole, or trimethoprim) versus placebo or versus no treatment.[8] Treatment duration varied from 2–5 weeks. Follow up was from 10–60 days. At 1 month, resolution of effusion (assessed by pneumatic otoscopy, tympanometry, and audiometry) was significantly more likely with antimicrobial treatment (pooled ARR for non-resolution versus placebo or no treatment 14%, 95% CI 4% to 24%; NNT 7). **Longer term outcomes:** The second systematic review (search date 1993, 8 RCTs, 2052 ears of children with OME) found no significant difference in presence of effusions between 6 weeks and 11 months after treatment (pooled ARR for presence of effusion compared with placebo +6%, 95% CI −3% to +14%).[9] The review also found no significant differences in effectiveness between antibiotics. A more recent meta-analysis based on eight RCTs (7 of 18 previously included RCTs and 1 newer RCT) compared antibiotics versus placebo in OME (1292 children) and found no significant effect (cure rate: 179/813 [22%] for antibiotics v 85/479 [18%] for placebo; ARI of cure +4.3%, 95% CI -0.3% to +8.8%; RR 1.24, 95% CI 0.99 to 1.54).[10]

Harms: The systematic reviews did not report rates of adverse events in children on placebo or no treatment. Adverse events on antibiotics were frequent. For amoxicillin, diarrhoea was reported in 20–30% and rashes in 3–5% of children. For co-amoxiclav, diarrhoea was reported in 9%, nausea and vomiting in 4%, and skin rashes and urticaria in 3% of children.[8,11] For antibiotics overall, nausea and vomiting, diarrhoea, or both were reported in 2–32% of children, and cutaneous reactions in less than 5%.[11] Adherence to lengthy courses of antibiotics is poor. Prescribing antibiotics for minor illness encourages further consultations[12] and antibiotic resistance.[13]

Comment: In the third meta-analysis the timing to outcomes was not clear.[10]

OPTION STEROIDS

One systematic review found no evidence of long term benefit from oral steroids in children with OME. We found no RCTs that adequately evaluated topical steroids.

Benefits: We found one systematic review (search date 2000).[14] **Oral steroids versus placebo:** The review identified three placebo controlled RCTs of oral steroids in 108 children with OME. Presence of effusion was assessed clinically by pneumatic otoscopy, tympanometry, and audiometry after 7–14 days of treatment. There was no significant difference in mean improvement at 2 weeks after treatment (AR of clearance compared with placebo 18%, 95% CI −3% to +39%). There were no available summary data beyond 6 weeks. **Added to antibiotic:** The systematic review identified four RCTs (292 children) comparing antibiotic plus oral steroids versus antibiotic alone. Time to measurement of results varied from 1 week to 2 months. There was a significant difference in clearance rates with combined treatment versus antibiotic alone (ARR for non-clearance versus antibiotic alone at 2 wks 0.32, 95% CI 0.2 to 0.5), but there was significant heterogeneity between studies (CI not provided; $P < 0.01$). **Topical steroids:** We found one RCT (61 children with chronic middle ear infection), which found that intra-nasal steroids plus antibiotics versus either antibiotics alone or placebo spray reduced effusions at 4 and 8 weeks (CI not provided; $P < 0.05$) and significantly improved middle ear pressure at 12 weeks (CI not provided; $P < 0.05$).[15]

Harms: Short courses of steroids can cause behavioural changes, increased appetite, and weight gain. Idiosyncratic reactions have been reported, such as avascular necrosis of the femoral head and fatal varicella infections.

Comment: The trials were small. Use of secondary care populations weakens the applicability of results to primary care.

OPTION ANTIHISTAMINES AND DECONGESTANTS

One systematic review found no benefit from antihistamines and decongestants versus placebo in children with OME.

Benefits: We found one systematic review (search date 1992, 4 placebo controlled RCTs, 1202 infants and older children).[8] Treatment lasted for 4 weeks. Meta-analysis found that combined antihistamine/decongestants versus placebo had no significant effect on effusion clearance rate, as assessed by history, otoscopy, and tympanometry (hierarchical Bayes meta-analysis: change in probability −0.009, 95% CI −0.036 to +0.054).

Harms: Adverse effects of antihistamines include hyperactivity, insomnia, drowsiness, behavioural change, blood pressure variability, and seizures. Decongestant nose drops given for 3 weeks or more can lead to iatrogenic rhinitis.[16]

Comment: The RCTs included clinically heterogeneous groups (e.g. infants and older children) and selected individuals from ambulatory care or waiting lists. There were too few children with allergies for subgroup analysis.

Otitis media with effusion

OPTION MUCOLYTICS

One systematic review found that 1–3 month courses of mucolytics compared with placebo or no treatment had no significant effect on resolution of effusion.

Benefits: We found one systematic review (search date 1993, 6 RCTs, 430 children) comparing S-carboxymethylcysteine, its lysine salt, or both, versus placebo or no treatment.[17] Treatment lasted for 15–90 days. Increased frequency of complete resolution with mucolytics did not quite reach significance (178 children; OR 2.25, 95% CI 0.97 to 5.22). Three small RCTs (155 children and 195 ears) comparing another mucolytic, bromhexine, versus placebo found conflicting results.

Harms: The review gave no information of adverse effects.[17] Reported adverse effects of S-carboxymethylcysteine include gastric irritation, nausea, and rashes.

Comment: The RCTs were heterogeneous in their clinical outcomes and treatment duration.

OPTION AUTOINFLATION

One systematic review has found benefit from autoinflation using a nasal balloon, although some children may find autoinflation difficult. The value of all methods of autoinflation has not yet been adequately evaluated.

Benefits: We found one systematic review (search date not stated, 6 RCTs) comparing autoinflation versus no treatment.[18] Improvement was variously defined as being effusion free, improved tympanogram, or improvement in hearing. The RCTs assessing different treatment effects yielded different results. However, trials evaluating nasal balloons in children found a homogeneous effect size (3 RCTs, 386 children). Children in the treatment group were more likely than control children to improve within 1 week to 3 months using tympanometric and audiometric criteria (RR 1.12, 95% CI 1.03 to 1.22).[18]

Harms: No serious adverse effects have been reported.

Comment: The Eustachian tubes can be inflated by several methods, including blowing up a balloon through a plastic tube inserted into the nostril. In one RCT, 12% of children aged 3–10 years were unable to use the balloon.[19] Most trials appeared not to use intention to treat analysis, and beneficial effects were noted only when adherence was 70% or greater. The evidence is suboptimal because different methods were used, outcome assessments were not blinded, and follow up was short. Other methods of autoinflation (such as inflating a carnival blower through the nostril or forcible exhalation through the nostrils, with closed mouth, into an anaesthetic mask with a flowmeter attachment) have not been adequately evaluated.

OPTION SURGERY

One systematic review has found that surgery (insertion of grommets, adenoidectomy, or both) results in short term hearing gain. Grommets and adenoidectomy alone were of similar effectiveness. A subsequent

RCT has found that grommets and adenoidectomy combined are more effective than adenotonsillectomy or grommets either alone or combined. Three subsequent RCTs found no benefit in language development with grommets. We found no good evidence of the effects of tonsillectomy.

Benefits: We found one systematic review (search date 1992, 19 RCTs) of surgery in children with OME.[20] Nine RCTs reported the data per child (1508 children) and 10 reported data per ear (1452 children). None were placebo controlled, although some used children as their own controls. Outcomes were mean change in audiometry, tympanometry, and clinical and otoscopic evidence of OME. The review concluded that evidence for the effectiveness of surgical interventions was still confused. **Grommets:** The review reported a mean 12 dB improvement in hearing after insertion of grommets (CI not provided).[20] However, the authors concluded that this was difficult to interpret clinically. Three subsequent RCTs (771 children) found that grommets do not improve language development in infants and young children.[21–23] However, one RCT (182 children) found that early insertion of bilateral grommets significantly reduced behavioural problems at 9 months compared with watchful waiting (24 withdrawals from watchful waiting, 8 from early surgery, no intention to treat analysis: Richman behaviour check list 25/84 [30%] v 31/66 [47%]; RR 0.63, 95% CI 0.30 to 0.96).[22] **Grommets plus adenoidectomy:** The review found that adenoidectomy gave little additional benefit over grommets alone in terms of mean hearing gain, which varied from 1.1–2.6 dB.[20] A subsequent RCT (228 children) compared adenotonsillectomy or adenoidectomy (analysed together) versus neither procedure.[24] All children had a grommet inserted into one ear. Outcomes were mean audiometric change, and tympanometric and otoscopic clearance assessed over 6 months to 10 years after treatment. The trial found benefit in combining adenoidectomy with grommets. Median duration of glue ear assessed tympanometrically was reduced from 7.8 years without treatment to 4.9 years with grommets, 4 years with adenoidectomy, and 2.8 years with adenoidectomy and grommets combined. The difference between duration for adenoidectomy alone and grommets alone was not significant (CI not provided; P = 0.2), but all other comparisons were significant. **Tonsillectomy:** The review found no good RCTs of tonsillectomy alone in OME.[20]

Harms: We found one systematic review (search date 1999), which found that transient otorrhea was common postoperatively (7 studies, 1522 children: incidence 16%, 95% CI 14% to 18%) and later (23 studies, 5491 people: incidence 26%, 95% CI 25% to 27%).[25] Recurrent ear discharge was also common (7 studies, 1144 children: incidence 7.4%, 95% CI 6% to 9%) and often became chronic (3 studies, 451 children: 3.8%, 95% CI 2% to 6%). A systematic review of observational and experimental studies (search date 1998) of the complications following grommet insertion found a reported prevalence of tympanosclerosis in 39–65% of ventilated ears as opposed to 0–10% of untreated ears.[26] Partial atrophy was noted in 16–73% of ears treated and in 5–31% of those untreated. Atelectasis ranged from 10–37% of ears treated as opposed to 1–20% untreated, and attic retraction between 10–52% and

29–40%, respectively. The average hearing loss associated with these abnormalities was less than 5 dB. **Adenoidectomy:** Deaths have been reported in one of 16 700–25 000 children when combined with tonsillectomy (no figures provided for adenoidectomy alone), and postoperative haemorrhage occurred in 0.5%.[27]

Comment: About half of children who have grommets inserted will undergo reinsertion within 5 years.[28] Resolution after surgery takes longer in younger children and in those whose parents smoke, irrespective of treatment.[22] The RCT of early insertion of grommets versus watchful waiting claims to use intention to treat analysis, because people randomised to watchful waiting who actually received early surgery were excluded from analysis rather than counted in the early surgery group.[22]

REFERENCES

1. Williamson IG, Dunleavey J, Bain J, Robinson D. The natural history of otitis media with effusion: a three year study of the incidence and prevalence of abnormal tympanograms in four SW Hampshire infant and first schools. *J Laryngol Otol* 1994;108: 930–934.

2. Strachan DP, Cook DG. Health effects of passive smoking. 4. Passive smoking, middle ear disease and adenotonsillectomy in children. *Thorax* 1998; 53:50–56. Search date 1997; primary sources Medline, and Embase.

3. Paradise JL, Rockette HE, Colborn DK, et al. Otitis media in 2253 Pittsburgh area infants: prevalence and risk factors during the first two years of life. *Pediatrics* 1997;99:318–333.

4. Haggard M, Hughes E. Objectives, values and methods of screening children's hearing – a review of the literature. London: HMSO, 1991.

5. Zeilhuis GA, Rach GH, Broek PV. Screening for otitis media with effusion in pre-school children. *Lancet* 1989;1:311–314.

6. Fiellau-Nikolajsen M. Tympanometry in three year old children: prevalence and spontaneous course of MEE. *Ann Otol Rhinol Laryngol* 1980;89(suppl 68):233–237.

7. Bennett KE, Haggard MP. Behaviour and cognitive outcomes in middle ear disease. *Arch Dis Child* 1999;80:28–35.

8. Stool SE, Berg SO, Berman S, et al. Otitis media with effusion in young children: clinical practice guideline number 12. AHCPR Publication 94–0622. Rockville, Maryland: Agency for Health Care Policy and Research, Public Health Service, United States Department of Health and Human Services, July, 1994. Search date 1992; primary sources online database of National Library of Medicine, and 10 specialised bibliographic databases.

9. Williams RL, Chalmers TC, Strange KC, Chalmers FT, Bowlin SJ. Use of antibiotics in preventing recurrent acute otitis media and in treating otitis media with effusion: a meta-analytic attempt to resolve the brouhaha. *JAMA* 1993;270: 1344–1351. Search date 1993; primary source Medline and Current Contents.

10. Cantekin EI, McGuire TW. Antibiotics are not effective for otitis media with effusion: reanalysis of meta-analysis. *Otorhinolaryngol Nova* 1998;8: 214–222.

11. Computerised clinical information system. Denver, Colorado: Micromedex Inc, June 1993.

12. Little P, Gould C, Williamson I, Warner G, Gantley M, Kinmonth AL. Reattendance and complications

in a randomised trial of prescribing strategies for sore throat: the medicalising effect of prescribing antibiotics. *BMJ* 1997;315:350–352.

13. Anonymous. Antimicrobial resistance is a major threat to public health [Editorial]. *BMJ* 1998;317: 609–610.

14. Butler CC, van der Voort JH. Oral or nasal steroids for hearing loss associated with otitis media with effusion in children. In: The Cochrane Library, Issue 4, 2000. Oxford: Update Software. Search date February 2000; primary sources Cochrane Controlled Trials Register, Embase, and Medline.

15. Tracy TM, Demain JG, Hoffman KM, Goetz DW. Intranasal beclomethasone as an adjunct to treatment of chronic middle ear effusion. *Ann Allergy Asthma Immunol* 1998;80:198–206.

16. Graf P. Rhinitis medicamentosa: aspects of pathophysiology and treatment. *Eur J Allergy Clin Immunol* 1997;52(Suppl 40):28–34.

17. Pignataro O, Pignataro LD, Gallus G, Calori G, Cordaro CI. Otitis media with effusion and S-carboxymethylcysteine and/or its lysine salt: a critical overview. *Int J Pediatr Otorhinolaryngol* 1996;35:231–241. Search date 1993; primary sources Medline, Embase, and Biosis.

18. Reidpath DD, Glasziou PP, Del Mar C. Systematic review of autoinflation for treatment of glue ear in children. *BMJ* 1999;318:1177–1178. Search date not stated; primary sources Medline, Cochrane Library, and pharmaceutical company database.

19. Blanshard JD, Maw AR, Bawden R. Conservative treatment of otitis media with effusion by autoinflation of the middle ear. *Clin Otolaryngol* 1993;18:188–192.

20. University of York. Centre for Reviews and Dissemination. 1992. The treatment of persistent glue ear in children. *Effective Health Care* 1(4). Search date 1992; primary sources BIDS, Medline, and Embase.

21. Rovers MM, Stratman H, Ingels K, van der Wilt GJ, van den Broek P, Zielhuis GA. The effect of ventilation tubes on language development in infants with otitis media with effusion: a randomised trial. *Pediatrics* 2000;106:3–42.

22. Wilks J, Maw R, Peters TJ, Harvey I, Golding J. Randomised controlled trial of early surgery versus watchful waiting for glue ear: The effect on behavioural problems in pre-school children. *Clin Otol Allied Sci* 2000;25:209–214.

23. Paradise J, Feldman HM, Campbell TF, et al. Effect of early or delayed insertion of tympanostomy tubes for persistent otitis media on developmental outcomes at the age of three years. *N Engl J Med* 2001;344:1179–1187.

24. Maw R, Bawden R. Spontaneous resolution of severe chronic glue ear in children and the effect of adenoidectomy, tonsillectomy, and insertion of ventilation tubes. *BMJ* 1993;306:756–760.

25. Kay DJ, Nelson M, Rosenfeld RM. Meta-analysis of tympanostomy tube sequelae. *Otolaryngol Head Neck Surg* 2001;124:374–380. Search date 1999; primary sources Medline and hand searches.

26. Schilder AG. Assessment of complications of the conditions and of the treatment of otitis media with effusion. *Int J Pediatr Otolaryngol* 1999; 49(Suppl 1):S247–S251. Search date 1998; primary sources not stated.

27. Yardley MP. Tonsillectomy, adenoidectomy and adenotonsillectomy; are they safe day case procedures. *J Laryngol Otol* 1992;106:299–300.

28. Maw AR. Development of tympanosclerosis in children with otitis media with effusion and ventilation tubes. *J Laryngol Otol* 1991;105:614–617.

Ian Williamson
Senior Lecturer in Primary Medical Care
Southampton University
Southampton
UK

Competing interests: None declared.

Reducing pain during blood sampling in infants

Search date January 2002

Linda Franck and Ruth Gilbert

INTERVENTIONS

Key Messages

Venepuncture versus heel puncture

- Three RCTs found that venepuncture versus heel puncture significantly reduced pain responses (particularly crying) during blood sampling and reduced the need for repeat punctures.

Sweet solutions

- Nineteen RCTs have found that oral sucrose, glucose, or other sweeteners versus water or no treatment in infants undergoing heel puncture or venepuncture significantly reduces pain responses, particularly the duration of crying.

- We found no clear evidence about the optimal concentration of sucrose or glucose for pain relief with heel puncture or venepuncture. We found no clear evidence about whether sucrose or glucose is more effective at reducing pain responses.
- One RCT found no significant difference between multiple and single doses of sucrose in pain scores for heel puncture.

Breast milk

- Four RCTs found no evidence that breast milk or breast feeding (1 RCT) versus water reduced pain responses or crying in neonates undergoing heel puncture.

Topical anaesthetic

- Systematic reviews and RCTs have found no clear evidence of reduced crying in infants who received either lidocaine or lidocaine–prilocaine cream (EMLA) versus placebo prior to heel puncture.
- Four RCTs reported limited evidence that EMLA reduced pain responses to venepuncture.
- Two RCTs found that tetracaine (amethocaine) gel versus placebo reduced pain scores and the number of infants who cried during venepuncture. One RCT found no evidence of benefit for heel puncture.

Other treatments

- RCTs found reduced pain responses in term and preterm infants given pacifiers compared with no treatment prior to heel puncture. Two RCTs found that pacifier plus sucrose versus pacifier alone had no significant effect on pain responses. One RCT found significant reduction in pain responses in term infants given a pacifier compared with water or no treatment during venepuncture.
- Two RCTs found term infants held during heel puncture had significantly reduced crying. One RCT found that sucrose did not appear to modify the effect of holding.
- One RCT comparing rocking versus no intervention in neonates undergoing heel puncture found limited evidence that rocking reduced pain. Another RCT found no significant difference in pain response.
- Three RCTs found limited evidence that pain responses were reduced by tucking the arms and legs into a mid-line flexed position during heel puncture, by providing multimodal sensory stimulation (massage, vocal, visual, sucking, or sweet solution), or by avoiding stressful handling before heel puncture. Two RCTs found no difference in pain responses from positioning or swaddling.
- One RCT found no effect of warming prior to heel puncture.
- Four RCTs in preterm and term infants have found that automated devices for heel puncture are less painful and cause less bruising than manual lancets, and that samples are obtained more quickly.

DEFINITION Methods of sampling blood in infants include heel puncture, venepuncture, and arterial puncture. Heel puncture involves lancing of the lateral aspect of the infant's heel, squeezing the heel, and collecting the pooled capillary blood. Venepuncture involves aspirating blood through a needle in a peripheral vein. Arterial blood sampling is not discussed in this review.

INCIDENCE/ Almost every infant in the developed world undergoes heel puncture
PREVALENCE to screen for metabolic disorders (e.g. phenylketonuria). Many

Reducing pain during blood sampling in infants

infants have repeated heel punctures or venepunctures to monitor blood glucose or haemoglobin. Preterm or ill neonates receiving intensive care may have 1–21 painful procedures a day.[1-3] Heel punctures comprise 61–87% and venepuncture comprise 8–13% of the invasive procedures performed on ill infants. Analgesics are rarely given specifically for blood sampling procedures, but 5–19% of infants receive analgesia for other indications.[2,3] In one study, comfort measures were provided during 63% of venepunctures and 75% of heel punctures.[3]

AETIOLOGY/ RISK FACTORS Blood sampling in infants can be difficult to perform, particularly in preterm or ill infants. Young infants may have increased sensitivity and more prolonged responses to pain than older age groups.[4] Factors that may affect the infant's pain responses include post-conceptional age, previous pain experience, and procedural technique.

PROGNOSIS Pain caused by blood sampling is associated with acute behavioural and physiological deterioration.[4] Other adverse effects of blood sampling include bleeding, bruising, haematoma, and infection. Extremely rarely, heel puncture can result in cellulitis, osteomyelitis, calcaneal spurs, and necrotising chondritis.[5-7]

AIMS To obtain an adequate blood sample with minimal pain for the infant and minimal adverse effects of treatments.

OUTCOMES We found no easily administered, widely accepted assessment of pain in infants. Where available, we have analysed the proportion of infants crying at all, or the duration of crying. Other pain related responses measured in the studies included facial expressions (the number of specific expressions, or the duration of those expressions), heart rate, and transcutaneous oxygen saturation levels. Studies used composite scales composed of behavioural and cardiorespiratory, or both, signs of pain related distress, only some of which have been validated. We have not pooled differences in pain related responses or for different pain scales.

METHODS *Clinical Evidence* search and appraisal January 2002, and additional hand searches to January 2002.

QUESTION **What are the effects of interventions to reduce pain related distress during blood sampling in infants?**

OPTION **VENEPUNCTURE VERSUS HEEL PUNCTURE**

Three RCTs have found that venepuncture versus heel puncture significantly reduces pain responses (particularly crying) during blood sampling, and also reduces the need for repeat punctures.

Benefits: We found one systematic review (search date 2001,[8] 3 RCTs;[9-11] 264 full term healthy neonates). All three RCTs found that venepuncture versus heel puncture significantly reduced pain responses, but each study used different measures of pain responses. Two of the RCTs found that fewer infants either cried after the procedure or had not stopped crying by 60 seconds with venepuncture compared with heel puncture (36/110 [33%] with venepuncture v 28/127 [22%] with heel puncture; RR 0.61, 95%

CI 0.50 to 0.76; NNT 4, 95% CI 3 to 7).[9,11] All three RCTs found that venepuncture versus heel puncture significantly reduced the number of repeat punctures required to obtain an adequate sample (16/93 [17%] with venepuncture v 64/111 [58%] with heel puncture; RR 0.30, 95% CI 0.18 to 0.49).[8]

Harms: One of the RCTs reported bruising in a single infant following heel puncture and higher maternal anxiety during venepuncture than during heel puncture.[10] Too few infants were studied to detect infection or rare complications.

Comment: Of the three RCTs, only one reported adequate concealment of randomisation and blinded assessment of pain responses.[9] All three RCTs compared blood sampling procedures performed by a single individual in each study. We also found one clinical controlled trial (66 children) comparing venepuncture versus heel puncture (with spring loaded lancet using blinded assessment of pain responses).[12] The study found that infants cried less after venepuncture than after heel puncture (mean difference 66 s, 95% CI 26 s to 107 s). Failure to obtain a sample was more frequent with venepuncture than with heel puncture (6/36 [17%] with venepuncture v 0/30 [0%] with heel puncture; ARR 17%, 95% CI 3% to 30%).[12] There was significant heterogeneity between studies for repeat punctures.

OPTION	ORAL SWEET SOLUTIONS

In term and preterm infants undergoing heel puncture or venepuncture, 19 RCTs have found that oral sucrose, glucose, or other sweeteners versus water or no treatment significantly reduce pain responses (particularly the duration of crying). One small RCT found no significant difference between multiple and single doses of sucrose in pain scores for heel puncture. We found no clear evidence that any one sugar is superior to the others, or evidence about the optimum concentration for pain relief.

Benefits: **Sucrose for heel puncture:** We found four systematic reviews (search dates 1995,[13] 2001,[14] 1998,[15] 2000;[16] 10 RCTs[17–26]) and 9 additional RCTs[27–35] of oral sucrose (0.05–2.00 mL of 7.5–70%) versus water or no treatment in newborns undergoing heel puncture. The 19 RCTs included 1209 term and preterm neonates.[17–35] All six RCTs in preterm neonates found that sucrose (24–70%) versus water significantly reduced pain responses and pain scores.[18,21,22,26,33,34] The time spent crying during the procedure was significantly reduced (by 30 s), and the total duration of crying was significantly reduced (by 39 s).[18,22] Of the 16 trials in term neonates, seven RCTs found that sucrose (12–70%) versus water significantly reduced pain scores.[19,23,26,31,32,34,35] Seven RCTs found that sucrose versus water decreased the percentage of time spent crying.[17,19,23,27–29,32] Seven RCTs found significantly reduced crying time (mean or median differences 16–90 s).[20,22,25,30–32,35] In one RCT, a significant difference was found only for neonates given 50% sucrose and not for those given lower concentrations.[20] One RCT used a low concentration of sucrose (2 mL of 7.5%) and found no significant difference in

Reducing pain during blood sampling in infants

duration of crying.[24] **Glucose for heel puncture:** We found four systematic reviews (search dates 1995,[13] 2001,[14] 1998,[15] 2000;[16] 2 RCTs[17,36]) and two additional RCTs.[11,37] Three RCTs included 412 term infants given 1–2 mL of 10–30% glucose versus water or no treatment prior to heel puncture.[11,17,36] Two RCTs found fewer infants cried at all with 30% glucose versus water,[11] no treatment,[36] or 10% glucose.[36] One RCT comparing glucose versus no treatment found that 30% glucose significantly reduced crying time (75% decrease) but 10% glucose did not significantly reduce crying time (50% decrease) compared with no treatment.[36] One RCT comparing 12% glucose versus water found no significant difference (mean crying time 56 s with glucose v 60 s with water).[17] One crossover trial of 17 preterm infants compared 10% glucose with no treatment. Mean pain scores were significantly reduced Premature Infant Pain Profile [see glossary, p 126] reduced by 2.5; P < 0.001).[37] **Other sweeteners for heel puncture:** We found three systematic reviews (search dates 1995,[13] 2001,[14] 1998;[15] 1 RCT[23]) and one additional RCT.[38] The RCT in the reviews comparing hydrogenated glucose versus water found significant decreases in pain score, duration of first cry and percentage of time spent crying, but no significant difference versus sucrose (25% or 50%).[23] The additional RCT (120 term infants) comparing an artificial sweetener (10 parts cyclamate and 1 part saccharin) versus water found small but significant differences in percentage of time crying and pain scores.[38] **Sucrose for venepuncture:** We found two systematic reviews (search dates 1995,[13] 2001;[14] 1 RCT[39]) and two additional RCTs[40,41] comparing sucrose versus water in 201 term neonates having venepuncture. The RCT from the reviews (28 preterm neonates) found that 24% sucrose versus water reduced mean crying time (mean duration of crying, 19 s in 8 preterm neonates given 24% sucrose v 73 s in 12 neonates given water). The study found that mean crying time was not significantly reduced with 12% sucrose versus water (8 neonates, 63 s).[39] The other RCTs found significantly reduced duration of crying and pain scores with 24–30% sucrose versus water or no treatment.[40,41] **Glucose for venepuncture:** We found two RCTs that compared 2 mL of 30% glucose versus water in term infants undergoing venepuncture.[11,40] One RCT (60 infants) found significantly reduced pain scores but no difference in the proportion of infants crying (46% with glucose v 39% with water).[11] The other RCT (75 infants) found significantly reduced median pain scores with glucose versus water or no treatment (median pain score difference 2, glucose 5, water 7, 95% CI 1 to 4; P = 0.005).[40] **Other sweeteners for venepuncture:** We found no RCTs of other sweeteners for venepuncture. **Concentration of glucose or sucrose for heel puncture and venepuncture:** We found two systematic reviews (search dates 2001[14] and 1998;[15] 1 RCT[36]) and six additional RCTs of the effects of glucose or sucrose concentration in heel puncture.[17,20,23,30,36,40] We found no studies of the effects of glucose or sucrose concentration in venepuncture. Three RCTs in term neonates compared different concentrations of sucrose during heel puncture.[17,20,23] One RCT (75 neonates) found that increasing concentrations of sucrose (2 mL of 12.5%, 25%, and 50%) produced significantly greater reductions in the duration of crying.[20]

The other two trials found no difference in crying duration with different sucrose concentrations (56 infants in total, given 2 mL of 25–50% or 12–25% sucrose).[17,23] Three RCTs compared different concentrations of glucose during heel puncture.[30,36,40] One RCT (60 term and preterm infants) compared 1 mL of 10% versus 1 mL of 30% glucose; the study found no significant difference in the duration of crying or the proportion of babies who cried at all (no crying in 40% with 10% glucose v 53% with 30% glucose; P > 0.05).[36] **Multiple doses of sweeteners:** We found one RCT (32 preterm neonates, mean gestation 31 wks) that compared a single dose (0.5 mL) of 24% sucrose 2 minutes before heel puncture versus three doses given 2 minutes prior, immediately before the procedure, and during the procedure.[33] Pain scores measured at five points during the procedure were significantly different only at the latest time. **Sucrose versus glucose for heel puncture and venepuncture:** We found one RCT (113 term infants undergoing heel puncture) comparing glucose versus sucrose. The study found that 30% sucrose versus 30% glucose reduced crying time by a mean of 30 seconds (P = 0.006).[30] Another RCT (150 term infants undergoing venepuncture) found no significant difference with 30% sucrose versus 30% glucose on pain scores.[40] **Repeated doses for repeated blood sampling:** We found no RCTs.

Harms: No adverse effects from oral sucrose or glucose administered to full term or preterm infants were reported in any of the RCTs. The safety of repeated oral administration of sucrose or glucose has not been adequately investigated. Theoretical adverse effects include hyperglycaemia and necrotising enterocolitis.

Comment: Some studies were crossover RCTs, which might produce biased estimates of the effect of sucrose if neonates become habituated to pain or if the washout period between interventions is too short.[18,22,34] Only some RCTs reported adequate allocation concealment.[11,18,19,21,31,33,40] In one study it was uncertain whether infants were randomly allocated.[28] Most had blinded measurement of at least some of the pain responses, particularly crying, on the basis of independent audio or video tape recordings. One RCT had no blinded outcome assessment.[22] We found inadequate evidence about the benefits or harms of repeated administration of sucrose or glucose for repeated blood sampling.

OPTION   BREAST MILK

Four RCTs found no evidence that breast milk or breast feeding (1 RCT) versus water reduced pain responses or crying in neonates undergoing heel puncture.

Benefits: We found one systematic review (search date 1998,[15] 2 RCTs,[25,36] 126 preterm and term neonates undergoing heel puncture) and two subsequent RCTs (147 term infants)[38,35] comparing breast milk (1–2 mL) versus water. None found a significant effect of breast milk on duration of crying[25,35,36,38] or proportion of infants not crying.[36] One RCT (62 term infants) found no significant effect of breastfeeding versus water on duration of crying.[35] We found no RCTs on the effects of breast milk during venepuncture.

Reducing pain during blood sampling in infants

Harms: None reported.

Comment: Concealment of allocation was not clearly stated in any RCT. Assessment of pain responses was blind in two RCTs[35,38] and not clearly stated in the other two.[25,36]

OPTION   **TOPICAL ANAESTHETICS**

Systematic reviews and additional RCTs found no evidence of reduced pain responses, particularly crying, in infants who received either lidocaine or lidocaine plus prilocaine cream (EMLA) versus placebo prior to heel puncture. Four RCTs found limited evidence that EMLA reduced pain responses to venepuncture. Two RCTs found that tetracaine (amethocaine) gel versus placebo reduced pain scores and the number of infants who cried during venepuncture; one RCT found no evidence of reduced crying for heel puncture.

Benefits: **Lidocaine or EMLA for heel puncture:** We found three systematic reviews (search dates 1996[42] and 1998,[15] 1998;[43] 5 RCTs[44–48]) and one additional RCT,[1] comparing lidocaine or EMLA versus placebo in neonates undergoing heel puncture. Treatments were usually given 30–60 minutes before heel puncture, with the exception of one RCT that randomised infants to eight application times (10–120 min before heel puncture).[47] The five studies used different assessments of pain responses. Three RCTs included 186 preterm neonates[1,44,45] and three RCTs included 192 infants who were mainly term neonates.[46–48] None of the RCTs found a significant difference with lidocaine or EMLA versus placebo on pain scores. One RCT found no significant difference with EMLA versus placebo in the proportion of infants who cried during the procedure (54/56 [96%] v 52/54 [96%]).[47] **EMLA for venepuncture:** We found two systematic reviews (search dates 1996[42] and 1998;[15] 2 RCTs[49,50]) and two additional RCTs[51,52] that compared EMLA versus placebo in infants having venepuncture. One RCT (120 term infants) found that EMLA versus placebo significantly reduced the duration of crying (median 12 s v 31 s; P < 0.05) and pain score at 15 seconds after venepuncture (NFCS score [see glossary, p 126] 287 v 374; P = 0.02), but found no significant difference in pain score 60 seconds after venepuncture.[49] The second RCT (60 children) found that 19/28 in the EMLA group and 14/28 in the placebo group did not cry at all during the procedure. The study did not measure duration of cry or pain score.[50] The third RCT (41 infants and toddlers) found a significant difference in mean behavioural pain score with EMLA versus placebo (P < 0.01).[51] The fourth RCT (19 preterm infants) found that EMLA versus placebo did not significantly reduce pain scores (NFCS score, mean difference 0, 95% CI –2.00 to +1.75) or the total duration of crying (median difference between EMLA and placebo –22 s, 95% CI –96 s to +24 s).[52] **Tetracaine (amethocaine) versus placebo:** We found three RCTs (in term and preterm infants reporting blinded assessments of pain scores and crying) comparing tetracaine (amethocaine) versus placebo.[53–55] Two RCTs involved 80 preterm and term neonates undergoing venepuncture.[53,54] Tetracaine significantly reduced the pain scores in infants having venepuncture and reduced the proportion who cried (4/19 [21%] with tetracaine v 15/20 [75%] with placebo; ARR 54% 95% CI 2% to 80%; NNT 2, 95% CI 1 to 4).[53,54] One RCT (60 neonates, median gestation 36 wks, undergoing heel puncture using an automated device) found that the tetracaine group had a lower pain score, and fewer infants cried with tetracaine than with placebo, but neither difference was significant (20/30 [67%] with tetracaine v 13/29 [45%]; ARI 22%, 95% CI −4% to +47%).[55] **Topical anaesthetic versus sucrose:** We found one RCT (55 venepunctures in 51 term neonates) that compared EMLA versus 24% sucrose versus EMLA plus sucrose versus water.[41] Crying was taped and assessed blind to treatment. Crying time was significantly higher in babies given water versus sucrose with or without EMLA (P = 0.001) or EMLA alone (P = 0.008). EMLA alone was reported to be less effective than sucrose alone or EMLA plus sucrose, but analyses were not presented. We found no studies of topical anaesthetic versus sweet solutions for heel puncture. **Topical anaesthetic versus pacifiers:** We found no RCTs.

Harms: We found six RCTs (250 infants) that reported the absence of adverse reactions to EMLA, or to placebo, or no difference in minor, transient local reactions.[1,46–48,51,52] One cohort study (500 neonates) found unusual cutaneous effects associated with EMLA in four neonates under 32 weeks' gestation.[56] Methaemoglobinaemia can occur with the prilocaine constituent of EMLA. Levels of methaemoglobin over 25–30% can cause clinical symptoms of hypoxia.[57] We found one systematic review (search date 1996, 12 RCTs or cohort studies, > 355 neonates)[42] and two subsequent RCTs (167 neonates)[1,57] of EMLA for heel puncture, venepuncture, circumcision, or lumbar puncture. All but one of these studies found mean methaemoglobin levels less than 1.5% in neonates given EMLA. The other RCT (47 preterm and term infants given EMLA) found that the highest mean methaemoglobin levels (2.3%, range 0.6–6.2%) occurred after 15 days of repeated doses of EMLA.[56] A systematic review found two case reports of neonates who were treated with oxygen at methaemoglobin levels of 12% and 16%.[42] No local skin reactions were seen after application of tetracaine or placebo in the 140 neonates studied.

Comment: Some of the studies reported adequate concealment of allocation.[46,47,49,52–55] Three RCTs used video taped recordings of pain responses to blind assessors to the intervention.[49,51–53,55] In the other RCTs, although placebo ointment was used, pain responses were assessed by observers at the time of the procedure, rather than by scoring of video film. Deduction of treatment allocation may have been possible in the EMLA studies because of the smell and skin blanching caused by EMLA. One study excluded 25% of children who had high behaviour scores before puncture, and presented results only for selected subgroups.[51] The findings of this study may be difficult to generalise.

Reducing pain during blood sampling in infants

OPTION **PACIFIERS**

Eight RCTs found reduced pain responses in term and preterm infants given pacifiers compared with no treatment prior to heel puncture. Three RCTs found that pacifiers plus sucrose or glucose versus pacifiers alone similarly reduced pain responses. One RCT found significant reduction in pain responses in term infants given a pacifier compared with water or no treatment during venepuncture.

Benefits: **Pacifier alone for heel puncture:** We found two systematic reviews (search dates 2001[14] and 1998;[15] 1 RCT[58]) and seven additional RCTs comparing pacifiers (see glossary, p 126) versus no treatment (445 infants of which 271 were preterm).[32,37,58–62] Pacifiers were given 2–5 minutes before heel puncture. Four RCTs were crossover trials.[37,58–60] All Four RCTs found that pacifiers versus no pacifiers significantly reduced pain responses[37,58,61] or the percentage of time spent in a distressed, fussy, or awake state.[60,61] In the three RCTs in term infants, those given a pacifier cried for significantly less time,[32,59,62] spent less time in fussy or awake states,[62] or had reduced pain score.[59] However, reductions were not significant for all measures of pain: in one study, grimacing was not significantly reduced by the pacifier[32] and in another, the pain score was similar during the procedure but fell more quickly in babies given pacifiers.[59] **Pacifier plus sucrose for heel puncture:** We found one RCT (crossover, 122 preterm neonates having heel puncture) that compared a pacifier dipped in 24% sucrose versus dipped in water.[58] The study found no significant difference in pain responses (mean Premature Infant Pain Profile [PIPP] score [see glossary, p 126]) between the interventions. **Pacifier plus glucose for heel puncture:** We found one RCT (crossover, 17 preterm infants) that compared a pacifier dipped in 10% glucose versus no treatment, 10% glucose alone, or pacifier alone.[37] Mean pain score was reduced (reduction in mean PIPP score: 3.6; P = 0.001) compared to no treatment, but was similar to glucose alone or pacifier alone. **Pacifier plus music for heel puncture:** One RCT (28 term and preterm infants) found no significant difference between pacifiers plus music versus pacifiers alone for pain score assessed at all time points except 4 minutes after heel puncture (P < 0.001).[59] **Pacifier plus multimodal sensory stimulation:** We found one RCT (crossover, 17 preterm infants) that found a pacifier plus multimodal sensory stimulation (pacifer plus glucose, massage, visual, and auditory stimulation) during heel puncture significantly reduced the pain score when compared with no treatment (mean PIPP score reduction: 7.15; P < 0.001) and when compared with glucose plus pacifer, pacifier alone, or glucose alone (mean PIPP score reduction: 2.6–4.55; P < 0.01 for each of the 3 comparisons).[37] **Pacifier for venepuncture:** We found one RCT (100 term infants undergoing venepuncture) comparing pacifiers in infants given pacifier or pacifier plus sucrose versus no treatment or 2 mL water orally.[39] The study found a significant reduction in the pain score during the procedure (median difference in 10 point pain score was 5 for pacifiers alone v water and 6 for pacifiers plus sucrose v water; P < 0.0001).

Harms: No adverse effects were reported in any of these studies.

Comment: None of the studies explicitly defined the method of allocation to pacifier or no treatment. Three RCTs blinded assessors to the intervention by analysing audio tapes of crying during the procedure.[37,60,62] Measurement of pain responses on the basis of facial expressions were not blinded to the pacifiers or music intervention.

OPTION **HOLDING**

Two RCTs found a significant reduction in crying in infants held during heel puncture. One RCT found that sucrose did not appear to modify the effect of holding.

Benefits: We found no systematic review but found two RCTs (124 term infants undergoing heel puncture).[19,63] One RCT (30 infants) compared holding the baby with skin to skin contact versus being swaddled in a crib.[63] Crying and grimacing were significantly reduced in the babies held skin to skin (proportion crying during procedure 8% v 45%; ARR 37%; CI not provided; NNT 3, 95% CI 2 to 13). The other RCT (94 term newborns) compared sucrose, sucrose plus holding, holding with water, and water alone for heel puncture.[19] Pain scores and duration of crying decreased in the holding group compared with no holding and in the sucrose groups compared with no sucrose, but the differences were of borderline significance. There was no evidence of an interaction between sucrose and holding (P = 0.37).

Harms: None reported.

Comment: Assessment of crying was based on analysis of audio or video tape recordings and was blind to the sucrose intervention but not to holding.[19,63] Assessments based on facial expressions were not blind to the intervention.

OPTION **ROCKING**

One RCT of rocking versus no intervention in neonates undergoing heel puncture found limited evidence that rocking reduced pain. Another RCT found no significant difference in pain response.

Benefits: We found no systematic review but found two RCTs, comparing rocking versus no intervention.[21,62] One RCT (44 preterm infants, 25–34 wks gestation) compared 0.05 mL water given before heel puncture versus simulated rocking using a respirator attached to an air mattress.[21] The study found no significant differences for facial expressions of pain. The other RCT (40 term neonates) compared no intervention with being held vertically and rocked by the examiner.[62] The study found that rocking reduced the duration of crying (P = 0.05) during the procedure and the risk of persistent crying (2/20 [10%] with rocking v 9/20 [45%] with no intervention; ARR 35%; CI not provided; NNT 3, 95% CI 2 to 10).

Harms: None reported.

Comment: The method of allocation to rocking or standard care was adequate in one study[21] and unclear in the other.[61] Both studies used blinded assessment of pain responses based on video[21] and audio tape[62] recordings.

Reducing pain during blood sampling in infants

| OPTION | POSITION, SWADDLING, AND PRIOR HANDLING |

Two RCTs found limited evidence that pain responses were reduced by tucking the arms and legs into a mid-line flexed position during heel puncture, or by avoiding stressful handling before heel puncture. Two RCTs found no difference in pain responses from positioning or swaddling.

Benefits: We found no systematic review but found four RCTs comparing positioning, swaddling, or stressful handling versus no intervention.[58,64–66] One crossover RCT (122 preterm infants, 25–34 wks gestation, undergoing heel puncture) compared prone position versus side or supine position. The study found no significant difference in the mean pain score.[58] One RCT (crossover, 15 preterm neonates) compared swaddling immediately after heel puncture versus standard care (no swaddling).[64] No significant difference in facial expressions of pain or arousal state were detected. Another RCT (crossover, 30 preterm neonates, 25–35 wks gestation) compared facilitative tucking during and after heel puncture (defined as the gentle containment of arms and legs in a flexed, mid-line position) with no intervention.[65] The study found a significant reduction in the total crying time and time to quietening (mean cry duration 2.2 v 0.3 min; P < 0.001). The fourth RCT (48 mainly preterm infants, mean gestation 35 wks) compared stressful handling (as if being prepared for a lumbar puncture) with avoidance of handling for 10 minutes prior to heel puncture.[66] The study found that prior handling increased facial expressions of pain, the proportion of time crying, and crying at all during the 2 minutes after heel puncture (21/21 [100%] handled babies cried v 21/27 [78%] non-handled babies; ARR 22%; CI not provided; NNT 5, 95% CI 3 to 17).

Harms: No adverse events were reported for any of these interventions.

Comment: None of the studies explicitly reported the method of allocation to the interventions and only the study comparing handling versus no handling assessed pain responses blind to the intervention.[66]

| OPTION | WARMING |

One RCT found no effect of warming prior to heel puncture

Benefits: We found one systematic review (search date 1998,[15] 1 RCT[67]) that compared 57 term infants undergoing heel puncture on 80 occasions with an automated lancet with (41 infants) or without (40 infants) prior warming of the heel. The heel was warmed for 10 minutes with a gel pack at 40°C. A slightly higher proportion of infants grimaced and cried with warming versus not warming (14/41 [34%] v 10/40 [25%]; RR 1.4, 95% CI 0.7 to 2.7). Sampling time was slightly longer in the warmed heels (median time 44 s, interquartile range 25–62 s v 40 s, interquartile range 28–72 s), but the number of repeat punctures was slightly lower (5/41 [12%] v 8/40 [20%]; RR 0.6, 0.2 to 1.7).

Harms: We found no evidence about harms.

Comment: Method of allocation was not reported and assessment of outcomes was not blind to the intervention.

| OPTION | DEVICES FOR HEEL PUNCTURE |

Four RCTs in preterm and term infants found that automated devices for heel puncture are less painful and cause less bruising than manual lancets and that samples are obtained more quickly. Two RCTs in preterm infants compared automated devices. One found no differences and the other found one device reduced sampling time and the need for repeat punctures.

Benefits: We found no systematic review but found four RCTs (70 preterm infants and 76 term infants) that compared spring loaded, automated devices with manual lancets.[68–71] One RCT (70 infants) found that fewer punctures occurred over 2–21 days in preterm infants randomised to repeated sampling using an automated device versus a manual lancet (mean difference in total number of punctures: 37, 95% CI 24 to 50).[68] The automated group had less bruising of the heel (27/32 [84%] with automated v 38/38 [100%] with manual; ARR 16%, 95% CI 4% to 28%; NNT 7), and inflammation of the heel (17/32 [53%] with automated v 30/38 [79%] with manual; ARR 26%, 95% CI 4% to 48%; NNT 4). One RCT (36 term infants) found a non-significant reduction in the risk of repeated puncture for a single sample (2/18 [11%] with automated v 3/18 [17%] with manual; ARR 6%, 95% CI −17% to +28%) and a significant increase in the proportion of infants who did not cry (5/18 [28%] with automated v 0/18 [0%] with manual; ARI 28%, 95% CI 5% to 50%; NNT 4).[69] One RCT found no difference in the time spent crying during a single procedure, but sampling was quicker with the automated device (mean difference 92 s, 95% CI 29 s to 154 s).[70] One RCT found a decreased duration of crying and sampling with the automated device than manual lancet (the results are being translated).[71] Two further RCTs in preterm infants compared two types of automated devices used on 344 occasions in 108 infants.[72,73] In one RCT (187 samplings), lack of pain assessed by facial expression was similar in both groups (32/87 [37%] with the Tenderfoot Preemie® v 33/83 [40%] with the Autolet®; ARR 3%, 95% CI −12% to +18%). The sampling time was similar (57 infants: median time 5.0 s with Tenderfoot Preemie® v 6.43 s with Autolet®; P < 0.05). The risk of haemolysis was similar (12/60 [20%] with the Tenderfoot Preemie® v 17/61 [28%] with the Autolet®; ARR 8%, 95% CI −7% to +23%). Fewer repeat samples were needed with the Tenderfoot Preemie® (17/90 [19%] v 40/97 [41%]; ARR 22%, 95% CI 10% to 35%). The other RCT found a shorter collection time with the Tenderfoot Preemie® versus the Monolet® (mean 3.9 s v 5.4 s), fewer punctures to obtain a sample (mean 1 v 2.1), and fewer repeat samples (0/49 [0%] v 6/40 [15%]; ARR 15%, 95% CI 5% to 25%).[73]

Harms: Manual lancets carry a risk of accidental injury to patients and staff.

Comment: Two RCTs allocated babies sealed envelopes with the device allocation.[71,73] Allocation method was not clearly reported in any of the other studies. Three RCTs attempted to blind some of the outcome measures to the procedure.[68,69,71]

Reducing pain during blood sampling in infants

Child health

GLOSSARY

Hydrogenated glucose syrup An aqueous solution of hydrogenated part hydrolysed starch composed of a mixture of mainly maltitol with sorbitol and hydrogenated oligosaccharides and polysaccharides. Preparations containing a minimum 98% maltitol are known as maltitol syrup.

NFCS score Facial Coding System used to evaluate pain responses in full term and preterm infants. Presence or absence is recorded of six facial actions (e.g. eyes squeezed shut, deepening of the naso-labial furrow).

Pacifier A device with a teat that a baby sucks on for comfort. Some pacifiers can deliver a liquid to the baby. Also known as a "dummy", "soother", or "plug" in some countries.

Premature Infant Pain Profile score A seven item composite scale that scores behavioural and cardiorespiratory pain responses coded 0 to 3 (maximum score 21).

Stressful handling A term used to describe the undressing of an infant and holding in a fixed position, as if being prepared for a lumbar puncture.

REFERENCES

1. Stevens B, Johnston C, Taddio A, et al. Management of pain from heel lance with lidocaine–prilocaine (EMLA) cream: is it safe and efficacious in preterm infants? *J Dev Behav Pediatr* 1999;20:216–221.

2. Johnston CC, Collinge JM, Henderson SJ, Anand KJ. A cross-sectional survey of pain and pharmacological analgesia in Canadian neonatal intensive care units. *Clin J Pain* 1997;13: 308–312.

3. Porter FL, Anand KJS. Epidemiology of pain in neonates. *Res Clin Forum* 1998;20:9–18.

4. Anand K, Stevens BJ, McGrath PJ. *Pain in neonates*. Amsterdam: Elsevier Science BV, 2000.

5. Meehan RM. Heel sticks in neonates for capillary blood sampling. *Neonatal Network* 1998;17: 17–24.

6. Lilien LD, Harris VJ, Ramamurthy RS, Pildes RS. Neonatal osteomyelitis of the calcaneus: complications of heel puncture. *J Pediatr* 1976; 88:478–480.

7. Blumenfeld TA, Turi GK, Blanc WA. Recommended site and depth of newborn heel skin punctures based on anatomical measurements and histopathology. *Lancet* 1979;1:230–233.

8. Shah V, Ohlsson A. Venepuncture versus heel lance for blood sampling in term neonates. In: The Cochrane Library, Issue 1, 2002. Oxford: Update Software. Search date 2001; primary sources Cochrane Library, Medline, Embase, and Cinahl.

9. Larsson BA, Tannfeldt G, Lagercrantz H, Olsson GL. Venepuncture is more effective and less painful than heel lancing for blood tests in neonates. *Pediatrics* 1998;101:882–886.

10. Shah VS, Taddio A, Bennett S, Speidel BD. Neonatal pain response to heel stick vs venepuncture for routine blood sampling. *Arch Dis Child Fetal Neonatal Ed* 1997;77:F143–F144.

11. Eriksson M, Gradin M, Schollin J. Oral glucose and venepuncture reduce blood sampling pain in newborns. *Early Hum Dev* 1999;55:211–218.

12. Logan PW. Venepuncture versus heel prick for the collection of the Newborn Screening Test. Australian. *Aust J Adv Nurs* 1999;17:30–36.

13. Stevens B, Taddio A, Ohlsson A, Einarson T. The efficacy of sucrose for relieving procedural pain in neonates: a systematic review and meta-analysis. *Acta Paediatr* 1997;86:837–842. Search date 1995; primary sources Medline, Embase, Reference Update, and hand searches of personal

files, bibliographies, most recent neonatal and pain journals, and conference proceedings.

14. Stevens B, Yamada J, Ohlsson A. Sucrose for analgesia in newborn infants undergoing painful procedures. In: The Cochrane Library, Issue 1, 2002. Oxford: Update Software. Search date 2001; primary sources Medline, Embase, Reference Update, Cochrane Library, and hand searches of personal files, bibliographies, recent neonatal and pain journals, and conference proceedings.

15. Ohlsson A, Taddio A, Jadad AR, Stevens B. Evidence-based decision making, systematic reviews and the Cochrane collaboration: implications for neonatal analgesia. In: Anand K, Stevens B, McGrath PJ, eds. *Pain in Neonates*. Amsterdam: Elsevier Science BV, 2000:251–268. Search date 1998; primary sources Medline, Cochrane Library, hand searches of personal files, and reference lists.

16. Bauer K, Versmold H. Oral sugar solutions in pain therapy of neonates and premature infants. *Z Geburtshilfe Neonatol* 2001;205:80–85 Search date 2000; primary source PubMed.

17. Abad Massanet F, Diaz Gomez NM, Domenech Martinez E, Robayna Curbelo M, Rico Sevillano J. Analgesic effect of oral sweet solution in newborns. *An Esp Pediatr* 1995;43:351–354.

18. Bucher HU, Moser T, von Siebenthal K, Keel M, Wolf M, Duc G. Sucrose reduces pain reaction to heel lancing in preterm infants: a placebo-controlled, randomized and masked study. *Pediatr Res* 1995;38:332–335.

19. Gormally S, Barr RG, Wertheim L, et al. Contact and nutrient caregiving effects on newborn infant pain responses. *Dev Med Child Neurol* 2001;43: 28–38.

20. Haouari N, Wood C, Griffiths G, Levene M. The analgesic effect of sucrose in full term infants: a randomised controlled trial. *BMJ* 1995;310: 1498–1500.

21. Johnston CC, Stremler RL, Stevens BJ, Horton LJ. Effectiveness of oral sucrose and simulated rocking on pain response in preterm neonates. *Pain* 1997;72:193–199.

22. Ramenghi LA, Wood CM, Griffith GC, Levene MI. Reduction of pain response in premature infants using intraoral sucrose. *Arch Dis Child Fetal Neonatal Ed* 1996;74:F126–F128.

23. Ramenghi LA, Griffith GC, Wood CM, Levene MI. Effect of non-sucrose sweet tasting solution on neonatal heel prick responses. *Arch Dis Child Fetal Neonatal Ed* 1996;74:F129–F131.

24. Rushforth JA, Levene MI. Effect of sucrose on crying in response to heel stab. *Arch Dis Child* 1993;69:388–389.

25. Ors R, Ozek E, Baysoy G, et al. Comparison of sucrose and human milk on pain response in newborns. *Eur J Pediatr* 1999;158:63–66.

26. Gibbins SA. Efficacy and safety of sucrose for procedural pain relief in preterm and term neonates. *Dissert Abstract Int* 2001;62–04B: 1804.

27. Blass EM, Hoffmeyer LB. Sucrose as an analgesic for newborn infants. *Pediatrics* 1991;87: 215–218.

28. Blass EM. Pain-reducing properties of sucrose in human newborns. *Chem Senses* 1995;20:29–35.

29. Blass EM. Milk-induced hypoalgesia in human newborns. *Pediatrics* 1997;99:825–829.

30. Isik U, Ozek E, Bilgen H, Cebeci, D. Comparison of oral glucose and sucrose solutions on pain response in neonates. *J Pain* 2000;1:275–278.

31. Overgaard C, Knudsen A. Pain-relieving effect of sucrose in newborns during heel prick. *Biol Neonate* 1999;75:279–284.

32. Blass EM, Watt LB. Suckling- and sucrose-induced analgesia in human newborns. *Pain* 1999;83: 611–623.

33. Johnston CC, Stremler R, Horton L, Friedman A. Effect of repeated doses of sucrose during heel stick procedure in preterm neonates. *Biol Neonate* 1999;75:160–166.

34. Mellah D, Gourrier E, Merbouche S, et al. Analgesia with saccharose during heel capillary prick. A randomized study in 37 newborns of over 33 weeks of amenorrhea. *Arch Pediatr* 1999;6: 610–616 [in French].

35. Bilgen H, Ozek E, Cebeci D, Ors R. Comparison of sucrose, expressed breast milk, and breast-feeding on the neonatal response to heel prick. *J Pain* 2001;2:301–305.

36. Skogsdal Y, Eriksson M, Schollin J. Analgesia in newborns given oral glucose. *Acta Paediatr* 1997; 86:217–220.

37. Bellieni CV, Buonocore G, Nenci A, et al. Sensorial saturation: an effective analgesic tool for heel-prick in preterm infants: a prospective randomized trial. *Biol Neonate* 2001;80:15–18.

38. Bucher HU, Baumgartner R, Bucher N, Seiler M, Fauchere JC. Artificial sweetener reduces nociceptive reaction in term newborn infants. *Early Hum Dev* 2000;59:51–60.

39. Abad F, Diaz NM, Domenech E, Robayna M, Rico J. Oral sweet solution reduces pain-related behaviour in preterm infants. *Acta Paediatr* 1996; 85:854–858.

40. Carbajal R, Chauvet X, Couderc S, Olivier-Martin M. Randomised trial of analgesic effects of sucrose, glucose, and pacifiers in term neonates. *BMJ* 1999;319:1393–1397.

41. Abad F, Diaz-Gomez NM, Domenech E, et al. Oral sucrose compares favourably with lidocaine–prilocaine cream for pain relief during venepuncture in neonates. *Acta Paediatr* 2001; 90:160–165.

42. Taddio A, Ohlsson A, Einarson TR, Stevens B, Koren G. A systematic review of lidocaine–prilocaine cream (EMLA) in the treatment of acute pain in neonates. *Pediatrics* 1998;101:E1. Search date 1996; primary sources Medline, Embase, Reference Update, and hand searches of personal files and meeting proceedings.

43. Essink-Tjebbes CM, Hekster YA, Liem KD, Van Dongen RTM. Topical use of local anesthetics in neonates. *Pharm World Sci* 1999;21:173–176. Search date 1998; primary source Medline.

44. Ramaioli F, Amice De D, Guzinska K, Ceriana P, Gasparoni A. EMLA cream and the premature infant. *Int Monitor Reg Anaesthesia* 1993;59. [Abstract]

45. Stevens B, Johnston C, Taddio A, Koren G, Aranda J. *The safety and efficacy of EMLA for heel lance in premature neonates.* International Association for the Study of Pain, 8th World Congress on Pain, Vancouver, Canada 1996;239:181–182.

46. Rushforth JA, Griffiths G, Thorpe H, Levene MI. Can topical lignocaine reduce behavioural response to heel prick? *Arch Dis Child Fetal Neonatal Ed* 1995;72:F49–F51.

47. Larsson BA, Jylli L, Lagercrantz H, Olsson GL. Does a local anaesthetic cream (EMLA) alleviate pain from heel-lancing in neonates? *Acta Anaesthesiol Scand* 1995;39:1028–1031.

48. Wester U. Analgesic effect of lidocaine ointment on intact skin in neonates. *Acta Paediatr* 1993; 82:791.

49. Larsson BA, Tannfeldt G, Lagercrantz H, Olsson GL. Alleviation of the pain of venepuncture in neonates. *Acta Paediatr* 1998;87:774–779.

50. Lindh V, Wiklund U, Hakansson S. Assessment of the effect of EMLA during venipuncture in the newborn by analysis of heart rate variability. *Pain* 2000;86:247–254.

51. Robieux I, Kumar R, Radhakrishnan S, Koren G. Assessing pain and analgesia with a lidocaine–prilocaine emulsion in infants and toddlers during venipuncture. *J Pediatr* 1991;118: 971–973.

52. Acharya AB, Bustani PC, Phillips JD, Taub NA, Beattie RM. Randomised controlled trial of eutectic mixture of local anaesthetics cream for venepuncture in healthy preterm infants. *Arch Dis Child Fetal Neonatal Ed* 1998;78:F138–F142.

53. Jain A, Rutter N. Does topical amethocaine gel reduce the pain of venepuncture in newborn infants? A randomised double blind controlled trial. *Arch Dis Child Fetal Neonatal Ed* 2000;83: F207–F210.

54. Moore J. No more tears: a randomized controlled double-blind trial of Amethocaine gel vs. placebo in the management of procedural pain in neonates. *J Adv Nurs* 2001;34:475–482.

55. Jain A, Rutter N, Ratnayaka M. Topical amethocaine gel for pain relief of heel prick blood sampling: a randomised double blind controlled trial. *Arch Dis Child Fetal Neonatal Ed* 2001;84: F56–F59.

56. Gourrier E, Karoubi P, el Hanache A, et al. Use of EMLA cream in a department of neonatology. *Pain* 1996;68:431–434.

57. Brisman M, Ljung BM, Otterbom I, Larsson LE, Andreasson SE. Methaemoglobin formation after the use of EMLA cream in term neonates. *Acta Paediatr* 1998;87:1191–1194.

58. Stevens B, Johnston C, Franck L, et al. The efficacy of developmentally sensitive interventions and sucrose for relieving procedural pain in very low birth weight neonates. *Nurs Res* 1999;48: 35–43.

59. Bo LK, Callaghan P. Soothing pain-elicited distress in Chinese neonates. *Pediatrics* 2000:105:E49.

60. Corbo MG, Mansi G, Stagni A, et al. Nonnutritive sucking during heelstick procedures decreases behavioral distress in the newborn infant. *Biol Neonate* 2000;77:162–167.

61. Field T, Goldson E. Pacifying effects of nonnutritive sucking on term and preterm neonates during heelstick procedures. *Pediatrics* 1984;74: 1012–1015.

Child health

62. Campos RG. Rocking and pacifiers: two comforting interventions for heelstick pain. *Res Nurs Health* 1994;17:321–331.

63. Gray L, Watt L, Blass EM. Skin-to-skin contact is analgesic in healthy newborns. *Pediatrics* 2000; 105(1):e14.

64. Fearon I, Kisilevsky BS, Hains SMJ, Muir DW, Tranmer J. Swaddling after heel lance: age-specific effects on behavioural recovery in preterm infants. *J Dev Behav Pediatr* 1997;18:222–232.

65. Corff KE, Seideman R, Venkataraman PS, Lutes L, Yates B. Facilitated tucking: a nonpharmacologic comfort measure for pain in preterm neonates. *J Obstet Gynecol Neonatal Nurs* 1995;24: 143–147.

66. Porter FL, Wolf CM, Miller JP. The effect of handling and immobilization on the response to acute pain in newborn infants. *Pediatrics* 1998; 102:1383–1389.

67. Barker DP, Willetts B, Cappendijk VC, Rutter N. Capillary blood sampling: should the heel be warmed? *Arch Dis Child Fetal Neonatal Ed* 1996; 74:F139–F140.

68. Vertanen H, Fellman V, Brommels M, Viinikka L. An automatic incision device for obtaining blood samples from the heels of preterm infants causes less damage than a conventional manual lancet. *Arch Dis Child Fetal Neonatal Ed* 2001;84: F53–F55.

69. Harpin VA, Rutter N. Making heel pricks less painful. *Arch Dis Child* 1983:226–228

70. Paes B, Janes M, Vegh P, LaDuca F, Andrew MA. Comparative study of heel-stick devices for infant blood collection. *Am J Dis Child* 1993;147: 346–348.

71. Cologna M, Sperandio L. The effect of two different methods of heel lancing on pain reaction in preterm neonates. *Assistenza Infermieristica e Ricerca:AIR* 1999;18:185–192.

72. Barker DP, Latty BW, Rutter N. Heel blood sampling in preterm infants: which technique? *Arch Dis Child Fetal Neonatal Ed* 1994;71: F206–F208.

73. Kellam B, Sacks LM, Waller et al. Tenderfoot Preemie vs. a manual lancet: a clinical evaluation. *Neonatal Network* 2001;20:31–36.

Linda Franck
Professor of Children's Nursing Research
King's College School of Nursing
and Midwifery
and Great Ormond Street Hospital
for Children NHS Trust
London
UK

Ruth Gilbert
Senior Lecturer in Clinical Epidemiology/Honorary Consultant Paediatrician
Centre for Evidence-Based Child Health
Institute of Child Health
London
UK

Competing interests: None declared.

Search date November 2001

David Creery and Angelo Mikrogianakis

INTERVENTIONS

Key Messages

- One non-systematic review and 11 observational studies found that campaigns involving advice to encourage non-prone sleeping positions were followed by a reduced incidence of sudden infant death syndrome (SIDS).

- One non-systematic review and three observational studies found that campaigns to reduce a number of SIDS risk factors, which included tobacco smoke exposure, were followed by a reduced incidence of SIDS.

- We found no evidence on advice to avoid soft sleeping surfaces in the prevention of SIDS.

- One non-systematic review and one observational study found that campaigns to reduce a number of SIDS risk factors, which included over wrapping, were followed by a reduced incidence of SIDS.

- One observational study found that a campaign to reduce a number of SIDS risk factors, which included advice to avoid bed sharing, was followed by a reduced incidence of SIDS.

- One non-systematic review and two observational studies found that campaigns to reduce a number of SIDS risk factors, which included advice to breast feed, were followed by a reduced incidence of SIDS.

- We found no evidence on advice to promote soother use in the prevention of SIDS.

Sudden infant death syndrome

DEFINITION Sudden infant death syndrome (SIDS) is the sudden death of an infant aged under 1 year that remains unexplained after review of the clinical history, examination of the scene of death, and post-mortem.

INCIDENCE/ PREVALENCE The incidence of SIDS has varied over time and among nations (incidence per 1000 live births of SIDS in 1996: Netherlands 0.3; Japan 0.4; Canada 0.5; England and Wales 0.7; USA 0.8; and Australia 0.9).[1]

AETIOLOGY/ RISK FACTORS By definition, the cause of SIDS is not known. Observational studies have found an association between SIDS and a number of risk factors including prone sleeping position,[2,3] prenatal or postnatal exposure to tobacco smoke,[4] soft sleeping surfaces,[5,6] hyperthermia/overwrapping (see web extra tables A, B, and C at www.clinicalevidence.com),[7,8] bed sharing (particularly with mothers who smoke),[9,10] lack of breastfeeding,[11,12] and soother use (see glossary, p 134).[7,13]

PROGNOSIS Although by definition prognosis is not applicable for an affected infant, the incidence of SIDS is increased in the siblings of that infant.[14,15]

AIMS To reduce the incidence of SIDS, with minimal adverse effects from interventions.

OUTCOMES The incidence of SIDS; the adverse effects of interventions, measured directly or by quality of life questionnaires.

METHODS *Clinical Evidence* search and appraisal November 2001.

QUESTION **What are the effects of interventions to reduce the risk of sudden infant death syndrome?**

OPTION **ADVICE TO AVOID PRONE SLEEPING**

One non-systematic review and 11 observational studies found that campaigns involving advice to encourage non-prone sleeping positions were followed by a reduced incidence of sudden infant death syndrome.

Benefits: **Randomised studies:** We found no systematic review and no RCTs comparing advice to avoid prone sleeping positions (see glossary, p 134) versus no such advice (see comment below). **Observational studies following national advice campaigns:** We found one non-systematic review (3 observational studies, one of which has also been reported separately[16]),[12] and 11 additional observational studies following national advice campaigns (see comment below).[9,17–27] The review and additional observational studies describe eight campaigns that delivered advice to avoid prone positioning alone (see table 1, p 136),[17-19,21,22,24-26] and six campaigns that provided advice to avoid a combination of different risk factors including prone positioning (see table 2, p 137).[9,12,16,20,23,27] The review and additional observational studies all found that the incidence of sudden infant death syndrome (SIDS) was reduced following the campaigns (see table 1, p 136 and table 2, p 137). One of the additional observational studies found that the incidence of prone positioning decreased significantly following the campaign (from 54% before campaign to 5% after campaign; P < 0.001).[27]

Harms: No frequencies of adverse effects of non-prone positioning were reported in 12 observational studies of advice to avoid prone sleeping.[9,12,16–27] One study found no increase in the risk of inhaling vomitus associated with non-prone positioning.[26] Two observational studies have documented a temporal relationship between advice to avoid prone sleeping and an increase in the incidence of occipital plagiocephaly without synostosis (see glossary, p 134), whereas the incidence of other forms of plagiocephaly with synostosis remained constant.[28,29]

Comment: The review of SIDS risk factor reduction campaigns in Norway, Denmark, and Sweden reported that the campaign in Norway provided advice to avoid prone sleeping plus advice to avoid tobacco smoke exposure.[12] However, the original paper describing the Norwegian campaign reported that this campaign only provided advice to avoid prone sleeping.[16] One of the additional observational studies reported that the incidence of SIDS was declining before the campaign started and, hence, the reduction attributable to advice provided by the campaign is not clear.[9,20] A second additional observational study did not report how advice was provided, exactly which SIDS risk factors were targeted, and did not describe details of the advice given to avoid exposure to cigarette smoke (i.e. prenatally, postnatally or both; maternal smoking alone or smoking by other household members as well).[23] A third additional observational study did not specify whether the advice to stop smoking was given to mothers or other family members and what advice was given regarding the avoidance of over heating.[27] Systematic reviews of observational studies have found an association between prone sleeping position and an increased risk of SIDS, leading to the initiation of non-prone sleep campaigns in several countries.[2,3] RCTs investigating the effects of advice to avoid prone positioning may be considered unethical given the existing observational evidence; they would also be difficult to conduct given the extremely large units of randomisation required and the high level of public awareness regarding the risks of prone positioning for sleep.

OPTION   **ADVICE TO AVOID TOBACCO SMOKE EXPOSURE**

One non-systematic review and three observational studies found that campaigns to reduce a number of sudden infant death syndrome risk factors, which included tobacco smoke exposure, were followed by a reduced incidence of sudden infant death syndrome.

Benefits: **Randomised studies:** We found no systematic review and no RCTs comparing advice to avoid tobacco smoke exposure versus no such advice (see comment below). **Observational studies following national advice campaigns:** We found one non-systematic review (3 observational studies, one of which has also been reported separately[16]),[12] and three additional observational studies following national advice campaigns (see table 2, p 137).[9,20,23,27] The review and additional observational studies found that the campaigns were all followed by a reduced incidence of sudden infant death syndrome during the data collection periods (see table 2, p 137). However, the campaigns included advice in addition to the avoidance of tobacco smoke exposure, and in some countries the incidence of sudden infant death syndrome had started to fall before the campaign started (see comment under advice to avoid prone sleeping, p 131). The first additional observational study found that the population attributable risk (see glossary, p 134) for sudden infant death syndrome associated with maternal smoking alone was 44% (prevalence 19%; OR 5.17), and for maternal smoking plus bed sharing was 33% (prevalence 5%; OR 11.1). The third additional observational study found that the percentage of mothers not smoking during pregnancy increased significantly following the campaign (from 77% before campaign to 82% after campaign; P < 0.01).[27]

Harms: We found no evidence on harms associated with a reduction in infant tobacco smoke exposure.

Comment: The sudden infant death syndrome reduction attributable to a reduction in maternal smoking is unclear. RCTs investigating the effects of advice to reduce infant tobacco smoke exposure would be difficult to conduct given the extremely large units of randomisation required and the high level of public awareness regarding the risks of tobacco smoke exposure.

OPTION   ADVICE TO AVOID SOFT SLEEPING SURFACES

We found no evidence on advice to avoid soft sleeping surfaces in the prevention of sudden infant death syndrome.

Benefits: We found no systematic review, RCTs, or observational studies (see comment below).

Harms: We found no evidence on harms associated with advice to avoid soft sleeping surfaces.

Comment: RCTs investigating the effects of advice to avoid soft sleeping surfaces would be difficult to conduct given the extremely large units of randomisation required.

OPTION   ADVICE TO AVOID OVER HEATING OR OVER WRAPPING

One non-systematic review and one observational study found that campaigns to reduce a number of sudden infant death syndrome risk factors, which included over wrapping, were followed by a reduced incidence of sudden infant death syndrome.

Benefits: **Randomised studies:** We found no systematic review and no RCTs comparing advice to avoid over heating or over wrapping (see glossary, p 134) versus no such advice (see comment below). **Observational studies following national advice campaigns:** We found one non-systematic review (3 observational studies, one of which has also been reported separately[16]),[12] and one additional observational study following national advice campaigns (see table 2, p 137).[27] Two of the national advice campaigns reported in the review and the additional observational study provided advice to avoid over heating or over wrapping plus advice to avoid other sudden infant death syndrome risk factors (see comment under advice to avoid prone sleeping, p 131).[12,27] The third campaign reported by the review did not provide advice on over heating or over wrapping.[12,16] The review and additional observational study found that the campaigns were all followed by a reduction in the incidence of sudden infant death syndrome during the data collection periods (see table 2, p 137).

Harms: We found no evidence on harms associated with advice to avoid over heating or over wrapping.

Comment: RCTs investigating the effects of advice to avoid over heating or over wrapping would be difficult to conduct given the extremely large units of randomisation required.

OPTION   ADVICE TO AVOID BED SHARING

One observational study found that a campaign to reduce a number of sudden infant death syndrome risk factors, which included advice to avoid bed sharing, was followed by a reduced incidence of sudden infant death syndrome.

Benefits: **Randomised studies:** We found no systematic review and no RCTs comparing advice to avoid bed sharing versus no such advice (see comment below). **Observational studies following national advice campaigns:** We found one observational study, which reported the results of a national campaign that provided advice to avoid bed sharing, to avoid prone sleeping (see glossary, p 134), to avoid exposing infants to tobacco smoke from any source either during pregnancy or for the first year of life, and to breast feed if possible (see comment below) (see table 2, p 137).[9,20] The observational study found that the incidence of sudden infant death syndrome reduced following the campaign, (see table 2, p 137) and that the population attributable risk (see glossary, p 134) for sudden infant death syndrome associated with maternal smoking plus bed sharing was 33% (prevalence 4.8%; OR 11.1).

Harms: We found no evidence on harms associated with advice to avoid bed sharing.

Comment: The observational study reported that advice to avoid bed sharing was introduced after the main campaign had started.[9,20] The study also reported that the incidence of sudden infant death syndrome was declining before the campaign started and, hence, the reduction attributable to advice provided by the campaign is not clear. RCTs investigating the effects of advice to avoid bed sharing would be difficult to conduct given the extremely large units of randomisation required.

OPTION   ADVICE TO BREAST FEED

One non-systematic review and two observational studies found that campaigns to reduce a number of sudden infant death syndrome risk factors, which included advice to breast feed, were followed by a reduced incidence of sudden infant death syndrome.

Sudden infant death syndrome

Benefits: **Randomised evidence:** We found no systematic review and no RCTs comparing advice to encourage breast feeding versus no such advice in order to reduce the incidence of sudden infant death syndrome (see comment below). **Observational studies following national advice campaigns:** We found one non-systematic review (3 observational studies, one of which has also been reported separately[16]),[12] and two additional observational studies following national advice campaigns (see table 2, p 137).[9,20,27] The review and additional observational studies found that the campaigns were all followed by a reduced incidence of sudden infant death syndrome during the data collection periods (see table 2, p 137). However, the campaigns included advice other than advice to encourage breast feeding, and in some countries the incidence of sudden infant death syndrome had started to fall before the campaign started (see comment under advice to avoid tobacco smoke exposure, p 132). The second additional observational study found that the incidence of no breastfeeding decreased significantly following the campaign (from 21% before campaign to 7% after campaign; $P < 0.001$).[27]

Harms: We found no evidence on harms associated with advice to encourage breast feeding.

Comment: RCTs investigating the effects of promotion of breast feeding would be unethical given the evidence of benefits associated with breast feeding.

| OPTION | ADVICE TO PROMOTE SOOTHER USE |

We found no evidence on advice to promote soother use in the prevention of sudden infant death syndrome.

Benefits: We found no systematic review, RCT, or observational studies (see comment below).

Harms: We found no evidence on harms associated with advice to promote soother use (see glossary, p 134).

Comment: RCTs investigating the effects of advice to promote soother use would be difficult to conduct given the extremely large units of randomisation required.

GLOSSARY

Occipital plagiocephaly with/without synostosis Flattening of the occipital bone with/without a malformation of the corresponding cranial suture line.

Over wrapping Wrapping/bundling of infants in excessive amounts of clothing or bedding as to result in sweating and/or significantly raised core temperatures.

Population attributable risk A measure of the disease rate in exposed people compared with that in unexposed people, multiplied by the prevalence of exposure to the risk factor in the population.

Prone sleeping Sleeping on one's front.

Soother (dummy, pacifier) An object placed in the infant's mouth for the sole purpose of providing comfort.

REFERENCES

1. Canadian Bureau of Reproductive and Child Health / Laboratory Centre for Disease Control / Canadian Perinatal Surveillance System (CPSS); Fact sheet: http://www.hc-sc.gc.ca/hpb/lcdc/brch/factshts/sids_e.html

2. Beal SM, Finch CF. An overview of retrospective case-control studies investigating the relationship between prone sleeping position and SIDS. *J Paediatr Child Health* 1991;27:334–339.

3. American Academy of Pediatrics AAP Task Force on Infant Positioning and SIDS. Positioning and SIDS. *Pediatrics* 1992;89(6 pt 1):1120–1126.

4. Anderson HR, Cook DG. Passive smoking and sudden infant death syndrome: review of the epidemiological evidence. *Thorax* 1997;52:1003–1009.

5. Mitchell EA, Thompson JM, Ford RP, Taylor BJ. Sheepskin bedding and the sudden infant death syndrome. New Z Cot Death Study Group. *J Pediatr* 1998;133:701–704.

6. Ponsonby AL, Dwyer T, Gibbons LE, Cochrane JA, Wang YG. Factors potentiating the risk of sudden infant death syndrome associated with the prone position. *N Engl J Med* 1993;329:377–382.

7. Fleming PJ, Blair PS, Bacon C, et al. Environment of infants during sleep and risk of the sudden infant death syndrome: results of the 1993–5 case-control study for confidential enquiry into stillbirths and deaths on infancy. Confidential Enquiry into Stillbirths and Deaths Regional Coordinators and Researchers. *BMJ* 1997;313:85–89.

8. Ponsonby AL, Dwyer T, Gibbons LE, Cochrane JA, Jones ME, McCall MJ. Thermal environment and sudden infant death syndrome: case-control study. *BMJ* 1992;304:277–282.

9. Mitchell EA, Tuohy PG, Brunt JM, et al. Risk factors for sudden infant death syndrome following the prevention campaign in New Zealand: a prospective study. *Pediatrics* 1997;100:835–840.

10. Scragg R, Mitchell EA, Taylor BJ, et al. Bed sharing, smoking, and alcohol in the sudden infant death syndrome. New Zealand Cot Death Study Group. *BMJ* 1993;307:1312–1318.

11. Mitchell EA, Taylor BJ, Ford RP, Stewart AW, Becroft DM, Thompson JM, et al. Four modifiable and other major risk factors for cot death: the New Zealand study. *J Paediatr Child Health* 1992;28(suppl 1):S3–S8.

12. Wennergren G, Alm B, Oyen N, et al. The decline in the incidence of SIDS in Scandinavia and its relation to risk-intervention campaigns. Nordic Epidemiological SIDS Study. *Acta Paediatrica* 1997;86:963–968.

13. L'Hoir MP, Engelberts AC, van Well GT, et al. Risk and preventive factors for cot death in The Netherlands, a low-incidence country. *Eur J Pediatr* 1998;157:681–688.

14. Oyen N, Skjaerven R, Irgens LM. Population-based recurrence risk of sudden

15. infant death syndrome compared with other infant and fetal deaths. *Am J Epidemiol* 1996;144:300–305.

16. Guntheroth WG, Lohmann R, Spiers PS. Risk of sudden infant death syndrome in

17. subsequent siblings. *J Pediatr* 1990;116:520–524.

18. Haaland K, Thoresen M. Crib death, sleeping position and temperature. *Tidsskr Nor Laegeforen* 1992;112:1466–1470. [Norwegian].

19. Schellscheidt J, Ott A, Jorch G. Epidemiological features of sudden infant death after a German intervention campaign in 1992. *Eur J Pediatr* 1997;156:655–660.

20. Skadberg BT, Morild I, Markestad T. Abandoning prone sleeping: Effect on the risk of sudden infant death syndrome. *J Pediatr* 1998;132:340–343.

21. Wigfield RE, Fleming PJ, Berry PJ, Rudd PT, Golding J. Can the fall in Avon's sudden infant death rate be explained by changes in sleeping position? *BMJ* 1992;304:282–283.

22. Mitchell EA, Aley P, Eastwood J. The national cot death prevention program in New Zealand. *Aust J Public Health* 16:158–161.

23. Markestad T, Skadberg B, Hordvik E, Morild I, Irgens LM. Sleeping position and sudden infant death syndrome (SIDS): effect of an intervention programme to avoid prone sleeping. *Acta Paediatr* 1995;84:375–378.

24. Vege A, Rognum TO, Opdal SH. SIDS – Changes in the epidemiological pattern in Eastern Norway 1984–1996. *Forensic Sci Int* 1998;93:155–166.

25. Adams EJ, Chavez GF, Steen D, Shah R, Iyasu S, Krous HF. Changes in the epidemiologic profile of sudden infant death syndrome as rates decline among California infants: 1990–1995. *Pediatrics* 1998;102:1445–1451.

26. Mitchell EA, Ford RP, Taylor BJ, et al. Further evidence supporting a causal relationship between prone sleeping position and SIDS. *J Paediatr Child Health* 1992;28(suppl 1):S9–12.

27. Dwyer T, Ponsonby AL, Blizzard L, Newman NM, Cochrane JA. The contribution of changes in the prevalence of prone sleeping position to the decline in sudden infant death syndrome in Tasmania. *JAMA* 1995;273:783–789.

28. Spiers PS, Guntheroth WG. Recommendations to avoid the prone sleeping position and recent statistics for sudden infant death syndrome in the United States. *Arch Pediatr Adolesc Med* 1994;148:141–146.

29. Kiechl-Kohlendorfer U, Peglow UP, Kiechl S, Oberaigner W, Sperl W. Epidemiology of sudden infant death syndrome (SIDS) in the Tyrol before and after an intervention campaign. *Wien Klin Wochenschr* 2001;113:27–32.

David Creery

Angelo Mikrogianakis

Children's Hospital of Eastern Ontario
Ottawa
Canada

Competing interests: None declared.

TABLE 1 Observational studies following national campaigns providing advice to avoid prone sleeping positions (see text, p 130–134).

Country/reference	Dissemination	SIDS incidence/1000 live births (95% CI)		Number of infants	Risk of prone sleeping after campaign (95% CI)
		From	To		
Germany (West) North Rhine Westphalia[17]	Not specified	1.56 2.17	0.92 1.33	59 cases, 156 controls	OR 11.7 (5.3 to 26.2)
Norway[18]	Health professional education Media campaign	3.5 (2.64 to 4.36)	0.3 (0.05 to 0.54)	6 cases, 493 controls	OR 42.0 (5 to 390)
UK, Avon[19]	Maternal education Health professional education	3.5	1.7	32 cases, 70 controls 152 population based controls	NA
Norway/Hordaland[21]	Health professional education Media campaign	3.5	1.6	30 cases, 123 controls	OR 11.3 (3.6 to 36.5)
Norway[22]	Health professional education Media campaign	2	0.6	200 cases	NA
New Zealand[24]	Maternal education Health professional education Media campaign	4	3.1	485 cases, 1800 controls	NA
Australia[25]	Maternal education Health professional education	3.8 (3.5 to 4.2)	1.5 (0.9 to 2.2)	449 cases	NA
USA[26]	Media campaign	2.36	2.02	233 cases	NA

SIDS, sudden infant death syndrome; NA, not available.

TABLE 2 Observational studies following national campaigns providing advice to avoid a number of sudden infant death syndrome risk factors including prone sleeping positions (see text, p 130–134).

Country/year of start	Data collection	Advice to: avoid or [encourage]	Dissemination	SIDS incidence/1000 live births (95% CI)		Number of infants	Risk (95% CI)
				From	To		
Norway 1989[12,16]	1992–1995	prone sleeping	Newspapers National media broadcasts Midwives Other healthcare professionals Presentation at a SIDS prevention conference	2.3	0.6	244 cases 869 controls	Adjusted OR prone sleeping 5.4 (2.8 to 10.5)
Denmark 1991[12]	1992–1995	prone sleeping tobacco smoke over wrapping	Not described	1.6	0.2	244 cases 869 controls	Adjusted OR prone sleeping 5.4 (2.8 to 10.5)
Sweden 1992[12]	1992–1995	prone sleeping tobacco smoke over wrapping [breastfeeding]	Not described	1.0	0.4		

TABLE 2   continued

| Country/year of start | Data collection | Advice to: avoid or [encourage] | Dissemination | SIDS incidence/1000 live births (95% CI) | | Number of infants | Risk (95% CI) |
				From	To		
New Zealand 1990[9,20]	1991–1993	*prone sleeping* *tobacco smoke (any source; during pregnancy/first year of life)* *bed sharing* *[breastfeeding]*	Parents antenatal classes Postnatal wards Healthcare professionals Conferences Journals Public newspapers TV programmes	4.1	2.1	127 cases 922 controls	Not reported
California, 1990–1995[23]		*prone sleeping* *cigarette smoking*	Public	2.69 (black infants) 1.04 (other infants)	2.15 (black infants) 0.61 (other infants)	3508 cases	Not reported
Austria 1994–1995[27]		*prone sleeping* *smoking* *over heating* *[breastfeeding]*	Parents antenatal classes, maternity wards, routine health checks Public newspapers Radio/TV	1984–1994: 1.83	1995: 0.4 1996–1998 unchanged	160 cases	Not reported

SIDS, sudden infant death syndrome.

INTERVENTIONS

PREVENTION
Likely to be beneficial
Prophylactic antibiotics after first or
    subsequent urinary tract
    infection 143
Immunotherapy 144

Unlikely to be beneficial
Surgical correction of minor
    functional anomalies 145
Surgical correction of moderate
    to severe vesicoureteric reflux
    (similar benefits to medical
    management) 145

INVESTIGATION
Unlikely to be beneficial
Routine diagnostic imaging in all
    children with first urinary tract
    infection 143

TREATMENT
Beneficial
7–10 days of antibiotics (better
    than shorter courses) 142

Likely to be beneficial
Oral (rather than intravenous)
    antibiotics for acute treatment of
    children 2 years or younger with
    normal renal tracts or mild
    vesicoureteric reflux 142

Unknown effectiveness
Giving early empirical antibiotic
    treatment instead of awaiting the
    results of microscopy or
    culture 141
Oral (rather than intravenous)
    antibiotics for the acute
    treatment of children 2 years or
    younger with moderate or severe
    vesicoureteric reflux 142

See glossary, p 146

Key Messages

- Antibiotic treatment is accepted clinical practice in children with acute urinary tract infection (UTI), and placebo controlled trials are considered unethical.

- We found little evidence on the effects of delaying treatment while results of microscopy or culture are awaited. Five retrospective studies found that medium to long term delays (4 days to 7 years) in treatment may be associated with an increased risk of renal scarring, but we found inconclusive evidence that shorter delays cause harm.

- Two RCTs have found higher cure rates (eradication of causative organism) with antibiotic treatment for 7 days or longer versus shorter courses.

- One RCT found no significant evidence of a difference between oral and intravenous antibiotics for acute treatment in children under the age of 2 years with an uncomplicated first UTI.

Urinary tract infection

- We found no evidence of benefit from routine diagnostic imaging of all children with a first UTI. We found indirect evidence suggesting that children at increased risk of morbidity may benefit from investigation.

- Two small RCTs found limited evidence that prophylactic antibiotic therapy (co-trimoxazole or nitrofurantoin) prevented recurrent UTI in children, particularly during the period of prophylaxis. We found inadequate evaluation of the long term benefits of prophylaxis, even in children with vesicoureteric reflux. We found insufficient evidence to comment on the optimum duration of prophylaxis.

- One systematic review has found that, in premature and in low birth weight neonates, intravenous immunoglobulins reduce the occurrence of serious infections, including UTIs.

- One RCT has found that an immunotherapeutic agent, pidotomid, reduces UTI recurrence in children.

- One systematic review and a later RCT found no evidence of differences between surgical and medical management (prophylactic antibiotic therapy) of vesicoureteric reflux in the prevention of recurrence of UTI or complications from UTI.

DEFINITION UTI is defined by the presence of a pure growth of more than 10^5 colony forming units of bacteria per ml. Lower counts of bacteria may be clinically important, especially in boys and in specimens obtained by urinary catheter. Any growth of typical urinary pathogens is considered clinically important if obtained by suprapubic aspiration. In practice, three age ranges are usually considered on the basis of differential risk and different approaches to management: children under 1 year; young children (1–4, 5, or 7 years, depending on the information source); and older children (up to 12–16 years). Recurrent UTI is defined as a further infection by a new organism. Relapsing UTI is defined as a further infection with the same organism.

INCIDENCE/ PREVALENCE Boys are more susceptible before the age of 3 months; thereafter the incidence is substantially higher in girls. Estimates of the true incidence of UTI depend on rates of diagnosis and investigation. At least 8% of girls and 2% of boys will have a UTI in childhood.[1]

AETIOLOGY/ RISK FACTORS The normal urinary tract is sterile. Contamination by bowel flora may result in urinary infection if a virulent organism is involved or if the child is immunosuppressed. In neonates, infection may originate from other sources. *Escherichia coli* accounts for about three quarters of all pathogens. *Proteus* is more common in boys (about 30% of infections). Obstructive anomalies are found in 0–4% and vesicoureteric reflux in 8–40% of children being investigated for their first UTI.[2] Although vesicoureteric reflux is a major risk factor for adverse outcome, other as yet unidentified triggers may also need to be present.

PROGNOSIS After first infection, about half of girls have a further infection in the first year and three quarters within 2 years.[3] We found no figures for boys, but a review suggests that recurrences are common under 1 year of age but rare subsequently.[4] Renal scarring occurs in 5–15% of children within 1–2 years of their first UTI, although 32–70% of these scars are noted at the time of initial assessment.[2] The incidence of renal scarring rises with each episode of infection in childhood.[5] An RCT comparing oral versus intravenous antibiotics found retrospectively that new renal scarring after a first UTI was more common in children with vesicoureteric reflux than in children without reflux (logistic regression model: AR of scarring 16/107 [15.0%] with reflux v 10/165 [6%] without reflux; RR 2.47, 95% CI 1.17 to 5.24).[6] A study (287 children with severe vesicoureteral reflux treated either medically or surgically for any UTI) evaluated the risk of renal scarring with serial DMSA (see glossary, p 146) scintigraphy over 5 years. It found that younger children (under 2 years) were at greater risk of renal scarring than older children regardless of treatment allocation for the infection (AR for deterioration in DMSA scan over 5 years 21/86 for younger children v 27/201 for older children; RR 1.82, 95% CI 1.09 to 3.03).[7] Renal scarring is associated with future complications: poor renal growth; recurrent adult pyelonephritis; impaired glomerular function; early hypertension; and end stage renal failure.[8–11] A combination of recurrent urinary infection, severe vesicoureteric reflux, and the presence of renal scarring at first presentation is associated with the worst prognosis.

AIMS	To relieve acute symptoms; to eliminate infection; and to prevent recurrence, renal damage, and long term complications.
OUTCOMES	**Short term:** clinical symptoms and signs (dysuria, frequency, fever); urine culture; incidence of new renal scars. **Long term:** incidence of recurrent infection; prevalence of renal scarring; renal size and growth; renal function; prevalence of hypertension and renal failure.
METHODS	*Clinical Evidence* search and appraisal May 2001.

QUESTION **What are the effects of treatment of acute urinary tract infection in children?**

Placebo controlled trials of antibiotics for symptomatic acute UTI in children are considered unethical. We found little evidence on the effects of giving early empirical treatment versus awaiting the results of microscopy or culture. Five retrospective studies found that delayed treatment may be associated with increased rates of renal scarring, but we found inconclusive evidence on the effects of shorter delays. Two RCTs have found higher cure rate (eradication of causative organism) with antibiotic treatment for 7 days or longer versus shorter courses. One RCT found no significant evidence of a difference between oral and intravenous antibiotics for acute treatment in children under the age of 2 years with an uncomplicated first UTI.

Benefits: **Versus placebo:** We found no RCTs. **Immediate empirical versus delayed treatment:** We found no RCTs comparing immediate empirical treatment versus treatment delayed while microscopy or culture results are awaited. Five retrospective observational studies found increased rates of scarring in children in whom diagnosis was delayed between 4 days (in acute UTI) to 7 years (when a child presented with chronic non-specific symptoms).[2] We found one RCT that compared oral cefixime for 14 days (double dose on day 1) versus intravenous cefotaxime for 3 days plus oral cefixime for 11 days for UTI in children under 2 years (see below). It found no evidence that children treated 24 hours after the onset of fever were at greater risk of renal scarring than children presenting within 24 hours (9/99 [9%] of children presenting before 24 h developed scarring v 19/159 [12%] of children presenting later; RR 1.3, 95% CI 0.6 to 2.7; P = 0.29). However, this incidental analysis was done retrospectively.[6] **Long versus short courses:** We found one systematic review (search date not stated, 14 RCTs) comparing short course (single dose to 4 days) versus longer courses (7–10 days) of a range of antibiotics.[12] It found two RCTs that were adequately powered to find an effect. One RCT (49 children) compared amoxicillin single dose versus 10 day regimen, and the other RCT compared cefadroxil 1 day versus 10 day regimen.[13,14] Both RCTs found that longer courses cured (eradication of causative organism on 4 days' follow up culture) significantly more children (results from the higher quality RCT:[13] AR of failure to cure 14/38 [37%] with short course v 2/27 [8%] with long course; ARI short v long course 29%; RR 4.6; no 95% CI provided; P < 0.01). The remaining 12 RCTs found no significant difference between long versus short courses but were too small to rule out a clinically important difference (see comment below). We found no RCTs comparing 5 day courses of antibiotics with other regimens. **Oral versus intravenous antibiotics:** We found one RCT (309 children, age ≤ 2 years, fever > 38.2 °C, first UTI confirmed from catheter specimen), which compared oral cefixime for 14 days (double dose on day 1) versus intravenous cefotaxime for 3 days plus 11 days of oral cefixime.[6] It found no significant difference between treatments in mean duration of fever (24.7 h with oral treatment v 23.9 h with iv; P = 0.76), re-infection rate (132/153 [86.3%] with oral treatment v 134/153 [87.6%] with iv treatment; P = 0.28), incidence of renal scarring (intention to treat analysis: 15/153 [10%] with oral treatment [21 children not scanned and counted as having no scarring] v 11/153 [7%] with iv treatment [13 children not scanned]; P = 0.21), and mean extent of scarring (8% of renal parenchyma with oral treatment v 9% with iv treatment).

Harms: **Long versus short courses:** The studies did not report comparative harms for long versus short courses of antibiotics nor for immediate versus delayed treatment. **Oral versus intravenous antibiotics:** One RCT found weak evidence from a post hoc subgroup analysis in children with grade III–IV reflux (see glossary, p 146) that renal scarring at 6 months may be more common with oral versus intravenous treatment (new renal scarring within 6 months: 8/24 [33%] after oral antibiotics v 1/22 [5%] after iv antibiotics; ARI 29%, 95% CI 8% to 49%; NNH 3, 95% CI 2 to 13).[6]

Comment: **Versus placebo:** Placebo controlled trials would be considered unethical because there is a strong consensus that antibiotics are likely to be beneficial. The improved response seen with longer versus shorter courses of antibiotics is indirect evidence that antibiotics are likely to be more effective than no treatment. **Long versus short courses:** The systematic review comparing long versus short courses of antibiotics rigorously evaluated the methods of the included studies. It found that few studies accounted for confounding factors such as age, sex, and previous UTI. Those that considered these did so by selecting one subgroup only and not by stratifying children according to these factors. This limits the generalisability of the results. The 12 trials that found no evidence of a difference between long and short courses were too small to exclude a clinically important effect. **Oral versus intravenous antibiotics:** The trial comparing oral versus intravenous antibiotics excluded three of 309 children because investigators considered that the severity of symptoms in these children warranted intravenous treatment.[6]

QUESTION **Which children benefit from diagnostic imaging?**

We found no evidence of benefit from routine diagnostic imaging of all children with a first UTI. We found indirect evidence suggesting that subgroups at increased risk of morbidity may benefit from investigation.

Benefits: We found no RCTs. One systematic review (search date 1994, 63 descriptive studies) found no direct evidence that routine diagnostic imaging in children with UTI was effective.[2] The quality of studies was generally poor, and none included clinically important long term outcome measures.

Harms: The studies reported no evidence of harms. Potential harms include those relating to radiation, invasive procedures, and allergic reactions to contrast media.

Comment: Subgroups of children at high risk of morbidity, including those with vesicoureteric reflux, may benefit from early investigation.[2] However, it may be difficult to identify such children clinically.[15] One prospective study found that the highest rates of renal scarring after pyelonephritis occurred between 1 and 5 years of age.[16] A further study found that presentation with pyelonephritic symptoms in children of all ages is associated with high rates of renal abnormalities (abnormal initial scans in 34/65 [52%] children).[17]

QUESTION **What are the effects of preventive interventions?**

OPTION **PROPHYLACTIC ANTIBIOTICS**

We found limited evidence from two small RCTs that prophylactic antibiotics (co-trimoxazole or nitrofurantoin) reduced UTI recurrence in children, particularly during the period of prophylaxis. We found inadequate evaluation of the long term benefits of prophylaxis, even in children with vesicoureteric reflux. We found insufficient evidence to comment on the optimum duration of prophylaxis.

Benefits: **Versus no prophylaxis:** We found one systematic review (search date 1999,[18] 2 RCTs,[19,3] 40 children without a neurogenic bladder — see glossary, p 146), which compared antibiotics versus no antibiotics to prevent UTIs. The first RCT (double blind, crossover trial, 18 girls [1 with vesicoureteric reflux], age 3–13 years) found fewer episodes of infection while taking antibiotics (nitrofurantoin) than while not taking antibiotics (2 episodes in 1 year with antibiotics v 35 without antibiotics; $P < 0.01$).[19] The second RCT (40 girls and 5 boys, first or subsequent acute UTI, radiologically normal urinary tracts, no vesicoureteric reflux) compared 10 months' treatment with prophylactic antibiotics (co-trimoxazole — see glossary, p 146, or nitrofurantoin) versus no treatment.[3] During the prophylaxis period, recurrent UTIs were less frequent in the intervention group (AR 0/25 [0%] with antibiotics v 11/22 [50%] with control; ARR 50%, 95% CI 26% to 74%). Twelve months after stopping prophylactic antibiotics, fewer children from the intervention group had experienced a UTI compared with those in the control group (AR 32% v 64%; ARR +27%, 95% CI −1.8% to +47%). **Duration of prophylaxis:** We found no RCTs evaluating the optimum length of prophylaxis even in children with vesicoureteric reflux (although 2 studies of prolonged acute treatment were identified).[20]

Harms: Potential harms include those of using long term antibiotics. In one study, although gut flora were affected by treatment, *E coli* cultured from rectal swabs from 70% of children remained sensitive to the prophylactic antibiotic (co-trimoxazole).[21]

Comment: The systematic review was thorough, but both RCTs that it identified had weak methods.[18] One was a crossover study that did not include a washout period and did not report separately the results for the period before the crossover.[19] The other RCT was not blinded, the control group received no treatment, and no criteria were given for the diagnosis of a UTI.[3] It may not be possible clinically to identify children who are at high risk of recurrent UTIs and long term damage.[22] Routine prophylaxis until the results of investigations are known may, therefore, be warranted, but we found no good evidence about the benefits or harms of antibiotic prophylaxis. The systematic review also found three other RCTs of antibiotic prophylaxis in children with a neurogenic bladder.[18]

OPTION   IMMUNOTHERAPY

One systematic review has found that, in premature and in low birth weight neonates, intravenous immunoglobulins reduce the occurrence of serious infections, including UTIs. One RCT has found that an immunotherapeutic agent, pidotomid, reduces UTI recurrence in children.

Benefits: **Intravenous immunoglobulin:** We found one systematic review (search date 1997, 15 RCTs), which compared intravenous immunoglobulin (see glossary, p 146) prophylaxis with placebo or no treatment.[23] It found that immunoglobulin prophylaxis significantly reduced serious infections, including UTIs, in preterm and in low birth weight neonates (RR 0.80, 95% CI 0.68 to 0.94; NNT 24, 95% CI 15 to 83).[23] The dose varied from 120 mg/kg to 1 g/kg. The number of treatments varied from one to seven. The specific effect on UTIs was not reported. **Other immunotherapeutic agents:** We found one RCT (60 children with recurrent UTIs) comparing pidotomid versus placebo.[24] It found that pidotomid reduced recovery time (recovery time 9.6 days with pidotomid v 12.3 days with placebo; P = 0.001) and recurrence rate for UTIs (RR recurrence 0.31). An open pilot study (40 children) compared nitrofurantoin with an antigenic extract of *E coli*.[25] No significant difference was found between the two treatments during active treatment or during the subsequent 6 months.

Harms: Parenteral treatment can cause pain, and there is an unquantified risk from the administration of blood products.[23] **Intravenous**

immunoglobulin: The systematic review found that prophylactic use of intravenous immunoglobulin was not associated with any short term serious adverse effects.[23] **Other immunotherapeutic agents:** In the RCT of pidotomid, the only adverse effects recorded were thought to be attributable to concomitant antibiotic therapy.[24] The open pilot study found no significant difference in withdrawal rates between the antigenic extract of E coli (1/22) and nitrofurantoin (1/18).[25]

Comment: **Intravenous immunoglobulin:** We found no evidence for or against the suggestion that preparations with specific antibodies against common pathogens are more beneficial.[26] The greatest benefits were noted in units with higher nosocomial infection rates (see glossary, p 146). It remains unclear whether intravenous immunoglobulin is only justified where infection control policies have failed to reduce the infection rate.[23] Preterm and low birth weight neonates might have greater immune deficiency than other neonates and might be expected to gain more from treatment with immunoglobulin. **Other immunotherapeutic agents:** The pidotomid study is being translated.[24] We also found one non-randomised age matched study in 10 otherwise healthy girls (aged 5–11 years) with recurrent UTI who were given intramuscular injections of inactivated uropathogenic bacteria (Solco-Urovac preparation). It found that the girls who had received the inactivated uropathogenic bacteria had significantly reduced frequency of subsequent UTI compared with 10 other age matched girls with UTI who had not received the inactivated bacteria preparation.[27] This study is limited by its non-randomised design and small sample size.

OPTION   **SURGICAL CORRECTION FOR ANOMALIES OBSTRUCTING MICTURITION**

We found no good studies evaluating surgical correction.

Benefits: We found no systematic review or RCTs.

Harms: Potential harms include the usual risks of surgery.

Comment: One small prospective study (271 children) suggested that children with minor anomalies do not develop renal scarring and therefore may not benefit from surgery.[28] Renal scars were present in more children with moderate degrees of vesicoureteric reflux than in children with minor anomalies (8/20 [40%] v 0/6 [0%]). In the presence of major anomalies, the prevention of UTIs is not the prime motive of surgical intervention.

OPTION   **SURGICAL CORRECTION FOR VESICOURETERIC REFLUX**

One systematic review and a later multicentre RCT found that, although surgery abolished reflux, there was no significant difference between surgery and medical management (prophylactic antibiotics) in the prevention of recurrence or complications from UTIs. We found no evidence on the long term effects of surgical versus medical treatment for clinical outcomes.

Benefits: **Versus medical management:** We found one systematic review[29] and one subsequent RCT.[30] The systematic review (search date 1988, 4 RCTs, 830 children with moderate/severe grade III–V vesicoureteric reflux — see glossary, p 146) compared surgical correction versus medical management (continuous prophylactic antibiotics).[29] It found that surgery abolished reflux, but found no significant differences in rates of subsequent UTIs, renal function, incidence of new renal scars, hypertension, or end stage renal failure among groups over a period of 6 months to 5 years. The subsequent RCT (132 children) found that surgery versus medical management reduced the incidence of pyelonephritis (pyelonephritis in 5/64 [8%] with surgery v 15/68 [22%] treated medically; ARR 14%, 95% CI 2% to 19%; RRR 65%, 95% CI 10% to 87%), although it found no significant difference in overall clinical outcome.[30] **Long term outcome:** We found no systematic review or RCTs.

Harms: **Versus medical management:** The review gave no information on surgical complications, and none of the individual studies were designed to compare rates of adverse effects.[29] In one arm of the subsequent RCT, seven of nine children who had postoperative obstruction developed evidence of renal scarring on DMSA (see glossary, p 146) scintigraphy. This may have negated an otherwise beneficial effect of surgery over medical management.[30]

Comment: The best results were obtained by centres handling the greatest number of children.[31] Surgery is usually considered only in children with more severe vesicoureteric reflux (grade III–V), who are less likely to experience spontaneous resolution.[4,32] **Long term outcome:** We found one prospective cohort study in 226 children aged 5 days to 12 years who presented with UTI and were found to have grade III–IV vesicoureteric reflux.[8] It found that surgery was associated with a higher rate of resolution of reflux compared with medical treatment (AR of resolution from age 8–14 years on micturating cystourethrography: 29/33 [88%] with surgery v 134/193 [69%] treated medically; ARI 19%, 95% CI 6% to 31%) but did not compare clinical outcomes.

GLOSSARY

Co-trimoxazole is the British Approved Name for a combination preparation containing trimethoprim and sulfamethoxazole.

DMSA Dimercaptosuccinic acid.

Intravenous immunoglobulins (normal immunoglobulins for intravenous use) Immunoglobulin preparations derived from donated human plasma containing antibodies prevalent in the general population.

Neurogenic bladder Loss of normal bladder function from damage to the nervous system (causing dysfunction of the nerves to and from the bladder or sphincters).

Nosocomial infection Definitions vary but typically an infection arising at least 48–72 hours after admission to hospital. The infection may have been acquired from other patients, hospital staff, the hospital environment, or from within people themselves.

Severity of vesicoureteric reflux:

Grade I Reflux into ureter only.

Grade II Reflux into ureter, pelvis, and calyces.

Grade III Mild/moderate dilatation or tortuosity of ureter and mild/moderate dilatation of pelvis, but little or no forniceal blunting.

Grade IV As grade III, but with complete obliteration of forniceal angles, yet maintenance of papillary impressions in calyces.

Grade V Gross dilatation of ureters, pelvis, and calyces, and papillary impressions in calyces obliterated.

REFERENCES

1. Stark H. Urinary tract infections in girls: the cost-effectiveness of currently recommended investigative routines. *Pediatr Nephrol* 1997;11: 174–177.
2. Dick PT, Feldman W. Routine diagnostic imaging for childhood urinary tract infections: a systematic overview. *J Pediatr* 1996;128:15–22. Search date 1994; primary sources Medline, Current Contents, and hand searches of article bibliographies.
3. Smellie JM, Katz G, Gruneberg RN. Controlled trial of prophylactic treatment in childhood urinary tract infection. *Lancet* 1978;ii:175–178.
4. Jodal U, Hansson S, Hjalmas K. Medical or surgical management for children with vesico-ureteric reflux? *Acta Paediatr Suppl* 1999;431: 53–61.
5. Jodal U. The natural history of bacteriuria in childhood. *Infect Dis Clin North Am* 1987;1: 713–729.
6. Hoberman A, Wald ER, Hickey RW, et al. Oral versus initial intravenous therapy for urinary tract infections in young febrile children. *Pediatrics* 1999;104:79–86.
7. Piepsz A, Tamminen-Mobius T, Reiners C, et al. Five-year study of medical and surgical treatment in children with severe vesico-ureteric reflux dimercaptosuccinic acid findings. International Reflux Study Group in Europe. *Eur J Pediatr* 1998; 157:753–758.
8. Smellie JM, Prescod NP, Shaw PJ, Risdon RA, Bryant TN. Childhood reflux and urinary infection: a follow-up of 10–41 years in 226 adults. *Pediatr Nephrol* 1998;12:727–736.
9. Berg UB. Long-term follow-up of renal morphology and function in children with recurrent pyelonephritis. *J Urol* 1992;148:1715–1720.
10. Martinell I, Claeson I, Lidin-Janson G, Jodal U. Urinary infection, reflux and renal scarring in females continuously followed for 13–38 years. *Pediatr Nephrol* 1995;9:131–136.
11. Jacobson S, Eklof O, Erikkson CG, Lins LE, Tidgren B. Development of hypertension and uraemia after pyelonephritis in childhood: 27 year follow up. *BMJ* 1989;299:703–706.
12. Moffatt M, Embree J, Grimm P, Law B. Short-course antibiotic therapy for urinary tract infections in children: a methodological review of the literature. *Am J Dis Child* 1988;142:57–61. Search date and primary sources not stated.
13. Avner ED, Ingelfinger JR, Herrin JT, et al. Single-dose amoxicillin therapy of uncomplicated pediatric urinary tract infections. *J Pediatr* 1983; 102:623–627.
14. McCracken GH, Ginsburg CM, Namasonthi V, et al. Evaluation of short-term antibiotic therapy in children with uncomplicated urinary tract infection. *Pediatrics* 1981;67:796–801.
15. Smellie JM, Normand ICS, Katz G. Children with urinary infection: a comparison of those with and those without vesicoureteric reflux. *Kidney Int* 1981;20:717–722.
16. Benador D, Benador N, Slozman D, Mermillod B, Girardin E. Are younger patients at higher risk of renal sequelae after pyelonephritis? *Lancet* 1997; 349:17–19.
17. Rosenberg AR, Rossleigh MA, Brydon MP, Bass SJ, Leighton DM, Farnsworth RH. Evaluation of acute urinary tract infection in children by dimercaptosuccinic acid scintography: a prospective study. *J Urol* 1992;148:1746–1749.
18. Le Saux N, Pham B, Moher D. Evaluating the benefits of antimicrobial prophylaxis to prevent urinary tract infections in children: a systematic review. *Can Med Assoc J* 2000;163:523–529 Search date 1999; primary sources Medline, Embase, Cochrane Library, textbooks, conference proceedings, experts; http://www.cma.ca/cmaj/vol-163/issue-5/0523.htm (last accessed 31 March 2001).
19. Lohr JA, Nunley DH, Howards SS, Ford RF. Prevention of recurrent urinary tract infections in girls. *Pediatrics* 1977;59:562–565.
20. Garin EH, Campos A, Homsy Y. Primary vesico-ureteral reflux: a review of current concepts. *Pediatr Nephrol* 1998;12:249–256.
21. Smellie JM, Gruneberg RN, Leakey A, Atkin WS. Long term low dose co-trimoxazole in prophylaxis of childhood urinary tract infection: clinical aspects/bacteriological aspects. *BMJ* 1976;2: 203–208.
22. Greenfield SP, Ng M, Gran J. Experience with vesicoureteric reflux in children: clinical characteristics. *J Urol* 1997;158:574–577.
23. Ohlsson A, Lacy JB. Intravenous immunoglobulin for preventing infection in pre-term and/or low-birth-weight infants. In: The Cochrane Library, Issue 3, 2000. Oxford: Update Software. Search date 1997; primary sources Medline, Embase, Cochrane Library, Reference Update, Science Citation Index, and hand searches of reference lists of identified RCTs and personal files.
24. Clemente E, Solli R, Mei V, et al. Therapeutic efficacy and safety of pidotomid in the treatment of urinary tract infections in children. *Arzneim Forsh* 1994;44:1490–1494.
25. Lettgen B. Prevention of urinary tract infections in female children. *Curr Ther Res* 1996;57:464–475.
26. Weisman LE, Cruess DF, Fischer GW. Opsonic activity of commercially available standard intravenous immunoglobulin preparations. *Paediatr Inf Dis J* 1994;13:1122–1125.
27. Nayir A, Emre S, Sirin A, Bulut A, Alpay H, Tanman F. The effects of vaccination with inactivated uropathogenic bacteria in recurrent urinary tract infections of children. *Vaccine* 1995;13:987–990.
28. Pylkannen J, Vilska J, Koskimies O. The value of childhood urinary tract infection in predicting renal injury. *Acta Paediatr Scand* 1981;70:879–883.
29. Shanon A, Feldman W. Methodological limitations in the literature on vesicoureteral reflux: a critical review. *J Pediatr* 1990;117:171–178. Search date 1988; primary source Medline.
30. Weiss R, Duckett J, Spitzer A. Results of a randomized clinical trial of medical versus surgical management of infants and children with grades III and IV primary vesico-ureteral reflux (United States): the international reflux study in children. *J Urol* 1992;148:1667–1673.
31. Smellie JM. Commentary: management of children with severe vesicoureteral reflux. *J Urol* 1992;148:1676–1678.
32. Sciagra R, Materassi M, Rossi V, et al. Alternative approaches to the prognostic stratification of mild to moderate primary vesicoureteral reflux in children. *J Urol* 1996;155:2052–2056.

James Larcombe
General Practitioner
Sedgefield, UK

Competing interests: None declared.

Middle ear pain and trauma during air travel

Search date March 2002

Simon Janvrin

INTERVENTIONS

Key Messages

- We found only limited evidence that oral decongestants are effective in reducing ear pain and hearing loss during air travel in adults. One small RCT found no evidence of benefit in children.

- We found insufficient evidence on the effects of topical decongestants in this setting.

DEFINITION The effects of air travel on the middle ear can include tympanic membrane pain, vertigo, hearing loss, and perforation.

INCIDENCE/ PREVALENCE The prevalence of symptoms depends on the altitude, type of aircraft, and characteristics of the passengers. One point prevalence study found that 20% of adult and 40% of child passengers had negative pressure in the middle ear after flight, and that 10% of adults and 22% of children had auroscopic evidence of damage to the tympanic membrane.[1] We found no data on the incidence of perforation, which seems to be extremely rare in commercial passengers.

AETIOLOGY/ RISK FACTORS During aircraft descent, the pressure in the middle ear drops relative to that in the ear canal. A narrow, inflamed, or poorly functioning Eustachian tube impedes the necessary influx of air. As the pressure difference between the middle and outer ear increases, the tympanic membrane is pulled inward.

PROGNOSIS In most people symptoms resolve spontaneously. Experience in military aviation shows that most ear drum perforations will heal spontaneously.[2]

AIMS To prevent ear pain and trauma during air travel.

OUTCOMES Incidence and severity of pain and hearing loss; incidence of perforation of tympanic membrane.

METHODS *Clinical Evidence* search and appraisal March 2002.

QUESTION What are the effects of preventive interventions?

OPTION ORAL DECONGESTANTS

We found limited evidence from two RCTs suggesting that oral pseudoephedrine may reduce the incidence of pain and hearing loss during flight in adult passengers prone to symptoms. One small RCT found no evidence of benefit in children.

Benefits: We found no systematic review. We found three RCTs. Two RCTs (350 adult passengers) compared oral pseudoephedrine (120 mg given 30 mins before flight) versus placebo.[3,4] All people had a history of ear pain during air travel. Those with acute or chronic ear problems were excluded. A total of 272 passengers completed the post flight questionnaires. The RCTs found that pseudoephedrine versus placebo significantly reduced pain and hearing loss (incidence of symptoms in combined treatment groups: 33% v 64%; RR 0.51, 95% CI 0.31 to 0.84). The third RCT (50 children up to the age of 6 years) compared oral pseudoephedrine versus placebo.[5] It found no significant difference in ear pain between children taking treatment versus placebo at either take off or landing.

Harms: "Dry mouth or drowsiness" was reported by 7–15% of adult participants taking pseudoephedrine versus 2% on placebo.[3,4] More children taking pseudoephedrine were drowsy on take off compared with placebo (60% v 13%).[5]

Comment: None.

Middle ear pain and trauma during air travel

OPTION	TOPICAL NASAL DECONGESTANTS

We found insufficient evidence on the effects of topical decongestants in this setting.

Benefits: We found no systematic review. We found one RCT comparing oxymetazoline nasal spray versus placebo nasal spray in 83 people during air travel.[3] It found no significant difference in reported ear pain between the two groups.

Harms: Nasal irritation was reported by 14% of people taking oxymetazoline. The rate in people taking placebo was not reported.

Comment: The RCT was too small to rule out an effect of topical decongestants.

REFERENCES

1. Stangerup S-E, Tjernstrom O, Klokke M, Harcourt J, Stokholm J. Point prevalence of barotitis in children and adults after flight, and the effect of autoinflation. *Aviat Space Environ Med* 1998;69: 45–49.

2. O'Reilly BJ. Otorhinolaryngology. In: Ernsting J, Nicholson AN, Rainford DJ, eds. *Aviation Medicine*. 3rd edition. Oxford: Butterworth-Heinemann, 1999:319–336.

3. Jones JS, Sheffield W, White LJ, Bloom MA. A double-blind comparison between oral

pseudoephedrine and topical oxymetazoline in the prevention of barotrauma during air travel. *Am J Emerg Med* 1998;16:262–264.

4. Csortan E, Jones J, Haan M, Brown M. Efficacy of pseudoephedrine for the prevention of barotrauma during air travel. *Ann Emerg Med* 1994;23: 1324–1327.

5. Buchanan BJ, Hoagland J, Fischer PR. Pseudoephedrine and air travel-associated ear pain in children. *Arch Pediatr Adolesc Med* 1999; 153:466–468.

Simon Janvrin
Civil Aviation Authority
West Sussex
UK

Competing interests: None declared.

Search date February 2002

Gerald McGarry

QUESTIONS

INTERVENTIONS

Key Messages

- One small RCT comparing chlorhexidine/neomycin cream versus silver nitrate cautery found no significant difference in reduction of nose bleeds. Some children found the smell and taste of the antiseptic cream unpleasant. All children found cautery painful despite the use of local anaesthesia.

- One small RCT compared silver nitrate cautery plus chlorhexidine/neomycin cream versus antiseptic cream alone. The study included too few children to allow conclusions to be drawn.

Recurrent idiopathic epistaxis (nosebleeds)

DEFINITION Recurrent idiopathic epistaxis is recurrent, self limiting, nasal bleeding in children for which no specific cause has been identified. There is no consensus on how frequent or severe recurrences need to be.

INCIDENCE/ PREVALENCE A cross sectional study of 1218 children (aged 11–14 years) found that 9% had frequent episodes of epistaxis.[1] It is likely that most epistaxis in children is not brought to the attention of health professionals, and that only the most severe episodes are considered for treatment.

AETIOLOGY/ RISK FACTORS In children, most epistaxis occurs from the anterior part of the septum in the region of Little's area.[2] Initiating factors include local inflammation, mucosal drying, and local trauma (including nose picking).[2] Epistaxis caused by other specific local (e.g. tumours) or systemic factors (e.g. clotting disorders) is not considered here.

PROGNOSIS Recurrent epistaxis is less common in adolescents over 14 years and many children "grow out" of this problem.

AIMS To reduce the number and severity of epistaxis episodes.

OUTCOMES Number and severity of epistaxis episodes.

METHODS *Clinical Evidence* search and appraisal February 2002.

QUESTION What are the effects of treatments in children with recurrent idiopathic epistaxis?

OPTION ANTISEPTIC CREAMS

We found no placebo controlled trials. One small RCT comparing chlorhexidine/neomycin cream versus silver nitrate cautery found no significant difference in reduction of nosebleeds. Some children found the smell and taste of antiseptic cream unpleasant. All children found cautery painful despite the use of local anaesthesia.

Benefits: We found no systematic review. **Versus other creams/ointments:** We found no RCTs. **Versus cautery:** We found one small RCT (48 children), which compared antiseptic cream (chlorhexidine hydrochloride 0.1%, neomycin sulphate 3250 U/g) applied to both nostrils twice daily for 4 weeks versus silver nitrate cautery.[3] Cautery was undertaken in secondary care using silver nitrate applied on a stick to prominent vessels or bleeding points. The children were aged 3–14 years, and had at least one episode of epistaxis in the previous 4 weeks and a "history of repeated epistaxis". After 8 weeks, the RCT found no significant difference between treatments. About half of the children in both groups had complete resolution (no bleeding in past 4 wks: 12/24 with antiseptic cream *v* 13/24 with cautery; RR 0.92, 95% CI 0.54 to 1.59). Rates of other outcomes were also similar between groups at 8 weeks: partial success (50% reduction in number of bleeds in past 4 wks: 4/24 with antiseptic cream *v* 3/24 with cautery), failure (less than 50% reduction in number of bleeds in past 4 wks: 7/24 with antiseptic cream *v* 6/24 with cautery), and lost to follow up at 8 weeks (1/24 with antiseptic cream *v* 2/24 with cautery). **Plus cautery:** See silver nitrate cautery, p 153.

Harms: No adverse reactions were observed with antiseptic cream, but some children found the smell and taste unpleasant (data not provided). Chlorhexidine/neomycin cream may cause occasional skin reactions. Some commercial antiseptic creams contain arachis (peanut) oil. All children undergoing cautery experienced pain even with the use of 5% cocaine as a local anaesthetic.[3]

Comment: See comment under silver nitrate cautery, p 153.

OPTION   SILVER NITRATE CAUTERY

We found no placebo controlled trials. One small RCT comparing cautery versus antiseptic cream found no significant difference in reduction of nosebleeds (see antiseptic creams, p 152). One small RCT compared silver nitrate cautery plus a cream containing chlorhexidine/neomycin versus antiseptic cream alone. The RCT included too few children to allow conclusions to be drawn.

Benefits: We found no systematic review. **Versus no treatment:** We found no RCTs. **Versus antiseptic cream:** See antiseptic creams, p 152. **Plus antiseptic cream:** One RCT (40 adults, 24 children) compared once only silver nitrate cautery plus chlorhexidine hydrochloride 0.1%/neomycin sulphate 3250 U/g cream twice daily for 2 weeks with antiseptic cream alone. The study included too few children to allow conclusions to be drawn.[4]

Harms: The RCT did not report harms.[4] Recognised complications of cautery include pain and septal perforation, although the incidence of septal perforation following unilateral cautery in children is not known (see harms of antiseptic creams, p 153).

Comment: Both trials involving silver nitrate cautery were undertaken in the context of secondary care.[3,4] Silver nitrate cautery is also used in primary care. It is unknown if complication rates differ. Simultaneous bilateral cautery in children is not recommended because of an expected increased risk of perforation.

REFERENCES

1. Rodeghiero F, Castaman G, Dini E. Epidemiological investigation of the prevalence of von Willebrand's disease. *Blood* 1987;69:454–459.

2. Watkinson JC. Epistaxis. In: Kerr AG, Mackay IS, Bull TR, eds. *Scott-Brown's Otolaryngology, Volume 4 Rhinology.* Oxford: Butterworth-Heinemann, 1997;18:1–19.

3. Ruddy J, Proops DW, Pearman K, Ruddy H. Management of epistaxis in children. *Int J Paediatr Otorhinolaryngol* 1991;21:139–142.

4. Murthy P, Nilssen ELK, Rao S, McClymont LG. A randomised clinical trial of antiseptic nasal carrier cream and silver nitrate cautery in the treatment of recurrent anterior epistaxis. *Clin Otolaryngol* 1999;228–231.

Gerald McGarry
Consultant Otorhinolaryngologist
Honorary Clinical Senior Lecturer
Glasgow Royal Infirmary
Glasgow
UK

Competing interests: None declared.

Recurrent tonsillitis

Search date December 2001

William McKerrow

Ear, nose, and throat disorders

QUESTIONS
Effects of tonsillectomy in severe tonsillitis in children and adults . . .155

INTERVENTIONS

Unknown effectiveness
Tonsillectomy versus
   antibiotics 155

Key Messages

- We found no RCTs evaluating tonsillectomy in adults, and we found inconclusive evidence from RCTs in children.

DEFINITION Tonsillitis is infection of the parenchyma of the palatine tonsils. Recurrent severe tonsillitis results in significant morbidity, including time lost from school or work. The definition of severe recurrent tonsillitis is arbitrary, but criteria used recently as a measure of severity were five or more episodes of true tonsillitis a year, symptoms for at least a year, and episodes that are disabling and prevent normal functioning.[1]

INCIDENCE/ PREVALENCE Recurrent sore throat has an incidence in general practice in the UK of 100/1000 population a year.[2] Acute tonsillitis is more common in childhood.

AETIOLOGY/ RISK FACTORS Common bacterial pathogens include β haemolytic and other streptococci. Bacteria are cultured successfully only from a minority of people with tonsillitis. The role of viruses is uncertain.

PROGNOSIS We found no good data on the natural history of tonsillitis or recurrent sore throat in children or adults. Participants in RCTs who were randomised to medical treatment (courses of antibiotics as required) have shown a tendency towards improvement over time.[3,4]

AIMS To abolish tonsillitis; to reduce the frequency and severity of recurrent throat infections; to improve general wellbeing, behaviour, and educational achievement, with minimal adverse effects.

OUTCOMES Number and severity of episodes of tonsillitis or sore throat; requirement for antibiotics and analgesics; time off work or school; behaviour, school performance, general wellbeing; morbidity and mortality of surgery; and adverse effects of drugs.

METHODS *Clinical Evidence* search and appraisal December 2001.

QUESTION **Is tonsillectomy effective in severe tonsillitis in children and adults?**

OPTION **TONSILLECTOMY VERSUS ANTIBIOTICS**

Limited evidence from one RCT suggests that tonsillectomy may benefit some children with severe tonsillitis. We found no good evidence on tonsillectomy in adults. We found that many important outcome measures have not been considered.

Benefits: We found two systematic reviews (search dates 1997[5] and 1998[6]). **Children:** Both reviews identified the same two RCTs as being the only ones that met quality inclusion criteria.[3,4] The smaller RCT involved 91 children who fulfilled criteria for "severe tonsillitis" (7 episodes in the preceding year, or 5 episodes/year in the preceding 2 years, or 3 episodes/year in the preceding 3 years).[3] The children were randomised to tonsillectomy alone (27 children), adenotonsillectomy (16 children), or intermittent courses of antibiotics as needed (48 children). Sixteen children were withdrawn from the non-surgical group by their parents and had surgery, and children who developed infections after surgery received antibiotics as necessary for each episode of infection. Secondary outcome measures such as time off school were also considered. The authors

Ear, nose, and throat disorders

concluded that children undergoing tonsillectomy experienced significantly fewer throat infections than those on antibiotics, amounting to an average of three fewer throat infections in the first 2 years, but by the third year the difference was no longer significant. The larger RCT (246 "less severely affected children") is published only in abstract form.[4] Some children in this study also underwent adenoidectomy. The limited data available provide no evidence of a difference between surgical and medical treatment. The second review concluded that it was not possible to determine the effectiveness of tonsillectomy from these RCTs.[6] **Adults:** The reviews found no RCTs that evaluated tonsillectomy in adults with recurrent tonsillitis or sore throats.

Harms: **Tonsillectomy:** The risks of tonsillectomy include those associated with general anaesthesia and those specific to the procedure. The overall complication rate in the smaller RCT[3] was 14% (all were "readily managed or self limiting") compared with 2–8% in one Scottish tonsillectomy audit.[7] Haemorrhage, either primary (in the immediate postoperative period) or secondary, occurred in 4% of children studied in the larger RCT[4] and fewer than 1% of children in the Scottish tonsillectomy audit.[7] **Antibiotics:** In the smaller RCT, erythematous rashes occurred in 4% of children in the non-surgical group while taking penicillin.[3] Other adverse effects of antibiotics include allergic reactions and the promotion of resistant bacteria. One RCT found that, for people with milder episodes of sore throat, the prescribing of antibiotics compared with no initial prescription increased the proportion of people who returned to see their physician in the short term because of sore throat (716 people with sore throat and an abnormal physical sign; return rate 38% with initial antibiotics v 27% without; adjusted HR for return 1.39, 95% CI 1.03 to 1.89).[8]

Comment: **Background:** Tonsillectomy is one of the most frequently performed surgical procedures in the UK, particularly in children, and accounts for about 20% of all operations performed by otolaryngologists.[7] Adenoidectomy is now performed with tonsillectomy only when there is a specific indication to remove the adenoids as well as the tonsils. **Quality of the evidence:** In the smaller RCT,[3] there were significant baseline differences between groups before treatment, and the authors pooled the results of tonsillectomy and adenotonsillectomy, making it impossible to assess the effectiveness of tonsillectomy alone. **Gaps in the evidence:** We found no RCT that found improved general wellbeing, development, or behaviour despite suggestions that these are influenced by tonsillectomy.[7] **New techniques:** Diathermy tonsillectomy and adjuvant treatment[9] may reduce adverse effects and are currently being studied.

REFERENCES

1. Management of Sore Throat and Indications for Tonsillectomy. National Clinical Guideline No 34. Scottish Intercollegiate Guidelines Network, Royal College of Physicians, 9 Queen Street, Edinburgh EH2 1JQ.

2. Shvartzman P. Careful prescribing is beneficial. BMJ 1994;309:1101–1102.

3. Paradise JL, Bluestone CD, Bachman RZ, et al. Efficacy of tonsillectomy for recurrent throat infection in severely affected children. N Engl J Med 1984;310:674–683.

4. Paradise JL, Bluestone CD, Rogers KD, et al. Comparative efficacy of tonsillectomy for recurrent throat infection in more versus less severely affected children [abstract]. Pediatric Res 1992; 31:126A.

5. Marshall T. A review of tonsillectomy for recurrent throat infection. Br J Gen Pract 1998;48: 1331–1335. Search date 1997; primary sources Cochrane Library and Medline.

6. Burton MJ, Towler B, Glasziou P. Tonsillectomy versus non-surgical treatment for chronic/recurrent

acute tonsillitis. In: The Cochrane Library, Issue 2, 2001. Oxford: Update Software. Search date 1998; primary sources Medline, Embase, Cochrane Controlled Trials Register, and hand searched references.

7. Blair RL, McKerrow WS, Carter NW, Fenton A. The Scottish tonsillectomy audit. *J Laryngol Otol* 1996; 110(suppl 20):1–25.

8. Little P, Gould C, Williamson I, Warner G, Gantley M, Kinmouth, AL. Reattendance and complications in a randomised trial of prescribing strategies for sore throat: the medicalising effect of prescribing antibiotics. *BMJ* 1997;315:350–352.

9. Steward DL, Chung SJ. The role of adjuvant therapies and techniques in tonsillectomy. *Curr Opin Otolaryngol Head Neck Surg* 2000;8:186–192.

William McKerrow
Raigmore Hospital
Inverness
UK

Competing interests: None declared.

Wax in ear

Search date December 2001

George Browning

QUESTIONS

INTERVENTIONS

Trade off between benefits and harms

Unknown effectiveness

*Although many practitioners consider these to be standard treatments, we found no RCTs of these interventions

See glossary, p 161

Key Messages

- One small RCT found that wax softeners were better than no treatment at completely removing ear wax without syringing. Five RCTs found no consistent evidence that any one type of wax softener was superior to the others. We found insufficient evidence to address the effects of wax softeners prior to syringing.
- We found no good evidence about mechanical methods of removing ear wax.

Ear, nose, and throat disorders

DEFINITION	Ear wax is normal and becomes a problem only if it produces deafness, pain, or other aural symptoms. Ear wax may also need to be removed if it prevents inspection of the ear drum. The term "impacted" is used in different ways, and can merely imply the co-existence of wax obscuring the ear drum with symptoms in that ear.[1,2]
INCIDENCE/ PREVALENCE	We found four surveys of the prevalence of impacted wax (see glossary, p 161) (see table 1, p 162).[3–6] The prevalence was higher in men than in women, in the elderly than in the young, and in people with intellectual impairment.[7] One survey found that 289 Scottish general practitioners each saw an average of nine people a month requesting removal of ear wax.[1]
AETIOLOGY/ RISK FACTORS	Factors that prevent the normal extrusion of wax from the ear canal (e.g. wearing a hearing aid, using cotton buds) increase the chance of ear wax accumulating.
PROGNOSIS	Most ear wax emerges from the external canal spontaneously. Without impaction or adherence to the drum, there is likely to be minimal, if any, hearing loss. One survey of 21 unselected out-patients with completely obstructing wax (see glossary, p 161) found that the average improvement in hearing following syringing was 5.5 dB (95% CI 0.6 to 10.5 dB).[1]
AIMS	To relieve symptoms or to allow examination by completely removing impacted wax or obstructing wax; and to soften impacted wax to ease mechanical removal.
OUTCOMES	Proportion of people (or ears) with relief of hearing loss or discomfort; total removal of wax; proportion of people requiring further intervention to improve symptoms; ease of mechanical removal measured, for example, by the volume of water used to accomplish successful syringing.
METHODS	*Clinical Evidence* search and appraisal December 2001. A search for surveys of the prevalence of ear wax was performed in Medline and Embase in July 2001.

QUESTION   What are the effects of methods to remove ear wax?

OPTION   WAX SOFTENERS

One RCT found limited evidence that using a wax softener for 5 days increased the chance of an ear being cleared of wax compared with no treatment. A third of untreated ears cleared in the same period. Five RCTs found no consistent evidence that any one type of wax softener was superior to the others. There is insufficient evidence to address the effects of wax softeners prior to syringing.

Benefits: We found no systematic review. **Versus placebo:** We found one RCT (113 people with impacted wax (see glossary, p 161) in one or both ears).[2] The ears were randomly allocated to treatment by the nursing staff with sterile water, sodium bicarbonate, a proprietary softening agent (arachis oil/chlorobutanol/p-dichlorobenzene), or no treatment. Participants and nurses were blinded to the active treatment allocation. The people were recruited from a hospital for the elderly. People already using ear drops and people with known pathology of the ear canal or ear drum were excluded. Of those recruited, 13 left hospital and three died before completing the trial. Analysis of the remaining 97 people (155 ears) found that the risk of persisting impaction at the end of the trial was reduced by any active form of treatment compared with no treatment (AR of persistent impaction: 26/38 [68%] ears with no treatment v 55/117 [47%] ears with any active treatment; ARR 21%, 95% CI 3% to 35%; RR 1.31, 95% CI 1.06 to 1.75; NNT 5, 95% CI 3 to 34). **Versus other wax softeners:** We found five trials comparing wax softeners (see table 2, p 163).[2,8-11] Only two were RCTs[2,11] and the other ones did not state allocation stereotypes or were quasi-randomised trials. The trials were conducted in a variety of settings. They varied in size from 35 people to 286 ears. The most common outcomes were a subjective assessment of the amount of wax remaining, the need for syringing, the perceived ease of syringing, or the result of syringing. The trials found no consistent evidence that any one type of wax softener was clinically superior to any other. **Prior to syringing:** We found four RCTs comparing wax softeners given prior to ear syringing[12-15] and one quasi-randomised trial.[16] All had design deficiencies that could lead to bias. Two of the RCTs found differences in effectiveness between wax softeners, and the other RCTs two found no overall difference (see table 3, p 165). One quasi-randomised trial found no difference between water instilled for 15 minutes and oil instilled nightly for 3 days.[16]

Harms: Seven RCTs did not report complications or adverse effects. Two found single cases of irritation, itch, or buzzing.[8,9] One RCT found that the frequency of adverse effects was similar in people using arachis oil/chlorobutanol/p-dichlorobenzene versus a proprietary agent (Otocerol® — the composition of which was not stated — see table 3, p 165).[11]

Comment: We found no good evidence about the optimal duration of treatment. Most trials did not use rigorous methods of randomisation, and did not include control for degree of occlusion at randomisation. Many trials were sponsored by companies that manufactured only one of the products being tested, but the possibility of publication bias has not been assessed. The inclusion criteria for the RCTs were not always clear: many stated that the participants had impacted wax without defining how this was assessed. The RCT that included a no treatment group found that 32% of ears with impacted wax showed spontaneous resolution after 5 days.[2]

| OPTION | MECHANICAL METHODS |

We found no good evidence about the benefits or harms of mechanical removal of wax.

Benefits: We found no systematic review and no RCTs comparing mechanical methods intended to remove ear wax with no treatment or alternative treatment.

Harms: A survey found that 38% of 274 general practitioners performing ear syringing reported complications, including otitis externa, perforation of the tympanic membrane, damage to the skin of the

Ear, nose, and throat disorders

external canal, tinnitus, pain, and vertigo.[1] We found no study of the incidence of these complications, or the effect of training and experience. People may experience dizziness during syringing or when wax is removed by suction.

Comment: There is consensus that syringing is effective and that training can reduce complications, but we found no evidence. Other mechanical techniques include manual removal under direct vision, with or without a microscope, using suction, probes, or forceps. These methods require specific training and access to appropriate equipment.

GLOSSARY

Impacted wax Wax that has been compressed in the ear canal, completely obstructing the lumen. In practice, many RCTs define impaction as the presence of symptoms associated with obstructing wax.

Obstructing wax Wax that obscures direct vision of the ear drum.

REFERENCES

1. Sharp JF, Wilson JA, Ross L, Barr-Hamilton RM. Ear wax removal: a survey of current practice. *BMJ* 1990;301:1251–1252.

2. Keane EM, Wilson H, McGrane D, Coakley D, Walsh JB. Use of solvents to disperse ear wax. *Br J Clin Pract* 1995;49:7–12.

3. Kalantan KA, Abdulghani H, Al-Taweel AA, Al-Serhani AM. Use of cotton tipped swab and cerumen impaction. *Ind J Otol* 1999;5:27–31.

4. Minja BM, Machemba A. Prevalence of otitis media, hearing impairment and cerumen impaction among school children in rural and urban Dar es Salaam, Tanzania. *Int J Pediatr Otorhinolaryngol* 1996;37:29–34.

5. Swart SM, Lemmer R, Parbhoo JN, Prescott CAJ. A survey of ear and hearing disorders amongst a representative sample of Grade 1 school children in Swaziland. *Int J Pediatr Otorhinolaryngol* 1995; 32:23–34.

6. Lewis-Cullinan C, Janken JK. Effect of cerumen removal on the hearing ability of geriatric patients. *J Adv Nurs* 1990;15:594–600.

7. Brister F, Fullwood HL, Ripp T, Blodgett C. Incidence of occlusion due to impacted cerumen among mentally retarded adolescents. *Am J Ment Defic* 1990;15:594–600.

8. Dummer DS, Sutherland IA, Murray JA. A single-blind, randomized study to compare the efficacy of two ear drop preparations ("Andax" and "Cerumol") in the softening of ear wax. *Curr Med Res Opin* 1992;13:26–30.

9. Lyndon S, Roy P, Grillage MG, Miller AJ. A comparison of the efficacy of two ear drop preparations ("Aurax" and "Earex") in the softening and removal of impacted ear wax. *Curr Med Res Opin* 1992;13:21–25.

10. Fahmy S, Whitefield M. Multicentre clinical trial of Exterol as a cerumenolytic. *Br J Clin Pract* 1982; 36:197–204.

11. Jaffe G, Grimshaw J. A multicentric clinical trial comparing Otocerol with Cerumol as cerumenolytics. *J Int Med Res* 1978;6:241–244.

12. Singer AJ, Sauris E, Viccellio AW. Ceruminolytic effects of docusate sodium: A randomized controlled trial. *Ann Emerg Med* 2000;36: 228–232.

13. Amjad AH, Scheer AA. Clinical evaluation of cerumenolytic agents. *Eye Ear Nose Throat Mon* 1975;54:76–77.

14. Chaput de Saintonge DM, Johnstone CI. A clinical comparison of triethanolamine polypeptide oleate-condensate ear drops with olive oil for the removal of impacted wax. *Br J Clin Pract* 1973;27: 454–455.

15. Fraser JG. The efficacy of wax solvents: in vitro studies and a clinical trial. *J Laryngol Otol* 1970; 84:1055–1064.

16. Eekhof JA, de Bock GH, Le Cessie S, Springer MP. A quasi-randomised controlled trial of water as a quick softening agent of persistent earwax in general practice. *Br J Gen Pract.* 2001;51: 635–637.

George Browning
Professor of Otorhinolaryngology
MRC Institute of Hearing Research
Glasgow
UK

Competing interests: None declared.

Wax in ear

| TABLE 1 | Surveys of the prevalence of impacted wax in specified populations (see text, p 159).[3–6] |

Reference	Where	Who	% with impacted wax
Kalantan et al[3]	Saudi Arabia	1278 people attending primary care centre (any reason)	25%
Minja et al[4]	Tanzania	802 primary school children	16%
Swart et al[5]	Swaziland	Infant school children	7%
Lewis-Cullinan et al[6]	USA	Hospitalised elderly people (all causes except intensive care)	35%

| TABLE 2 | Effects of wax softeners: results of comparative RCTs (see text, p 160). |

Ref	Wax softener	Administration	Selection characteristic; setting	Number of people (ears)	Randomisation; blinding	Outcome	Results	Adverse effects
2	(a) Arachis oil Chlorobutanol p-dichlorobenzene (Cerumol®) (b) Sodium bicarbonate (in glycerol) (c) Sterile water (d) Nothing	4 drops twice a day for 5 days	Impacted ear(s); hospital	113 recruited; 97 completed (155)	Randomisation (technique not described) Double blind (active treatments)	Residual wax; 3 tiered clinical rating scale	Treatment better than no treatment; no difference between agents	None
8	(a) Ethyleneoxide-polyoxypropylene glycol Choline salicylate (b) Arachis oil Chlorobutanol p-dichlorobenzene (Cerumol®)	Drops to fill ear twice a day for 4 days	Impacted or hardened wax; general practice	50 (100)	Not stated; single blind	Wax amount, colour, and consistency; objective hearing; global impression of efficiency	No difference	Two irritation with (a); one itch, one buzzing with (b)
9	(a) Ethyleneoxide-polyoxypropylene glycol Choline salicylate (b) Arachis oil Almond oil Rectified camphor oil		Symptoms requiring wax softener; general practice	36 (72)	Not stated; not blind	Need for syringing; ease of syringing; global impression of efficiency	(a) better than (b); easy removal: 37/38 v 19/30	One irritation with (b); one disliked smell
10	(a) 5% urea hydrogen peroxide in glycerol (b) Glycerol	5–10 drops twice a day for a week	Ear wax problems; ENT dept	40 (80)	Alternation; double blind	Need for syringing; ease of syringing	(a) better than glycerol; success: 35/40 v 20/40	None

Ear, nose, and throat disorders

TABLE 2   continued

Ref	Wax softener	Administration	Selection characteristic; setting	Number of people (ears)	Randomisation; blinding	Outcome	Results	Adverse effects
10	(a) 5% urea hydrogen peroxide in glycerol (b) Arachis oil Chlorobutanol p-dichlorobenzene (Cerumol®)	5–10 drops twice a day for a week	Ear wax problems; ENT department	50 (100)	Alternation; double blind	Need for syringing; ease of syringing	(a) better than (b); success: 47/50 v 24/50	None
11	(a) 5% urea hydrogen peroxide in glycerol (b) Arachis oil Chlorobutanol p-dichlorobenzene	5–10 drops twice a day for a week	Ear wax problems; general practice	160 (286)	Alternation; double blind	Need for syringing; ease of syringing	(a) better than (b); success: 146/157 v 93/129	None
11	(a) Otocerol® (b) Arachis oil Chlorobutanol p-dichlorobenzene (Cerumol®)	Three consecutive nights	For whom a wax softener would normally be prescribed; general practice	106 (not stated)	Random allocation; double blind	3 tiered clinical rating scale	No difference overall; 38/53 v 33/53	Pain; irritation; giddiness; smell (Otocerol® 7/53 Cerumol® 10/53)
12	(a) Triethalonamine polypeptide (b) Docusate sodium (Waxol®)							

ENT, ear, nose and throat; ref, reference.

TABLE 3 Effects of wax softeners prior to syringing: results of comparative RCTs (see text, p 160).

Ref	Wax softener	Administration	Selection characteristic; setting	Number of people (ears)	Randomisation; blind	Outcome	Results	Adverse effects
13	(a) Triethanolamine polypeptide oleate condensate (b) Carbamide peroxide	One dose 30 minutes before syringing	Hard or impacted wax; setting unclear	80 (not stated)	Random allocation; double blind	Result of syringing; 4 tiered clinical rating scale	(a) better than (b); success: 33/40 v 7/40 but (b) normally used as multiple installations	Not reported
14	(a) Triethanolamine polypeptide oleate condensate (b) Olive oil	One dose 20 minutes before syringing	Impacted wax suitable for syringing; hospital outpatient dept	67 (not stated)	Random order; double blind	3 tiered clinical rating scale	No difference overall (20/32 v 21/35); (a) needed less water	None
12	(a) Triethylamine polypeptide (b) Docusate sodium (Waxol®)	One dose 15 minutes before syringing	Partial or totally accluding wax	50 (50)	Random order; non-blinded	Visualisation of tympanic membrane	(b) better than (a) (22/27 v 8/23)	None
16	(a) Water, cotton ear plug® (b) Oil, cotton ear plug	(a) 15 minutes® (b) nightly for 3 days	Persistent wax after five syringing attempts; general practice	130 (224)	Quasi-randomised (year of birth); not blind	Number of attempts needed to clear	No difference; however, statistical tests performed may have been inadequate	Not addressed
15	(a) Arachis oil Chlorobutanol p-dichlorobenzene (Cerumol®) (b) Docusate sodium (Waxsol®) (c) Olive oil v (d) Sodium bicarbonate (in glycerol) (c) Olive oil (d) Sodium bicarbonate (in glycerol)	Ear canal filled for 15 minutes, once daily every 3 days	Bilateral hard and occluding wax; geriatric hospital	124 (248)	Each participant was allocated (d) in one randomly chosen ear and treatment in the other ear. Double blind.	Failed forceful syringing	(a) better than (d), 1/24 v 5/24	Red canals

Bacterial conjunctivitis

Search date February 2002

Christine Chung, Elisabeth Cohen and Justine Smith

Key Messages

Empirical antibiotic treatment of suspected bacterial conjunctivitis

- One systematic review found limited evidence that topical norfloxacin versus placebo significantly increased rates of clinical and microbiological improvement or cure after 5 days. RCTs comparing different topical antibiotics versus each other found no significant difference in rates of clinical or microbiological cure. One RCT found no significant difference with topical polymyxin–bacitracin ointment versus oral cefixime in the number of people who improved clinically or in bacteriological failure rates.

Antibiotic treatment in culture positive bacterial conjunctivitis

- One systematic review has found that antibiotics (polymyxin–bacitracin, ciprofloxacin, or ofloxacin) versus placebo significantly increase rates of both clinical and microbiological cure. RCTs comparing different antibiotics versus each other found conflicting results for rates of clinical and microbiological cure.

DEFINITION Conjunctivitis is any inflammation of the conjunctiva, generally characterised by irritation, itching, foreign body sensation, and tearing or discharge. Bacterial conjunctivitis may usually be distinguished from other types of conjunctivitis by the presence of a yellow–white mucopurulent discharge. There is also usually a papillary reaction (small bumps with fibrovascular cores on the palpebral conjunctiva, appearing grossly as a fine velvety surface). Bacterial conjunctivitis is usually bilateral. This review covers only non-gonococcal bacterial conjunctivitis.

INCIDENCE/ PREVALENCE We found no good evidence on the incidence or prevalence of bacterial conjunctivitis.

AETIOLOGY/ RISK FACTORS Conjunctivitis may be infectious (caused by bacteria or viruses) or allergic. In adults, bacterial conjunctivitis is less common than viral conjunctivitis, although estimates vary widely (viral conjunctivitis has been reported to account for 8–75% of acute conjunctivitis).[1–3] *Staphylococcus* species are the most common pathogens for bacterial conjunctivitis in adults, followed by *Streptococcus pneumoniae* and *Haemophilus influenzae*.[4,5] In children, bacterial conjunctivitis is more common than viral, and is mainly caused by *H influenzae*, *S pneumoniae*, and *Moraxella catarrhalis*.[6,7]

PROGNOSIS Most bacterial conjunctivitis is self limiting. One systematic review (search date 2002) found clinical cure or significant improvement with placebo within 2–5 days in 64% of people (99% CI 54% to 73%).[8] Some organisms cause corneal or systemic complications, or both; otitis may develop in 25% of children with *H influenzae* conjunctivitis,[9] and systemic meningitis may complicate primary meningococcal conjunctivitis in 18% of people.[10]

AIMS To achieve rapid cure of inflammation, and to prevent complications, with minimum adverse effects of treatment.

OUTCOMES Time to cure or improvement. **Clinical signs/symptoms:** hyperaemia, discharge, papillae, follicles, chemosis, itching, pain, photophobia. Most studies used a numbered scale to grade signs and symptoms. Some studies also included evaluation by investigators and patients regarding success of treatment. **Culture results:** These are proxy outcomes usually expressed as the number of colonies, sometimes with reference to a threshold level. Results were often classified into categories such as eradication, reduction, persistence, and proliferation.

METHODS *Clinical Evidence* search and appraisal February 2002.

QUESTION **What are the effects of empirical treatment with antibiotics in adults and children with suspected bacterial conjunctivitis?**

One systematic review found limited evidence that topical norfloxacin versus placebo significantly increased rates of clinical and microbiological improvement or cure after 5 days. RCTs comparing different topical antibiotics versus each other found no significant

difference in rates of clinical or microbiological cure. One RCT found no significant difference with topical polymyxin–bacitracin ointment versus oral cefixime in the number of people who improved clinically or in bacteriological failure rates.

Benefits: **Versus placebo:** We found one systematic review (search date 2000, 1 RCT, 284 adults; 50% of participants were culture positive) comparing topical norfloxacin versus placebo.[8] It found that nor-floxacin significantly increased rates of clinical and microbiological improvement or cure after 5 days (88%, 95% CI 81% to 93% with norfloxacin v 72%, 95% CI 63% to 79% with placebo; P < 0.01; see comment below). **Versus each other:** We found no systematic review but found 20 RCTs in adults and children (see web extra table A at www.clinicalevidence.com). These RCTs found no significant difference between different topical antibiotics versus each other in rates of clinical or microbiological cure. Six of the RCTs (evaluating lomefloxacin, fusidic acid, rifamycin, chloramphenicol, and tobramycin) found no significant difference between different anti-biotics in effectiveness or tolerability (grading by patients). [11–16] One of the RCTs found no significant difference with polymyxin–bacitracin ointment plus oral placebo versus topical placebo plus oral cefixime in the number of people who improved clinically or in bacteriological failure rates.[17]

Harms: The placebo controlled RCT identified by the review reported minor adverse events in 4.2% of people using norfloxacin and 7.1% using placebo (no statistical analysis available).[5] Placebo contained higher proportions of benzalkonium chloride (0.01% with placebo v 0.0025% with norfloxacin). One non-systematic review described complications of topical antibiotics.[18] These included four reported cases of idiosyncratic aplastic anaemia associated with topical chloramphenicol and three cases of Stevens–Johnson syndrome associated with topical sulphonamides. However, the review did not report the number of people using these drugs, making it difficult to exclude other possible causes of aplastic anaemia.

Comment: The placebo controlled RCT identified by the review did not address the effect of using topical antibiotics on antibiotic resistance, which would be of interest given the self limiting nature of the disease.[5] None of the trials specified their methods for selecting participants. The findings may not be generalisable to primary care populations. Most trials included children as well as adults, and the ratio of children to adults was usually not specified. The comparisons of lomefloxacin versus chloramphenicol and fusidic acid, and the comparison of norfloxacin versus fusidic acid, were single blind. Lomefloxacin and fusidic acid are not available in the USA, and chloramphenicol is rarely used in the USA because of reports of idiosyncratic aplastic anaemia.

QUESTION   **What are the effects of topical antibiotics in adults and children with culture positive bacterial conjunctivitis?**

One systematic review has found that antibiotics (polymyxin–bacitracin, ciprofloxacin, or ofloxacin) versus placebo significantly increase rates of both clinical and microbiological cure. RCTs comparing different antibiotics versus each other found conflicting results for rates of clinical and microbiological cure.

Benefits: **Versus placebo:** We found one systematic review (search date 2000, 3 RCTs) in people with culture positive bacterial conjunctivitis, which compared antibiotics (polymyxin–bacitracin, ciprofloxacin, and ofloxacin) versus placebo.[8] The review identified no trials of gentamicin that included only culture proven conjunctivitis. The first RCT (84 children) identified by the review found that in children with culture proven *H influenzae* and *S pneumoniae* bacterial conjunctivitis topical polymyxin–bacitracin versus placebo significantly increased clinical cure after 3–5 days (62% with antibiotic *v* 28% with placebo; P < 0.02), but found no significant difference after 8–10 days (91% with antibiotic *v* 72% with placebo; P > 0.05).[19] The RCT found that topical polymyxin–bacitracin versus placebo significantly increased microbiological cure rates after both 3–5 days and 8–10 days. The RCT also found that when systemic antibiotics were given for concurrent problems, there was no significant difference in outcomes between treatments, although the numbers were too small to rule out a clinically important effect (see web extra table A at www.clinicalevidence.com). The second and third RCTs identified by the review did not specify the ages of participants. The second RCT (177 people) identified by the review found that ciprofloxacin versus placebo significantly improved microbiological cure rates after 3 days (132/140 [94%] with antibiotic *v* 22/37 [59%] with placebo; RR 1.59, 95% CI 1.21 to 2.08).[20] The third RCT (132 people) identified by the review found that ofloxacin versus placebo significantly increased clinical and microbiological improvement after 2 days (64% with ofloxacin *v* 22% with placebo; P < 0.001).[21] **Versus each other:** We found no systematic review but found six RCTs.[20,22-26] The first RCT (139 children) found that fusidic acid versus chloramphenicol significantly increased the number of children judged to have been clinically cured (85% with fusidic acid *v* 48% with chloramphenicol; P < 0.0001).[22] The second RCT (251 people) found no significant difference between ciprofloxacin versus tobramycin in reduction or eradication of bacteria after 7 days (94.5% with ciprofloxacin *v* 91.9% with tobramycin; P > 0.5).[20] The third RCT (141 children) found no significant difference between ciprofloxacin versus tobramycin in the number of children judged to have been clinically cured (87% with ciprofloxacin *v* 90% with tobramycin; P > 0.05) or in the number of children in whom microbiological eradication was achieved (90% with ciprofloxacin *v* 84% with tobramycin; P = 0.29) after 7 days.[23] The fourth RCT (156 children) compared three treatments: trimethoprim–polymyxin, gentamicin, and sulfacetamide.[24] It found no significant difference between any of the treatments in the number of children judged to have been clinically cured (84% with trimethoprim–polymyxin *v* 88% with gentamicin *v* 89% with sulfacetamide; P > 0.1), or in the number of children in whom microbiological eradication was achieved (83% with trimethoprim–polymyxin *v* 68% with gentamicin *v* 72% with sulfacetamide; P > 0.1) after 2–7 days. The fifth RCT (40 people) found no significant difference between lomefloxacin versus ofloxacin in the number of people whose symptoms and signs had resolved after 7 days (88% with lomefloxacin *v* 75% ofloxacin; P < 0.08).[25] The sixth RCT (121 people) found that topical netilmicin (0.3%) versus topical gentamicin (0.3%) administered as one or two drops to affected eyes four times daily significantly increased the number of people whose infections were judged to have resolved after both 5 and 10 days (P = 0.01 after 5 days; P = 0.001 after 10 days; other results presented graphically).

Harms: Of the 116 children initially enrolled in the first placebo controlled RCT identified by the review, one was excluded because of possible allergic reaction to the ointment; the other exclusions were unrelated to adverse effects.[19] In RCTs that included people with both culture proved and suspected bacterial conjunctivitis, minor adverse events were reported with antibiotics: burning, bitter taste, pruritus, or punctate epithelial erosions (35% with tobramycin v 20% with ciprofloxacin; no statistical detail available),[27] bad taste (20% with norfloxacin v 6% with fusidic acid),[28] stinging (50% with norfloxacin v 37% with fusidic acid),[28] and burning (33% with gentamicin v 20% with lomefloxacin).[13] The RCT comparing topical netilmicin versus topical gentamicin found no significant difference in the number of people reporting adverse reactions to either drug (redness, itching, and burning).[26]

Comment: The third RCT identified by the review, which compared antibiotics versus placebo, is published only in abstract form.[21] A fourth RCT identified by the review is published in Japanese and is awaiting translation.[29] None of the RCTs addressed the effect on antibiotic resistance of using topical antibiotics in bacterial conjunctivitis, which would be of interest given the self limiting nature of the disease. Furthermore, they did not report on patient oriented outcomes or look at rates of reinfection.

REFERENCES

1. Wishart PK, James C, Wishart MS, Darougar S. Prevalence of acute conjunctivitis caused by chlamydia, adenovirus, and herpes simplex virus in an ophthalmic casualty department. *Br J Ophthalmol* 1984;68:653–655.

2. Fitch CP, Rapoza PA, Owens S, et al. Epidemiology and diagnosis of acute conjunctivitis at an inner-city hospital. *Ophthalmology* 1989;96:1215–1220.

3. Woodland RM, Darougar S, Thaker U, et al. Causes of conjunctivitis and keratoconjunctivitis in Karachi, Pakistan. *Trans R Soc Trop Med Hygiene* 1992;86:317–320.

4. Seal DV, Barrett SP, McGill JI. Aetiology and treatment of acute bacterial infection of the external eye. *Br J Ophthalmol* 1982;66:357–360.

5. Miller IM, Wittreich J, Vogel R, Cook TJ, for the Norfloxacin-Placebo Ocular Study Group. The safety and efficacy of topical norfloxacin compared with placebo in the treatment of acute bacterial conjunctivitis. *Eur J Ophthalmol* 1992;2:58–66.

6. Gigliotti F, Williams WT, Hayden FG, et al. Etiology of acute conjunctivitis in children. *J Pediatr* 1981; 98:531–536.

7. Weiss A, Brinser JH, Nazar-Stewart V. Acute conjunctivitis in childhood. *J Pediatr* 1993;122:10–14.

8. Sheikh A, Hurwitz B, Cave J. Antibiotics versus placebo for acute bacterial conjunctivitis. In: The Cochrane Library, Issue 3, 2001. Oxford: Update Software. Search date 2000; primary sources Cochrane Controlled Trials Register, Medline, bibliographies of identified trials, Science Citation Index, and personal contacts with investigators and pharmaceutical companies.

9. Bodor FF. Conjunctivitis-otitis media syndrome: more than meets the eye. *Contemp Pediatr* 1989; 6:55–60.

10. Barquet N, Gasser I, Domingo P, et al. Primary meningococcal conjunctivitis: report of 21 patients and review. *Rev Infect Dis* 1990;12:838–847.

11. Kettenmeyer A, Jauch A, Boscher M, et al. A double-blind double-dummy multicenter equivalence study comparing topical lomefloxacin 0.3% twice daily with norfloxacin 0.3% four times daily in the treatment of acute bacterial conjunctivitis. *J Clin Res* 1998;1:75–86.

12. Agius-Fernandez A, Patterson A, Fsadni M, et al. Topical lomefloxacin versus topical chloramphenicol in the treatment of acute bacterial conjunctivitis. *Clin Drug Invest* 1998;15:263–269.

13. Montero J, Casado A, Perea E, et al. A double-blind double-dummy comparison of topical lomefloxacin 0.3% twice daily with topical gentamicin 0.3% four times daily in the treatment of acute bacterial conjunctivitis. *J Clin Res* 1998; 1:29–39.

14. Adenis JP, Arrata M, Gastaud P, et al. Etude randomisee multicentrique acide fusidique gel ophtalmique et rifamycine collyre dans les conjonctivites aigues. *J Fr Ophtalmol* 1989;12: 317–322.

15. Huerva V, Ascaso FJ, Latre B, et al. Tolerancia y eficacia de la tobramicina topica vs cloranfenicol en el tratamiento de las conjunctivitis bacterianas. *Ciencia Pharmaceutica* 1991;1:221–224.

16. Gallenga PE, Lobefalo L, Colangelo L, et al. Topical lomefloxacin 0.3% twice daily versus tobramycin

0.3% in acute bacterial conjunctivitis: a multicenter double-blind phase III study. *Ophthalmologica* 1999;213:250–257.

17. Wald ER, Greenberg D, Hoberman A.. Short term oral cefixime therapy for treatment of bacterial conjunctivitis. *Pediatr Infect Dis Jl* 2001;20: 1039–1042.

18. Stern GA, Killingsworth DW. Complications of topical antimicrobial agents. *Int Ophthalmol Clin* 1989;29:137–142.

19. Gigliotti G, Hendley JO, Morgan J, et al. Efficacy of topical antibiotic therapy in acute conjunctivitis in children. *J Pediatr* 1984;104:623–626.

20. Leibowitz HM. Antibacterial effectiveness of ciprofloxacin 0.3% ophthalmic solution in the treatment of bacterial conjunctivitis. *Am J Ophthalmol* 1991;112:29S–33S.

21. Ofloxacin Study Group III. A placebo-controlled clinical study of the fluoroquinolone ofloxacin in patients with external infection. *Invest Ophthalmol Vis Sci* 1990;31:572.

22. Van Bijsterveld OP, El Batawi Y, Sobhi FS, et al. Fusidic acid in infections of the external eye. *Infection* 1987;15:16–19.

23. Gross RD, Hoffman RO, Lindsay RN. A comparison of ciprofloxacin and tobramycin in bacterial conjunctivitis is children. *Clin Pediatr* 1997;36: 435–444.

24. Lohr JA, Austin RD, Grossman M, et al. Comparison of three topical antimicrobials for acute bacterial conjunctivitis. *Pediatr Infect Dis J* 1988;7:626–629.

25. Tabbara KF, El-Sheik HF, Monowarul Islam SM, Hammouda E. Treatment of acute bacterial conjunctivitis with topical lomefloxacin 0.3% compared to topical ofloxacin 0.3%. *Eur J Ophthalmol* 1999; 9:269–275.

26. Papa V, Aragona P, Scuderi AC, et al. Treatment of acute bacterial conjunctivitis with topical netilmicin. *Cornea* 2002;21:43–47.

27. Alves MR, Kara JN. Evaluation of the clinical and microbiological efficacy of 0.3% ciprofloxacin drops and 0.3% tobramycin drops in the treatment of acute bacterial conjunctivitis. *Revista Brasiliera de Oftalmol* 1993;52:371–377.

28. Wall AR, Sinclair N, Adenis JP. Comparison of Fucithalmic (fusidic acid viscous eye drops 1%) and Noroxin (norfloxacin ophthalmic solution 0.3%) in the treatment of acute bacterial conjunctivitis. *J Clin Res* 1998;1:316–325.

29. Mitsui Y, Matsuda H, Miyajima T, et al. Therapeutic effects of ofloxacin eye drops (DE-055) on external infection of the eye: multicentral double blind test. *J Rev Clin Ophthalmol* 1986;80: 1813–1828.

30. The Trimethoprim-Polymyxin B Sulphate Ophthalmic Ointment Study Group. Trimethoprim-polymyxin B sulphate ophthalmic ointment versus chloramphenicol ophthalmic ointment in the treatment of bacterial conjunctivitis — a review of four clinical studies. *J Antimicrob Chemother* 1989;23:261–266.

31. Behrens-Baumann W, Quentin CD, Gibson JR, et al. Trimethoprim-polymyxin B sulphate ophthalmic ointment in the treatment of bacterial conjunctivitis: a double-blind study versus chloramphenicol ophthalmic ointment. *Curr Med Res Opin* 1988;11:227–231.

32. Van-Rensburg SF, Gibson JR, Harvey SG, Burke CA. Trimethoprim-polymyxin ophthalmic solution versus chloramphenicol ophthalmic solution in the treatment of bacterial conjunctivitis. *Pharmatherapeutica* 1982;3:274–277.

33. Gibson JR. Trimethoprim-polymyxin B ophthalmic solution in the treatment of presumptive bacterial conjunctivitis — a multicentre trial of its efficacy versus neomycin-polymyxin B-gramicidin and chloramphenicol ophthalmic solutions. *J Antimicrob Chemother* 1983;11:217–221.

34. Genee E, Schlechtweg C, Bauerreiss P, Gibson JR. Trimethoprim-polymyxin eye drops versus neomycin-polymyxin-gramicidin eye drops in the treatment of presumptive bacterial conjunctivitis — a double-blind study. *Ophthalmologica* 1982;184:92–96.

35. Malminiemi K, Kari O, Latvala M-L, et al. Topical lomefloxacin twice daily compared with fusidic acid in acute bacterial conjunctivitis. *Acta Ophthalmol Scand* 1996;74:280–284.

36. Carr WD. Comparison of Fucithalmic (fusidic acid viscous eye drops 1%) and Chloromycetin Redidrops (chloramphenicol eye drops 0.5%) in the treatment of acute bacterial conjunctivitis. *J Clin Res* 1998;1:403–411.

37. Horven I. Acute conjunctivitis. A comparison of fusidic acid viscous eye drops and chloramphenicol. *Acta Ophthalmol* 1993;71: 165–168.

38. Hvidberg J. Fusidic acid in acute conjunctivitis. Single-blind, randomized comparison of fusidic acid and chloramphenicol viscous eye drops. *Acta Ophthalmol* 1987;65:43–47.

39. Uchida Y. Clinical efficacy of topical lomefloxacin (NY-198) in bacterial infections of the external eye. *Folia Ophthalmologica* 1991;42:59–70.

Christine Chung
Cornea Fellow

Elisabeth Cohen
Director

Cornea Service, Wills Eye Hospital
Jefferson Medical College
Philadelphia
USA

Justine Smith
Assistant Professor of Ophthalmology
Casey Eye Institute
Oregon Health & Science University
Portland
USA

Competing interests: None declared.

Ocular herpes simplex

Search date August 2001

Nigel Barker

INTERVENTIONS

Key Messages

Treating epithelial disease

- One systematic review has found that idoxuridine or vidarabine versus placebo significantly increases the number of people healed after 14 days and that trifluridine or aciclovir (acyclovir) versus idoxuridine significantly increases the number of people healed after 7 and 14 days.

- One systematic review has found no significant difference between debridement versus placebo in the number of people healed, but that debridement plus antiviral treatment versus debridement alone significantly increases the number of people healed after 7 and 14 days.

- One systematic review has found that topical interferon versus placebo significantly increases the number of people healed after both 7 and 14 days. The review found no significant difference between topical interferon versus a topical antiviral agent in the number of people healed after 7 days, but found that topical interferon significantly increases the number of people healed after 14 days.

Treating stromal keratitis

- One RCT found that topical corticosteroids versus placebo significantly reduced the progression and shortened the duration of stromal keratitis.

- One RCT in people with stromal keratitis found no significant difference between oral aciclovir versus placebo in rates of treatment failure.

Preventing ocular herpes simplex

- One large RCT in people with at least one previous episode of epithelial or stromal keratitis found that long term oral aciclovir versus placebo significantly reduced the risk of recurrences.

- One RCT in people with epithelial keratitis receiving topical trifluorothymidine found no significant difference between short term prophylaxis with oral aciclovir versus placebo in the rate of stromal keratitis or iritis.

Preventing ocular herpes simplex in people with corneal grafts

- One small RCT in people who had undergone corneal transplantation performed for herpes simplex virus infection found limited evidence that prophylactic use of oral aciclovir significantly reduced recurrences and improved graft survival.

DEFINITION	Ocular herpes simplex is usually caused by herpes simplex virus type 1 (HSV-1), but also occasionally by type 2 virus (HSV-2). Ocular manifestations of HSV are varied and include blepharitis, canalicular obstruction, conjunctivitis, epithelial keratitis, stromal keratitis (see glossary, p 179), iritis, and retinitis. HSV infections are classified as neonatal, primary (HSV in a person with no previous viral exposure), and recurrent (previous viral exposure with humoral and cellular immunity present).
INCIDENCE/ PREVALENCE	Infections with HSV are usually acquired in early life. A US study found antibodies against HSV-1 in about 50% of people with high socioeconomic status and 80% of people with low socioeconomic status by the age of 30 years.[1] However, only about 20–25% of people with HSV antibodies had any history of clinical manifestations of ocular or cutaneous herpetic disease.[2] Ocular HSV is the most common cause of corneal blindness in high income countries and the most common cause of unilateral corneal blindness in the world.[3] A 33 year study of the population of Rochester, Minnesota, found the annual incidence of new cases of ocular herpes simplex to be 8.4/100 000 (95% CI 6.9 to 9.9) and the annual incidence of all episodes (new and recurrent) to be 20.7/100 000 (95% CI 18.3 to 23.1).[4] The prevalence of ocular herpes was 149 cases/ 100 000 population (95% CI 115 to 183). Twelve per cent had bilateral disease.
AETIOLOGY/ RISK FACTORS	Epithelial keratitis (see glossary, p 179) results from productive, lytic viral infection of the corneal epithelial cells. Stromal keratitis (see glossary, p 179) and iritis are thought to result from a combination of viral infection and compromised immune mechanisms. We found no quantified measures of risk.
PROGNOSIS	HSV epithelial keratitis tends to resolve within 1–2 weeks. In a trial of 271 people treated with topical trifluorothymidine and randomly assigned to receive either oral aciclovir or placebo, the epithelial lesion had resolved completely or was at least less than 1 mm after 1 week of treatment with placebo in 89% of people and after 2 weeks in 99% of people.[5] Stromal keratitis or iritis occurs in about 25% of people following epithelial keratitis.[6] The effects of HSV

stromal keratitis include scarring, tissue destruction, neovascularisation, glaucoma, and persistent epithelial defects. Rate of recurrence of ocular herpes for people with one episode is 10% at 1 year, 23% at 2 years, and 50% at 10 years.[7] Five per cent of corneal grafts performed in Australia over a 10 year period were in people with visual disability or with actual or impending corneal perforation following stromal ocular herpes simplex. The recurrence of HSV in a corneal graft has a major effect on graft survival. The Australian Corneal Graft Registry has found that, in corneal grafts performed for HSV keratitis, there was at least one HSV recurrence in 58% of corneal grafts that failed over a follow up period of 9 years.[8]

AIMS   To reduce the morbidity of HSV keratitis and iritis; to reduce the risk of recurrent disease after a first episode; to reduce the risk of recurrent disease; and to improve corneal graft survival after penetrating keratoplasty.

OUTCOMES   Healing time; severity and duration of symptoms; severity of complications; rates of recurrence; corneal graft survival.

METHODS   *Clinical Evidence* search and appraisal August 2001.

QUESTION   **What are the effects of treatments for epithelial ocular herpes simplex?**

OPTION   **TOPICAL ANTIVIRAL AGENTS**

One systematic review has found that antiviral treatment (idoxuridine or vidarabine) versus placebo significantly increases the number of people healed after 14 days. The review also found that either trifluridine or aciclovir (acyclovir) versus idoxuridine significantly increases the number of people healed after 7 and 14 days, but found no significant difference with vidarabine versus idoxuridine in the number of people healed after 7 or 14 days. The review included "healed" as an outcome measure without clearly defining this term.

Benefits: We found one systematic review (search date 2000, 96 RCTs, 4991 people; see comment below).[9] **Versus placebo:** The review found that idoxuridine versus placebo significantly increased the number of people healed after 7 days (10 RCTs; OR 4.05, 95% CI 2.60 to 6.30; see comment below) and after 14 days (2 RCTs; OR 4.17, 95% CI 1.33 to 13.00).[9] The review also compared vidarabine versus placebo and found no significant difference in the number of people healed after 7 days (numerical data not provided), but found that vidarabine significantly increased the number of people healed after 14 days (1 RCT; OR 5.40, 95% CI 1.42 to 20.5). **Versus each other:** The review found that trifluridine versus idoxuridine significantly increased the number of people healed after 7 days (3 RCTs; OR 4.74, 95% CI 2.52 to 8.91) and after 14 days (4 RCTs; OR 6.83, 95% CI 3.02 to 15.5).[9] The review also found that aciclovir versus idoxuridine significantly increased the number of people healed after 7 days (8 RCTs; OR 5.33, 95% CI 3.33 to 8.53) and after 14 days (11 RCTs; OR 3.71, 95% CI 2.27 to 6.08), but that there was no significant difference with vidarabine versus idoxuridine in the number of people healed after 7 days (3

RCTs; OR 1.24, 95% CI 0.72 to 2.00) or after 14 days (3 RCTs; OR 1.24, 95% CI 0.65 to 2.37). **Antiviral treatment plus physical debridement:** See benefits of debridement, p 175.

Harms: The review did not report harms.

Comment: The review included healed as an outcome measure without clearly defining this term.[9] The review reported that the number of people involved in the comparison of vidarabine versus placebo was small, although it did not provide any absolute numbers.

OPTION   DEBRIDEMENT

One systematic review has found no significant difference between debridement versus placebo in the number of people healed after 7 or 14 days. The review found that debridement plus antiviral treatment versus debridement alone significantly increases the number of people healed after both 7 and 14 days, and that debridement plus antiviral treatment versus antiviral treatment alone significantly increases the number of people healed after 7 days but not after 14 days. The review included healed as an outcome measure without clearly defining this term.

Benefits: We found one systematic review (search date 2000, 96 RCTs, 4991 people).[9] **Debridement alone:** The review compared different types of physicochemical debridement versus placebo and found no significant difference in the number of people healed after 7 days (2 RCTs; OR 1.62, 95% CI 0.72 to 3.61; see comment below) or after 14 days (1 RCT; OR 2.12, 95% CI 0.38 to 12.0).[9] **Debridement plus antiviral treatment:** The review found that physicochemical debridement plus an antiviral agent versus physicochemical debridement alone significantly increased the number of people healed after 7 days (7 RCTs; OR 2.08, 95% CI 1.17 to 3.71) and after 14 days (2 RCTs; OR 10.81, 95% CI 1.81 to 64.5).[9] The review also found that physicochemical debridement plus an antiviral agent versus antiviral treatment alone significantly increased the number of people healed after 7 days (7 RCTs; OR 2.01, 95% CI 1.21 to 3.34), but found no significant difference in the number of people healed after 14 days (significance testing not provided). One RCT identified by the review compared debridement plus aciclovir versus debridement plus idoxuridine and found no significant difference in the number of people healed after 7 or 14 days (significance testing not provided).

Harms: The review reported that epithelial keratitis (see glossary, p 179) occurred in some people after physicochemical debridement alone (absolute numbers not provided) and limited the use of this treatment.[9]

Comment: The review found that all methods of debriding the corneal epithelium produced similar rates of re-epithelialisation.[9] The variety of treatments used in the review limits the applicability of the summary results.

OPTION   INTERFERON

One systematic review has found that topical interferon versus placebo significantly increases the number of people healed after both 7 and 14 days. The review found no significant difference between topical

Ocular herpes simplex

interferon versus a topical antiviral agent in the number of people healed after 7 days, but found that topical interferon significantly increases the number of people healed after 14 days. The review also found that topical interferon plus a topical antiviral agent versus a topical antiviral agent alone significantly increases the number of people healed after 14 days. The review included "healed" as an outcome without clearly defining this term.

Benefits: We found one systematic review (search date 2000, 96 RCTs, 4991 people).[9] **Versus placebo:** The review found that topical interferon versus placebo significantly increased the number of people healed after 7 days (3 RCTs; OR 2.09, 95% CI 1.15 to 3.81; see comment below) and after 14 days (2 RCTs; OR 3.43, 95% CI 1.30 to 9.02).[9] **Different concentrations:** The review found no significant difference with low concentration interferon (less than 1 MU/mL) versus higher concentrations of interferon in the number of people healed after 7 days (1 RCT; OR 0.21, 95% CI 0.02 to 2.42).[9] **Versus topical antivirals:** The review found no significant difference with topical interferon versus topical antiviral agents in the number of people healed after 7 days (2 RCTs; OR 1.18, 95% CI 0.29 to 4.75), but found that topical interferon versus a topical antiviral agent significantly increased the number of people healed after 14 days (3 RCTs; OR 3.48, 95% CI 1.06 to 11.4).[9] **Topical interferons plus antiviral agents:** The review found that topical interferon plus a topical antiviral agent versus a topical antiviral agent alone (usually trifluridine) significantly increased the number of people healed after 7 days (8 RCTs; OR 13.3, 95% CI 7.41 to 23.9) but found no significant difference in the number of people healed after 14 days (5 RCTs; OR 2.62, 95% CI 0.91 to 7.57).[9]

Harms: The review did not report data on harms.

Comment: The review included healed as an outcome measure without clearly defining this term.[9]

QUESTION What are the effects of treatments for stromal ocular herpes simplex?

OPTION TOPICAL CORTICOSTEROIDS

One RCT found that topical corticosteroids significantly reduced the progression and shortened the duration of stromal keratitis.

Benefits: We found one RCT (106 people) comparing topical prednisolone sodium phosphate (in decreasing concentrations over 10 wks) versus placebo.[10] All participants received topical trifluorothymidine. It found that prednisolone versus placebo significantly reduced the persistence or progression of stromal inflammation and shortened the duration of stromal keratitis (see glossary, p 179) (median 26 days with corticosteroid v median 72 days with placebo; difference in medians 46 days, 95% CI 14 to 58 days).[10]

Harms: The RCT found that adverse events were recorded in nine people given steroids.[10] Four people developed dendritic epithelial keratitis (see glossary, p 179) and were removed from the trial. Four people developed toxic responses to trifluorothymidine after week 5. These people were not withdrawn but the trifluorothymidine was stopped.

One person developed an epithelial defect and was withdrawn. Adverse events were reported in six people receiving placebo. All six were withdrawn from the study (1 person developed dendritic keratitis, 3 people developed an epithelial defect, and 2 people developed allergic conjunctivitis attributed to trifluorothymidine within the first 9 days of the trial).

Comment: The trial did not specify whether intention to treat analysis was performed or if people who withdrew from the trial were excluded from the analysis.

OPTION   ORAL ACICLOVIR

One RCT in people with stromal keratitis found no significant difference with oral aciclovir versus placebo in median time to treatment failure or in rates of treatment failure.

Benefits: We found one RCT (104 people with herpes simplex virus stromal keratitis [see glossary, p 179] receiving concomitant topical cortico-steroids and trifluorothymidine) of oral aciclovir versus placebo.[11] The primary outcome was time to treatment failure (assessed by 8 criteria). The RCT found no significant difference between aciclovir versus placebo in median time to treatment failure (84 days with aciclovir *v* 62 days with placebo; P = 0.46), and no significant difference in reported rates of treatment failure by week 16 (38/51 [75%] with aciclovir *v* 39/53 [74%] with placebo; RR 1.01, 95% CI 0.78 to 1.24).

Harms: The RCT found that two people in the placebo group developed adverse effects attributed to trifluorothymidine (epithelial keratopa-thy in 1 person and an allergic reaction in the other).[11] Other adverse effects reported included pneumonia with possible pulmo-nary embolus (1 person), congestive heart failure (1 person), diarrhoea (1 person), oedema of the lower extremities (1 person), and anaemia (1 person). Adverse reactions reported in the aciclovir group included toxicity to trifluorothymidine (1 person) and head-ache (1 person).

Comment: None.

QUESTION   What are the effects of interventions used as prophylaxis for people with ocular herpes simplex?

OPTION   ORAL ACICLOVIR

One large RCT in people with previous ocular herpes simplex found that long term prophylaxis (1 year) with oral aciclovir versus placebo significantly reduced the risk of recurrences. One RCT in people with epithelial keratitis receiving topical trifluorothymidine found no significant difference in the rate of stromal keratitis or iritis between short term prophylaxis with oral aciclovir versus placebo.

Benefits: We found no systematic review. We found two RCTs.[5,12] The first RCT (703 immunocompetent people aged ≥ 12 years who had epithelial or stromal ocular herpes simplex virus in one or both eyes within the preceding 12 months) compared oral aciclovir (400 mg

Eye disorders

Ocular herpes simplex

twice daily for 1 year) versus placebo.[12] It found that aciclovir treatment significantly reduced the risk of any type of recurrence after 1 year (19% with aciclovir v 32% with placebo; RR 0.55, 95% CI 0.41 to 0.75). Prespecified subgroup analysis (337 people with at least 1 previous episode of stromal keratitis) found that aciclovir versus placebo significantly reduced the risk of stromal keratitis (see glossary, p 179), but only in people who had at least one prior episode (14% with aciclovir v 28% with placebo; RR 0.48, 95% CI 0.29 to 0.80). The RCT found no rebound in the rate of ocular herpes simplex virus in the 6 months after stopping treatment with aciclovir. The second RCT (287 people with epithelial keratitis all treated with topical trifluorothymidine) compared a 3 week course of oral aciclovir versus placebo.[5] It found no significant difference in the rate of stromal keratitis or iritis (11% with aciclovir v 10% with placebo; RR 1.04, 95% CI 0.52 to 2.10), and no significant difference in the cumulative probability of developing stromal keratitis or iritis at 1 year follow up (12% with aciclovir v 11% with placebo; P = 0.92).

Harms: The RCT found that adverse effects (mostly gastrointestinal problems) were uncommon and occurred with similar frequency in both groups.[12] Thirty two people (15 aciclovir v 17 placebo) discontinued treatment because of adverse effects. The most common adverse effect reported was gastrointestinal upset (7 aciclovir v 9 placebo).

Comment: None.

| QUESTION | What are the effects of antiviral prophylaxis on corneal graft survival? |

| OPTION | ORAL ACICLOVIR |

One small RCT (in people who had undergone corneal transplantation performed for herpes simplex virus infection) found limited evidence that prophylactic use of oral aciclovir significantly reduced recurrences and improved graft survival.

Benefits: We found no systematic review. We found one small non-blinded RCT (22 people, 23 eyes, who had received keratoplasty — see glossary, p 179), which compared oral aciclovir (800 or 1000 mg, 4 or 5 times orally daily, tapered during the first 12 months, for a maximum of 15 months) versus usual care.[13] Oral aciclovir was started before surgery or on the first day after surgery. The RCT found that oral aciclovir versus usual care significantly reduced the number of recurrences of ocular herpes simplex after a mean follow up of 17 months in people receiving aciclovir and 21 months in those receiving placebo (0% with aciclovir v 44% with placebo; P < 0.01), and also that aciclovir versus usual care significantly reduced the number of eyes with graft failure (14% with aciclovir treated eyes v 56% with placebo; P < 0.05).

Harms: None reported.

Comment: None.

GLOSSARY

Epithelial keratitis Inflammation of the cells that form the surface layer of the cornea.

Keratoplasty A procedure in which diseased corneal tissue is removed and replaced by donor corneal material.

Stromal keratitis Inflammation of the middle layer of the cornea. The stroma forms 90% of the corneal substance. It lies between the epithelium and Bowman's membrane anteriorly and Desçemet's membrane and the endothelium posteriorly.

REFERENCES

1. Nahmias AJ, Lee FK, Beckman-Nahmias S. Sero-epidemiological and sociological patterns of herpes simplex virus infection in the world. *Scand J Infect Dis Suppl* 1990;69:19–36.
2. Kaufman HE, Rayfield MA, Gebhardt BM. Herpes simplex viral infections. In: Kaufman HE, Baron BA, McDonald MB, eds. *The Cornea.* 2nd ed. Butterworth-Heinemann, 1997.
3. Dawson CR, Togni B. Herpes simplex eye infections: clinical manifestations, pathogenesis, and management. *Surv Ophthalmol* 1976;21: 121–135.
4. Liesegang TJ, Melton LJ III, Daly PJ, et al. Epidemiology of ocular herpes simplex. Incidence in Rochester, Minnesota, 1950 through 1982. *Arch Ophthalmol* 1989;107:1155–1159.
5. The Herpetic Eye Disease Study Group. A controlled trial of oral acyclovir for the prevention of stromal keratitis or iritis in patients with herpes simplex virus epithelial keratitis. The Epithelial Keratitis Trial. *Arch Ophthalmol* 1997;115: 703–712.
6. Wilhelmus KR, Coster DJ, Donovan HC, Falcon MG, Jones BR. Prognosis indicators of herpetic keratitis. Analysis of a five-year observation period after corneal ulceration. *Arch Ophthalmol* 1981; 99:1578–1582.
7. Liesegang TJ. Epidemiology of ocular herpes simplex. Natural history in Rochester, Minnesota, 1950 through 1982. *Arch Ophthalmol* 1989;107: 1160–1165.
8. Williams KA, Muehlberg SM, Lewis RF, Giles LC, Coster DJ. *The Australian Corneal Graft Registry: 1996 Report.* Adelaide: Mercury Press, 1997.
9. Wilhelmus KR. Interventions for herpes simplex virus epithelial keratitis (Cochrane Review). In: The Cochrane Library, Issue 3, 2001. Oxford: Update Software. Search date November 2000; primary sources Medline, Central, Embase, Index medicus, Excerpta Medica Ophthalmology, Cochrane Eyes and Vision Group specialised register, The Cochrane Controlled Trials Register, hand searching of reference lists of primary reports, review articles, and corneal textbooks, and conference proceedings pertaining to ocular virology.
10. Wilhelmus KR, Gee L, Hauck WW, et al. Herpetic Eye Disease Study. A controlled trial of topical corticosteroids for herpes simplex stromal keratitis. *Ophthalmology* 1994;101:1883–1895.
11. Barron BA, Gee L, Hauck WW, et al. Herpetic Eye Disease Study. A controlled trial of oral acyclovir for herpes simplex stromal keratitis. *Ophthalmology* 1994;101:1871–1882.
12. Herpetic Eye Disease Study Group. Acyclovir for the prevention of recurrent herpes simplex virus eye disease. *N Engl J Med* 1998;339:300–306.
13. Barney NP, Foster CS. A prospective randomized trial of oral acyclovir after penetrating keratoplasty for herpes simplex keratitis. *Cornea* 1994;13: 232–236.

Nigel Barker
Consultant Ophthalmologist
Specialist Eye Centre
Christ Church
Barbados

Competing interests: None declared.

Eye disorders

Search date October 2001

Denise Mabey and Nicole Fraser-Hurt

INTERVENTIONS

Key Messages

Prevention of scarring trachoma by reducing active trachoma

- One RCT identified by two systematic reviews found that promotion of face washing plus topical tetracycline versus topical tetracycline alone significantly reduced the rate of severe trachoma after 1 year, but found no significant difference in the overall rate of trachoma. However, the RCT was too small to rule out a clinically important effect. One additional RCT found that face washing alone versus no intervention did not significantly reduce the number of children with trachoma, although face washing plus topical tetracycline versus no intervention significantly reduced the number of children with trachoma. A pilot study for an RCT included in the systematic reviews found that fly control using insecticide versus no intervention significantly reduced the incidence of trachoma.

- One unpublished systematic review found limited evidence from low powered RCTs that antibiotics versus control significantly reduced active trachoma after 3 and 12 months. One additional RCT found that topical tetracycline plus face washing versus no intervention significantly reduced the number of children with trachoma after 3 months. The same review found limited evidence from three RCTs that oral azithromycin versus topical tetracycline significantly reduced active trachoma after 3 months. These RCTs were low powered or of unusual design and at 12 months the difference between treatments disappeared. One subsequent RCT found that oral azithromycin versus topical tetracycline significantly increased clinical resolution of trachoma at 10 and 6 months.

Treatment of scarring trachoma

- We found no good evidence on the effects of surgery to improve visual acuity in people with scarring trachoma. In people with major trichiasis, one RCT found that tarsal rotation versus eversion splinting, tarsal advance, and tarsal grooving significantly increased operative success, but found no significant difference between tarsal rotation versus tarsal advance and rotation in operative success. A second RCT found that tarsal rotation versus tarsal advance and rotation significantly increased operative success. In people with minor trichiasis, one RCT found that tarsal rotation versus cryoablation or electrolysis significantly increased operative success. In people with major trichiasis, one RCT found no significant difference between village versus health centre based tarsal rotation surgery in operative success.

DEFINITION	**Active trachoma** is chronic inflammation of the conjunctiva caused by infection with *Chlamydia trachomatis*. The World Health Organization classification for active trachoma defines mild trachoma (grade TF) as the presence of five or more follicles in the upper tarsal conjunctiva of at least 0.5 mm diameter. Severe trachoma (grade TI) is defined as pronounced inflammatory thickening of the upper tarsal conjunctiva that obscures more than half of the normal deep vessels. **Scarring trachoma** is caused by repeated active infection by *C trachomatis* in which the upper eyelid is shortened and distorted (entropion) and the lashes abrade the eye (trichiasis). Blindness results from corneal opacification, which is related to the degree of entropion/trichiasis.
INCIDENCE/ PREVALENCE	Trachoma is the world's leading cause of preventable blindness and is second only to cataract as an overall cause of blindness.[1] Globally, active trachoma affects an estimated 150 million people, most of them children. About 5.5 million people are blind or at risk of blindness as a consequence of trachoma. Trachoma is a disease of poverty regardless of geographical region. Scarring trachoma is prevalent in large regions of Africa, the Middle East, south-west Asia, the Indian subcontinent, and Aboriginal communities in Australia, and there are also small foci in Central and South America.[1] In areas where trachoma is constantly present at high prevalence, active disease is found in more than 50% of preschool children and may have a prevalence of 60–90%.[2] The prevalence of active trachoma decreases with increasing age, with less than 5% of adults showing signs of active disease.[2] Although similar rates of active disease are observed in male and female children, the later sequelae of trichiasis, entropion, and corneal opacification are more common in women than men.[2] As many as 75% of women and 50% of men over the age of 45 years may show signs of scarring disease.[3]
AETIOLOGY/ RISK FACTORS	Active trachoma is associated with young age and with situations in which there is close contact between people. Discharge from the eyes and nose may be a source of further reinfection.[4] Sharing a bedroom with someone who has active trachoma is a risk factor for infection.[5] Facial contact with flies is held to be associated with active trachoma, but studies reporting this relationship employed weak methods.[6]
PROGNOSIS	Corneal damage from trachoma is caused by multiple processes. Scarring may cause an inadequate tear film and a dry eye may be

more susceptible to damage from inturned lashes, leading to corneal opacification. The prevalence of scarring and consequent blindness increases with age and, therefore, is most commonly seen in older adults.[7]

AIMS   To prevent active trachoma; to reduce the rate of progression to scarring; to relieve entropion and trichiasis in people with scarring trachoma; to minimise side effects of treatment.

OUTCOMES   Rates of active trachoma; clinical signs of active trachoma using the World Health Organization grading scale; laboratory evidence of *C trachomatis* infection; eyelid position; degree of entropion/trichiasis.

METHODS   *Clinical Evidence* search and appraisal October 2001.

QUESTION   What are the effects of interventions to prevent scarring trachoma by reducing active trachoma?

OPTION   PUBLIC HEALTH INTERVENTIONS

One RCT identified by two systematic reviews found that promotion of face washing plus topical tetracycline versus topical tetracycline alone significantly reduced the rate of severe trachoma after 1 year, but found no significant difference in the overall rate of trachoma. However, the RCT was too small to rule out a clinically important effect. One additional RCT found that face washing alone versus no intervention did not significantly reduce the number of children with trachoma, although face washing plus topical tetracycline versus no intervention significantly reduced the number of children with trachoma. A pilot study for an RCT included in the systematic reviews found that fly control using insecticide versus no intervention significantly reduced the incidence of trachoma.

Benefits: We found two systematic reviews[8,9] and one additional RCT.[10] The first systematic review (search date 1999) identified one RCT and one pilot study for an RCT.[8] The second systematic review (search date 1999) identified the same RCT and pilot study as the first review plus two subsequent RCTs (see comment below).[9]
Promotion of face washing: Both reviews identified one RCT (1417 children aged 1–7 years in 6 villages) that compared promotion of face washing plus 30 days of daily topical tetracycline (ointment) versus 30 days of daily topical tetracycline alone.[11] It found that promotion of face washing plus topical tetracycline increased the likelihood of children having a clean face on at least two of three follow up visits, although the result was not significant (OR for having a clean face with face washing plus topical tetracycline v topical tetracycline alone 1.6, 95% CI 0.94 to 2.74). The RCT also found that promotion of face washing plus topical tetracycline versus topical tetracycline alone significantly reduced the risk of severe trachoma after 1 year (OR for severe trachoma 0.62, 95% CI 0.40 to 0.97), but found that this reduction was not significant for all grades of trachoma combined (OR for mild and severe trachoma 0.81, 95% CI 0.42 to 1.59). The RCT found that when all participants from intervention and control villages were pooled, children who had a sustained clean face were significantly less likely to have active trachoma than those who had ever had a

dirty face (OR 0.58, 95% CI 0.47 to 0.72). The additional RCT (1143 children in 36 communities) compared three groups: daily face washing (performed by a teacher); daily face washing (performed by a teacher) plus daily topical tetracycline (as drops for 1 wk each month); and no intervention.[10] Trachoma was defined as the presence of at least one follicle or some papillae on the upper tarsal plate (this study predated the present World Health Organization definition of trachoma). Losses to follow up were treated as being trachoma positive. The RCT found no significant difference between face washing alone versus no intervention in the number of children with trachoma after 3 months (191/246 [78%] with face washing alone v 160/211 [76%] with no intervention; RR 1.0; CI not provided). It also found that face washing plus tetracycline drops versus no intervention significantly reduced the number of children with trachoma after 3 months (215/312 [69%] with face washing plus topical tetracycline v 160/211 [78%] with no intervention; RR 0.9; CI not provided).[10] **Fly control using insecticide:** The reviews identified one pilot study for an RCT (414 children < 10 years) that compared spraying of deltamethrin for 3 months versus no intervention in two pairs of villages.[6] One pair received the intervention or none in the wet season and one pair received the intervention or none in the dry season. There were a total of 191 children under 10 years of age in the control villages and 223 children in the intervention villages. The pilot study found that spraying of deltamethrin significantly reduced the number of new cases of trachoma (World Health Organization classification) after 3 months (RR 0.25, 95% CI 0.09 to 0.64).

Harms: The reviews and additional RCT did not report adverse effects.[8–10]

Comment: Cluster randomisation used in the RCTs and the pilot study limits the power to detect differences between groups, and makes interpretation of the results for individual children difficult.[6,10,11] The RCT comparing promotion of face washing plus topical tetracycline versus topical tetracycline alone was too small to rule out a clinically important effect.[11] The two subsequent RCTs identified by the second systematic review compared antibiotics versus health education plus face washing, and it was not possible to extract data relating to the health education and face washing interventions separately.[9] The additional RCT predates the simplified World Health Organization classification of trachoma, limiting the applicability of the results.[10]

OPTION   ANTIBIOTICS

One unpublished systematic review found limited evidence from low powered RCTs that antibiotics versus control significantly reduced active trachoma after 3 and 12 months. One additional RCT found that topical tetracycline plus face washing versus no intervention significantly reduced the number of children with trachoma after 3 months. The same review found limited evidence from three RCTs that oral azithromycin versus topical tetracycline significantly reduced active trachoma after 3 months. Those RCTs were low powered or of unusual design, and at

12 months the difference between treatments disappeared. One subsequent RCT found that oral azithromycin versus topical tetracycline significantly increased clinical resolution of trachoma at 10 weeks and 6 months.

Benefits: **Versus placebo or no treatment:** We found one unpublished systematic review (search date 1999, 11 RCTs)[12] and one additional RCT.[10] The review identified eight RCTs that compared antibiotics (topical or oral) versus control (no treatment, placebo, or a monthly vitamin tablet)(see table 1, p 188). [13-20] The review found that antibiotics versus control significantly reduced active trachoma (assessed clinically) after 3 months (8 RCTs; OR 0.43, 95% CI 0.35 to 0.52) and after 12 months (5 RCTs; OR 0.47, 95% CI 0.38 to 0.60; see comment below). The review found no significant difference between treatments in C trachomatis infection rates based on bacteriological testing after 3 months (3 RCTs; OR 0.63, 95% CI 0.38 to 1.05), but found that antibiotics significantly reduced infection rates after 12 months (1 RCT; OR 0.27, 95% CI 0.11 to 0.67). For the additional RCT see benefits of public health interventions, p 182. **Oral versus topical antibiotics:** We found one unpublished systematic review (search date 1999, 3 RCTs, 6226 people; see comment below)[12] and one subsequent RCT.[21] The review found that oral azithromycin versus topical tetracycline significantly reduced active trachoma after 3 months (3 RCTs, 6226 people; OR 0.82, 95% CI 0.71 to 0.94), but found no significant difference between treatments in rates of active trachoma after 12 months (1 RCT; 5573 people; OR 0.88, 95% CI 0.77 to 1.01) (see table 2, p 189).[12] The review also found that oral azithromycin versus topical tetracycline significantly reduced bacteriologically defined infection after both 3 months (OR 0.49, 95% CI 0.39 to 0.62) and 12 months (OR 0.70, 95% CI 0.57 to 0.87) (see table 2, p 189). The subsequent RCT (314 children) compared a single dose of oral azithromycin versus topical tetracycline and found that oral azithromycin significantly increased the cure rate (defined as clinical resolution of trachoma) after 10 weeks (104/152 [68%] with azithromycin v 71/139 [51%] with tetracycline; RR 1.31, 95% CI 1.08 to 1.59) and after 6 months (135/154 [88%] v 103/141 [73%] with tetracycline; RR 1.19, 95% CI 1.06 to 1.34).[21]

Harms: None reported.

Comment: RCTs conducted prior to 1987 may use definitions of trachoma that differ from the present World Health Organization definition.[10,13-19] **Versus placebo or no treatment:** The trials were undertaken in various settings, and most were in children attending boarding schools.[10,12] Several unusual study designs were used, for example family based treatment. The trials were all of moderate or poor quality and many had no intention to treat analysis. Antibiotic treatments included topical and oral doses. **Oral versus topical treatment:** Two of the RCTs were small (total 224 people) and low powered.[12] The third RCT compared mass treatment, in which people were treated irrespective of disease status and were randomly allocated by village (cluster randomisation).[12] Correlation analysis found some similarity between individuals within a cluster, limiting the validity of results. We found no evidence regarding the development of bacterial resistance.

QUESTION What are the effects of surgical treatments for scarring trachoma (entropion and trichiasis)?

We found no good evidence on the effects of surgery to improve visual acuity in people with scarring trachoma. In people with major trichiasis, one RCT found that tarsal rotation versus eversion splinting, tarsal advance, and tarsal grooving significantly increased operative success, but found no significant difference between tarsal rotation versus tarsal advance and rotation in operative success. A second RCT found that tarsal rotation versus tarsal advance and rotation significantly increased operative success. In people with minor trichiasis, one RCT found that tarsal rotation versus cryoablation or electrolysis significantly increased operative success. In people with major trichiasis, one RCT found no significant difference between village versus health centre based tarsal rotation surgery in operative success.

Benefits: We found no systematic review but found three RCTs.[25–27] In the two RCTs that compared surgical interventions versus each other, one experienced surgeon performed most of the operations.[25,26] Both of these RCTs defined operative success as no lashes in contact with the globe in primary position of gaze and complete lid closure with gentle voluntary effort. **Major trichiasis:** See glossary, p 186. The first RCT (165 Omani villagers, 165 eyelids) compared five surgical techniques: bilamellar tarsal rotation; eversion splinting; tarsal advance; tarsal grooving; and tarsal advance and rotation (see glossary, p 186).[25] It found that tarsal rotation versus eversion splinting, tarsal advance, and tarsal grooving significantly increased operative success after 2 weeks (30/44 [68%] with tarsal rotation v 8/25 [32%] with eversion splinting; RR 2.13, 95% CI 1.16 to 3.91; 30/44 [68%] with tarsal rotation v 11/41 [27%] with tarsal advance; RR 2.5, 95% CI 1.5 to 4.4; 30/44 [68%] with tarsal rotation v 3/32 [9%] with tarsal grooving; RR 7.3, 95% CI 2.4 to 21.8), but found no significant difference between tarsal rotation versus tarsal advance and rotation in operative success after 2 weeks (30/44 [68%] with tarsal rotation v 10/23 [43%] with tarsal advance and rotation; RR 1.57, 95% CI 0.94 to 2.6). However, analysis was not by intention to treat and the power of the trial was low. The second RCT (Omani villagers, 200 eyelids) compared bilamellar tarsal rotation versus tarsal advance and rotation.[26] It found that tarsal rotation significantly increased operative success after 25 months (HR for failure, tarsal advance and rotation v tarsal rotation 3.1, 95% CI 1.9 to 5.2). **Minor trichiasis:** See glossary, p 186. The second RCT (172 eyelids) compared three treatments: tarsal rotation; cryoablation; and electrolysis.[26] It found that tarsal rotation versus both treatments significantly increased operative success after 25 months (HR of failure, electrolysis v tarsal rotation 6.1, 95% CI 2.9 to 12.8; HR of failure, cryoablation v tarsal rotation 7.5, 95% CI 3.6 to 15.4). **Location of surgery:** We found one RCT (158 people with major trichiasis), which compared village versus health centre based tarsal rotation surgery for major trichiasis.[27] It found that attendance rates were not significantly different between interventions (57/86 [66%] v 32/72 [44%]; RR 1.5, 95% CI not provided). The RCT also found that there was also no significant difference between interventions in operative success rate (defined as no evidence of trichiasis) after 3 months (intention to treat analysis by *Clinical Evidence*; 52/86 [60%] with village surgery v 30/72 [42%] with health centre surgery; RR 1.4, 95% CI not available).[27]

Harms: Adverse outcomes of interventions were corneal exposure, ulceration, phthisis bulbi (see glossary, p 186), and severe recurrent trichiasis.[25,28] In the two RCTs that compared different surgical techniques versus each other, major trichiasis and defective closure after surgical procedures for scarring trachoma were more common after eversion splinting, tarsal advance, and tarsal grooving than after bilamellar tarsal rotation and tarsal advance and rotation.[25,26] Cryoablation of the eyelashes can cause necrosis of the lid margin, corneal ulcers, and in the RCT in which cryoablation was used it was the only procedure associated with onset of phthisis bulbi (2 cases out of 57).[26] Further details of harms are summarised in table 3, p 190.

Comment: The pragmatic definitions of major trichiasis and minor trichiasis are limited to use in these trials.[25,26] In both RCTs comparing surgical interventions, one experienced operator performed most of the surgery. The evidence of both benefits and harms may not be applicable to different operators, or where the quality of surgical equipment does not match those in the trials. In the RCT comparing village based versus health centre based surgery, problems with the unit of randomisation prevented the calculation of confidence limits for the relative risks stated.

GLOSSARY

Bilamellar tarsal rotation The upper lid is cut full thickness horizontally in a line parallel and 3 mm from the eyelid margin and running from just lateral to the lacrimal punctum to the lateral canthus. Everting sutures are then placed through all layers of the lid to prevent the margin from turning inwards.

Eversion splinting The lid margin is split posterior to the lashes, the eversion of the anterior section is maintained by sutures tied over a roll of paraffin gauze.

Major trichiasis Lid closure complete; six or more lashes in contact with eyeball.

Minor trichiasis Lid closure complete; one to five lashes in contact with eyeball.

Phthisis bulbi A disorganised, shrunken eye that has no perception of light.

Tarsal advance The lid margin is split posterior to the lashes. The skin, lashes, and orbicularis are freed from the tarsal plate and retracted away from the cornea and are sutured back on to the tarsal plate, leaving a bare area of tarsus to act as the lid margin.

Tarsal advance and rotation The upper lid is everted over a speculum. The tarsal plate is fractured parallel to and 3 mm from the lid margin. In this operation the skin and orbicularis are not cut. The short portion of tarsal plate attached to the lid margin is then rotated through 180° and sutured into place to form the new lid margin.

Tarsal grooving A wedge of skin, orbicularis, and tarsus is removed parallel to the lid margin. Sutures through all layers act to evert the lid margin.

REFERENCES

1. Thylefors B, Negrel AD, Pararajasegaram R, et al. Global data on blindness. *Bull World Health Organ* 1995;73:115–121.

2. West SK, Munoz B, Turner VM, et al. The epidemiology of trachoma in central Tanzania. *Int J Epidemiol* 1991;20:1088–1092.

3. Courtright P, Sheppard J, Schachter J, et al. Trachoma and blindness in the Nile Delta: current patterns and projections for the future in the rural Egyptian population. *Br J Ophthalmol* 1989;73:536–540.

4. Bobo L, Munoz B, Viscidi R, et al. Diagnosis of *Chlamydia trachomatis* eye infection in Tanzania by polymerase chain reaction/enzyme immunoassay. *Lancet* 1991;338:847–850.

5. Bailey R, Osmond C, Mabey DCW, et al. Analysis of the household pattern of trachoma in a Gambian village using a Monte Carlo simulation procedure. *Int J Epidemiol* 1989;18:944–951.

6. Emerson PM, Lindsay SW, Walraven GE, et al. Effect of fly control on trachoma and diarrhoea. *Lancet* 1999;353:1401–1403.

7. Munoz B, West SK. The forgotten cause of blindness. *Epidemiol Rev* 1997;19:205–217.

8. Emerson PM, Cairncross S, Bailey RL, Mabey DC. Review of the evidence base for the "F" and "E" components of the SAFE strategy for trachoma control. *Trop Med Int Health* 2000;5:515–527. Search date 1999; primary sources Medline, BIDS, and hand searches of reference lists.

9. Pruss A, Mariotti SP. Preventing trachoma through environmental sanitation: a review of the evidence base. *Bull World Health Organ* 2000;78:258–266. Search date 1999; primary sources Medline, Healthstar, and hand searches of reference lists and selected conference proceedings.

10. Peach H, Piper S, Devanesen D, et al. Trial of antibiotic drops for the prevention of trachoma in school-age Aboriginal children. *Annual Report Menzies School for Health Research* 1986;74–76.

11. West S, Munoz B, Lynch M, et al. Impact of facewashing on trachoma in Kongwa, Tanzania. *Lancet* 1995;345:155–158.

12. Mabey D, Fraser-Hurt N. Antibiotics for trachoma (Protocol for a Cochrane Review). In: The Cochrane Library, Issue 4, 2000. Oxford: Update Software. Search date 1999; primary sources Medline, Embase, Cinalh, Science Citation Index, and personal contacts.

13. Attiah MA, el Kohly AM. Clinical assessment of the comparative effect of terramycin and GS 2989 in the mass treatment of trachoma. *Rev Int Trach Pathol Ocul Trop Subtrop Sante Publique* 1973;50:11–20.

14. Darougar S, Jones BR, Viswalingam N, et al. Family-based suppressive intermittent therapy of hyperendemic trachoma with topical oxytetracycline or oral doxycycline. *Br J Ophthalmol* 1980;64:291–295.

15. Dawson CR, Hanna L, Wood TR, et al. Controlled trials with trisulphapyrimidines in the treatment of chronic trachoma. *J Infect Dis* 1969;119:581–590.

16. Foster SO, Powers DK, Thygeson P. Trachoma therapy: a controlled study. *Am J Ophthalmol* 1966;61:451–455.

17. Hoshiwara I, Ostler HB, Hanna L, et al. Doxycycline treatment of chronic trachoma. *JAMA* 1973;224:220–223.

18. Shukla BR, Nema HV, Mathur JS, et al. Gantrisin and madribon in trachoma. *Br J Ophthalmol* 1966;50:218–221.

19. Woolridge RL, Cheng KH, Chang IH, et al. Failure of trachoma treatment with ophthalmic antibiotics and systemic sulphonamides used alone or in combination with trachoma vaccine. *Am J Ophthalmol* 1967;63(suppl):1577–1586.

20. Tabbara KF, Summanen P, Taylor PB, et al. Minocycline effects in patients with active trachoma. *Int Ophthalmol* 1988;12:59–63.

21. Bowman RJC, Sillah A, Van Dehn C, et al. Operational comparison of single-dose azithromycin and topical tetracycline for trachoma. *Investig Ophthalmol Visu Sci* 2000;41:4074–4079.

22. Dawson CR, Schachter J, Sallam S, et al. A comparison of oral azithromycin with topical oxytetracycline/polymyxin for the treatment of trachoma in children. *Clin Infect Dis* 1997;24:363–368.

23. Schachter J, West SK, Mabey D, et al. Azithromycin in control of trachoma. *Lancet* 1999;354:630–635.

24. Tabbara KF, Abu el Asrar A, al Omar O, et al. Single-dose azithromycin in the treatment of trachoma. A randomized, controlled study. *Ophthalmology* 1996;103:842–846.

25. Reacher MH, Huber MJE, Canagaratnam R, et al. A trial of surgery for trichiasis of the upper lid from trachoma. *Br J Ophthalmol* 1990;74:109–113.

26. Reacher MH, Munoz B, Alghassany A, et al. A controlled trial of surgery for trachomatous trichiasis of the upper lid. *Arch Ophthalmol* 1992;110:667–674.

27. Bowman RJ, Soma OS, Alexander N, et al. Should trichiasis surgery be offered in the village? A community randomised trial of village vs. health centre-based surgery. *Trop Med Internat Health* 2000;5:528–533.

28. Reacher MH, Taylor HR. The management of trachomatous trichiasis. *Rev Int Trach Pathol Ocul Trop Subtrop Sante Publique* 1990;67:233–262.

Nicole Fraser-Hurt
Epiconsult Ltd
Nhlangano
Swaziland

Denise Mabey
Guy's and St Thomas' Hospital Trust
London
UK

Competing interests: None declared.

TABLE 1 Interventions to prevent scarring trachoma by reducing active trachoma: RCTs of antibiotics compared with no treatment, placebo, or a monthly vitamin tablet in people with active trachoma (see text, p 184).

Study	Treatment	Route	Dose	Duration	Comparison
13	Tetracycline derivative GS2989	Topical	0.25%	Once every school day for 11 weeks	No treatment
13	Oxytetracycline	Topical	Not stated	Once every school day for 11 weeks	No treatment
14	Oxytetracycline	Topical	1%	Twice daily for 7 consecutive days every month for 12 months	Vitamin pills, orally, 1 dose every month for 12 months
14	Doxycycline	Oral	5 mg/kg	1 dose every month for 12 months	Vitamin pills, orally, 1 dose every month for 12 months
15	Trisulfapyrimidine	Oral	3.5 g/day	3 daily during 3 consecutive weeks	Lactose, orally, 3 daily for 3 weeks
15	Trisulfapyrimidine	Oral	3.5 g/day	3 daily during 3 consecutive weeks	Lactose, orally, 3 daily for 3 weeks
16	Sulfametopyridazine	Oral	0.5 g	Once daily for 5 consecutive days every week for 3 weeks	No treatment
16	Tetracycline	Topical	1%	3 times daily on 5 consecutive days every week for 6 weeks	No treatment
17	Doxycycline	Oral	2.5–4.0 mg/kg	Once daily for 5 consecutive days every week up to 28 doses in 40 days	Placebo once daily for 5 consecutive days every week up to 28 doses in 40 days
18	Sulfafurazole plus sulfadimethoxine	Topical plus oral	15%/100 mg/kg	Twice daily for 5 consecutive days every month for 5 months/biweekly for 5 months	No treatment
18	Sulfadimethoxine	Oral	100 mg/kg	Twice weekly or weekly dose for 5 months	No treatment
18	Sulfafurazole	Topical	15%	Twice daily for 5 consecutive days every month for 5 months	No treatment
19	Tetracycline	Topical	1%	Twice daily for 6 consecutive days every week for 6 weeks	No treatment
20	Minocycline	Oral	100 mg	Once daily on 5 consecutive days every week for 5 weeks	Placebo topically twice daily on 5 consecutive days every week for 5 weeks
20	Tetracycline	Topical	1%	Twice daily on 5 consecutive days every week for 5 weeks	Placebo topically twice daily on 5 consecutive days every week for 5 weeks

TABLE 2 Interventions to prevent scarring trachoma by reducing active trachoma and bacteriological infection following oral azithromycin or topical tetracycline (see text, p 184).

Study	Treatment	Dose	Duration	Comparison	Dose/duration
22	Azithromycin orally	20 mg/kg	1 dose, or 3 times 1 dose at weekly intervals, or 6 times 1 dose at 28 day intervals	1% topical oxytet/polymyxin plus oral placebo	Ointment once daily for 5 consecutive days monthly for 6 months
23	Azithromycin orally	20 mg/kg up to 1 g	Once a week for 3 weeks	1% topical oxytetracycline	Once daily for 6 weeks
	Women of childbearing age; erythromycin	500 mg twice daily or 250 mg four times daily	14 days	ND	ND
24	Azithromycin orally	20 mg/kg	1 dose	1% topical tetracycline	Twice daily for 5 consecutive days every week for 6 weeks

ND, no data.

Trachoma

TABLE 3 Summary of harms following surgery for scarring trachoma (see text, p 186).

	Bilamellar tarsal rotation	Tarsal advance and rotation	Eversion splinting	Tarsal advance	Tarsal grooving
Reference[26]					
Major trichiasis	4/150	4/101	ND	ND	ND
Defective closure	2/150	1/101	ND	ND	ND
Reference[28]					
Major trichiasis	1/44	1/23	7/25	10/41	11/32
Defective closure	2/44	0/23	0/25	0/41	5/32

ND, no data.

Search date July 2001

George Swingler and Jimmy Volmink

INTERVENTIONS

Key Messages

Prevention

■ Two RCTs have found that live attenuated varicella vaccine significantly reduces
  clinical chickenpox in healthy children, with no significant increase in adverse
  effects. We found no evidence in immunocompromised people.

■ One systematic review has found that high dose aciclovir (at least 3200 mg/
  day) significantly reduces clinical chickenpox and reduces all cause mortality in
  people with human immunodeficiency virus (HIV) infection.

■ One small RCT in healthy children has found that zoster immune globulin (ZIG)
  versus human immune serum globulin (ISG) significantly reduces the number
  of children with clinical chickenpox. In immunocompromised children, one RCT
  found no significant difference between ZIG versus varicella zoster immune
  globulin (VZIG) in clinical chickenpox.

Chickenpox

Treatment

- RCTs have found that oral aciclovir versus placebo significantly reduces the symptoms of chickenpox in healthy people when given within 24 hours of onset of the rash, but found no significant difference if started after 24 hours. Two RCTs compared intravenous aciclovir versus placebo in children with cancer; one found that aciclovir significantly reduced clinical deterioration, and the other small RCT found no significant difference.

DEFINITION	Chickenpox is due to primary infection with varicella zoster virus (VZV). In healthy people, it is usually a mild self limiting illness, characterised by low grade fever, malaise, and a generalised, itchy vesicular rash.
INCIDENCE/ PREVALENCE	Chickenpox is extremely contagious. Over 90% of unvaccinated people become infected, but at different ages in different parts of the world. Over 80% of people have been infected by the age of 10 years in the USA, UK, and Japan, but only by 30 years of age or older in India, Southeast Asia, and the West Indies.[1,2]
AETIOLOGY/ RISK FACTORS	Chickenpox is caused by exposure to VZV.
PROGNOSIS	**Infants and children:** In healthy children, the illness is usually mild and self limited. In the USA, the death rate in children aged 1–14 years with chickenpox is about 1.4/100 000 and 7/100 000 in infants.[3] In Australia, mortality in children aged between 1 and 11 years with chickenpox is about 0.5–0.6/100 000 and 1.2/ 100 000 in infants.[4] Bacterial skin sepsis is the most common complication in children under 5 years, and acute cerebellar ataxia is the most common complication in older children; both cause hospital admission in 2–3/10 000 children.[5] **Adults:** Mortality in adults is higher, about 31/100 000.[3] Varicella pneumonia is the most common complication, causing 20–30 hospital admissions/ 10 000 adults.[5] Activation of latent VZV infection can cause shingles, also know as acute herpes zoster. **Cancer chemotherapy:** One case series (77 children with cancer and chickenpox) found that more children receiving chemotherapy versus those in remission developed progressive chickenpox with multiple organ involvement (19/60 [32%] v 0/17 [0%]), and more children died (4/60 [7%] v 0/17 [0%]).[6] **HIV infection:** One retrospective case series found that one in four children with HIV who acquired chickenpox in hospital developed pneumonia and 5% died.[7] In a retrospective cohort study (73 children with HIV and chickenpox), infection beyond 2 months occurred in 10 children (14%), and recurrent VZV infections occurred in 38 children (55%).[8] Half of recurrent infections involved generalised rashes and the other half had zoster. **Newborns:** We found no cohort studies of untreated children with perinatal exposure to chickenpox. One cohort study (281 neonates receiving VZIG (see glossary, p 196) because their mothers had developed a chickenpox rash in the month before or after delivery) found that 134 (48%) developed a chickenpox rash and 19 (14%) developed severe chickenpox. Severe chickenpox occurred in neonates of mothers whose rash had started in the 7 days before delivery.[9]

AIMS	To prevent clinical chickenpox (characterised by a rash); to reduce the duration of illness and complications of chickenpox.
OUTCOMES	Development of clinical chickenpox; duration of illness (onset of last new lesions, disappearance of fever); complications of chickenpox; mortality.
METHODS	*Clinical Evidence* search and appraisal July 2001. All identified RCTs with English abstracts were reviewed.

QUESTION **What are the effects of treatments to prevent chickenpox?**

OPTION **LIVE ATTENUATED VARICELLA VACCINE**

Two RCTs have found that live attenuated varicella vaccine significantly reduces chickenpox in healthy children, with no significant increase in adverse effects. We found no RCTs in immunocompromised people.

Benefits:	We found no systematic review. **In healthy people:** We found two RCTs. The first RCT (914 healthy children aged 1–14 years) found that live attenuated varicella vaccine versus placebo significantly reduced clinical chickenpox at 9 months (0/468 [0%] with vaccine *v* 38/446 [8.5%] with placebo; OR 0.0, 95% CI 0.0 to 0.09) and at 2 years (1/163 [1%] with vaccine *v* 21/161 [13%] with placebo; OR 0.05, 95% CI 0.01 to 0.35).[10,11] The second RCT (327 healthy children aged 10–30 months) also found that live attenuated varicella vaccine versus placebo significantly reduced clinical chickenpox after a mean of 29 months (AR 5/166 [3.0%] *v* 41/161 [25%]; RR 0.12, 95% CI 0.05 to 0.29).[12] **In immunocompromised people:** We found no RCTs assessing clinical outcomes in people receiving cancer chemotherapy, in people with HIV, or in those aged under 1 month or over 65 years.
Harms:	**In healthy people:** In the second RCT, the only reported adverse effect with varicella vaccine was a non-significant increase in varicella like papules or vesicles (AR 5.4% with vaccine *v* 3.7% with placebo; RR 1.45, 95% CI 0.53 to 4.0).[12] No children had fever or constitutional symptoms. Postmarketing analysis of a database of 89 753 vaccinated adults and children failed to find associations with any rare serious adverse events.[13] **In immunocompromised people:** One RCT found that, of 22 children vaccinated at the start of cancer chemotherapy, three (14%) developed mild maculopapular rashes and fever 16, 24, and 40 days after vaccination, and one had an isolated fever 7 days after vaccination.[14]
Comment:	A systematic review of vaccines for preventing varicella in children and adults is under way.[15]

Chickenpox

OPTION	ACICLOVIR

One systematic review has found that high dose aciclovir (at least 3200 mg/day) significantly reduces the risk of clinical chickenpox and reduces all cause mortality in people with HIV infection. We found no RCTs in people with other forms of immunocompromise.

Benefits: **In people with HIV:** We found one systematic review (search date not stated, 8 RCTs, 1792 people with different stages of HIV, median CD4 count 34–607/mm^3) comparing high dose aciclovir versus placebo.[16] Three of the RCTs were unpublished, including two pharmaceutical company trials. It found that aciclovir (at least 3200 mg/day) versus placebo taken for up to 22 months significantly reduced clinical chickenpox (AR 14/895 [2%] with aciclovir v 54/897 [6%] with placebo; OR 0.29, 95% CI 0.13 to 0.63; NNT 23, 95% CI 17 to 39). All cause mortality was also reduced (HR 0.78, 95% CI 0.65 to 0.93; OR 0.75, 95% CI 0.57 to 1.00). We found no RCTs of lower doses of aciclovir in people with HIV. **In other immunocompromised people:** We found no RCTs of aciclovir in people with other forms of immunocompromise.

Harms: The systematic review did not assess adverse effects (see harms under aciclovir for treatment, p 196).

Comment: None.

OPTION	ZOSTER IMMUNE GLOBULIN

One small RCT in healthy children has found that zoster immune globulin (ZIG) versus immune serum globulin (ISG) significantly reduced the number of children with clinical chickenpox. We found no RCTs of ZIG versus varicella zoster immune globulin (VZIG) in healthy children. In immunocompromised children, one RCT found no significant difference between ZIG versus VZIG in the risk of clinical chickenpox.

Benefits: We found no systematic review. **Versus placebo:** We found no RCTs. **Versus ISG in healthy children:** We found one small RCT (12 healthy susceptible children exposed to a sibling with recent onset of chickenpox) comparing ZIG (see glossary, p 196) (2 ml/10 kg) versus ISG (see glossary, p 196) (2 ml/10 kg).[17] It found that ZIG significantly reduced the number of children with clinical chickenpox at 20 days (AR 0/6 [0%] v 6/6 [100%]; OR 0.0, 95% CI 0 to 0.28). **Versus ISG in immunocompromised children:** We found no RCTs. **Versus VZIG in healthy children:** We found no RCTs. **Versus VZIG in immunocompromised children:** We found one RCT (164 immunocompromised children, mostly with leukaemia, exposed to a sibling with chickenpox) comparing ZIG (1.25 ml/10 kg) versus VZIG (see glossary, p 196) (1.25 ml/10 kg).[18] It found no significant difference in number of children with clinical chickenpox at 12 weeks (AR 31/88 [37%] with ZIG v 36/81 [44%] with VZIG; RR 0.84, 95% CI 0.58 to 1.22). A second RCT compared high dose VZIG (2.5 ml/10 kg) versus low dose VZIG (1.25 ml/10 kg). It found no significant difference in the number of children with clinical chickenpox at 12 weeks (AR 19/40 [47.5%] with low dose v 22/46 [48%] with high dose; RR 1.00, 95% CI 0.61 to 1.65).[18]

Harms: None of the RCTs assessed adverse effects.

Comment: The imprecise estimates might not exclude clinically important differences, especially in the comparison of high dose versus low dose VZIG.[18]

QUESTION What are the effects of treatments for chickenpox?

OPTION ACICLOVIR

RCTs have found that oral aciclovir versus placebo significantly reduces the symptoms of chickenpox in healthy people when given within 24 hours of onset of the rash, but found no significant difference if started after 24 hours. Two RCTs compared intravenous aciclovir versus placebo in children with cancer; one has found that aciclovir significantly reduces clinical deterioration, the other small RCT found no significant difference.

Benefits: We found no systematic reviews. **In healthy people:** We found six RCTs (total of 1136 people) comparing oral aciclovir versus placebo in healthy people.[19-24] In the first four RCTs, aciclovir was given within 24 hours of the onset of the rash, and in the last two RCTs after 24 hours. The largest RCT (724 children) found that aciclovir (20 mg/kg 4 times daily) versus placebo significantly reduced the time to the last new lesions (median 1 day with aciclovir v 2 days with placebo; P < 0.001), and reduced the time to cessation of fever (median 1 day with aciclovir v 2 days with placebo; P < 0.001).[20] The second RCT (62 adolescents) found that aciclovir (800 mg 4 times daily) versus placebo significantly reduced the time to last new lesions (median 2.2 days with aciclovir v 3.2 days with placebo; P < 0.001).[19] The third RCT (102 children) found no significant difference between aciclovir (10–20 mg/kg 4 times daily) versus placebo in the time to last new lesions, but aciclovir significantly reduced the time to cessation of fever (median 1 day with aciclovir v 2 days with placebo; P = 0.001).[21] The fourth RCT (76 adults) compared aciclovir (800 mg 5 times daily) given within 24 hours of the rash versus 24–72 hours after the rash versus placebo.[23] It found that aciclovir given within 24 hours versus placebo significantly reduced the maximum number of lesions and the time to full crusting of lesions, but found no difference in time to full crusting of lesions if aciclovir was given after 24 hours. The two remaining RCTs (total of 168 healthy people)[22,24] compared aciclovir versus placebo given to people more than 24 hours after the onset of the rash. Neither found a significant difference in the time to last new lesions, and did not provide numerical information on the time to cessation of fever. **In immunocompromised people:** We found two placebo controlled RCTs of intravenous aciclovir in children with cancer and receiving chemotherapy. The largest RCT (50 children aged 1–14 years with chickenpox, 60% of whom had a rash for > 24 h) found that significantly more children receiving placebo versus aciclovir 500 mg/m^2 clinically deteriorated, and were transferred to open aciclovir (1/25 [4%] with aciclovir v 12/25

[48%] with placebo; RR 0.08, 95% CI 0.01 to 0.59; NNT 3, 95% CI 2 to 4).[25] Analysis of the remaining children not moved to open aciclovir treatment found that aciclovir significantly reduced the time to full crusting of lesions (mean 5.7 v 7.1 days; P < 0.013), but found no significant difference in cessation of fever. The second RCT (20 children, mean age 6.4 years) comparing aciclovir 500 mg/m^2 versus placebo found no significant difference in the number of children who clinically deteriorated, and who subsequently needed to receive open aciclovir (AR 1/8 [12.5%] with aciclovir v 5/12 [42%]; RR 0.30, 95% CI 0.04 to 2.1). However, the RCT was too small to exclude a clinically important difference.[26]

Harms: No serious harms were reported in any of the six RCTs in healthy people, except for one child taking placebo who developed cerebellar ataxia. Of the three RCTs (total of 889 people) reporting possible adverse effects, none found significant differences between treatment and control groups, or unfavourable trends in children taking aciclovir.[19-21] Adverse effects assessed included gastrointestinal symptoms, leukopoenia, thrombocytopoenia, and abnormalities of liver enzymes.

Comment: The effect on the measured outcomes was small and of questionable clinical importance in healthy people who make an uneventful recovery without treatment. In the first RCT in immunocompromised children, the exclusion of the children taking placebo who clinically deteriorated from the subsequent analysis means that the effect of placebo may have been overestimated, diminishing the significance of differences between treatments.[25]

GLOSSARY

Immune serum globulin (ISG) Immunoglobulin prepared from pooled human plasma.
Varicella zoster immune globulin (VZIG) Is prepared from units of donor plasma selected for high titres of antibodies to VZV.
Zoster immune globulin (ZIG) Is prepared from the plasma of donors convalescing from *Herpes zoster* (sustainable supplies are difficult to obtain).

REFERENCES

1. Lee BW. Review of varicella zoster seroepidemiology in India and Southeast Asia. *Trop Med Int Health* 1998;3:886–890.
2. Garnett GP, Cox MJ, Bundy DA, Didier JM, St Catharine J. The age of infection with varicella-zoster virus in St Lucia, West Indies. *Epidemiol Infect* 1993;110:361–372.
3. Preblud SR. Varicella: complications and costs. *Pediatrics* 1986;78:728–735.
4. Scuffman PA, Lowin AV, Burgess MA. The cost effectiveness of varicella vaccine programs for Australia. *Vaccine* 1999;18:407–415.
5. Guess HA, Broughton DD, Melton LJ, Kurland LT. Population-based studies of varicella complications. *Pediatrics* 1986;78:723–727.
6. Feldman S, Hughes WT, Daniel CB. Varicella in children with cancer: seventy-seven cases. *Pediatrics* 1975;56:388–397.
7. Leibovitz E, Cooper D, Giurgiutiu D, et al. Varicella-zoster virus infection in Romanian children infected with the human immunodeficiency virus. *Pediatrics* 1993;92:838–842.

8. von Seidlein L, Gillette SG, Bryson Y, et al. Frequent recurrence and persistence of varicella-zoster virus infections in children infected with human immunodeficiency virus type 1. *J Pediatr* 1996;128:52–57.
9. Miller E, Cradock-Watson JE, Ridehalgh MK. Outcome in newborn babies given anti-varicella-zoster immunoglobulin after perinatal maternal infection with varicella-zoster virus. *Lancet* 1989; 2:371–373.
10. Weibel RE, Neff BJ, Kuter BJ, et al. Live attenuated varicella virus vaccine. Efficacy trial in healthy children. *N Engl J Med* 1984;310: 1409–1415.
11. Kuter BJ, Weibel RE, Guess HA, et al. Oka/Merck varicella vaccine in healthy children: final report of a 2-year efficacy study and 7-year follow-up studies. *Vaccine* 1991;9:643–647.
12. Varis T, Vesikari T. Efficacy of high-titer live attenuated varicella vaccine in healthy young children. *J Infect Dis* 1996;174:S330–S334.

13. Black S, Shinefield H, Ray P, et al. Postmarketing evaluation of the safety and effectiveness of varicella vaccine. *Pediatr Infect Dis J* 1999;18: 1041–1046.

14. Cristofani LM, Weinberg A, Peixoto V, et al. Administration of live attenuated varicella vaccine to children with cancer before starting chemotherapy. *Vaccine* 1991;9:873–876.

15. Coole L, Law B, McIntyre P. Vaccines for preventing varicella in children and adults. (Protocol for a Cochrane Review). In: The Cochrane Library, Issue 3, 2001. Oxford: Update Software.

16. Ioannidis JP, Collier AC, Cooper DA, et al. Clinical efficacy of high-dose aciclovir in patients with human immunodeficiency virus infection: a meta-analysis of randomized individual patient data. *J Infect Dis* 1998;178:349–359. Search date not stated; primary sources Medline, handsearching of abstracts from meetings, trial directories, and communication with experts.

17. Brunell PA, Ross A, Miller LH, Kuo B. Prevention of varicella by zoster immune globulin. *N Engl J Med* 1969;280:1191–1194.

18. Zaia JA, Levin MJ, Preblud SR, et al. Evaluation of varicella-zoster immune globulin: protection of immunosuppressed children after household exposure to varicella. *J Infect Dis* 1983;147: 737–743.

19. Balfour HH Jr, Rotbart HA, Feldman S, et al. Aciclovir treatment of varicella in otherwise healthy adolescents. The Collaborative Aciclovir Varicella Study Group. *J Pediatr* 1992;120:627–633.

20. Dunkle LM, Arvin AM, Whitley RJ, et al. A controlled trial of aciclovir for chickenpox in normal children. *N Engl J Med* 1991;325:1539–1544.

21. Balfour HH Jr, Kelly JM, Suarez CS, et al. Aciclovir treatment of varicella in otherwise healthy children. *J Pediatr* 1990;116:633–639.

22. Al Nakib W, Al Kandari S, El Khalik DM, El Shirbiny AM. A randomised controlled study of intravenous aciclovir (Zovirax) against placebo in adults with chickenpox. *J Infect* 1983;6:49–56.

23. Wallace MR, Bowler WA, Murray NB, Brodine SK, Oldfield EC. Treatment of adult varicella with oral aciclovir. A randomized, placebo-controlled trial. *Ann Intern Med* 1992;117:358–363.

24. Andreoni M, Canfarini M, Grint PC, Martorelli M, Di Luzio Paparatti U, Rocchi G. A double blind, placebo controlled trial of efficacy and safety of oral aciclovir (Zovirax) in the treatment of chickenpox in adults. *Riv Eur Sci Med Farmacol* 1992;14:63–69.

25. Nyerges G, Meszner Z, Gyarmati E, Kerpel-Fronius S. Aciclovir prevents dissemination of varicella in immunocompromised children. *J Infect Dis* 1988; 157:309–313.

26. Prober CG, Kirk LE, Keeney RE. Aciclovir therapy of chickenpox in immunosuppressed children: a collaborative study. *J Pediatr* 1982;101:622–625.

George Swingler

South African Cochrane Centre and
School of Child and Adolescent Health,
Red Cross Children's Hospital and
University of Cape Town
Cape Town
South Africa

Jimmy Volmink

Director of Research and Analysis
Global Health Council
Washington DC
USA

Competing interests: None declared.

Mammalian bites

Infectious diseases *(vertical, left margin)*

Search date November 2001

Iara Marques de Medeiros and Humberto Saconato

Key Messages

- We found no RCTs on the effect of educational programmes to prevent mammalian bites. One RCT found that an educational programme versus no education in school children significantly increased precautionary behaviour around dogs. We found no RCTs of education to prevent bites in specific occupational groups.

- We found no evidence on tetanus toxoid after human or animal bites.

- Limited evidence from one systematic review found no significant difference between antibiotics versus control in the infection rate in people with dog, cat, or human bites. Subgroup analysis in people with infections of the hand found that antibiotics significantly reduced infections. One small RCT in the review found that in people with human bites, antibiotics versus control significantly reduced the rate of infection.

- One poor quality RCT comparing primary wound closure versus no closure in people with dog bites found no significant difference in the incidence of infection.

- We found no systematic review, RCTs, or good cohort studies assessing debridement, irrigation, decontamination measures, or serum infiltration in the wound. There is consensus that such measures are likely to be beneficial.

■ We found no RCTs of antibiotics versus placebo for the treatment of infectious complications of mammalian bites. One RCT in people with infected and uninfected animal or human bites comparing penicillin with or without dicloxacillin versus amoxicillin/clavulanic acid found no significant difference in failure rate (which was undefined).

DEFINITION Bite wounds are mainly caused by humans, dogs, or cats. They include superficial abrasions (30–43%), lacerations (31–45%), and puncture (see glossary, p 203) wounds (13–34%).[1]

INCIDENCE/ PREVALENCE In the USA, 17–18% of people with dog bites seek medical attention, and 1% require hospitalisation;[2,3] the incidence of dog bites is 3.5–4.7 million bites a year.[4] Children constitute 30–50% of all mammalian bite injuries.[5] In areas where domestic animal rabies has not been controlled, dogs account for 90% of the reported animal bites in humans. In contrast, in areas where domestic animal rabies is well controlled, dogs account for less than 5% of the reported animal bites.

AETIOLOGY/ RISK FACTORS Over 70% of cases, people are bitten by their own pets or by an animal known to them. Males are more likely to be bitten than females, and males are most likely to be bitten by dogs whereas females are more likely to be bitten by cats.[4] One study found that children under 5 years old were significantly more likely than older children to provoke animals prior to being bitten.[6] One study of infected dog and cat bites found that the most commonly isolated bacteria was *Pasteurella*, followed by *Streptococci*, *Staphylococci*, *Moraxella*, *Corynebacterium*, and *Neisseria*.[7] Mixed aerobic and anaerobic infection was more common than anaerobic infection alone.

PROGNOSIS In the USA, dog bites cause about 20 deaths a year.[8] In children, dog bites frequently involve the face, potentially resulting in severe lacerations, and scarring.[9] Rabies, a life threatening viral encephalitis, may be contracted as a consequence of being bitten or scratched by a rabid animal. More than 99% of human rabies is in developing countries where canine rabies is endemic.[10] In people bitten by a rabid animal and not treated, the risk of contracting rabies has been estimated to be 5–80%, depending on the animal species, severity of the bite, infectivity of the animal saliva, virus inoculum, host factors, and possibly the strain of rabies virus.[11,12] One study in the USA reported that the risk of rabies in 21 people with proven rabies exposure was between 5–15%.[13]

AIMS To reduce mammalian bites; to reduce complications after mammalian bites, with minimal adverse effects.

OUTCOMES Prevention of mammalian bites; prevention of infection after mammalian bites; cure rate of infection due to mammalian bites.

METHODS *Clinical Evidence* search and appraisal November 2001. In addition, we searched Web of Science (Science Citation Index to October 2001). Observational studies were used when systematic reviews or RCTs were not found.

Mammalian bites

QUESTION	What are the effects of interventions to prevent mammalian bites?

OPTION	EDUCATION

We found no RCTs of the effect of education programmes on the incidence of mammalian bites. One RCT found that an educational programme versus no education in school children significantly increased precautionary behaviour around dogs. We found no RCTs of education to prevent bites in specific occupational groups.

Benefits: We found no systematic review. **In the general population:** We found no RCTs on the effect of education programmes on the incidence of mammalian bites. One RCT (346 school children aged 7–8 years in 8 primary schools in Sydney, Australia) cluster randomised schools to either an educational programme or no education.[14] The educational programme consisted of one 30 minute lesson demonstrating behavioural techniques around dogs, such as how to recognise friendly, angry, or frightened dogs; how to approach dogs and owners when they wanted to pat a dog; and how to adopt a precautionary and protective body posture when approached or knocked over by a dog. After 10 days, children were videotaped for 10 minutes whilst playing in school grounds where a dog was leashed. The trial found that children in schools receiving education versus no education were significantly less likely to pat the dog without hesitation and try to excite it (118/149 [79%] v 18/197 [9%]; RR 0.16, 95% CI 0.064 to 0.20), and if they did it was only after considerable period of careful assessment. **In specific occupational groups:** We found no RCTs.

Harms: The RCT did not report on adverse effects.[14]

Comment: The trial was brief and reported only the proxy outcome of behaviour modification. The effect of such a programme on the incidence of dog bites in the long term is unclear.

QUESTION	What are the effects of measures to prevent complications from mammalian bites?

OPTION	TETANUS TOXOID

We found no evidence on the effects of tetanus toxoid in preventing tetanus after human or animal bites.

Benefits: We found no systematic review, RCTs, or cohort studies in human or animal bites.

Harms: We found no evidence.

Comment: General measures to prevent tetanus may be beneficial (cleaning the wound, removing debris, excision [except on the face], irrigation, and excision and removal of skin flaps around puncture wounds), but we found no RCTs to confirm or refute this view. We found no studies of the effects of passive immunisation using tetanus immunoglobulin.[15]

OPTION ANTIBIOTIC PROPHYLAXIS

Limited evidence from one systematic review found no significant difference between antibiotics versus control in the infection rate in people with dog, cat, or human bites. Meta-analysis according to the site of the wound found that antibiotics significantly reduced infections of the hand. One small RCT in the review found that in people with human bites, antibiotics versus control significantly reduced the rate of infection.

Benefits:
We found one systematic review (search date 2000, 7 RCTs, 1 quasi-randomised controlled trial, 522 people bitten by dogs, cats, or humans in the preceding 24 h) comparing prophylactic antibiotics versus placebo or no treatment.[16] There was significant heterogeneity between trials. It found no significant difference between antibiotics versus placebo in the infection rate after dog, cat, and human bites (timescale not specified: OR 0.49, 95% CI 0.15 to 1.58). When the results were analysed for each wound site (hands, trunk, arms, or head/neck), antibiotics significantly reduced only infections of the hand (3 RCTs: 2% with antibiotics v 28% with control; OR 0.10, 95% CI 0.01 to 0.86; NNT 4, 95% CI 2 to 50). **Animal bites:** The review identified six RCTs (463 people) of dog bites, and found no significant difference between antibiotics versus control in the rate of infection (10/225 [4%] with antibiotics v 13/238 [5%] with control; OR 0.74, 95% CI 0.30 to 1.85). The review identified one small RCT of cat bites (12 people), which found no significant difference in the rate of infection between antibiotics versus control reduced (4/6 [67%] with antibiotics v 0/5 with control; P < 0.06).[16] **Human bites:** The review included one RCT of human bites (48 people with uncomplicated bites on the hand in the preceding 24 h) comparing oral cephalosporin versus intravenous cephalosporin plus penicillin versus placebo. All participants received debridement, irrigation, and sterile dressing and remained in hospital for 5 days. It found that antibiotics by either route versus placebo significantly reduced the number of people with wound infection (0/33 with oral or intravenous antibiotics v 7/15 [47%]; P < 0.05, timescale not stated).[16]

Harms:
The review did not report on adverse effects.[16]

Comment:
Most of the RCTs were small, and gave insufficient information about allocation concealment and randomisation. Some studies were not double blind, and four studies had withdrawal rates of greater than 10%.[16] The effects of antibiotic prophylaxis in preventing complications of mammalian bites remains unclear. Only a few studies analysed the effect of antibiotics on specific wound types (lacerations, puncture [see glossary, p 203], or avulsions).[16]

OPTION PRIMARY WOUND CLOSURE

One poor quality RCT comparing primary wound closure versus no closure in people with dog bites found no significant difference in the incidence of infection, but the RCT was too small to exclude clinically important effects.

Benefits:
We found no systematic review. We found one RCT (96 people bitten by dogs in the preceding 30 mins to 24 h) comparing primary

Mammalian bites

wound closure versus no closure.[17] All wounds were debrided and irrigated, and tetanus immunisation was updated but no antibiotics were given. In uncomplicated lacerations, closure was performed by an experienced nurse; in complicated lacerations closure was performed by a specialist. The RCT found no difference between closed versus open wounds in the incidence of infection (timescale not stated: 7/92 [8%] with closed v 6/77 [8%] with open; RR 0.98, 95% CI 0.33 to 2.62). There were significantly more infections of the hand compared with the rest of the body (69% with hand v 31% with rest of body), but there was no difference between closure and non-closure groups in hand infections (5/9 [56%] with closure v 4/9 [44%] with non-closure). The rabies risk was not assessed.

Harms: The RCT did not report on adverse effects.[17]

Comment: Although the RCT found no increased risk of infection with primary wound closure, further RCTs are required to confirm this conclusion, and also to evaluate if wound closure may increase the risk of rabies.

OPTION   **DEBRIDEMENT, IRRIGATION, AND DECONTAMINATION**

We found no systematic review, RCTs, or good cohort studies assessing debridement, irrigation, decontamination measures, and serum infiltration in the wound. However, there is consensus that such measures are likely to be beneficial.

Benefits: We found no systematic review, RCTs, or good cohort studies.

Harms: We found no evidence.

Comment: It would be regarded as unethical to conduct an RCT comparing debridement, irrigation, and decontamination versus no treatment.

QUESTION   **What are the effects of treatments for the infectious complications of mammalian bites?**

OPTION   **ANTIBIOTICS**

We found no RCTs of antibiotics versus placebo for the treatment of infectious complications of mammalian bites. One RCT in people with infected and uninfected animal and human bites comparing penicillin with or without dicloxacillin versus amoxicillin/clavulanic acid found no significant difference in failure rate (which was undefined).

Benefits: We found no systematic review. **Versus placebo:** We found no RCTs. **Versus other antibiotics:** We found one RCT (61 people bitten in the preceding 30 mins to 10 days; 48 by animals, 13 by humans) comparing penicillin with or without dicloxacillin versus amoxicillin/clavulanic acid.[10] Treatment was given for 5 days in people bitten less than 8 hours previously without clinical infection (34 people), and for 10 days in people bitten more than 8 hours previously or with clinical infection (27 people). All wounds received usual care, and were left closed or open at the discretion of the attending physician. Before inclusion, 27 people already had clinical signs of infection (see comment below). The RCT found no significant difference in failure rate (which was undefined) between penicillin/dicloxacillin versus amoxicillin/clavulanic acid (timescale not stated: 1/31 [3%] v 3/30 [10%]; RR 0.32, 95% CI 0.03 to 2.54).

Harms: Adverse effects were significantly more common in people using amoxicillin/clavulanic acid versus penicillin/dicloxacillin (13/31 [42%] v 3/30 [10%]; RR 4.2, 95% CI 1.5 to 7.4; NNH 3, 95% CI 2 to 19). Diarrhoea was the most common adverse event (9/31 [29%] with amoxicillin/clavulanic acid v 1/30 [3%] with penicillin/dicloxacillin; RR 8.71, 95% CI 1.34 to 23.3; NNH 4, 95% CI 1 to 79).[10]

Comment: Interpretation of the results is difficult as the main outcome measure of "failure rate" was not defined. Also, failure rates were not separated according to whether people had infected or uninfected wounds at inclusion.

GLOSSARY

Abrasion The scraping or rubbing away of a small area of skin or mucous membrane.

Laceration Occurs when the skin and/or soft tissues are torn by the crushing and shearing forces produced on impact; characterised by ragged, irregular margins, surrounding contusion, marginal abrasion, and tissue bridging in the wound depths.

Puncture A wound caused by perforation of the skin with a sharp point.

REFERENCES

1. Dire DJ. Emergency management of dog and cat bite wounds. *Emerg Med Clin North Am* 1992;10: 719–736.
2. Sacks JJ, Kresnow M, Houston B. Dog bites: how big a problem? *Injury Prev* 1996;2:52–54.
3. Quinlan KP, Sacks JJ. Hospitalizations for dog bite injuries. *JAMA* 1999;281:232–233.
4. Overall KL, Love M. Dog bites to humans–demography, epidemiology, injury and risk. *JAMA* 2001;218:1923–1934.
5. Fishbein DB, Bernard KW. Rabies virus. In: *Mandell, Douglas and Bennett's Principles and practice of Infectious Diseases*. 4th ed. Vol 2:1527–1543.
6. Avner JR, Baker MD. Dog bites in urban children. *Pedriatrics* 1991;88:55–57.
7. Talan DA, Citron DM, Abrahamian FM, Moran GJ, Goldstein EJ. Bacteriologic analysis of infected dog and cat bites. Emergency Medicine Animal Bite Infection Study Group. *N Engl J Med* 1999;340: 85–92.
8. Sacks JJ, Sattin RW, Bonzo SE. Dog bite-related fatalities from 1979 through 1988. *JAMA* 1989; 262:1489–1492.
9. Karlson TA. The incidence of facial injuries from dog bites. *JAMA* 1984;251:3265–3267.
10. Goldstein EJC, Reinhardt JF, Murray PM, Finegold SM. Outpatient therapy of bite wounds. Demographic data, bacteriology, and prospective, randomized trial of amoxicillin/clavulanic acid versus penicillin +/- dicloxacillin. *Int J Dermatol* 1987;26:123–127.
11. Hattwick M, Gregg MB. The disease in man. In: Baer GM, ed. *The natural history of rabies*. New York: Academic Press, 1975:281–304.
12. Suntharasamai P, Warrell DA, Warrell MJ, et al. New purified Vero-cell vaccine prevents rabies in patients bitten by rabid animals. *Lancet* 1986;2: 129–131.
13. Anderson LJ, Sikes RK, Langkop CW. Postexposure trial of a human diploid cell strain rabies vaccine. *J Infect Dis* 1980;142:133–138.
14. Chapman S, Cornwall J, Righetti J, Sung L. Preventing dog bites in children: randomised controlled trial of an educational intervention. *BMJ* 2000;320:1512–1513.
15. De Melker HE, De Melker RA. Dog bites: publications on risk factors, infections, antibiotics and primary wound closure. *Ned Tijdschr Geneesd* 1996;140:709–713.
16. Medeiros I, Saconato H. Antibiotic prophylaxis for mammalian bites (Cochrane Review). In: The Cochrane Library, Issue 2, 2001. Oxford: Update Software. Search date 2000; primary sources Medline, Embase, Lilacs, and the Cochrane Controlled Trials Register.
17. Maimaris C, Quinton DN. Dog-bite lacerations: a controlled trial of primary wound closure. *Arch Emerg Med* 1988;5:156–161.

Iara Marques de Medeiros

Humberto Saconato

Universidade Federal do Rio Grande do Norte, Natal, Brazil

Competing interests: None declared.

Measles

Search date November 2001

Anna Donald and Vivek Muthu

INTERVENTIONS	

Key Messages

Benefits of treatment

- Measles is a serious, highly contagious, yet preventable disease. In healthy people who have not been vaccinated against it, measles infection causes pneumonia, brain damage, dementia, or death in about 6% of cases and requires hospital admission in up to 20%. Severity and frequency of complications are higher in people who are ill or malnourished.

- Large cohort studies, large cross-sectional time series, and population surveillance data from different countries have all found that combined measles, mumps, and rubella (MMR) and live monovalent measles vaccination programmes reduce risk of measles infection to near zero, especially in populations in which vaccine coverage is high.

- We found no RCTs comparing clinical effects of MMR versus no vaccination or placebo on measles infection rates. Such trials are likely to be considered unethical because of the large body of whole-population evidence finding benefit from vaccination.

- Unlike live monovalent measles vaccine, MMR additionally vaccinates against mumps and rubella, which themselves cause serious complications (mumps causes orchitis, pancreatitis, meningoencephalitis, deafness, and congenital fetal abnormalities; congenital infection with rubella causes deafness, blindness, heart defects, liver, spleen, and brain damage, and stillbirth).

Harms of treatment

- One systematic review, one RCT, one large population based survey, and one population based study found no evidence of MMR being associated with developmental regression or autism compared with placebo or no vaccine. Large cross-sectional time series have consistently found no evidence of MMR or live monovalent measles vaccine being associated with autism.

- One large, long term population surveillance study and one population based case control study found no evidence that either the monovalent measles vaccine or MMR was associated with inflammatory bowel disease. One large cohort study and two population based case control studies found no association of inflammatory bowel disease with the monovalent vaccine.

- One systematic review and one additional RCT have found that MMR and monovalent measles vaccine are associated with a small and similar risk of self limiting fever within 3 weeks of vaccination compared with 100% risk of acute fever in people with measles.

DEFINITION Measles is an infectious disease caused by a ribonucleic acid (RNA) paramyxomavirus. The illness is characterised by an incubation period of 10–12 days; a prodromal period of 2–4 days with upper respiratory tract symptoms; Koplik's spots on mucosal membranes and high fever; followed by further fever; and a widespread maculo-papular rash that persists for 5–6 days.[1]

INCIDENCE/ Measles incidence varies widely according to vaccination coverage.
PREVALENCE Worldwide, there are an estimated 30 million cases of measles each year,[2] but an incidence of only 0–10/100 000 people in countries with widespread vaccination programmes such as the USA, UK, Mexico, India, China, Brazil, and Australia.[3] In the USA, before licensure of effective vaccines, greater than 90% of people were infected by the age of 15 years, whereas after licensure in 1963, incidence fell by about 98%.[1] Mean annual incidence in Finland was 366/100 000 in 1970,[4] but declined to about zero by the late 1990s.[5] Similarly, annual incidence declined to about zero in Chile, the English speaking Caribbean, and Cuba during the 1990s with introduction of vaccination programmes.[6,7]

AETIOLOGY/ Measles is spread through airborne droplets that persist for up to
RISK FACTORS 2 hours in closed areas following the presence of an infected person. Measles is highly contagious. As with other infectious diseases, other risk factors include overcrowding, low herd immunity, and immunosuppression. People with immunosuppression, children of less than 5 years of age, and adults of more than 20 years of age have a higher risk of severe complications and death, although these also occur in healthy people (see prognosis below).[1] Newborn babies have a lower risk of measles than older infants because of the presence of protective maternal antibodies, although in recent US outbreaks, maternal antibody protection was lower than expected.[1]

PROGNOSIS The World Health Organization estimated that in the year 2000, measles caused 777 000 deaths and a burden of disease of 27.5 million disability adjusted life years.[8] **Disease in healthy people:** In developed countries, most prognostic data come from the pre-vaccination era and from subsequent outbreaks in non-vaccinated populations. In the USA, measles is complicated in about 30% of reported cases. From 1989–1991 in the USA, measles resurgence among young children (< 5 years) who had not been immunised led to 55 622 cases with more than 11 000 hospital admissions and 125 deaths.[1] Measles complications include diarrhoea (8%), otitis media (7%), pneumonia (6%), death (0.1–0.2%), acute encephalitis (about 0.1% followed by death in 15% and permanent neurological damage in about 25%), seizures (with or without fever in 0.6–0.7%), idiopathic thrombocytopenia (1/6000 reported cases), and subacute sclerosing panencephalitis causing degeneration of the central nervous system and death 7 years after measles infection (range 1 month to 27 years; 0.5–1.0/100 000 reported cases).[1,9] Measles during pregnancy

Infectious diseases

results in higher risk of premature labour, spontaneous abortion, and low birth weight infants. An association with birth defects remains uncertain.[1] **Disease in malnourished or immunocompromised people:** In malnourished or immuno-compromised people, particularly those with vitamin A deficiency, measles case fatality can be as high as 25%. Worldwide, measles is a major cause of blindness and causes 5% of deaths in young children (< 5 years).[1,10]

AIMS	Preventing measles with minimum adverse effects.
OUTCOMES	**Prevention, benefits:** Clinically apparent measles and measles related complications, including death. We have included a proxy outcome (seroconversion — see glossary, p 212) because it is so highly correlated with vaccine efficacy.[11] **Prevention, harms:** Acute fever, febrile seizures, inflammatory bowel disease, developmental regression, autism and clinical measles after seroconversion.
METHODS	*Clinical Evidence* search and appraisal November 2001. The authors also searched World Health Organization, US Communicable Disease Control, and UK Public Health Laboratory Service websites and hand searched national and international policy documents. In the benefits section, we have included RCTs and stronger observational studies, given that RCTs have long been considered unethical for assessing the clinical efficacy of measles vaccines (see benefits, p 206). In the harms section, we have included RCTs and robust observational studies (see harms, p 208). In the comments section we have included weaker studies (see comment, p 211). We have included only those studies of the combined measles, mumps, and rubella vaccine (see glossary, p 212) that used the Schwarz strain of the measles virus and only those studies of the monovalent measles vaccine (see glossary, p 212) that considered live attenuated strains of the virus, because of the relative inefficacy of measles vaccines using killed strains.

QUESTION What are the effects of interventions to prevent measles infection?

OPTION MEASLES VACCINATION

We found no RCTs comparing measles infection rates following the combined measles, mumps, and rubella (MMR) vaccine versus placebo or versus monovalent vaccine alone. We found strong evidence from national population surveillance that both MMR and monovalent measles vaccination virtually eliminate risk of measles and measles complications. We found no evidence that MMR or live monovalent measles vaccines are associated with autism or inflammatory bowel disease. We found consistent evidence from RCTs and cohort studies that MMR and live monovalent measles vaccines are associated with small, similar risks of self limiting fever within 3 weeks of vaccination. Measles causes acute fever in 100% of infected children.

Benefits:	**Monovalent measles vaccine or combined MMR vaccine versus placebo or no vaccine:** See glossary, p 212. We found two early RCTs of monovalent measles vaccine versus placebo or no vaccine in the UK[12] and USA.[13] Both found efficacy rates of 95% or

greater for vaccines using live attenuated Schwarz[12] and Edmonston[13] strains of the measles virus (Schwarz RCT: 9538 children received live vaccine, 16 239 unvaccinated; Edmonston RCT: 1308 live vaccine, 1271 placebo). We found no RCTs comparing the clinical effects of MMR versus no vaccine or placebo. Such studies have been considered unethical because of previous evidence of the efficacy of measles vaccine and harms of measles infection. We found two RCTs that compared seroconversion (see glossary, p 212) rates of MMR versus placebo.[14,15] The first compared MMR versus placebo in 282 previously non-immune children (92% of whom were ≤1 year old). At 8 weeks, almost all children receiving MMR seroconverted for measles, whereas none of the children receiving placebo seroconverted (measles seroconversion rate 99%–100% with MMR, depending on vaccine batch used).[14] The second trial examined seroconversion with MMR vaccine in 1481 children (1232 MMR, 249 placebo), of whom 446 in the vaccine group were naïve to measles, mumps, and rubella.[15] In this subgroup, seroconversion rates at 8 weeks approached 100%, whereas none of the previously non-immune placebo group seroconverted for measles. One large, retrospective cohort study of the entire US population from 1985–1992 compared measles infection rates in children who were vaccinated versus children whose parents had declined vaccination (17 390 cases from a vaccinated population of 51 264 140 to 52 377 192 from 1985–1992; 2827 cases from an unvaccinated population of 234 040 to 245 887 from 1985–1992).[16] The study did not state what proportion of vaccinated children received monovalent versus MMR vaccine, although MMR was already widely used in the USA by 1985. The study found that although overall measles incidence was low because of herd immunity (see glossary, p 212), vaccination reduced measles infection compared with no vaccination (RR unvaccinated v vaccinated 4–170, depending on age group and year of survey). One large, prospective cohort study followed up 9274 children who had been enrolled in a placebo controlled trial of live monovalent measles vaccine in 1964 (36 530 children aged 10 months to 2 years; Schwarz strain vaccine).[17] The cohort study found that by 1990, over a period of 15 years (12–27 years after the trial) and after controlling for subsequent vaccination in initial placebo groups, but not controlling for growing herd immunity following mass vaccination, measles incidence was higher in the unvaccinated group (AR 0.3/1000 person years with vaccine v 1/1000 person years with no vaccine; $P < 0.001$). One systematic review (search date not stated, 10 cohort studies, 2 case control) and one subsequent cohort study examined effects of live monovalent measles vaccination on mortality. The review found that live, standard titre monovalent measles vaccination in seven developing countries reduced all-cause mortality by 30–80%, depending on follow up period and country.[18] The more recent study compared a group of children in Bangladesh vaccinated with live, Schwarz strain monovalent measles vaccine versus age matched, unvaccinated children (8135 matched pairs).[19] It found similar results (16 270 children aged 9–60 months; RR for death at 3 years' follow up vaccinated v unvaccinated 0.54, 95% CI 0.45 to 0.65). We found many population based studies from different countries with different healthcare systems and different socioeconomic and demographic distributions. These studies have consistently found measles vaccination coverage to be associated with a steep decline in measles. One cross-sectional time series from the World Health Organization found a global decline in reported measles incidence (which underestimates true incidence) from about 4 500 000 a year in 1980 to about 1 000 000 a year in 2000.[20] The decline was associated with the rise in reported measles vaccination coverage from about 10% in 1980 to about 80% in 2000. One population-based time series of measles incidence from Finland found that in a population of about 5 million people following the introduction of a live monovalent vaccination programme (1975–1981), the number of new measles cases each year fell from an average of 2074 cases in 1977–1981 to 44 cases in 1985. New cases declined to about zero by the mid 1990s. Shortly after introducing the MMR programme in Finland in 1982, rubella and mumps incidence also fell to about zero.[4] One cross-sectional study in a Brazilian city, which was repeated before and after a measles vaccination campaign in 1987 (8163 people, strain not stated) found that reported measles incidence fell from 222/100 000 in 1987 to 2.7/100 000 in 1988.[21] **MMR versus monovalent measles vaccine:** We found no RCTs comparing clinical effects of MMR versus monovalent vaccine in children of the same age. We found one RCT that compared live Schwarz strain monovalent measles vaccine given at 9 months of age followed by MMR at 15 months (442 children) versus MMR only (no prior vaccination) at 12 months (495 children).[22] Pre-vaccination measles seropositivity was higher in the younger, monovalent vaccine group, perhaps because of maternal antibody persistence (prevaccine, 8.1% seropositive in monovalent group v 1.4% in MMR group; P < 0.0001). After 60 months' follow up, measles infection rates were higher with monovalent vaccination followed by MMR compared with MMR alone (AR for infection 2.7% with monovalent plus MMR v 0% with MMR; ARR 2.7%; CI not stated; P < 0.0001); however, effects may be confounded by the different timing of the vaccinations. We found two RCTs that compared seroconversion rates following live MMR versus Schwarz strain monovalent measles vaccine. The first trial (420 children with no clinical history of measles or mumps, mean age about 15 months) found similar seroconversion rates in both groups after 6 weeks (96.8% with monovalent measles v 92.6% with MMR).[23] The second RCT (319 children, mean age 13 months) also found similar seroconversion rates in both groups at 6 weeks (92% with Schwarz strain monovalent measles vaccine v 93% with MMR).[24]

Harms: **Acute fever and febrile convulsions:** We found one systematic review and four RCTs examining fever as an outcome of vaccination in otherwise healthy children. Results should be interpreted in light of the 100% prevalence of acute fever in children with measles infection. The systematic review (search date 1998) reported that up to 5% of non-immune people develop moderate to high fever (≥ 38.6°C) within 7–21 days of vaccination.[25] The first RCT (crossover design) compared the acute harms of MMR versus placebo in 1162 homozygous and heterozygous twins (460 children aged

1 year, of whom 1.3% had been previously vaccinated; 702 aged ≥ 2 years, 95% of whom had been previously vaccinated or experienced measles).[26] One member of each twin pair was randomly selected and allocated to MMR vaccination followed 3 weeks later by placebo, or vice versa. The other twin was allocated to the opposite combination. The trial found that among children aged 14–18 months, MMR was more likely to cause fever than placebo within 21 days (AR fever, 12% in MMR group v 4% in placebo group; OR for fever ≥ 39.5°C 2.83, 95% CI 1.47 to 5.45; OR for fever ≥ 38.5°C 3.28, 95% CI 2.23 to 4.82; OR for fever ≥ 37.5°C 2.66, 95% CI 1.66 to 3.08). The second and third RCTs, which compared MMR versus Schwarz strain monovalent measles vaccine in infants with no history of measles, found no difference in fever rates between the two groups.[23,24] The fourth RCT compared Schwarz strain monovalent measles vaccine given at 9 months followed by MMR at 15 months versus MMR alone at 12 months.[22] It found similar rates of fever for monovalent measles vaccine and initial MMR, although results may be confounded by the age difference between the two groups (AR for fever 8.7% with monovalent vaccine v 11.2% with MMR; P value not provided). One retrospective cohort study in 679 942 children from four US health maintenance organisations found that children who had received MMR were more likely to experience febrile convulsions at 1–2 weeks after MMR than children of the same age who had not been vaccinated, although the estimated increase in absolute risk was small (RR for febrile seizure 8–14 days after vaccination 2.83, 95% CI 1.44 to 5.55; ARI of febrile seizure, estimated by comparison with background seizure risk in all children aged 12–24 months, 0.025%; NNH 4000; CI not provided).[27] However, the study found no increase in risk within the first week or from 2–4 weeks following vaccination (RR for first wk 1.73, 95% CI 0.72 to 4.15; RR for 15–30 days 0.97, 95% CI 0.49 to 1.95). Seven years' follow up of 543 children with febrile convulsions in the initial month of follow up (22 following MMR, 521 who had not been vaccinated) found no difference between MMR versus no vaccination for subsequent seizure (RR 0.56, 95% CI 0.07 to 4.20). Similarly, among 271 children with febrile convulsion in one of the four participating health maintenance organisations, the study found no evidence that MMR vaccination prior to seizure increased risk of learning disability or developmental delay compared with no vaccination prior to seizure (RR after adjusting for age at first febrile seizure 0.56, 95% CI 0.07 to 4.20). We found one study that reported results of population based surveillance of harms of MMR in all 1.8 million people vaccinated over a 14 year period in Finland.[28] Surveillance was passive, relying on healthcare personnel to be aware of the surveillance programme and to report adverse events that they felt might be associated with MMR. Throughout the surveillance period, the programme was advertised in seminars, the media, and medical press. Acute reactions were more likely to have been reported than long term effects. The study found that fever was associated with MMR in 277 children (AR 0.02%). Children with fever not brought to the attention of health professionals would have escaped detection. Febrile seizure was reported in 52 cases (AR 0.003%), of which 28 cases could have been caused by MMR according to predefined clinical and

Infectious diseases

serological criteria (AR 0.002%). **Developmental regression or autism:** The RCT comparing harms of MMR versus placebo found no evidence that MMR was associated with acute developmental regression (see glossary, p 212).[26] We found one systematic review of observational studies of different kinds that found no association between MMR and autism.[29] The review included two large cross-sectional time series. Neither found evidence that MMR is associated with autism, but that incidence of autism has been increasing independently of MMR coverage. The first study examined MMR vaccine coverage (see glossary, p 212) among children aged 14–17 months enrolled in Californian kindergartens and born between 1980 and 1994, and autism caseloads referred to the state developmental services department over the same period.[30] The study found that MMR coverage at 24 months rose slightly (from 72% in 1980 to 82% in 1994; 14% proportional rise); however, referral rates for new autism cases increased disproportionately in the same period (from 44/100 000 births in 1980 to 208/100 000 live births in 1994; 373% proportional rise). Referral rates to the department may not accurately reflect incidence of autistic syndromes. The second study, which took its data from a national UK general practice registry, found that the risk of autism among boys increased in the period from 1988–1993, whereas MMR coverage remained almost constant at about 97% over the same period (AR of first diagnosis of autism aged 2–5 years 0.008%, 95% CI 0.004% to 0.014% for cohort born in 1988 v 0.029%, 95% CI 0.020% to 0.043% for cohort born in 1993).[31] A third population based study identified 498 children diagnosed with autism born in eight health districts in the UK between 1979 and 1988.[32] The study found that incidence of autism increased over this period. However, there was no step increase or change in the rate of increase of incidence following the start of the MMR vaccination programme or after MMR coverage levelled off at almost 100%. The long term population based passive surveillance study from Finland similarly reported no cases of developmental regression in 1.8 million people vaccinated with MMR.[28] It also reported no cases of autism in the long term, although the study may have limited reliability for detecting long term adverse effects. **Inflammatory bowel disease:** We found one systematic review (search date 1998) of six large observational studies from different developed countries.[25] The review found no evidence of an association between inflammatory bowel disease and MMR and measles vaccines. We found three additional studies. The first was a retrospective cohort study comparing rates of ulcerative colitis, Crohn's disease, and inflammatory bowel disease (assessed by postal questionnaire) in 7616 people who had received live monovalent measles vaccination versus those who had not received measles vaccination by the age of 5 years (mean age at vaccination 17.6 months, standard deviation 7.4 months). People were those available from an original population based cohort of 16 000 children born in the first week of 1970 in the UK.[33] The study found no difference for risk of ulcerative colitis, Crohn's disease, or inflammatory bowel disease between people (aged 26 years at the time of the study) who had received monovalent measles vaccine and those who had not, whether or not the result was adjusted for sex, socioeconomic status, and crowding (AR for Crohn's disease 0.25% with vaccine v 0.31% without, adjusted OR 0.7, 95% CI 0.3 to 1.6; AR for ulcerative colitis 0.16% with vaccine v 0.27% without, adjusted OR 0.6, 95% CI 0.2 to 1.6; AR for inflammatory bowel disease 0.41% with vaccine v 0.58% without, adjusted OR 0.6, 95% CI 0.3 to 1.2). The second (the long term, prospective population based passive surveillance study from Finland) reported no cases of inflammatory bowel disease associated with vaccination in 1.8 million people vaccinated with MMR followed up for 14 years.[28] The third was a case control study of 142 people with definite or probable inflammatory bowel disease from members of four US health maintenance organisations (67 people with ulcerative colitis and 75 with Crohn's disease).[34] Cases were identified by computerised search of electronic records and manual abstraction of medical records (from 1958–1989 for 3 organisations and from 1979–1989 for 1; people who were not organisation members between 6 months of age and disease onset were excluded). The study found that people with inflammatory bowel disease were not more likely to have received MMR than people without inflammatory bowel disease taken from the same health maintenance organisation and matched for sex and year of birth (OR for Crohn's disease 0.40, 95% CI 0.08 to 2.00; OR for ulcerative colitis 0.80, 95% CI 0.18 to 3.56; OR for all inflammatory bowel disease 0.59, 95% CI 0.21 to 1.69). The study similarly found no evidence of an association between all measles containing vaccines, Crohn's disease, ulcerative colitis, or all inflammatory bowel disease. **Measles risk after seroconversion:** One systematic review of cohort studies (search date 1995) examined risk of measles infection at least 21 days after vaccine induced seroconversion (monovalent or polyvalent vaccine).[11] It identified 10 studies that met inclusion criteria. In the subset of six cohort studies examining live vaccine, where vaccination status was cross checked against medical records, risk of clinical measles infection in children who had seroconverted after vaccination was about zero (0 infections out of 2061 people exposed; 95% CI not provided).

Comment: **Benefits:** Many case control studies conducted during measles outbreaks have found that live measles vaccination (monovalent or MMR) protects against infection, with protective efficacy of about 95% or higher. Given the evidence for benefit already described, we have not included further details of these studies. In addition, and although not the focus of this topic, it should be noted that the MMR vaccine also protects people from mumps and rubella, which cause serious complications in non-immune people (mumps causes orchitis, pancreatitis, meningoencephalitis, deafness, and congential fetal abnormalities; congenital rubella infection causes deafness, blindness, heart defects, liver, spleen and brain damage, and stillbirth). **Harms:** In addition to the more reliable evidence described above, we found two case series. The first was a time sensitive, population based series of 473 children with childhood autism (see glossary, p 212) or atypical autism (see glossary, p 212) born between 1979 and 1998 and registered in five health districts in London, UK.[35] Of these children, 118 had documented evidence of developmental regression. The study found no trends for risk of developmental regression with respect to year of birth

Infectious diseases

from 1979–1998, although MMR vaccination was introduced in 1988. The study found that MMR vaccination was just as likely to precede or follow documented parental concerns about development, suggesting that the temporal relation of vaccination and onset of developmental problems was not compatible with a causal association (443 children with autism in whom timing of first parental concerns recorded; 26% vaccinated prior to parental concern about development v 26% vaccinated after parental concerns expressed; P = 0.83). The second series raised the question of a possible relation between MMR and developmental disorder in 12 children with bowel symptoms.[36] The series was retrospective (parents surveyed up to 8 years after vaccination), small; lacked a control group; and was selective in its sample. For these reasons, we found that the study does not establish MMR as a cause of inflammatory bowel disease, autism, or development regression, and that its hypothesis has been satisfactorily tested by scientifically reliable studies (see harms above).

GLOSSARY

Acute developmental regression Rapid loss of acquired developmental skills.

Atypical autism shares clinical features with autism but does not meet ICD-10 or DSM-IV diagnostic criteria.

Childhood autism ICD-10 or DSM-IV autism (comprising communication difficulties, problems with social interaction, and behavioural problems) in children aged under 3 years.

Combined measles, mumps, and rubella (MMR) vaccine Vaccine with components that aim to raise immunity to measles, mumps, and rubella infections. Contains live attenuated measles virus (Schwarz strain).

Herd immunity Background level of immunity in the community. A high level of herd immunity reduces risk of infection even in non-immune individuals, because there is no pool of at risk individuals who may transmit the infectious agent.

Live monovalent vaccine Commonly known as the single measles vaccine. Uses live, attenuated virus (most commonly Schwarz strain), and only to bring about measles immunity.

Seroconversion Development in the blood of specific antimeasles antibody. Seroconversion is a proxy for clinical efficacy.

Vaccine coverage Prevalence of vaccination in the community.

REFERENCES

1. Center for Disease Control. Epidemiology and Prevention of Vaccine-preventable Diseases. Atlanta: CDC, 2000.

2. http://www.unicef.org/programme/health/document/meastrat.pdf

3. http://www.who.int/vaccines-surveillance/graphics/htmls/meainc.htm

4. Peltola H, Heinonen P, Valle M, et al. The elimination of indigenous measles, mumps and rubella from Finland by a 12-year, two-dose vaccination program. N Eng J Med 1994;331:1397–1402.

5. Peltola H, Davidkin I, Valle M, et al. No measles in Finland. Lancet 1997;350:1364–1365.

6. de Quadros CA, Olive J, Hersh BS, et al. Measles elimination in the Americas: evolving strategies. JAMA 1996;275:224–229.

7. Pan American Health Organization. Surveillance in the Americas. Weekly Bulletin 1995;1.

8. World Health Report, 2001: Statistical annex. Geneva: WHO, 2001.

9. Miller E, Waight P, Farrington CP, Andrews N, Stowe J, Taylor B. Idiopathic thrombocytopenic purpura and MMR vaccine. Arch Dis Child 2001; 84:227–229.

10. http://www.who.int/child-adolescent-health/OVERVIEW/Child_Health/child_epidemiology.htm

11. Anders J, Jacobson R, Poland G, Jacobson RSJ, Wollan PC. Secondary failure rates of measles vaccines: a metaanalysis of published studies. Pediatr Infect Dis J 1996;15:62–66. Search date 1995; primary sources Medline (English language only) and hand searching of references cited in initial search and references cited within first generation references.

12. Measles Vaccination subcommittee of the Committee on Development of Vaccines and Immunisation Procedures. Clinical trial of live measles vaccine given alone and live vaccine preceded by killed vaccine. Fourth report to the Medical Research Council. Lancet 1977;2: 571–575.

13. Guinee VF, Henderson DA, Casey HL, et al. Cooperative measles vaccine field trial. I. Clinical efficacy. *Pediatrics* 1966;37:649–665.

14. Bloom JL, Schiff GM, Graubarth H, et al. Evaluation of a trivalent measles, mumps, rubella vaccine in children. *J Pediatr* 1975;87:85–87.

15. Schwarz AJ, Jackson JE, Ehrenkranz J, Ventura A, Schiff GM, Walters VW. Clinical evaluation of a new measles–mumps–rubella trivalent vaccine. *Am J Dis Child* 1975;129:1408–1412.

16. Salmon DA Haber M, Gangarosa E, Phillips L, Smith NJ, Chen RT. Health consequences of religious and philosophical exemptions from immunization laws: individual and societal risk of measles. *JAMA* 1999;282:47–53.

17. Ramsay ME, Moffatt D, O'Connor M. Measles vaccine: a 27-year follow up. *Epidemiol Infect* 1994;112:409–412.

18. Aaby P, Samb B, Simondon F, Seck AM, Knudsen K, Whittle H. Non-specific beneficial effect of measles immunisation: analysis of mortality studies from developing countries. *BMJ* 1995; 311:481–485. Search date not stated; primary source Medline.

19. Koenig MA, Khan B, Wojtynak B. Impact of measles vaccination on childhood mortality in rural Bangladesh. *Bull World Health Organization* 1990; 68:441–447.

20. http://www.who.int/vaccines-surveillance/graphics/htmls/IncMeas.htm

21. Pannuti CS, Moraes JC, Souza VA, Camargo MC, Hidalgo NT. Measles antibody prevalence after mass immunization in Sao Paulo, Brazil. *Bull World Health Organization* 1991;69:557–560.

22. Ceyhan M, Kanra G, Erdem G, Kanra B. Immunogenicity and efficacy of one dose measles–mumps–rubella (MMR) vaccine at twelve months of age as compared to monovalent measles vaccination at nine months followed by MMR revaccination at fifteen months of age. *Vaccine* 2001;19:4473–4478.

23. Edees S, Pullan CR, Hull D. A randomised single blind trial of a combined mumps measles rubella vaccine to evaluate serological response and reactions in the UK population. *Public Health* 1991;105:91–97.

24. Robertson CM, Bennet VJ, Jefferson N, Mayon-White RT. Serological evaluation of a measles, mumps, and rubella vaccine. *Arch Dis Child* 1988; 63:612–616.

25. Duclos P, Ward BJ. Measles vaccines: a review of adverse events. *Drug Safety* 1998;6:435–454. Search date 1998; primary sources Stratton RS, Howe CJ, Johnston Jr RB. Adverse events associated with childhood vaccines: evidence bearing on causality. Washington DC: National Academy Press 1994 for papers published before 1994; for articles published after 1994 primary sources WHO Collaborating Centre for International Drug Monitoring Database; discussion groups; advisory committee documents and other unspecified databases.

26. Virtanen M, Peltola H, Paunio M, Heinonen OP. Day-to-day reactogenicity and the healthy vaccinee effect of measles–mumps–rubella vaccination. *Pediatrics* 2000;106:e62.

27. Barlow WE, Davis RL, Glasser JW. The risk of seizures after receipt of whole cell pertussins or measles mumps and rubella vaccine. *N Eng J Med* 2001;345:656–661.

28. Patja A, Davidkin I, Kurki T, Kallio MJ, Valle M, Peltola H. Serious adverse events after measles–mumps–rubella vaccination during a fourteen year prospective follow up. *Pediatr Infect Dis J* 2000;19:1127–1134.

29. Institute of Medicine. Immunization safety review: measles–mumps–rubella vaccine and autism. Washington DC: National Academy Press, 2001.

30. Dales L, Hammer SJ, Smith N. Time trends in autism and in MMR immunization coverage in California. *JAMA* 2001;285:1183–1185.

31. Kaye JA, del Mar Melero-Montes M, Jick H. Mumps, measles, and rubella vaccine and the incidence of autism recorded by general practitioners: a time trend analysis. *BMJ* 2001; 322:460–463.

32. Taylor B, Miller E, Farrington CP, et al. Autism and measles, mumps, and rubella vaccine: no epidemiological evidence for a causal association. *Lancet* 1999;353:2026–

33. Morris DL, Montgomery SM, Thompson NP. Measles vaccination and inflammatory bowel disease: A National British Cohort study. *Am J Gastroenterol* 2000;95:3507–3512.

34. Davis RL, Kramarz P, Bohlke K, et al. Measles–mumps–rubella and other measles containing vaccines do not increase risk for inflammatory bowel disease: A case control study from the Vaccine Safety Datalink project. *Arch Pediatr Adolesc Med* 2001;155:354–359.

35. Taylor B, Miller E, Lingam R, Andrews N, Simmons A, Stowe J. Measles, mumps, and rubella vaccination and bowel problems or developmental regression in children with autism: a population study. *BMJ* 2002;324:393–396.

36. Wakefield AJ, Murch SH, Anthony A, et al. Ileal–lymphoid–nodular hyperplasia, non-specific colitis, and pervasive developmental disorder in children. *Lancet* 1998; 351:637–641.

Anna Donald

Vivek Muthu

Bazian Ltd
London
UK

Competing interests: None declared.

Meningococcal disease

Search date October 2001

J Correia and C A Hart

INTERVENTIONS

Likely to be beneficial
Prophylactic antibiotics in
  contacts* 216

Unknown effectiveness
Antibiotics for throat carriage
  (reduce carriage but unknown
  effect on risk of disease) . . .216

Pre-admission parenteral
  antibiotics in suspected
  cases* 217

* Based on observational evidence.
  RCTs unlikely to be conducted.

Key Messages

- We found no randomised evidence regarding the effects of prophylactic antibiotics on the incidence of meningococcal disease among contacts. Observational evidence suggests that antibiotics reduce the risk of disease. We found no good evidence to address the question of which contacts should be treated.

- RCTs have found that antibiotics reduce throat carriage of the meningococcus. We found no evidence that eradicating throat carriage reduces the risk of meningococcal disease.

- We found no RCTs on the effect of pre-admission antibiotics in meningococcal disease. Most observational studies we found show a trend toward benefit with antibiotics, but at least one found contradictory results.

DEFINITION   Meningococcal disease is any clinical condition caused by *Neisseria meningitidis* (the meningococcus) groups A, B, C, or other serogroups. These conditions include purulent conjunctivitis, septic arthritis, meningitis, and septicaemia with or without meningitis.

INCIDENCE/   Meningococcal disease is sporadic in temperate countries, and is
PREVALENCE   most commonly caused by group B or C meningococci. The incidence in the UK varies from 2–8 cases/100 000 people a year,[1] and in the USA from 0.6–1.5/100 000 people.[2] Occasional outbreaks occur among close family contacts, secondary school pupils, and students living in halls of residence. Sub-Saharan Africa has regular epidemics due to serogroup A, particularly in countries lying between Gambia in the west and Ethiopia in the east (the "meningitis belt"), where incidence during epidemics reaches 500/100 000 people.[3]

AETIOLOGY/   The meningococcus infects healthy people and is transmitted by
RISK FACTORS   close contact: probably by exchange of upper respiratory tract secretions (see table 1, p 221).[4–12] Risk of transmission is greatest during the first week of contact.[7] Risk factors include crowding and exposure to cigarette smoke.[13] Children younger than 2 years have the highest incidence, with a second peak between ages 15–24 years. There is currently an increased incidence of meningococcal disease among university students, especially among those in their first term and living in catered accommodation,[14] although we found no accurate numerical estimate of risk from close contact in, for example, halls of residence. Close contacts of an index case have a much higher risk of infection than do people in the general population.[7,10,11] The risk of epidemic spread is higher with groups A and C meningococci than with group B meningococci.[4-6,8] It is not known what makes a meningococcus virulent, but certain clones tend to predominate at different times and in different groups. Carriage of meningococcus in the throat has been reported in 10–15% of people; recent acquisition of a virulent meningococcus is more likely to be associated with invasive disease.

PROGNOSIS   Mortality is highest in infants and adolescents, and is related to disease presentation: case fatality rates are 19–25% in septicaemia, 10–12% in meningitis plus septicaemia, and less than 1% in meningitis alone.[15–17]

AIMS   To prevent disease in contacts.

OUTCOMES   Rates of infection; rates of eradication of throat carriage; adverse effects of treatment.

METHODS   *Clinical Evidence* search and appraisal October 2001. In addition, the author drew from a collection of references from the preelectronic data era.

QUESTION What are the effects of prophylactic antibiotics on risk of disease in people exposed to someone with meningococcal disease?

We found no randomised evidence on the effects of prophylactic antibiotics on the incidence of meningococcal disease among contacts. Observational studies suggest that antibiotics reduce the risk of disease. We found no good evidence to address the question of which contacts should be treated.

Benefits: We found no systematic review and no RCTs examining the effect of prophylactic antibiotics in people who have been in contact with someone with meningococcal disease. **Rifampicin:** We found only anecdotal data. **Phenoxymethylpenicillin:** We found one retrospective study, but the results of that study cannot be generalised beyond the sample tested.[18] **Sulfadiazine:** One observational cohort study of soldiers in temporary troop camps in the 1940s compared the incidence of meningococcal disease in camps where sulfadiazine was given to everyone after a meningococcal outbreak, versus incidence in camps where no prophylaxis was given. The study reported a higher incidence of meningococcal disease in soldiers not given prophylaxis (approximate figures 17/9500 [0.18%] v 2/7000 [0.03%] over 8 wks).[19]

Harms: **Rifampicin:** No excess adverse effects compared with placebo were found in RCTs on throat carriage of meningococcal disease.[20,21] However, rifampicin is known to turn urine and contact lenses orange, and to induce hepatic microsomal enzymes, potentially rendering oral contraception ineffective. Rifampicin prophylaxis may be associated with emergence of resistant strains.[22] **Sulfadiazine:** One in 10 soldiers experienced minor adverse events, including headache, dizziness, tinnitus, and nausea.[19]

Comment: RCTs addressing this question are unlikely to be performed, because the intervention has few associated risks whereas meningococcal disease has high associated risks. RCTs would also need to be large to find a difference in incidence of meningococcal disease. In the sulfadiazine cohort study, the two infected people in the treatment group only became infected after leaving the camp.[19]

QUESTION What are the effects of antibiotics in people with throat carriage of meningococcal disease?

RCTs have found that antibiotics reduce throat carriage of meningococcus. We found no evidence that eradicating throat carriage reduces the risk of meningococcal disease.

Benefits: We found no systematic review. **Incidence of disease:** We found no RCTs or observational studies that examined whether eradicating throat carriage of meningococcus reduces the risk of meningococcal disease. **Throat carriage:** We found five placebo controlled RCTs that examined the effect of antibiotics on carriage of meningococcus in the throat (see table 2, p 222).[20,21,23-25] All trials reported that antibiotics (rifampicin, minocycline, or ciprofloxacin) achieved high rates of eradication (ranging from 90–97%), except one trial of rifampicin in students with heavy growth on culture, in which the rate of eradication was 73%.[20] Eradication rates on placebo ranged from 9–29%. We found seven RCTs that compared different antibiotic regimens (see table 3, p 223).[26–32] Three RCTs found no significant difference between rifampicin and minocycline, ciprofloxacin, or intramuscular ceftriaxone.[27,30,32] A fourth RCT randomised households to different treatments and found that intramuscular ceftriaxone versus rifampicin increased eradication rates.[29] However, that trial used cluster randomisation, and therefore the results should be interpreted with caution. Another trial found no significant difference between oral azithromycin versus rifampicin in eradicating meningococcal throat carriage.[31]

Harms: **Minocycline:** One RCT reported adverse effects (1 or more of nausea, anorexia, dizziness, and abdominal cramps) in 36% of participants.[23] **Rifampicin:** See harms of postexposure antibiotic prophylaxis, p 216. **Ciprofloxacin:** Trials of single dose prophylactic regimens reported no more adverse effects than comparators or placebo.[24,25,30] Ciprofloxacin is contraindicated in pregnancy and in children because animal studies have indicated a possibility of articular cartilage damage in developing joints.[33] **Ceftriaxone:** Two trials of ceftriaxone found no significant adverse effects.[29,30] In one trial, 12% of participants complained of headache.[31] Ceftriaxone is given as a single intramuscular injection. **Azithromycin:** No serious or moderate adverse effects were reported, but nausea, abdominal pain, and headache of short duration were reported equally in the azithromycin and rifampicin treated groups.[29]

Comment: Eradication of meningococcal throat carriage is a well accepted surrogate for prevention of meningococcal disease. It is unlikely that any RCT will be conducted on the efficacy of prophylactic antibiotics in preventing secondary community acquired meningococcal disease in household contacts, because the number of participants required would be large.

QUESTION **What are the effects of pre-admission antibiotics in people with suspected meningococcal disease?**

We found no RCTs on the effect of pre-admission antibiotics in meningococcal disease. Most observational studies we found show a trend toward benefit with antibiotics, but at least one found contradictory results.

Benefits: We found no systematic review and no RCTs on pre-admission antibiotics for suspected meningococcal disease. **Penicillin:** We found seven observational studies on the effect of pre-admission parenteral penicillin in people of all ages with confirmed, probable, or suspected meningococcal disease (see table 4, p 224).[34–40] We also found two reports of pooled data from six of the observational studies.[41,42] The first report (3 English observational studies,[34–36] 487 people) found that antibiotics significantly reduced mortality (OR 2.61, 95% CI 1.04 to 7.18).[41] However, the second report (664 people; the same people in the English studies[34–36] plus partial data from a Danish cohort[43]) found no significant benefit with antibiotics (outcomes not specified; OR 0.82, 95% CI 0.43 to 1.56).[42] We found one additional observational study that assessed the effect of antibiotics in people with suspected meningitis in an

Meningococcal disease

epidemic setting in sub-Saharan Africa.[44] The results were difficult to interpret and no conclusions can be drawn. **Other antibiotics:** We found six observational studies on the effect of giving pre-admission antibiotics other than penicillin to people with suspected meningococcal disease.[45–50] All described disease outcomes when a range of antibiotics (including both oral and parenteral drugs) were given to individuals (mainly children) from a few hours up to a week before being admitted to hospital to treat meningococcal disease. One large case series (667 people)[45] found no significant benefit with pre-admission antibiotics in terms of mortality or sequelae, but found that the duration of symptoms before admission was significantly longer in people receiving pre-admission antibiotics (P < 0.001; CI not provided). Other studies have found that prior antibiotics significantly reduced mortality (P < 0.01;[46] OR 0.06, 95% CI 0.01 to 0.024[47]), sequelae (OR 0.16, 95% CI 0.04 to 0.58),[47] and the risk of developing invasive disease in unsuspected cases (OR 0.26, 95% CI 0.08 to 0.81).[49] One study (288 children aged 3–36 months) found no significant benefit with antibiotics for meningitis caused by N meningitidis, but found significantly fewer complications (neurological or hearing problems, death) in children with pneumococcal meningitis (OR 0.14, 95% CI 0.02 to 0.79).[50] However, all of these results need careful interpretation (see comment below).

Harms:
One study about the harms of penicillin found that anaphylaxis occurred in about 0.04% of cases, and fatal anaphylaxis occurred in about 0.002% of cases.[51] One of the studies reported a death from penicillin anaphylaxis.[47]

Comment:
We found no studies about the relationship between early treatment with antibiotics and development of subsequent antibiotic resistance. Given the limitations of observational studies, the confounding effects of increased disease awareness (following media coverage or official recommendations) leading to early suspicion and diagnosis (by parents and doctors) and earlier referral, the evaluation of the effect of pre-admission penicillin on mortality is problematic. However, it is unlikely that RCTs on pre-admission antibiotics will be performed because of the unpredictably rapid course of disease in some people, the intuitive risks involved in delaying treatment, combined with a relatively low risk of causing harm. A systematic review of the effects of pre-admission antibiotics is under way.

REFERENCES

1. www.phls.co.uk/facts/meni.htm. Disease Facts: Meningococcal Disease.

2. Centers for Disease Control. Summary of notifiable diseases United States, 1997. *MMWR Morb Mortal Wkly Rep* 1998;46:1–87.

3. Hart CA, Cuevas LE. Meningococcal disease in Africa. *Ann Trop Med Parasitol* 1997;91: 777–785.

4. French MR. Epidemiological study of 383 cases of meningococcus meningitis in the city of Milwaukee, 1927–1928 and 1929. *Am J Public Health* 1931;21:130–137.

5. Pizzi M. A severe epidemic of meningococcus meningitis in 1941–1942, Chile. *Am J Public Health* 1944;34:231–239.

6. Lee WW. Epidemic meningitis in Indianapolis 1929–1930. *J Prev Med* 1931;5:203–210.

7. De Wals P, Herthoge L, Borlée-Grimée I, et al. Meningococcal disease in Belgium. Secondary attack rate among household, day-care nursery and pre-elementary school contacts. *J Infect* 1981;3(suppl 1):53–61.

8. Kaiser AB, Hennekens CH, Saslaw MS, Hayes PS, Bennett JV. Seroepidemiology and chemoprophylaxis of disease due to sulphonamide resistant Neisseria meningitidis in a civilian population. *J Infect Dis* 1974;130:217–221.

9. Zangwill KM, Schuchat A, Riedo FX, et al. School-based clusters of meningococcal disease in the United States. *JAMA* 1997;277:389–395.

10. The Meningococcal Disease Surveillance Group. Meningococcal disease secondary attack rate and chemoprophylaxis in the United States. *JAMA* 1976;235:261–265.

11. Olcen P, Kjellander J, Danielson D, Linquist BC. Epidemiology of *Neisseria meningitidis*: prevalence and symptoms from the upper respiratory tract in family members to patients with meningococcal disease. *Scand J Infect Dis* 1981;13:105–109.

12. Hudson, PJ, Vogt PL, Heun EM, et al. Evidence for school transmission of *Neisseria meningitidis* during a Vermont outbreak. *Pediatr Infect Dis* 1986;5:213–217.

13. Stanwell-Smith RE, Stuart JM, Hughes AO, et al. Smoking, the environment and meningococcal disease: a case control study. *Epidemiol Infect* 1994;112:315–328.

14. Communicable Disease Surveillance Centre. Meningococcal disease in university students. *Commun Dis Rep CDR Wkly* 1998;8:49.

15. Andersen BM. Mortality in meningococcal infections. *Scand J Infect Dis* 1978;10:277–282.

16. Thomson APJ, Sills JA, Hart CA. Validation of the Glasgow meningococcal septicaemia prognostic score: a 10 year retrospective survey. *Crit Care Med* 1991;19:26–30.

17. Riordan FAI, Marzouk O, Thomson APJ, Sills JA, Hart CA. The changing presentation of meningococcal disease. *Eur J Pediatr* 1995;154: 472–474.

18. Hoiby EA, Moe PJ, Lystad A, Froholm LO, Bovre K. Phenoxymethyl-penicillin treatment of household contacts of meningococcal disease patients. *Antonie Van Leeuwenhoek* 1986;52:255–257.

19. Kuhns DW, Nelson CT, Feldman HA, Kuhns LR. The prophylactic value of sulfadiazine in the control of meningococcic meningitis. *JAMA* 1943;123: 335–339.

20. Deal WB, Sanders E. Efficacy of rifampicin in treatment of meningococcal carriers. *N Engl J Med* 1969;281:641–645.

21. Eickhoff TC. In vitro and in vivo studies of resistance to rifampicin in meningococci. *J Infect Dis* 1971;123:414–420.

22. Weidmer CE, Dunkel TB, Pettyjohn FS, Smith CD, Leibowitz A. Effectiveness of rifampin in eradicating the meningococcal carrier state in a relatively closed population: emergence of resistant strains. *J Infect Dis* 1971;124:172–178.

23. Devine LF, Johnson DP, Hagerman CR, Pierce WE, Rhode SL, Peckinpaugh RO. The effect of minocycline on meningococcal nasopharyngeal carrier state in naval personnel. *Am J Epidemiol* 1971;93:337–345.

24. Renkonen OV, Sivonen A, Visakorpi R. Effect of ciproflaxacin on carrier rate of *Neisseria meningitidis* in army recruits in Finland. *Antimicrob Agents Chemother* 1987;31:962–963.

25. Dworzack DL, Sanders CC, Horowitz EA, et al. Evaluation of single dose ciprofloxacin in the eradication of *Neisseria meningitidis* from nasopharyngeal carriers. *Antimicrob Agents Chemother* 1988;32:1740–1741.

26. Artenstein MS, Lamson TH, Evans JR. Attempted prophylaxis against meningococcal infection using intramuscular penicillin. *Mil Med* 1967;132: 1009–1011.

27. Guttler RB, Counts GW, Avent CK, Beaty HN. Effect of rifampicin and minocycline on meningococcal carrier rates. *J Infect Dis* 1971; 124:199–205.

28. Blakebrough IS, Gilles HM. The effect of rifampicin on meningococcal carriage in family contacts in northern Nigeria. *J Infect* 1980;2:137–143.

29. Schwartz B, Al-Tobaiqi A, Al-Ruwais A, et al. Comparative efficacy of ceftriaxone and rifampicin in eradicating pharyngeal carriage of Group A *Neisseria meningitidis*. *Lancet* 1988;1: 1239–1242.

30. Cuevas LE, Kazembe P, Mughogho GK, Tillotson GS, Hart CA. Eradication of nasopharyngeal carriage of *Neisseria meningitidis* in children and adults in rural Africa: A comparison of ciprofloxacin and rifampicin. *J Infect Dis* 1995;171:728–731.

31. Girgis N, Sultan Y, Frenck RW Jr, et al. Azithromycin compared with rifampin for eradication of masopharyngeal colonization by *Neisseria meningitidis*. *Pediatr Infect Dis* J 1998; 17:816–819.

32. Simmons G, Jones N, Calder L. Equivalence of ceftriaxone and rifampicin in eliminating nasopharyngeal carriage of serogroup B *Neisseria meningitidis*. *J Antimicrob Chemother* 2000;45: 909–911.

33. Schulter G. Ciprofloxacin: a review of its potential toxicologic effects. *Am J Med* 1987(suppl 4A):82: 91–93.

34. Strang JR, Pugh EJ. Meningococcal infections: reducing the case fatality rate by giving penicillin before admission to hospital. *BMJ* 1992;305: 141–143.

35. Cartwright K, Reilly S, White D, Stuart J. Early treatment with parenteral penicillin in meningococcal disease. *BMJ* 1992;305: 143–147.

36. Gossain S, Constantine CE, Webberley JM. Early parenteral penicillin in meningococcal disease. *BMJ* 1992;305:523–524.

37. Woodward CM, Jessop EG, Wale MCJ. Early management of meningococcal disease. *Commun Dis Rep CDR Rev* 1995;5:R135–R137.

38. Sorensen HT, Nielsen GL, Schonheyder HC, et al. Outcome of pre-hospital antibiotic treatment of meningococcal disease. *J Clin Epidemiol* 1998; 51:717–721.

39. Jolly K, Stewart G. Epidemiology and diagnosis of meningitis: results of a five-year prospective, population-based study. *Commun Dis Public Health* 2001;4:124–129.

40. Jefferies C, Lennon D, Stewart J, Martin D. Meningococcal disease in Auckland, July 1992 – June 1994. *N Z Med J* 1999;112: 115–117.

41. Cartwright K, Strang J, Gossain S, Begg N. Early treatment of meningococcal disease [letter]. *BMJ* 1992;305:774.

42. Sorensen HT, Steffensen FH, Schonheyder HC, Nielsen GL, Olsen J. Clinical management of meningococcal disease. Prospective international registration of patients may be needed. *BMJ* 1998;316:1016–1017.

43. Sorensen HT, Moller-Petersen J, Krarup HB, Pedersen H, Hansen H, Hamburger H. Early treatment of meningococcal disease. *BMJ* 1992; 305:774.

44. Wall RA, Hassan-King M, Thomas H, Greenwood BM. Meningococcal bacteraemia in febrile contacts of patients with meningococcal disease. *Lancet* 1986;2:624.

45. Bohr V, Rasmussen N, Hansen B, et al. 875 cases of bacterial meningitis: diagnostic procedures and the impact of preadmission antibiotic therapy. Part III of a three-part series. *J Infect* 1983;7: 193–202.

46. Goldacre MJ. Acute bacterial meningitis in childhood: aspects of pre-hospital care in 687 cases. *Arch Dis Child* 1977;52:501–503.

47. Barquet N, Domingo P, Cayla JA, et al. Meningococcal disease in a large urban population (Barcelona, 1987–1992): predictors of dismal prognosis. Barcelona Meningococcal Disease Surveillance Group. *Arch Intern Med* 1999;159:2329–2340.

Meningococcal disease

Infectious diseases

48. Morant GA, Diez DJ, Gimeno CC, Pereiro BI, Brines SJ, Sauri M. [An analysis of prior antibiotic treatment on the impact of meningococcal disease in children of the Valencian Community. The Study Group of Invasive Diseases]. *Anales Espanoles de Pediatria* 1999; 50;17–20.
49. Wang VJ, Malley R, Fleisher GR, Inkelis SH, Kuppermann N. Antibiotic treatment of children with unsuspected meningococcal disease. *Arch Pediatr Adolesc Med* 2000;154:556–560.
50. Bonsu BK, Harper MB. Fever interval before diagnosis, prior antibiotic treatment, and clinical outcome for young children with bacterial meningitis. *Clin Infect Dis* 2001;32: 566–572.
51. Idsoe O, Guthe T, Willcox RR, de Weck AL. Nature and extent of penicillin side-reactions, with particular reference to fatalities from anaphylactic shock. *Bull World Health Organ* 1968;38: 159–188.

J Correia
Dr
Instituto Materno Infantil de Pernambuco
Recife
Brazil

C A Hart
Professor
Department of Medical Microbiology and
Genitourinary Medicine
University of Liverpool
Liverpool
UK

Competing interests: None declared.

TABLE 1 Risk of infection among contacts (see text, p 215).

Group of meningococcus	Setting	Risk
A	Household contacts in Milwaukee, USA[4]	AR 1100/100 000; RR not possible to estimate.
	General population in Santiago province, Chile	Attack rate in general population 23–262/100 000 (1941 and 1942).
	Household contacts[5]	Attack rate in household contacts 250/100 000 (2.5%) over both years.
	General population in Indianapolis, USA[6]	AR 4500/100 000; RR not possible to estimate.
B	Household contacts in Belgium[7]	RR 1245*
	Nursery schools[7]	RR 23*
	Day care centres[7]	RR 76*
C	Household contacts from two lower socioeconomic groups Dade County, Florida, USA[8]	Attack rate in two communities 13/100 000 population. Attack rate in household contacts 5/85 (582/100 000).
Unspecified	School based clusters in USA. Predominant meningococcal types: 13 clusters of Gp C, 7 Gp B, 1 Gp Y, 1 GpC/W135 (impossible to distinguish)[9]	RR 2.3*
	Household contacts from several states in USA, meningococcus types B and C predominantly[10]	RR 500–800*
	Household contact in Norway. Meningococcus types A, B, and C predominantly[11]	RR up to 4000*
	Schools. Predominant meningococcus type C[12]	OR 14.1 (95% CI 1.6 to 127)

*Compared with the risk in the general population.

Meningococcal disease

TABLE 2 Effect of antibiotics on throat carriage: results of placebo controlled RCTs (see text, p 216).

Antibiotic	Group of meningococcus	Participants	Eradication		RR (95% CI)
			Treatment (%)	Placebo (%)	
Rifampicin (oral)[20]	B, X, Z	30 students with heavy growth on culture	11/15 (73)	2/15 (13)	5.5 (1.5 to 21)
Rifampicin (oral)[21]	B, C, Y, Z29 E, W 135, NT	76 airforce recruits	36/38* (95)	3/22‡ (14)	7.0 (5.8 to 8.1)
Minocycline (oral)[23]	Predominantly Y (63%)	149 naval recruits	37/41 (90)†	14/48 (29)§	3.1 (2.6 to 3.6)
Ciprofloxacin (oral)[24]	Non-groupable (61%), B (17.5%)	120 army recruits in Finland	54/56 (97) 5 second samples missing	7/53 (13) 6 second samples missing or not a carrier	7.3 (6.5 to 8.1)
Ciprofloxacin (oral)[25]	B (41%), Z (33%)	46 healthy volunteers	22/23 (96) (one did not adhere to treatment)	2/22 (9)	10.5 (8.9 to 12.1)

*9 lost to follow up. †37 either did not have meningococci prior to treatment or did not provide a full set of cultures. ‡7 lost to follow up. §23 either did not have meningococci prior to treatment or did not provide a full set of cultures.

TABLE 3 Effects of antibiotics on throat carriage: results of comparative RCTs (see text, p 217).

Antibiotic	Group of meningococcus	Participants	Rate of eradication (%)	RR (95% CI)
Phenoxymethylpenicillin (im)[26]	C (49%), B (33%), NG (17%)	Adults	41/118 (35)	No data
Erythromycin (oral)[26]	C	Adults	0/7 (0)	No data
Rifampicin (oral)[27]	B + C (31%), NG (69%)	Adults	43/51 (84)	0.89 (0.76 to 1.02)
Minocycline (oral)[27]	B + C (31%), NG (69%)	Adults	36/38 (95)	No data
Rifampicin (oral)[27]	A	Children	37/48 (77)	No data
Sulfadimidine (oral)[28]	A	Children	0/34 (0)	No data
Ceftriaxone (im)[29]	A	Adults and children	66/68 (97)	1.29 (1.10 to 1.49)
Rifampicin (oral)[29]	A	Adults and children	27/36 (75)	No data
Ceftriaxone (im)[30]	A	Adults and children	39/41 (95)	No data
Ciprofloxacin (oral)[30]	A	Adults and children	70/79 (89)	No data
Rifampicin (oral)[30]	A	Adults and children	85/88 (97)	No data
Azithromycin (oral)[31]	B (63%), A (37%)	Adults	56/60 (93)	No data
Rifampicin (oral)[31]	B (63%), A (37%)	Adults	56/59 (95)	No data
Ceftriaxone (im)[32]	B (54%), other serogroups (46%)	Adults and children	97/100 (97)	No data
Rifampicin (oral)[32]	B (51%), other serogroups (49%)	Adults and children	78/82 (95.1)	No data

im, intramuscular.

Meningococcal disease

TABLE 4 Effects of early (pre-admission) parenteral penicillin: results of observational studies (see text, p 217).

Setting	Group of meningococcus	Participants	Parenteral penicillin (number of deaths/ number of people[%])		RR (95% CI)
			Given	Not given	
District general hospital in Darlington, UK (from 1986 to 1991)[34]	NR	46 patients admitted to hospital with confirmed, probable and possible MD, all age groups (52% under 5 years of age)	0/13 (0)	8/33 (24.3)	Incalculable
Three health districts in south-west England, UK (from 1982 to 1991)[35]	Mostly B and C	340* confirmed, probable and possible cases of MD, all age groups (36% under 5 years of age)	5/93 (5.4)	22/246 (8.9)	RR 0.6 (0.23 to 1.54)
Worcester health district, England, UK (1986–1992)[36]	NR	102† confirmed, probable and possible patients with MD; age distribution not reported	1/23 (4.4)	11/79 (13.9)	RR 0.31 (0.04 to 2.29)
District hospital in Wessex, England, UK (1990 to 1993)[37]	NR	68 cases of MD, all age groups (44% under 5 years of age)	0/13 (0)	3/55 (5.5)	Not calculated
County of North Jutland, Denmark‡[38]	NR	302 patients with MD seen by GPs before admission to hospital. All age groups.	9/44 (20.5)	16/258 (6.2)	Adjusted OR 3.2 (95% CI 0.9–10.6)§
Hospitals in Auckland, New Zealand (1992–1997)[40]	Predominantly B	106** confirmed or probable cases of MD, all age groups.	1/24 (4.2)	2/42 (4.9)	RR 0.85 (0.08 to 8.93)
Health district in England, UK (from 1994 to 1998)[39]‡‡	Mostly B (53%) and C (30%)	258†† confirmed, probable and possible cases of MD; all age groups (49% under 5 years of age)	2/72 (2.8)	16/186 (8.6)	RR 0.32 (0.08 to 1.37)

*Number of individuals seen by their general practitioners (GPs) before admission; in one case of a patient who died, there was no information on previous antibiotic use. †A total of 109 patients had their records reviewed, but seven were excluded from analysis because they had received oral penicillin. ‡A partial series of 177 cases from the Danish historical cohort was reported in 1992.[43] showing similar trends of excess mortality in the treated group OR 9.3 (95% CI 3.1 to 27.9). §Adjusted OR, multivariate analysis. **The only prospective study found; all others in the table are retrospective. ††The paper also reports meningitis of other aetiologies. Only those regarded as meningococcal disease are described here. ‡‡The only prospective study found. All others in the table are retrospective CI, confidence interval; MD, meningococcal disease; NR, not reported.

Search date May 2001

Jimmy Volmink

INTERVENTIONS

Key Messages

- One systematic review has found that, in mothers with human immuno-deficiency virus (HIV), zidovudine versus placebo given to mothers significantly reduces the incidence of HIV in infants.

- One RCT has found that nevirapine versus zidovudine given to mothers with HIV and to their newborns significantly reduces the incidence of HIV in infants.

- One RCT has found that a longer versus a shorter course of zidovudine given to mother and infant significantly reduces the incidence of HIV in infants.

- One RCT found limited evidence that elective caesarean section versus vaginal delivery in women with HIV reduced the incidence of HIV in infants.

- One RCT, in women with HIV who had access to clean water and health education, has found that formula feeding versus breast feeding significantly reduces the incidence of HIV in infants, without increasing infant mortality. However, in countries with high infant mortality, avoiding breast feeding may further increase infant morbidity and mortality.

- We found insufficient evidence about the effects of vaginal microbicides on the transmission of HIV to infants.

- One RCT found no significant difference in the incidence of HIV in infants of mothers taking hyperimmune globulin (HIVIG) versus immunoglobulin without HIV antibody (IVIG), in addition to a standard zidovudine regimen.

- RCTs found no significant difference in the incidence of HIV in the infants of pregnant women given vitamin A or multivitamins versus placebo.

Mother to child transmission of HIV

DEFINITION Mother to child transmission of HIV type 1 (see glossary, p 230) infection can occur during pregnancy, in the intrapartum period, or postnatally through breast feeding.[1] In contrast, HIV type 2 (see glossary, p 230) is rarely transmitted from mother to child.[2] Infected children usually have no symptoms and signs of HIV at birth, but develop them over subsequent months or years.[3]

INCIDENCE/ PREVALENCE A review of 13 cohorts found that the risk of mother to child transmission of HIV is about 15–20% in Europe, 15–30% in the USA, and 25–35% in Africa.[4] One global report estimated that 620 000 children below the age of 15 years were infected with HIV during 1999, bringing the total number of children with HIV/AIDS to 1.3 million worldwide.[5] Most of these children were infected from their mother, and 90% live in sub-Saharan Africa.

AETIOLOGY/ RISK FACTORS Transmission of HIV to children is more likely if the mother has a high viral load.[1,6,7] Women with detectable viraemia (by p24 antigen or culture) have double the risk of transmitting HIV-1 to their infants than those who do not.[1] Breast feeding has also been shown in prospective studies to be a risk factor.[8,9] Other risk factors include sexually transmitted diseases, chorioamnionitis, prolonged rupture of membranes, and vaginal mode of delivery.[5,10-13]

PROGNOSIS About 25% of infants infected with HIV progress rapidly to AIDS or death in the first year. Some survive beyond 12 years of age.[3] One European study found a mortality of 15% in the first year of life, and a mortality of 28% by the age of 5 years.[14]

AIMS To reduce mother to child transmission of HIV and improve infant survival, with minimal adverse effects.

OUTCOMES HIV infection status of the child; infant morbidity and mortality; maternal morbidity and mortality; adverse effects of treatment.

METHODS *Clinical Evidence* search and appraisal May 2001.

QUESTION **What are the effects of measures to reduce mother to child transmission of HIV?**

OPTION **ANTIRETROVIRAL DRUGS**

One systematic review has found that zidovudine versus placebo significantly reduces the incidence of HIV in infants. One RCT has found that nevirapine versus zidovudine given to the mother and to her newborn significantly reduces the risk of HIV transmission. One RCT has found that longer versus shorter courses of zidovudine given to mother and infant significantly reduces the incidence of HIV in infants.

Benefits: **Zidovudine versus placebo:** We found one systematic review (search date not stated, 4 RCTs, 1585 women), which compared zidovudine versus placebo given to the mother before, during, or after labour (see table 1, p 232).[19] In one of the included RCTs, infants of mothers receiving zidovudine were also given zidovudine for 6 weeks after birth.[15] Overall, zidovudine versus placebo significantly reduced the incidence of HIV in infants (AR 79/616 [13%] with zidovudine v 150/634 [24%]; RR 0.54, 95% CI 0.42 to 0.69; NNT 9, 95% CI 7 to 14). The results were still significant when the

RCT of zidovudine that used the most intensive regimen[15] was excluded from the analysis (combined results for less intensive regimens versus placebo: AR 70/495 [14%] v 119/507 [23%]; RR 0.60, 95% CI 0.46 to 0.79; NNT 11, 95% CI 8 to 20).[16–18] The effect of zidovudine versus placebo was similar in reducing the incidence of HIV in infants from breast feeding and non-breast feeding mothers (breast feeding RR 0.62, 95% CI 0.46 to 0.85; non-breast feeding RR 0.50, 95% CI 0.30 to 0.85). **Zidovudine versus nevirapine:** The systematic review[19] identified one unblinded RCT (626 women from a predominantly breast feeding population in Uganda), which compared zidovudine versus nevirapine.[20] It found that nevirapine given to mothers as a single oral dose at the onset of labour and to infants as a single dose within 72 hours of birth versus zidovudine given orally to women during labour and to their newborns for 7 days after birth, significantly reduced the number of infants with HIV at 14–16 weeks (RR 0.58, 95% CI 0.40 to 0.83). **Alternative zidovudine regimens:** One RCT (1437 women) compared four different zidovudine regimens; zidovudine was given to mothers from a specific time in gestation until delivery and to the infant until a specific age: "short–short" course (mother from 35 wks, infant for up to 3 days); "long–long" (mother from 28 wks, infant for up to 6 wks); "short–long" (mother from 35 wks, infant for up to 6 wks); and "long–short" (mother from 28 wks, infant for up to 3 days). The RCT found that a "long–long" course versus a "short–short" course significantly reduced the number of infants with HIV (AR 9/220 [4%] v 24/229 [10%]; RR 2.56, 95% CI 1.22 to 5.39). It found no significant difference between a "long–long" versus a "short–long" course (RR 1.32, 95% CI 0.80 to 2.20), or versus a "long–short" course (RR 0.73, 95% CI 0.40 to 1.33).[21]

Harms: **Zidovudine versus placebo:** The review found that intensive zidovudine versus placebo significantly increased the risk of neonatal haematological toxicity (RR 1.86, 95% CI 1.18 to 2.94; specific effects undefined), whereas no significant difference was found for less intensive regimens versus placebo (RR 0.77, 95% CI 0.44 to 1.35).[19] Infants who received the most intensive regimen, who were followed for 18 months had mild reversible anaemia, which resolved by 12 weeks of age.[22] The same trial in uninfected infants followed for a median of 4.2 years found no significant difference between zidovudine versus placebo in growth patterns, immunological parameters, or the occurrence of childhood cancers.[23] The RCT of combination antiretroviral therapy has reported no serious adverse drug reactions to date.[19] **Zidovudine versus nevirapine:** The RCT found no significant difference in serious adverse effects in mothers and infants (4.0% v 4.7% in mothers; 19.8% v 20.5% in infants up to 18 months of age).[23] **Alternative zidovudine regimens:** The RCT found that the rate of serious adverse events in mothers and infants was similar for all regimens. The rates of severe anaemia in infants were "long–long" (1%); "long–short" (0%); "short–long" (0.3%); and "short–short" (1.3%).[21]

Comment: The review[19] identified one RCT currently in progress in South Africa, Uganda, and Tanzania, comparing zidovudine plus lamivudine versus placebo. Preliminary results suggest that zidovudine plus lamivudine reduces the risk of HIV transmission at 6 weeks of age when administered in the antenatal, intrapartum, and postpartum period (RR 0.52, 95% CI 0.35 to 0.76), and during the intrapartum and postpartum period (RR 0.66, 95% CI 0.46 to 0.94). The RCT found that zidovudine plus lamivudine given during the intrapartum period alone did not significantly reduce the risk of transmission (RR 1.01, 95% CI 0.74 to 1.38). Other RCTs evaluating alternative anti-retroviral drug regimens are currently in progress.

OPTION **ELECTIVE CAESAREAN SECTION**

One RCT found limited evidence that elective caesarean section versus vaginal delivery significantly reduced the incidence of HIV in infants.

Benefits:
We found one systematic review (search date not stated, 1 RCT, 436 women), which compared elective caesarean section at 38 weeks versus vaginal delivery.[19] It found that caesarean section significantly reduced the number of infants with HIV at 18 months (AR 3/170 [2%] with caesarean section v 21/200 [11%] with vaginal delivery; RR 0.16, 95% CI 0.05 to 0.55; NNT 11, 95% CI 10 to 21).

Harms:
No serious adverse effects were reported in either group. Postpartum fever was significantly more common in women having caesarean section versus vaginal delivery (AR 2/183 [1%] v 15/225 [7%]; RRI 6.1, 95% CI 1.45 to 22; NNH 18, 95% CI 16 to 50). Postpartum bleeding, intravascular coagulation, or severe anaemia occurred rarely in either group.

Comment:
A total of 15% of the women withdrew from the trial or were lost to follow up. None of the women analysed breast fed, although this was not stated as specific exclusion criterion. More women who gave birth by caesarean section versus vaginal delivery had received zidovudine during pregnancy (70% v 58%); this means that the observed difference between groups may not have been due exclusively to the different delivery methods.

OPTION **AVOIDING BREAST FEEDING**

One RCT in women with HIV, who had access to clean water and health education, has found that formula feeding versus breast feeding significantly reduces the incidence of HIV in infants, without increasing mortality.

Benefits:
We found no systematic review. We found one RCT (425 HIV-1 seropositive women with access to clean water and health education in Kenya), which found that breast feeding versus formula feeding significantly increased the number of infants with HIV at 24 months (AR 61/197 [31%] with breast feeding v 31/205 [15%]; RR 2.0, 95% CI 1.4 to 3.0; NNT 6, 95% CI 4 to 13).[23] Although infants were breast fed throughout the trial duration, the greatest exposure to breast milk occurred during the first 6 months of life. The trial found no significant difference in the mortality rate at 24 months with breast feeding versus formula feeding (AR 45/197 [23%] with breast feeding v 39/204 [19%] with formula feeding; RR 1.2, 95% CI 0.82 to 1.75).[24]

Harms: The RCT did not report on adverse effects (see comment below).

Comment: In countries with high infant mortality, avoiding breast feeding may further increase infant morbidity and mortality through its effect on nutrition, immunity, maternal fertility, and birth spacing. Access to clean water and education when using formula feeds may explain the similar mortality rates in breast fed and formula fed infants.

OPTION   VAGINAL MICROBICIDES

We found insufficient evidence about the effects of vaginal microbicides on the incidence of HIV in infants.

Benefits: We found no systematic review or RCTs.

Harms: One non-randomised trial (see comment below) reported no adverse effects in mothers or in infants.

Comment: We found one non-randomised trial (2094 women), which compared vaginal cleansing (with 0.25% chlorhexidine) from admission in labour to delivery versus no vaginal cleansing.[25] Women were allocated to the treatment or control group on the basis of months of the year. The trial found no significant difference in the transmission of HIV after vaginal cleansing versus no cleansing (AR 136/505 [26.9%] v 133/477 [27.9%]; RR 0.95, 95% CI 0.8 to 1.2). The results should be interpreted with caution because HIV status was not determined in the 41% of infants who were lost to follow up, and the trial was not randomised and was, therefore, potentially biased.

OPTION   IMMUNOTHERAPY

One RCT found no significant difference in the incidence of HIV in infants of mothers taking HIV hyperimmune globulin (HIVIG) versus immunoglobulin without HIV antibody (IVIG) in addition to a standard zidovudine regimen.

Benefits: We found one systematic review (search date not stated, 1 RCT, 501 women),[19] which compared HIVIG versus IVIG given to women during pregnancy, the intrapartum period, and to their infants at birth. Women in both groups received a standard course of zidovudine and no infants were breast fed. The RCT found no significant difference in transmission of HIV between HIVIG versus IVIG regimens at 6 months of age (4.1% v 6.0%; 95% CI for difference not provided; P = 0.36).

Harms: The trial reported no significant adverse effects.

Comment: The low overall transmission rate (5%) in this study was much lower than the anticipated rate of greater than 15% used to calculate the appropriate sample size. The trial is unable to exclude a clinically important effect of HIVIG on the number of children with HIV.

OPTION   VITAMIN SUPPLEMENTS

Two RCTs found that vitamin supplements versus placebo given to pregnant women had no significant effect on the incidence of HIV in their infants.

Mother to child transmission of HIV

Benefits: We found no systematic review but found two RCTs.[26,27] The first RCT (1083 women with HIV-1 between 12 and 27 weeks' gestation in Tanzania) compared vitamin A and/or multivitamin supplements (excluding vitamin A) versus placebo, using a factorial design.[26] It found no significant difference in the number of infants with HIV in women taking multivitamins or vitamin A versus placebo at birth (multivitamins v placebo: AR 38/376 [10%] v 24/363 [7%], RR 1.54, 95% CI 0.94 to 2.51; vitamin A v placebo: AR 38/380 [10%] v 24/358 [6.7%], RR 1.49, 95% CI 0.91 to 2.43), or at 6 weeks among infants free of infection at birth (multivitamins v placebo: 31/191 [16%] v 28/179 [16%], RR 1.04, 95% CI 0.65 to 1.66; vitamin A v placebo: 35/196 [18%] v 24/174 [14%], RR 1.30, 95% CI 0.80 to 2.09).[28] The second RCT (728 pregnant women with HIV in South Africa) compared vitamin A with placebo.[27] It found no significant difference in the number of children with HIV infection at 3 months (20% with vitamin A v 22% with placebo; 95% CI for difference not provided). Mortality rates were similar in vitamin A and placebo groups at 1 month, 3 months, and 13 months of age.

Harms: Neither RCT reported adverse effects.[26,27]

Comment: The RCTs were performed because observational studies have found an association in pregnant women between transmission of HIV and low serum levels of vitamin A.[28]

GLOSSARY

Human immunodeficiency virus type 1 (HIV-1) is the most common cause of HIV disease throughout the world.

Human immunodeficiency virus type 2 (HIV-2) is predominantly found in West Africa and is more closely related to the simian immunodeficiency virus than to HIV-1.

REFERENCES

1. John GC, Kreiss J. Mother-to-child transmission of human immunodeficiency virus type 1. *Epidemiol Rev* 1996;18:149–157.

2. Adjorlolo-Johnson G, De Cock KM, Ekpini E, et al. Prospective comparison of mother-to-child transmission of HIV-1 and HIV-2 in Abidjan, Ivory Coast. *JAMA* 1994;272:462–466.

3. Peckham C, Gibb D. Mother-to-child transmission of the human immunodeficiency virus. *N Engl J Med* 1995;333:298–302.

4. The Working Group on MTCT of HIV. Rates of mother-to-child transmission of HIV-1 in Africa, America and Europe: results of 13 perinatal studies. *J Acquir Immune Defic Syndr* 1995;8:506–510.

5. UNAIDS (Joint United Nations Programme on HIV/AIDS). *Report of the global HIV/AIDS epidemic.* June 2000. Geneva: UNAIDS; 2000. UNAIDS/00.13E.

6. Mofenson LM. Epidemiology and determinants of vertical HIV transmission. *Semin Pediatr Infect Dis* 1994;5:252–256.

7. Khouri YF, McIntosh K, Cavacini L, et al. Vertical transmission of HIV-1: correlation with maternal viral load and plasma levels of CD4 binding site anti-gp 120 antibodies. *J Clin Invest* 1995;95:732–737.

8. Dunn DT, Newell ML, Ades AE, Peckham CS. Risk of human immunodeficiency virus type-1 transmission through breastfeeding. *Lancet* 1992;240:585–588.

9. Miotti PG, Taha ET, Newton I, et al. HIV transmission through breastfeeding: a study in Malawi. *JAMA* 1999;282:744–749.

10. Nair P, Alger L, Hines S, Seiden S, Hebel R, Johnson JP. Maternal and neonatal characteristics associated with HIV infection in infants of seropositive women. *J Acquir Immune Defic Syndr* 1993;6:298–302.

11. Minkoff H, Burns DN, Landesman S, et al. The relationship of the duration of ruptured membranes to vertical transmission of human immunodeficiency virus. *Am J Obstet Gynecol* 1995;173:585–589.

12. European Collaborative Study. Risk factors for mother-to-child transmission of HIV-1. *Lancet* 1992;339:1007–1012.

13. Mofenson LM. A critical review of studies evaluating the relationship of mode of delivery to perinatal transmission of human immunodeficiency virus. *Pediatr Infect Dis J* 1995;14:169–176.

14. The European Collaborative Study. Natural history of vertically acquired human immunodeficiency virus-1 infection. *Pediatrics* 1994;94:815–819.

15. Connor EM, Sperling RS, Gelber RD, et al. Reduction of maternal-infant transmission of human immunodeficiency virus type 1 with zidovudine treatment. *N Engl J Med* 1994;311:1173–1180.

16. Shaffer N, Chuachoowong R, Mock PA, et al. Short-course zidovudine for perinatal HIV-1 transmission in Bangkok, Thailand: a randomised

controlled trial. Bangkok Collaborative Perinatal HIV Transmission Study Group. *Lancet* 1999;353: 773–780.

17. Wiktor SZ, Ekpini E, Karon JM, et al. Short-course oral zidovudine for prevention of mother-to-child transmission of HIV-1 in Abidjan, Cote d'Ivoire: a randomised trial. *Lancet* 1999;353:781–785.

18. Dabis F, Msellati P, Meda N, et al. Six-month efficacy, tolerance, and acceptability of a short regimen of oral zidovudine to reduce vertical transmission of HIV in breastfed children in Cote d'Ivoire and Burkina Faso: a double-blind placebo-controlled multicentre trial. DITRAME Study Group. Diminution de la Transmission Mere-Enfant. *Lancet* 1999;353:786–792.

19. Brocklehurst P. Interventions aimed at decreasing the risk of mother-to-child transmission of HIV infection. In: The Cochrane Library, Issue 3, 2000. Oxford: Update Software. Search date not stated; primary sources Cochrane Pregnancy and Childbirth Group Trials Register, and Cochrane Controlled Trials Register.

20. Guay LA, Musoke P, Fleming T, et al. Intrapartum and neonatal single-dose nevirapine compared with zidovudine for prevention of mother-to-child transmission of HIV-1 in Kampala, Uganda: HIVNET 012 randomised trial. *Lancet* 1999;354: 795–802.

21. Lallemant M, Jourdain G, Le Couer S, et al. A trial of shortened zidovudine regimens to prevent mother-to-child transmission of human immunodeficiency virus type 1. *N Engl J Med* 2000;343:982–991.

22. Sperling RS, Shapiro DE, McSherry GD, et al. Safety of the maternal-infant zidovudine regimen utilized in the Pediatric AIDS Clinical Trial Group 076 Study. *AIDS* 1998;12: 1805–1813.

23. Culnane M, Fowler MG, Lee S, et al. Lack of long term effects of in utero exposure to zidovudine among uninfected children born to HIV-infected women. *JAMA* 1999;281: 151–157.

24. Nduati R, John G, Mbori-Ngacha D, et al. Effect of breastfeeding and formula feeding on transmission of HIV-1: a randomized clinical trial. *JAMA* 2000; 283:1167–1174.

25. Biggar RJ, Miotti PG, Taha TE, et al. Perinatal intervention trial in Africa: effect of a birth canal cleansing intervention to prevent HIV transmission. *Lancet* 1996;347:1647–1650.

26. Fawzi WW, Msamanga G, Hunter D, et al. Randomized trial of vitamin supplements in relation to vertical transmission of HIV-1 in Tanzania. *J Acquir Immune Defic Syndr* 2000;23: 246–254.

27. Coutsoudis A, Pillay K, Spooner E, Kuhn L, Coovadia HM. Randomized trial testing the effect of vitamin A supplementation on pregnancy outcomes and early, mother-to-child HIV-1 transmission in Durban, South Africa. *AIDS* 1999; 13:1517–1524.

28. Fawzi WW, Hunter DJ. Vitamins in HIV disease progression and vertical transmission. *Epidemiology* 1998;9:457–466.

Jimmy Volmink
Director of Research and Analysis
Global Health Council
Washington, DC
USA

Competing interests: None declared.

Mother to child transmission of HIV

TABLE 1 Placebo controlled trials of zidovudine to reduce mother to child transmission of HIV (see text, p 226).

Ref	Participants	Maternal treatment	Infant treatment	Transmission rate	RRR (95% CI)
Infants not breast fed					
15	477 women with confirmed HIV (60 centres in USA and France)	*Antepartum* Orally 1 mg 5 times daily starting at 14–34 weeks gestation *Intrapartum* 2 mg/kg iv over 1 hour then 1 mg/kg/hour until delivery	Orally 2 mg/kg every 6 hours for 6 weeks (given only to babies of mothers treated with ZDV)	At 18 months: placebo 26% ZDV 8%	70% (39% to 85%)
16	397 women with confirmed HIV-1 (2 centres in Bangkok, Thailand)	*Antepartum* Orally 3 mg twice daily from 36 weeks' gestation *Intrapartum* Orally 300 mg every 3 hours until delivery	Nil	At 6 months: placebo 19% ZDV 9%	50% (15% to 70%)
Infants breast fed					
17	280 women with confirmed HIV-1 (1 hospital in Cote d'Ivoire)	*Antepartum* Orally 3 mg twice daily from 36 weeks' gestation *Intrapartum* Orally 300 mg every 3 hours until delivery	Nil	At 3 months: placebo 25% ZDV 16%	37% (−6% to +62%)
18	431 women with confirmed HIV-1 (Cote d'Ivoire and Burkina Faso)	*Antepartum* Orally 250 or 3 mg twice daily from 36 to 38 weeks gestation *Intrapartum* Orally single dose of 500 or 600 mg at onset of labour *Postpartum* Orally 250 or 3 mg twice daily for 7 days	Nil	At 6 months: placebo 28% ZDV 18%	35% (4% to 56%)

iv, intravenously; ref, reference; ZDV, zidovudine.

Infectious diseases

Key Messages

Treating newly diagnosed tuberculosis

- RCTs found no evidence of a difference in relapse rates between standard short course (6 months) and longer term (8–9 months) chemotherapy in people with pulmonary tuberculosis. RCTs suggest that taking pyrazinamide in the first 2 months speeds up sputum clearance but that there is conflicting evidence relating to its effect on relapse rates.

- Limited evidence from two RCTs found no significant difference between daily versus twice or three times weekly short course regimens.

- One systematic review has found evidence that reducing treatment from 6–4 months' significantly increases relapse rates.

Tuberculosis

- We found no good evidence comparing regimens containing quinolones versus existing regimens.

Treating multidrug resistant tuberculosis

- We found no good evidence comparing different drug regimens for multidrug resistant tuberculosis.

Improving adherence and reattendance

- We found insufficient evidence on the effects of training health staff, health education by a doctor, routine prompts to attend, or sanctions for failure to attend to treatment.
- We found limited evidence suggesting that adherence to treatment may be improved by defaulter actions, cash incentives, health education by a nurse, or community health advisers.
- RCTs found conflicting evidence about the effects of direct observation on treatment adherence.
- Two RCTs found conflicting evidence on the effects of prompts and contracts on reattendance for Mantoux test reading.

DEFINITION　Tuberculosis is caused by *Mycobacterium tuberculosis* and can affect many organs. Specific symptoms relate to site of infection and are generally accompanied by fever, sweats, and weight loss.

INCIDENCE/ About a third of the world's population is infected with *M tubercu-*
PREVALENCE *losis*. The organism kills more people than any other infectious agent. The World Health Organization estimates that 95% of cases are in developing countries, and that 25% of avoidable deaths in developing countries are caused by tuberculosis.[1]

AETIOLOGY/ Social factors include poverty, overcrowding, homelessness, and
RISK FACTORS inadequate health services. Medical factors include HIV and immunosuppression.

PROGNOSIS　Prognosis varies widely and depends on treatment.[2]

AIMS　To cure tuberculosis; eliminate risk of relapse; reduce infectivity; avoid emergence of drug resistance; and prevent death.

OUTCOMES　*M tuberculosis* in sputum (smear examination and culture), symptoms, weight, cure, relapse rates, attendance, and completion of treatment.

METHODS　*Clinical Evidence* search and appraisal August 2001. Key words: tuberculosis, pulmonary, isoniazid, pyrazinamide, and rifampicin. We included all Cochrane systematic reviews and studies that were randomised or used alternate allocation, and had at least 1 year follow up after completion of treatment.

OPTION   SHORT COURSE CHEMOTHERAPY (6 MONTHS)

RCTs found no evidence of a difference in relapse rates between standard short course (6 months) and longer term (8–9 months) chemotherapy in people with pulmonary tuberculosis. RCTs suggest that treatment with pyrazinamide in the first 2 months speeds up sputum clearance, but the evidence relating to its effect on relapse rates is conflicting.

Benefits: We found no systematic review, but found four RCTs.[3–6] **Versus longer courses:** We found two RCTs (1295 people with untreated, culture/smear positive pulmonary tuberculosis), which compared 6 versus 8–9 months of chemotherapy.[3,4] Participants were followed up for at least 1 year after treatment was completed. The trials were performed in the UK and in East and Central Africa, and used different combinations of isoniazid, rifampicin, ethambutol, streptomycin, and pyrazinamide for initial (first 2 months) and continuation treatment. The RCTs found no significant difference in relapse rates between short course and longer regimens. **Different short course regimens:** The second RCT found no significant difference between regimens using ethambutol or streptomycin as the fourth drug in the initial phase.[4] A 6 month regimen using rifampicin and isoniazid throughout was highly effective (relapse rate 2%) and significantly better than isoniazid alone in the 4 month continuation phase (relapse rate 9%). When treatment with isoniazid alone was prolonged in a 6 month continuation phase, the relapse rate was not significantly better than with 4 months' continuation.[3] **Pyrazinamide:** The second RCT found that sputum conversion was faster with regimens containing pyrazinamide for the first 2 months, but there was no significant difference in relapse rates at 3 years' follow up.[4] The third RCT (833 people) compared four different 6 month regimens and found that bacterial relapse was higher for those not receiving pyrazinamide in the 12 months after chemotherapy (12/160 [7.5%] v 8/625 [1.3%]).[5] The fourth RCT (497 people) of ongoing pyrazinamide found that relapse at 18 months was more likely in those not receiving pyrazinamide, but the difference was not significant (3.1% v 1.0%).[6]

Harms: In the largest RCT, possible adverse reactions were reported in 24/851 people (3%), with six requiring modification of treatment.[3] Two people in the trial developed jaundice, one of whom died. **Pyrazinamide:** Adding pyrazinamide did not increase the incidence of hepatitis (4% with and without pyrazinamide).[4] However, mild adverse effects were more common, including arthralgia, skin rashes, flu-like symptoms, mild gastrointestinal disturbance, vestibular disturbance, peripheral neuropathy, and confusion. Arthralgia was the most common adverse effect, reported in about 1% of people on pyrazinamide, but was mild and never required modification of treatment.[3,4]

Comment: In people treated previously, the organisms may have acquired drug resistance so short course chemotherapy may not be effective.

| OPTION | INTERMITTENT SHORT COURSE CHEMOTHERAPY |

Two RCTs found no significant difference in cure rates between daily versus twice or three times weekly short course regimens, but the limited data available did not exclude a clinically important difference.

Benefits: We found one systematic review (search date 2001, 1 RCT, 399 people)[7] and one subsequent RCT (206 children).[8] The review compared three times weekly versus daily chemotherapy for 6 months in people with newly diagnosed pulmonary tuberculosis. One month after treatment was completed there was no significant difference in rates of bacteriological cure (defined as negative sputum culture, 99.9% v 100.0%) or relapse (5/186 [2.7%] people v 1/192 [0.5%] people; RR 4.0, 95% CI 0.7 to 24.1).[7] The subsequent RCT comparing twice weekly versus daily chemotherapy found no significant difference in cure rates (85/89 [95%] v 114/117 [97%]; RR 0.98, 95% CI 0.84 to 1.02).[8] At least 12 cohort studies have found cure rates of 80–100% with three times weekly regimens taken over 6–9 months.[7]

Harms: Intermittent treatment has the potential to contribute to drug resistance, but this was not shown in the studies.[7]

Comment: The RCTs had low event rates and were too small to exclude a clinically significant difference between the dosing regimens.

| OPTION | CHEMOTHERAPY FOR LESS THAN 6 MONTHS |

One systematic review found limited evidence suggesting that reducing duration of treatment to less than 6 months significantly increased relapse rates.

Benefits: We found one systematic review (search date 1999, 7 RCTs, 2248 outpatients with newly diagnosed pulmonary tuberculosis), which compared a variety of shorter (minimum 2 months) and longer (maximum 12 months) drug regimens.[9] The trials included people in India, Hong Kong, Singapore, and Germany. The review found that a 3 month versus a 12 month regimen significantly increased relapse rates (5 RCTs: RR 3.03, 95% CI 2.08 to 4.40). One of the RCTs found that people given a 2 month regimen were significantly less likely to change or discontinue drugs than those given a 12 month regimen (6/299 [2.6%] v 17/299 [5.7%]; RR 0.35; 95% CI 0.14 to 0.88).[9]

Harms: The review found similar rates of adverse events or toxicity with both shorter and longer regimens.

Comment: The treatments were given under optimal conditions. In clinical practice adherence is likely to be lower, so relapse rates associated with the shorter regimens are likely to be higher than those in clinical trials.

OPTION   REGIMENS CONTAINING QUINOLONES

We found insufficient evidence on regimens containing quinolones.

Benefits: We found no systematic review, but found two RCTs.[10,11] One RCT in Tanzania (200 people) comparing a regimen containing ciprofloxacin versus a regimen not containing a quinolone found that more people relapsed after the ciprofloxacin regimen, but the difference was not significant (RR of relapse at 6 months 16.0, 95% CI 0.9 to 278.0).[10] A relatively low dosage of ciprofloxacin was used (750 mg daily). The second RCT (160 people) compared a regimen containing ciprofloxacin versus a regimen without, and focused only on adverse effects (see harms below).[11]

Harms: Adverse effects, which were mild and responsive to symptomatic treatment, were similar in people taking quinolone regimens versus controls.[11]

Comment: Quinolones have good bactericidal activity *in vitro*. Some of the newer quinolones have enhanced antimycobacterial activity compared with ciprofloxacin.

QUESTION   What are the effects of different drug regimens in people with multidrug resistant tuberculosis?

We found no RCTs comparing different drug regimens for multidrug resistant tuberculosis.

Benefits: We found no systematic review and no RCTs comparing different regimens in people with multidrug resistant tuberculosis.

Harms: We found no evidence.

Comment: Current clinical practice in multidrug resistant tuberculosis is to include at least three drugs to which the particular strain of tuberculosis is sensitive, using as many bactericidal agents as possible. People are observed directly and managed by a specialised clinician.

QUESTION   Which interventions improve adherence to treatment?

We found insufficient evidence on the effects of staff training on adherence to treatment.

Benefits: We found one systematic review (search date 2000, 1 poorly randomised RCT [see comment below]) comparing intensive staff supervision versus routine supervision at centres in Korea performing tuberculosis extension activities.[12] Centres were paired and randomised, and supervision was carried out by senior doctors. The review found that higher completion rates were achieved with intensive supervision (RR 1.2, CIs not estimated because of cluster design).

Harms: None reported.

Comment: The trial used cluster randomisation, but the unit of analysis was the individual.

OPTION	PROMPTS

We found no RCTs about the effects of prompts on reattendance.

Benefits: We found one systematic review (search date 2000), which found no RCTs of prompts to return for treatment.[12]

Harms: None.

Comment: None.

OPTION	DEFAULTER ACTIONS

One systematic review has found that intensive action for defaulter actions (see glossary, p 241) improves completion of treatment.

Benefits: We found one systematic review (search date 2000, 2 RCTs conducted in India).[12] The first RCT in the review found that up to four home visits to defaulters significantly improved completion of treatment compared with the routine policy of a reminder letter followed by one home visit (RR 1.32, 95% CI 1.02 to 1.71). The second RCT found that up to two reminder letters significantly improved completion of treatment (RR 1.21, 95% CI 1.05 to 1.39), even in people who were illiterate.

Harms: None reported.

Comment: None.

OPTION	CASH INCENTIVES

One systematic review has found that cash incentives versus usual care improve attendance among people living in deprived circumstances. One subsequent RCT found that cash incentives improved treatment completion in intravenous drug abusers. Another subsequent RCT found no significant difference in treatment completion with immediate versus deferred cash incentives.

Benefits: **Versus no cash incentive:** We found one systematic review (search date 2000, 2 RCTs conducted in the USA)[12] and one subsequent RCT.[13] The first RCT in the review found that in homeless men, money ($5) versus usual care improved attendance at the first appointment (RR 1.6, 95% CI 1.3 to 2.0). The second RCT in the review, in migrants, found that combining cash ($10) with health education versus usual care improved attendance (RR 2.4, 95% CI 1.5 to 3.7).[12] The subsequent RCT (163 iv drug users) compared three groups: direct observation at a participant chosen site plus a $5 per visit incentive; direct observation at a designated site plus $5 per visit; and direct observation at a participant chosen site without a cash incentive. It found that both groups given cash incentives versus the group given no incentive were significantly more likely to complete treatment (28/53 [53%] with chosen site plus $5 v 2/55 [4%] with no cash incentive; OR 29.7, 95% CI 6.5 to 134.5; 33/55 [60%] with designated site plus $5 v 2/55 [4%] with no cash incentive; OR 39.7, 95% CI 8.7 to 134.5).[13] **Immediate versus deferred cash incentive:** We found one RCT (300 iv drug users), which compared three groups: treatment with direct observation by a nurse; treatment with self administration plus peer counselling and education; and routine care (see direct patient observation, p 240). Participants were further randomised to receive a $10 immediate versus deferred cash incentive.[14] The immediate payment was given at the end of each month when people completed a routine assessment for adherence and drug toxicity. The deferred payment was given either after the 6 months' treatment period, or when the person withdrew from the study. The RCT found no difference between immediate versus deferred payments in treatment completion (125/150 [83%] v 112/150 [75%]; P = 0.09).[14]

Harms: None measured.

Comment: None.

OPTION   HEALTH EDUCATION

One RCT found that health education by a nurse improved treatment completion, with no evidence of benefit from health education by a doctor. One RCT in drug users found no significant effect of health education.

Benefits: We found one systematic review (search date 2000, 2 RCTs conducted in the USA).[12] The first RCT in the review compared three methods of health education versus an educational leaflet. Health education consisted of telephoning by a nurse, visiting by a nurse, or consultation by a clinic doctor. The trial found that treatment completion was significantly increased by the nurse telephone call versus the leaflet (75/80 [94%] v 55/77 [71%]; RR 1.30, 95% CI 1.18 to 1.37) and by the nurse visit versus the leaflet (75/79 [95%] v 55/77 [71%]; RR 1.33, 95% CI 1.20 to 1.38). However, consultation by the clinic doctor was not significantly better than the education leaflet (64/82 [78%] v 55/77 [71%]; RR 1.09, 95% CI 0.89 to 1.23). The second RCT in drug users found that 5–10 minutes of health education had no significant effect on whether people kept a scheduled appointment (RR 1.04, 95% CI 0.70 to 1.54).[12]

Harms: None measured.

Comment: Education is often part of a package of care that includes prompts and incentives, which makes it difficult to evaluate the independent effects of education.

OPTION   SANCTIONS

We found no RCTs on the effect of sanctions.

Benefits: We found one systematic review (search date 2000), which identified no RCTs of sanctions.[12]

Harms: The use of sanctions may be ethically dubious.

Comment: In New York (USA), incarcerating people who did not comply with treatment was thought to increase compliance with the Department of Health's community tuberculosis treatment programme.[15]

Tuberculosis

OPTION   COMMUNITY HEALTH WORKERS

One RCT has found that health advisors recruited from the community increased attendance for treatment.

Benefits: We found one systematic review (search date 2000, 1 RCT in homeless people).[12] It found that health advisors recruited from the community increased the number of people who kept their appointments (62/83 [75%] attended v 42/79 [53%]; RR 1.4, 95% CI 1.1 to 1.8).

Harms: None reported.

Comment: None.

OPTION   DIRECT PATIENT OBSERVATION

RCTs found conflicting evidence about the effects of direct observation on treatment adherence.

Benefits: We found one systematic review (search date 2000, 2 RCTs, 1052 people),[12] two subsequent RCTs,[16,17] and one additional RCT.[14] The two RCTs in the review compared direct observation of people as they took their drugs versus self administered treatment at home. The first RCT in the review (216 people in South Africa) found no significant difference between the two strategies, although overall adherence in the study was low.[18] The second RCT in the review (836 people in Thailand) compared direct observation (either from health centre staff, community members, or a family member) versus self treatment. It found that direct observation versus self treatment improved treatment completion (347/414 [84%] v 320/422 [76%]; RR 1.11, 95% CI 1.04 to 1.16; NNT 13, 95% CI 8 to 36) and cure rate (RR 1.64, 95% CI 1.17 to 2.30).[19] The first subsequent RCT (156 people conducted in South Africa) compared direct observation by lay health workers versus direct observation by clinic nurse versus self treatment. It found no significant difference in cure rates.[16] The second subsequent RCT (497 adults) compared treatment with direct observation by health workers versus direct observation by family members versus self administered treatment. It found no significant difference in cure rates with observation by health workers versus self administered treatment (108/170 [64%] with health worker observation v 100/162 [62%] with self administration; ARI 2.0%, 95% CI –8.6% to +12.2%) or with observation by family members versus self administration (91/165 [55%] with observation by family members v 100/162 [62%] with self administration; ARR 7.0%, 95% CI –4.1% to 17.3%). It found no significant difference between interventions in treatment completion.[17] The additional RCT (300 iv drug users) compared three groups: treatment with direct observation by nurse; treatment with self administration plus peer counselling and education; and routine care. Participants were further randomised to receive a $10 immediate versus deferred cash incentive (see cash incentives, p 238).[14] It found no significant difference between observation or peer support versus self administration alone in treatment completion (observation v self administration alone, P = 0.86; peer support v self administration alone, P value not stated).[14]

Harms: Potential harms include reduced co-operation between patient and doctor, removal of individual responsibility, detriment to long term sustainability of antituberculosis programmes, and increased burden on health services to the detriment of care for other diseases. None of these have been adequately investigated.

Comment: Numerous observational studies have evaluated interventions described as directly observed treatment, but all were packages of interventions that included specific investment in antituberculosis programmes, such as strengthened drug supplies, improved microscopy services, and numerous incentives, sanctions, and other co-interventions that were likely to influence adherence.[20,21]

QUESTION Which interventions improve reattendance for Mantoux test reading?

OPTION PROMPTS AND CONTRACTS TO IMPROVE REATTENDANCE FOR MANTOUX TEST READING

Two RCTs found conflicting evidence on the effects of prompts and contracts on reattendance for Mantoux test reading.

Benefits: **Prompts:** We found one systematic review (search date 2000, 1 RCT, 701 healthy people).[12] The RCT compared an automatic telephone message prompt to return for Mantoux reading versus no prompt. It found that people were slightly more likely to return in the intervention group, but the difference was not significant (93% v 88%; RR 1.05, 95% CI 1.00 to 1.10).[12] **Contracts:** We found no systematic review. One RCT in healthy students in the USA found that, compared with no commitment, reattendance for Mantoux reading was significantly improved by verbal commitments (RR 1.10, 95% CI 1.03 to 1.18) and by written commitments (RR 1.12, 95% CI 1.05 to 1.19).[22]

Harms: None reported.

Comment: None.

GLOSSARY

Defaulter actions Actions taken by health workers when people fail to attend for treatment of their tuberculosis.

REFERENCES

1. Global Tuberculosis Programme. *Treatment of tuberculosis*. Geneva: World Health Organization, 1997:WHO/TB/97.220.
2. Enarson D, Rouillon A. Epidemiological basis of tuberculosis control. In: Davis PD, ed. *Clinical tuberculosis*. 2nd ed. London: Chapman and Hall Medical, 1998.
3. East and Central African/British Medical Research Council Fifth Collaborative Study. Controlled clinical trial of 4 short-course regimens of chemotherapy (three 6-month and one 8-month) for pulmonary tuberculosis. *Tubercle* 1983;64:153–166.
4. British Thoracic Society. A controlled trial of 6 months chemotherapy in pulmonary tuberculosis, final report: results during the 36 months after the end of chemotherapy and beyond. *Br J Dis Chest* 1984;78:330–336.
5. Hong Kong Chest Service/British Medical Research Council. Controlled trial of four thrice weekly regimens and a daily regimen given for 6 months for pulmonary tuberculosis. *Lancet* 1981; 1:171–174.
6. Farga V, Valenzuela P, Valenzuela MT, et al. Short-term chemotherapy of tuberculosis with 5-month regimens with and without pyrazinamide in the second phase (TA-82) [in Spanish]. *Rev Med Chil* 1986;114:701–705.
7. Mwandumba HC, Squire SB. Fully intermittent dosing with drugs for tuberculosis. In: The Cochrane Library, Issue 3, 2001. Oxford: Update Software. Search date 2001; primary sources Cochrane Infectious Diseases Group Trials Register, Cochrane Controlled Trials Register,

Infectious diseases

Medline, Embase, reference lists of article, researchers contacted for unpublished trials.

8. Naude JMTW, Donald PR, Huseey GD, et al. Twice weekly vs. daily chemotherapy for childhood tuberculosis. *Pediatr Infect Dis* 2000;19: 405–410.

9. Gelband H. Regimens of less than six months treatment for TB. In: The Cochrane Library, Issue 4, 2000. Oxford: Update Software. Search date 1999; primary sources Medline, Cochrane Parasitic Diseases Trials Register, contact with researchers, and hand searched references.

10. Kennedy N, Berger L, Curran J, et al. Randomized controlled trial of a drug regimen that includes ciprofloxacin for the treatment of pulmonary tuberculosis. *Clin Infect Dis* 1996;22:827–833.

11. Kennedy N, Fox R, Uiso L, Ngowi FI, Gillespie SH. Safety profile of ciprofloxacin during long-term therapy for pulmonary tuberculosis. *J Antimicrob Chemother* 1993;32:897–902.

12. Volmink J, Garner P. Interventions for prompting adherence to tuberculosis treatment. In: The Cochrane Library, Issue 3, 2001. Oxford: Update Software. Search date 2000; primary sources Medline, Embase, Cochrane Controlled Trials Register 1998, Issue 3, Cochrane Collaboration Effective Professional Practice (CCEPP) Registry Trials, LILACS to 2000, hand searched journals and references, and contact with authors.

13. Malotte CK, Hollingshead JR, Larro M. Incentives vs. outreach workers for latent tuberculosis treatment in drug users. *Am J Prev Med* 2001;20:103–107.

14. Chaisson R, Barnes GL, Hackman JR, et al. A randomized, controlled trial of interventions to improve adherence to isoniazid therapy to prevent tuberculosis in injection drug users. *Am J Med* 2001;110:610–615.

15. Fujiwara PI, Larkin C, Frieden TR. Directly observed therapy in New York history, implementation, results and challenges. *Tuberculosis* 1997;18: 135–148.

16. Zwarenstein M, Schoeman JH, Vundule C, Lombard CJ, Tatley M. A randomised controlled trial of lay health workers as direct observers of tuberculosis. *Int J Tuberc Lung Dis* 2000;4: 550–554.

17. Walley JD, Khan MA, Newell JN, Khan MH. Effectiveness of the direct observation component of DOTS for tuberculosis: a randomised controlled trial in Pakistan. *Lancet* 2001;357:664–669.

18. Zwarenstein M, Schoeman JH, Vundule C, Lombard C, Tatley M. Randomised controlled trial of self-supervised and directly observed treatment of tuberculosis. *Lancet* 1998;352: 1340–1343.

19. Kamolratanakul P, Sawert H, Lertmaharit S, et al. Randomized controlled trial of directly observed treatment (DOT) for patients with pulmonary tuberculosis in Thailand. *Trans R Soc Trop Med Hyg* 1999;93:552–557.

20. Garner P. What makes DOT work? *Lancet* 1998; 352:1326–1327.

21. Volmink J, Matchaba P, Garner P. Directly observed therapy and treatment adherence. *Lancet* 2000; 355:1345–1350. Search date 1999; primary sources Medline, Embase, Cochrane Controlled Trials Register, and hand searches of reference lists.

22. Wurtele SK, Galanos AN, Roberts MC. Increasing return compliance in a tuberculosis detection drive. *J Behav Med* 1980;3:311–318.

Paul Garner
Professor
Liverpool School of Tropical Medicine
Liverpool
UK

Alison Holmes
Senior Lecturer
Hammersmith Hospital
Imperial College
London
UK

Competing interests: None declared.

QUESTIONS

INTERVENTIONS

Key Messages

- One small RCT found limited evidence that various psychotherapies were more effective than treatment as usual. One other small RCT found no significant difference between psychotherapy and dietary advice. One small RCT found a 100% withdrawal rate with dietary advice. Seven small RCTs found no overall significant differences between different psychotherapies. However, all the RCTs were small and were unlikely to have been powered to detect a difference between treatments.

- Four RCTs found no evidence that the addition of an antidepressant to treatment improved outcomes.

- Three RCTs found no evidence that cyproheptadine increased weight gain compared with placebo.

- Limited evidence from one small RCT found outpatient treatment was as effective as inpatient treatment in those individuals not so severely ill as to warrant emergency intervention.

- One small RCT found no benefit from zinc in the treatment of anorexia nervosa.

- One small RCT found no benefit from cisapride in the treatment of anorexia nervosa.

- We found no good evidence of the effect of hormonal treatment on fracture rates. One small RCT found no effect of oestrogen on bone mineral density.

- We found no RCTs to support the use of neuroleptic medication in anorexia nervosa.

DEFINITION Anorexia nervosa is characterised by a refusal to maintain weight at or above a minimally normal weight (< 85% of expected weight for age and height, or body mass index [BMI — see glossary, p 250] < 17.5 kg/m^2), or a failure to show the expected weight gain during growth. In association with this, there is often an intense fear of gaining weight, preoccupation with weight, denial of the current low weight and its adverse impact on health, and amenorrhoea. Two subtypes of anorexia nervosa, binge–purge and restricting, have been defined.[1]

INCIDENCE/ A mean incidence in the general population of 19/100 000 a year
PREVALENCE in females and 2/100 000 a year in males has been estimated from 12 cumulative studies.[2] The highest rate was in female teenagers (age 13–19 years), where there were 50.8 cases/100 000 a year. A large cohort study of Swedish school children (4291 people, age 16 years) were screened by weighing and subsequent interview, and the prevalence of anorexia nervosa cases (defined using DSM-III and DSM-III-R criterita) was found to be 7/1000 for girls and 1/1000 for boys.[3] Little is known of the incidence or prevalence in Asia, South America, or Africa.

AETIOLOGY/ The aetiology of anorexia nervosa has been related to family,
RISK FACTORS biological, social, and cultural factors.[4] Studies have found that anorexia nervosa is associated with a family history of anorexia nervosa (HR 11.4, 95% CI 1.1 to 89), of bulimia nervosa (adjusted HR 3.5, 955 CI 1.1 to 14),[5] depression, generalised anxiety disorder, obsessive complusive disorder, or obsessive compulsive personality disorder (adjusted RR 3.6, 95% CI 1.6 to 8).[6] A twin study estimated the heritability to be 58% (95% CI 33% to 77%), with the remaining variance apparently due to non-shared environment. However, the study was unable to completely rule out a contribution of a non-shared environment. Specific aspects of childhood temperament thought to be related include perfectionism, negative self-evaluation, and extreme compliance.[7] Perinatal factors include prematurity (OR 3.2, 95% CI 1.6 to 6.2), particularly if the baby was small for gestational age (OR 5.7, 95% CI 1.4 to 4.1).

PROGNOSIS We found no good evidence on the prognosis of people with anorexia nervosa who do not access formal medical care. A summary of treatment studies (68 studies published between 1953 and 1989, 3104 people, length of follow up 1–33 years) found that 43% of people recover completely (range 7–86%), 36% improve (range 1–69%), 20% develop a chronic eating disorder (range 0–43%), and 5% die from anorexia nervosa (range 0–21%).[8] Favourable prognostic factors include an early age at onset and a short interval between onset of symptoms and the beginning of treatment. Unfavourable prognostic factors include vomiting, bulimia, profound weight loss, chronicity, and a history of premorbid developmental or clinical abnormalities. The all cause standardised mortality ratio of eating disorders (anorexia nervosa and bulimia nervosa) has been estimated at 538, about three times higher than other psychiatric illness.[9] The average annual risk of mortality was 0.59% a year in females in 10 eating disorder populations (1322 people) with a minimum follow up of 6 years.[10] The mortality risk was higher for people with lower weight and with older age at presentation. Young women with anorexia nervosa are at an increased risk of fractures later in life.[11]

AIMS   To restore physical health (weight within the normal range and no sequelae of starvation, e.g. regular menstruation, normal bone mass), normal patterns of eating and attitudes towards weight and shape, and no additional psychiatric comorbidity (e.g. depression, anxiety, obsessive compulsive disorder); to reduce the impact of the illness on social functioning and quality of life.

OUTCOMES   The most widely used measure of outcome is the Morgan and Russell scale (see glossary, p 250),[12] which includes nutritional status, menstrual function, mental state, and sexual and social adjustment. Biological outcome criteria alone such as weight (BMI or in relation to matched population weight) and menstrual function are used infrequently as outcome measures. RCTs do not usually have sufficient power or long enough follow up periods to address mortality. Other validated outcome measures used include eating symptom measures.[13–16]

METHODS   *Clinical Evidence* search and appraisal April 2001, and hand search of reference lists of identified reviews. To be included, an RCT had to have at least 30 people and follow up greater than 75%. Results from each of the identified trials were extracted independently by the two reviewers. Any disagreements were discussed until a consensus was reached. A systematic review (in German) was identified through direct contact with the author and is being translated.[17]

QUESTION   What are the effects of treatments in anorexia nervosa?

OPTION   PSYCHOTHERAPY

One small RCT found limited evidence that various psychotherapies were more effective than treatment as usual. One other small RCT found no significant difference between psychotherapy and dietary advice. One small RCT found a 100% withdrawal rate with dietary advice. Seven small RCTs found no significant difference between different psychotherapies.

Benefits: We found no systematic review. We found nine small RCTs. Three small RCTs of limited quality compared different psychotherapies (see glossary, p 250) versus dietary advice (see glossary, p 250) or treatment as usual (see web extra table A at www.clinicalevidence. com). All three RCTs were carried out in an outpatient setting in people with a late age of onset and long duration of illness.[18–20] The largest RCT found significant improvements in weight gain for some psychotherapies versus treatment as usual and for the number of people classified as recovered.[18] The second RCT found a significant improvement for cognitive therapy versus baseline.[20] All people treated with dietary advice withdrew from treatment and refused release of their results, making it impossible to compare the two groups. The third RCT found no difference in outcomes between the groups (see web extra table A at www.clinicalevidence.com).[19] Seven small RCTs of limited quality compared different psychotherapies. Three of these were undertaken in an outpatient

Anorexia nervosa

setting,[21–23] and one was carried out in an inpatient setting[24] in people with an early age of onset and short illness duration. Two of the RCTs were carried out in an outpatient setting in people with a later age of onset and longer duration of illness.[18,25] One RCT included people with early and late onset anorexia nervosa and with long and short duration of illness.[26,27] No RCT found an overall significant difference between different psychotherapies.

Harms: The acceptability of the treatment varied between RCTs. Failure to engage or early withdrawal from treatment ranged from 5–33% between RCTs (4/84 [5%];[18] 7/33 [21%];[23] 19/56 [33%];[24] 8/54 [14%];[26] 7/43 [16%][21]), but this may have been caused by different methods of case ascertainment. The number of people admitted for inpatient treatment (see glossary, p 250) also varied between RCTs, ranging from 0–36% (12/84 [14%];[18] 3/30 [10%];[19] 0/30 [0%];[25] 4/40 [10%];[21] 16/41 [36%];[22] 8/33 [24%];[23] 6/25 [24%][24]). One death was attributed to anorexia nervosa in the control group in one outpatient RCT with a 1 year follow up.[18] Three deaths attributed to anorexia nervosa occurred in the 5 year follow up period in one inpatient based RCT.[27]

Comment: All the RCTs were small and had limited power to detect clinically important differences if they existed. The amount of therapeutic input varied considerably between and within the RCTs. There was variation in methods of recruitment, reporting of key results (e.g. withdrawal rates), and the description of participants' characteristics and selection. The people in the inpatient RCTs covered a broad range of severity.[26]

OPTION   **ANTIDEPRESSANT MEDICATION**

Three small RCTs found no evidence of beneficial effects from the use of amitriptyline or fluoxetine.

Benefits: We found no systematic review. We found three small RCTs. The first RCT allocated 42 people with early onset and short duration anorexia nervosa (mean age 16.6 years, mean 27% below average weight, 1.5 years duration of anorexia nervosa) from two centres (5 outpatients) to amitriptyline or placebo.[28] Eighteen people refused to participate and two more in the amitriptyline group had low amitriptyline blood levels suggesting poor treatment adherence. The RCT found no difference between the groups on any outcome variable measured at 5 weeks. The second RCT (33 women; mean age 26.2 years; mean BMI (see glossary, p 250) 15.0 kg/m^2; mean duration of anorexia nervosa 8.0 years) compared fluoxetine 60 mg versus placebo for the duration (mean 36 days) of inpatient treatment (see glossary, p 250) (which included individual and group psychotherapy [see glossary, p. 250]).[29] There were two early withdrawals from the fluoxetine group. The RCT found no significant differences in weight gain, eating symptoms, or depressive symptoms between the groups. The third RCT[30] compared amitriptyline, cyproheptadine, and placebo, and found no significant difference between treatments (see benefits under cyproheptadine, p 248).

Harms: None reported. The QT interval may be prolonged in people with anorexia nervosa,[31] and tricyclic antidepressants (amitriptyline, protriptyline, nortriptyline, doxepin, maprotiline) also increase the QT interval.[32–34] In an observational study (495 people with mental illness and 101 healthy controls), an increased risk of QTc was seen with tricyclic use, adjusting for age and other drug use (adjusted OR 2.6, 95% CI 1.2 to 5.6).[35]

Comment: The RCTs were all of short duration. Prolongation of the QT interval may be associated with increased risk of ventricular tachycardia, torsades de pointes, and sudden death.[33,34]

OPTION	NEUROLEPTIC MEDICATION

We found no good evidence.

Benefits: We found no systematic review and no RCTs.

Harms: The QT interval may be prolonged in people with anorexia nervosa,[31,32] and many neuroleptics (haloperidol, pimozide, sertindole, thioridazine, chlorpromazine, and others) may also increase the QT interval.[33,34] An observational study (495 people with mental illness and 101 healthy controls) found an increased risk of QTc with high and very high dose neuroleptic use after adjusting for age and other drug use (high dose: adjusted OR 3.4, 95% CI 1.2 to 10.1; very high dose: adjusted OR 5.6, 95% CI 1.6 to 19.3).[35]

Comment: Prolongation of the QT interval may be associated with increased risk of ventricular tachycardia, torsades de pointes, and sudden death.[33,34]

OPTION	ZINC

One RCT found no improvement in daily weight gain with the addition of zinc to an inpatient regime.

Benefits: We found no systematic review. We found one RCT (54 people aged > 15 years, mean BMI (see glossary, p 250) 15.8 kg/m^2, mean duration of anorexia nervosa 3.7 years, admitted to 2 eating disorder units), which compared 100 mg zinc gluconate versus placebo.[36] All but three of the people had normal zinc levels at pretreatment. Treatment was continued until the individual had gained 10% of weight over the admission weight on two consecutive weeks. Ten people in the zinc group and nine in the placebo group did not complete the study. There was no difference in average daily weight gain (zinc 0.079 kg v placebo 0.039 kg; difference 0.04 kg, 95% CI −0.005 to +0.08).

Harms: None reported.

Comment: None.

Anorexia nervosa

OPTION	CYPROHEPTADINE

One RCT in outpatients and two RCTs in inpatients found no significant difference between cyproheptadine and placebo in weight gain.

Benefits: We found no systematic review. We found three small RCTs. The first RCT (24 women in an outpatient setting) compared cyproheptadine versus placebo.[37] The trial found no significant difference in response to treatment after 2 months. The second RCT (81 women in 3 specialised inpatient centres) compared cyproheptadine versus placebo, and behaviour therapy versus no behaviour therapy.[38] The effect of behaviour therapy was not reported. There were no significant differences in weight gain between the cyproheptadine and placebo groups. The third RCT (72 women, mean age 20.6 years, mean 77% of target weight, mean duration of anorexia 2.9 years, at 2 specialised inpatient units) compared amitriptyline (up to a maximum of 160 mg) versus cyproheptadine (up to a maximum of 32 mg) versus placebo.[30] The drug treatment had no significant effect on treatment efficiency, i.e. the reciprocal of days to reach target weight times 90 (a dummy figure of 120 was used if people failed to reach target weight).

Harms: No harms were reported in the first two RCTs.[37,38] In the third RCT, on both day 7 and day 21, placebo exceeded the amitriptyline group in number of physical adverse events rated moderate or severe. Cyproheptadine had the lowest number of adverse effects. No one had to be withdrawn from the protocol because of adverse experiences.[30]

Comment: All three RCTs were of short duration.

OPTION	INPATIENT VERSUS OUTPATIENT TREATMENT SETTING IN ANOREXIA NERVOSA

We found weak evidence from one systematic review that outpatient treatment was as effective as inpatient treatment in those people not so severely ill as to warrant emergency intervention.

Benefits: We found one systematic review (search date 1999)[39] comparing inpatient (see glossary, p 250) with outpatient care. The review identified one RCT, which had a 5 year follow up.[40,41] Ninety people referred with anorexia nervosa (mean age 22 years, weight loss 26% of matched population mean weight, mean duration 3.2 years) were randomised to four treatment groups: inpatient treatment, outpatient treatment (individual and family therapy [see glossary, p 250]), outpatient group therapy, and assessment only. Assessors were not blind to treatment allocation. Adherence to allocated treatment (defined as accepting allocation and at least 1 attendance at a treatment group or individual treatment session) differed significantly between groups: inpatient treatment 18 of 30 (60%); outpatient treatment (individual and family therapy) 18 of 20 (90%); outpatient group psychotherapy (see glossary, p 250) 17 of 20 (85%); and assessment interview only 20 of 20 (100%). Treatment adherence differed significantly between outpatient and inpatient treatment (RR 1.46, 95% CI 1.06 to 2.0). Average acceptance of therapeutic input also varied between groups

(20 weeks inpatient treatment, 9 outpatient sessions, and 5 group sessions). In the assessment only group, six people had no treatment of any kind in the first year, and the others had treatment elsewhere (6 had inpatient treatment, 5 had outpatient hospital treatment, and 3 had at least weekly contact with their general practitioners). Six people in this group spent almost the entire year in treatment. There were no significant differences between any of the four groups at 1, 2, and 5 years mean weight or in the Morgan and Russell global scores (see glossary, p 250). The proportion of people with a good outcome with inpatient treatment was five of 29 (17%) at 2 years and nine of 27 (33%) at 5 years; with outpatient treatment (individual and family therapy) four of 20 (20%) at 2 years and eight of 17 (47%) at 5 years; with outpatient group psychotherapy five of 19 (26%) at 2 years and 10 of 19 (53%) at 5 years; and with assessment interview only two of 20 (10%) at 2 years and six of 19 (32%) at 5 years.

Harms: One person died as a result of anorexia nervosa between the assessment and the start of outpatient group treatment, and one of the people allocated to inpatient treatment died as a result of anorexia nervosa by 5 years.[40,41]

Comment: The systematic review[39] was unable to draw meaningful conclusions from numerous case series as participant characteristics, treatments, mortality, and outcomes varied widely. Individuals admitted for inpatient treatment had a lower mean weight than those treated as outpatients. One subsequent observational study (355 people with anorexia nervosa; 169 with anorexia nervosa bulimic type; mean age 25 years; mean duration of illness 5.7 years; 75% available for 2.5 years' follow up) found that people with longer duration of illness had a higher likelihood of good outcome with longer than with briefer duration of inpatient treatment, and those with a shorter duration of illness had a higher likelihood of good outcome with briefer inpatient treatment.[42] Median duration of inpatient treatment was 11.6 weeks for anorexia nervosa and 10.6 weeks for anorexia nervosa/bulimia nervosa.

OPTION CISAPRIDE

One small RCT found no clear benefit from cisapride.

Benefits: We found no systematic review. We found one small RCT (34 inpatients aged 18–40 years at 2 hospitals; mean duration 2.7 years; BMI (see glossary, p 250) 15.1 kg/m^2) comparing cisapride (30 mg) versus placebo for 8 weeks.[43] The trial found no significant difference in weight gain (placebo 5.7 kg v cisapride 5.1 kg; P = NS).

Harms: No adverse events were noted in this RCT. The QT interval in anorexia nervosa is prolonged even in the absence of medication; therefore, cisapride is not recommended in anorexia nervosa. Cisapride has now been withdrawn in many countries because of an increased risk of cardiac irregularities, including ventricular tachycardia, torsades de pointes, and sudden death.[33,34]

Comment: Five people withdrew from the RCT and were not included in the analysis.

Anorexia nervosa

| QUESTION | What are the effects of interventions to prevent or treat complications of anorexia? |

| OPTION | HORMONAL TREATMENT |

We found no good evidence on the effects of hormonal treatment on fracture rates. One small RCT found no effect of oestrogen administration on bone mineral density.

Benefits: We found no systematic review. We found one RCT (48 women, mean age 23.7 years, mean duration of anorexia nervosa 4.0 years) of hormone replacement therapy (Premarin 0.625 mg on days 1–25 plus Provera 5 mg on days 16–25) versus an oral contraceptive containing 35 μg ethinyl oestradiol versus no medication.[44] All women maintained a calcium intake of 1500 mg using oral calcium carbonate. Spinal bone mineral density was measured at 6 monthly intervals. There was no significant difference in the final bone density at follow up of 0.5–3 years.

Harms: Three women withdrew from the oestrogen treatment; two because of adverse effects, and one woman withdrew from the control treatment.

Comment: Improvements in bone mineral density would not necessarily lead to reductions in risk of fractures.

GLOSSARY

Body mass index Weight (kg) divided by height (m) squared.

Dietary advice Dieticians with experience of eating disorders discuss diet, mood, and daily behaviours.

Family therapy Treatment that includes members of the family of origin or the constituted family, and that addresses the eating disorder as a problem of family life.

Inpatient treatment This has been regarded as the standard approach to the management of anorexia nervosa.[45] One of the key components of inpatient treatment is refeeding, which is achieved through structured, supervised meals. Psychotherapy (of a variety of different types) and pharmacotherapy are included in many programmes.

Morgan Russell scales A widely used measure of outcome for anorexia nervosa that consists of two scores: an average outcome score and a general outcome score. The average outcome score is based on the outcome in five areas: nutritional status, menstrual function, mental state, sexual adjustment, and socioeconomic status.

Psychotherapy Different types of psychological treatments given individually or in groups are included here. These use psychodynamic, cognitive behavioural, or supportive techniques, or combinations of these.

REFERENCES

1. American Psychiatric Association. *Diagnostic and Statistical Manual of Mental Disorders (DSM-IV)*. 4th ed. Washington DC: APA, 1994.

2. Pawluck DE, Gorey KM. Secular trends in the incidence of anorexia nervosa: integrative review of population-based studies. *Int J Eat Disord* 1998;23:347–352.

3. Råstam M, Gillberg C, Garton M. Anorexia nervosa in a Swedish urban region. A population-based study. *Br J Psychiatry* 1989;155:642–646.

4. Strober M, Freeman R, Lampert C, et al. Controlled family study of anorexia nervosa and

bulimia nervosa: evidence of shared liability and transmission of partial syndromes. *Am J Psychiatry* 2000;157:393–401.

5. Lilenfeld LR, Kaye WH, Greeno CG, et al. A controlled family study of anorexia nervosa and bulimia nervosa: psychiatric disorders in first-degree relatives and effects of proband comorbidity. *Arch Gen Psychiatry* 1998;55:603–610.

6. Wade TD, Bulik CM, Neale M, et al. Anorexia nervosa and major depression: shared genetic and environmental risk factors. *Am J Psychiatry* 2000;157:469–471.

7. Fairburn CG, Cooper Z, Doll HA, Welch SL. Risk factors for anorexia nervosa: three integrated case-control comparisons. *Arch Gen Psychiatry* 1999;56:468–476.

8. Steinhausen, H-C. The course and outcome of anorexia nervosa. In: Brownell K, Fairburn CG, eds. *Eating Disorders and Obesity: a comprehensive handbook*. New York: The Guilford Press,1995:234–237.

9. Harri, EC, Barraclough B. Excess mortality of mental disorder. *Br J Psychiatry* 1998;173: 11–53.

10. Nielsen S, Møller-Madsen S, Isager T, Jørgensen J, Pagsberg K, Theander S. Standardized mortality in eating disorders: a quantitative summary of previously published and new evidence. *J Psychosom Res* 1998;44: 413–434.

11. Lucas A, Melton L, Crowson C, O'Fallon WM. Long term fracture risk among women with anorexia nervosa: a population-based cohort study. *Mayo Clin Proc* 1999;74:972–977.

12. Morgan HG, Russell GF. Value of family background and clinical features as predictors of long-term outcome in anorexia nervosa: four-year follow-up study of 41 patients. *Psychol Med* 1975;5:355–371.

13. Cooper Z, Fairburn CG. The Eating Disorders Examination. A semi-structured interview for the assessment of the specific psychopathology of eating disorders. *Int J Eat Disord* 1987;6:1–8.

14. Garner DM. *Eating Disorder Inventory-2 (EDI-2): professional manual*. Odessa FL: Psychological Assessment Resources Inc., 1991.

15. Garner DM, Garfinkel PE. The eating attitudes test: an index of the symptoms of anorexia nervosa. *Psychol Med* 1979;10:647–656.

16. Henderson M, Freeman CPL. A self-rating scale for bulimia: the 'BITE'. *Br J Psychiatry* 1987;150: 18–24.

17. Herzog T (in press). Stand der vergleichenden Therapieforschung bei Anorexia nervosa. Ergebnisse einer Systematischen Literaturübersicht. In: Gastpar M, Remschmidt HJ, Senf W, eds. *Forschungsperspektiven bei Essstorungen*. Berlin: Verlag Wissenschaft und Praxis.

18. Dare C, Eisler I, Russell G, Treasure J, Dodge L. Psychological therapies for adult patients with anorexia nervosa: a randomised controlled trial of outpatient treatments. *Br J Psychiatry* 2001;178: 216–221.

19. Hall A, Crisp AH. Brief psychotherapy in the treatment of anorexia nervosa. Outcome at one year. *Br J Psychiatry* 1987;151:185–191.

20. Serfaty MA. Cognitive therapy versus dietary counselling in the outpatient treatment of anorexia nervosa: effects of the treatment phase. *Eur Eat Dis Rev* 1999;7:334–350.

21. Eisler I, Dare C, Hodes M, Russell GFM, Dodge E, Le Grange D. Family therapy for adolescent anorexia nervosa: the results of a controlled comparison of two family interventions. *J Child Psychol Psychiatry* 2000;41: 727–736.

22. Robin AL, Siegel PT, Moye AW, et al. A controlled comparison of family versus individual therapy for adolescents with anorexia nervosa. *J Am Acad Child Adolesc Psychiatry* 1999;38:1482–1489.

23. Wallin U, Kronvall P, Majewski M-L. Body awareness therapy in teenage anorexia nervosa: outcome after 2 years. *Eur Eat Dis Rev* 2000;8: 19–30.

24. Geist R, Heinmaa M, Stephens D, et al. Comparison of family therapy and family group psychoeducation in adolescents with anorexia nervosa. *Can J Psychiatry* 2000;45: 173–178.

25. Treasure JL, Todd G, Brolly M, Tiller J, Nehmed A, Denman F. A pilot study of a randomized trial of cognitive analytical therapy vs educational behavioral therapy for adult anorexia nervosa. *Behav Res Ther* 1995;33:363–367.

26. Russell GFM, Szmukler G, Dare C, Eisler I. An evaluation of family therapy in anorexia nervosa and bulimia nervosa. *Arch Gen Psychiatry* 1987; 44:1047–1056.

27. Eisler I, Dare C, Russell GFM, Szmukler GI, Le Grange D, Dodge E. Family and individual therapy in anorexia nervosa. A 5-year follow-up. *Arch Gen Psychiatry* 1997;54:1025–1030.

28. Biederman J, Herzog DB, Rivinus TM, et al. Amitriptyline in the treatment of anorexia nervosa: a double-blind, placebo-controlled study. *J Clin Psychopharmacol* 1985;5:10–16.

29. Attia E, Haiman C, Walsh BT, et al. Does fluoxetine augment the inpatient treatment of anorexia nervosa? *Am J Psychiatry* 1998;155: 548–551.

30. Halmi KA, Eckert E, LaDu TJ, et al. Anorexia nervosa. Treatment efficacy of cyproheptadine and amitriptyline. *Arch Gen Psychiatry* 1986;43: 177–181.

31. Ackerman MJ. The long QT syndrome: ion channel diseases of the heart. *Mayo Clin Proc* 1998;73: 250–269.

32. Becker A, Grinspoon SK, Klibanski A, Herzog DB. Current concepts: eating disorders. *N Engl J Med* 1999;340:1092–1098.

33. Yap Y, Camm J. Risk of torsades de pointes with non-cardiac drugs: doctors need to be aware that many drugs can cause QT prolongation. *BMJ* 2000;320:1158–1159.

34. Sheridan DJ. Drug-induced proarrhythmic effects: assessment of changes in QT interval. *Br J Clin Pharm* 2000;50:297–302.

35. Reilly JG, Ayis SA, Ferrier IN, Jones SJ, Thomas SHL. QTc interval abnormalities and psychotropic drug therapy in psychiatric patients. *Lancet* 2000; 355:1048–1052.

36. Birmingham CL, Goldner EM, Bakan R. Controlled trial of zinc supplementation in anorexia nervosa. *Int J Eat Disord* 1994;15:251–255.

37. Vigersky RA, Loriaux L. The effect of cyproheptadine in anorexia nervosa: a double blind trial. In: Vigersky RA, ed. *Anorexia Nervosa*. New York: Raven Press,1977:349–356.

38. Goldberg SC, Halmi KA, Eckert RC, Casper RC, Davis JM. Cyproheptadine in anorexia nervosa. *Br J Psychiatry* 1979;134:67–70.

39. West Midlands Development and Evaluation Service. *In-patient Versus Out-patient Care for Eating Disorders*. DPHE 1999 Report No. 17. Birmingham: University of Birmingham, 1999. Search date 1999; primary sources Medline, Psychlit, Cochrane Library, variety of internet sites, and hand searches of relevant editions of relevant journals and references from identified articles.

40. Crisp AH, Norton K, Gowers S, et al. A controlled study of the effect of therapies aimed at adolescent and family psychopathology in anorexia nervosa. *Br J Psychiatry* 1991;159: 325–333.

41. Gowers S, Norton K, Halek C, Crisp AH. Outcome of outpatient psychotherapy in a random allocation treatment study of anorexia nervosa. *Int J Eat Disord* 1994;15:65–177.

Anorexia nervosa

42. Kächele H for the study group MZ-ESS. Eine multizentrische Studie zu Aufwand und Erfolg bei psychodynamischer Therapie von Eβstörungen. *Psychother Med Psychol (Stuttg)* 1999;49:100–108.

43. Szmukler GI, Young GP, Miller G, et al. A controlled trial of cisapride in anorexia nervosa. *Int J Eat Disord* 1995;17:347–357.

44. Klibanski A, Biller BMK, Schoenfeld DA, Herzog DB, Saxe VC. The effects of estrogen administration on trabecular bone loss in young women with anorexia nervosa. *J Clin Endocrinol Metab* 1995;80:898–904.

45. American Psychiatric Association. Practice guideline for the treatment of patients with eating disorders (revision). *Am J Psychiatry* 157:1(suppl):1–39.

Janet Treasure
Psychiatrist
Institute of Psychiatry Kings College London
London
UK

Ulrike Schmidt
Psychiatrist
South London and Maudsley NHS Trust
London
UK

Competing interests: None declared.

Search date May 2001

Philip Hazell

INTERVENTIONS

Key Messages

- One systematic review found no evidence of benefit from tricyclic antidepressants in prepubertal children and no clear benefit in adolescents. We found limited evidence on the use of fluoxetine and no evidence to support the use of other serotonin reuptake inhibitor drugs. We found limited evidence to support the use of the reversible monoamine oxidase inhibitor moclobemide, and no evidence to support the use of the non-reversible monoamine oxidase inhibitors, venlafaxine or lithium.

- We found insufficient evidence on the effects of St John's Wort *(Hypericum perforatum)* in children and adolescents with depression.

- We found insufficient evidence on the use of electroconvulsive therapy in children and adolescents with depression.

- One systematic review has found cognitive behavioural therapy to be superior to non-specific supportive therapies for mild to moderate depression in children and adolescents. Two RCTs of interpersonal therapy also suggested benefit compared with no treatment. We found insufficient evidence to conclude that family therapy or group treatments other than cognitive behavioural therapy are effective treatments for depression in children and adolescents. We found no systematic reviews or RCTs looking at long term outcomes for psychological or pharmacological treatments.

DEFINITION Compared with adult depression, depression in children and adolescents may have a more insidious onset, may be characterised more by irritability than sadness, and occurs more often in association with other conditions such as anxiety, conduct disorder, hyperkinesis, and learning problems.[1]

INCIDENCE/ PREVALENCE Estimates of prevalence of depression among children and adolescents in the community range from 2–6%.[2,3] Prevalence tends to increase with age, with a sharp rise around onset of puberty. Pre-adolescent boys and girls are affected equally by the condition, but depression is seen more frequently among adolescent girls than boys.[4]

AETIOLOGY/ RISK FACTORS Uncertain, but may include childhood events and current psychosocial adversity.

PROGNOSIS In children and adolescents, the recurrence rate of depressive episodes first occurring in childhood or adolescence is 70% by 5 years, which is similar to the recurrence rate in adults.[5] Young people experiencing a moderate to severe depressive episode may be more likely than adults to have a manic episode within the next few years.[4] Trials of treatment for child and adolescent depression have found high rates of spontaneous remission (as much as two thirds of people in some inpatient studies).

AIMS To improve mood, social and occupational functioning, and quality of life; to reduce morbidity and mortality; to prevent recurrence of depressive disorder; and to minimise adverse effects of treatment.

OUTCOMES In children and adolescents there are developmentally specific continuous measures such as the Children's Depression Rating Scale and the Children's Depression Inventory. Categorical outcomes are sometimes expressed as people no longer meeting specified criteria for depression on a structured psychiatric interview such as the Kiddie-SADS.

METHODS *Clinical Evidence search and appraisal May 2001.*

QUESTION What are the effects of treatments?

OPTION PRESCRIPTION ANTIDEPRESSANT DRUGS

Two systematic reviews found no evidence of benefit from tricyclic antidepressants in prepubertal children and no clear benefit in adolescents. We found limited evidence that fluoxetine may be of some benefit for child and adolescent depression. We found no evidence about other serotonin reuptake inhibitor drugs. We found little high quality evidence regarding moclobemide. We found no evidence on the effectiveness of non-reversible monoamine oxidase inhibitors. We found no evidence that venlafaxine or lithium are beneficial, although the power of the RCTs was too low to rule out a clinically important difference.

Benefits: **Tricyclic antidepressants:** We found two systematic reviews (search date 2000[6] and search date 1999[7], 9 RCTs, 357 children and adolescents) that overlapped in their inclusion of seven RCTs.

The first systematic review found no significant reduction in non-response with active drug versus placebo (273 people; OR 0.83, 95% CI 0.48 to 1.42).[6] The second review found similar results (330 people; OR 0.92, 95% CI 0.57 to 1.47).[7] Analyses for children (2 RCTs) and adolescents (5 RCTs) also found no significant benefit of treatment (children RR of failure to recover 0.9, 95% CI 0.7 to 1.2; adolescents RR of failure to recover 0.9, 95% CI 0.7 to 1.3), but found a significant difference using the weighted mean difference in adolescents (WMD in depression checklist scores −2.3, 95% CI −3.3 to −1.4) but not in children.[6] **Pulsed intravenous clomipramine:** See glossary, p 258. We found no systematic review. One small RCT (including 16 non-suicidal adolescent outpatients with major depression) found that significantly more people (7/8) responded to intravenous clomipramine 200 mg than to saline (3/8).[8] **Monoamine oxidase inhibitors:** We found no systematic review. In one small RCT, 20 adolescents treated with moclobemide showed greater improvement on one clinician rated scale than those treated with placebo, but not on other clinician rated and self-reported measures.[9] We found no RCTs of non-reversible monoamine oxidase inhibitors. **Selective serotonin reuptake inhibitors:** We found one systematic review (search date 1998, 2 RCTs, 126 children) addressing both adults and children.[10] The first RCT in the systematic review (40 adolescents, of whom 30 completed the trial) found no benefit on the Clinical Global Impressions scale. The second RCT (96 children and adolescents) found significantly more children and adolescents improved with fluoxetine (27/48) than with placebo (16/48) on the Clinical Global Impressions scale (RR of failure to recover 0.66, 95% CI 0.45 to 0.96), and there was greater mean improvement with active treatment on the self report Children's Depressive Rating Scale (34% v 18%; P < 0.01) but not on other measures. The systematic review did not pool results from the two RCTs. However, combination of the results for clinician global rating, using a fixed effects model, found an insignificant/borderline significant relative risk for non-improvement (0.7, 95% CI 0.49 to 1.00). **Selective noradrenergic reuptake inhibitors:** We found one systematic review (search date 1998, 1 RCT, 33 children).[10] The one small RCT compared a combination of venlafaxine and psychotherapy with a combination of placebo and psychotherapy. It found no significant difference with regard to improvement. **Lithium:** We found no systematic review. One small placebo controlled RCT compared lithium versus placebo in 30 depressed prepubertal children with a family history of bipolar affective disorder.[11] It found no significant difference of global assessment or of depression scores at follow up.

Harms: We found one unpublished systematic review (see comment below). We found single case reports and case series of toxicity and death from tricyclic antidepressants in overdose and therapeutic doses. Of the 17 children randomised to lithium treatment, four were withdrawn because of adverse effects (3 had confusion, 1 had nausea and vomiting).[11]

Comment: One systematic review awaiting publication found that tricyclic antidepressants were more commonly associated with vertigo

(OR 8.47, 95% CI 1.40 to 51.0), orthostatic hypotension (OR 4.77, 95% CI 1.11 to 20.5), and dry mouth (OR 5.19, 95% CI 1.15 to 23.5) than placebo.[6] It found no significant differences for other adverse effects (tiredness, sleep problems, headache, palpitations, tremor, perspiration, constipation, or problems with micturition). Further research is needed to determine long term effects of intravenous clomipramine.

OPTION ST JOHN'S WORT (*HYPERICUM PERFORATUM*)

We found no evidence on the effects of St John's Wort (*H perforatum*) in children and adolescents with depression.

Benefits: We found no systematic review and no RCTs in children or adolescents.

Harms: We found no evidence on adverse effects in children and adolescents.

Comment: None.

OPTION ELECTROCONVULSIVE THERAPY

We found insufficient evidence about the use of electroconvulsive therapy in children and adolescents with depression.

Benefits: We found no systematic reviews or RCTs.

Harms: We found no evidence on specific harms in children or adolescents.

Comment: None.

OPTION SPECIFIC PSYCHOLOGICAL TREATMENTS

One systematic review has found that cognitive behavioural therapy increases the rate of resolution of the symptoms of depression compared with non-specific supportive therapies for children and adolescents with mild to moderate depression. We found limited evidence from two small RCTs of interpersonal therapy versus clinical monitoring alone or placement on a waiting list. We found insufficient evidence that family therapy or group treatments other than cognitive behavioural therapy are effective treatments for depression in children and adolescents.

Benefits: **Cognitive behavioural therapy:** See glossary, p 258. We found one systematic review (search date 1997, 6 RCTs, 376 people) of cognitive behavioural therapy compared with "inactive" treatment that ranged from waiting list control to supportive psychotherapy.[12] Cognitive behavioural therapy was associated with increased rate of resolution of symptoms of depression (OR 3.2, 95% CI 1.9 to 5.2; NNT 4, 95% CI 3 to 5): a finding consistent with three non-systematic meta-analytic studies.[13–15] **Interpersonal therapy:** See glossary, p 258. We found no systematic review. We found two RCTs, which compared 12 weekly sessions of interpersonal therapy versus clinical monitoring or waiting list control in adolescents with depression. In the first RCT, 18 of 24 adolescents receiving interpersonal therapy recovered versus 11 of 24 adolescents receiving clinical monitoring alone (RR 1.64, 95% CI 1.00 to 2.68; ARR 0.29, 95% CI 0.03 to 0.56).[16] In the second RCT, 17 of 19 adolescents receiving interpersonal therapy recovered versus 12 of 18 adolescents on the waiting list (RR 1.33, 95% CI 0.94 to 1.93; ARR 0.22, 95% CI −0.03 to +0.49).[17] **Systemic behavioural family therapy:** See glossary, p 258. We found no systematic review. One RCT of family therapy versus non-specific supportive therapy did not find a significant difference in remission rates (29% v 34%).[18] **Group administered cognitive behavioural therapy:** We found no systematic review. One RCT group that administered cognitive behavioural therapy for adolescents with depression produced a significantly higher remission rate among those receiving treatment (67%) compared with those on a waiting list (48%).[19] **Group therapeutic support versus group social skills training:** We found no systematic review. One RCT (47 adolescents) comparing group therapeutic support versus group social skills training found no significant difference in remission rates (50% v 40%).[20]

Harms: We found no report of harms specifically for children and adolescents.

Comment: In the first RCT of interpersonal therapy, sessions were augmented by telephone contact.

QUESTION **Which treatments are most effective at improving long term outcome?**

We found no systematic reviews and no RCTs looking at long term outcomes.

Benefits: We found no systematic reviews and no RCTs. We found no RCTs comparing structured psychotherapy with pharmacotherapy in children and adolescents. We found no RCTs comparing combined pharmacotherapy and psychotherapy with either treatment alone. We found no RCTs comparing different psychotherapies.

Harms: See harms of prescription antidepressant drugs, p 255.

Comment: We found one prospective cohort study in which adolescents with depression, randomised to cognitive behavioural therapy, systemic behavioural family therapy (see glossary, p 258), or non-directive supportive therapy were assessed at 3 monthly intervals for the first 12 months and then once again at 24 months. The study found no significant difference between the groups. Of 106 adolescents, 38% experienced sustained recovery, 21% experienced persistent depression, and 41% had a relapsing course.[21]

Depression in children and adolescents

GLOSSARY

Cognitive behavioural therapy A brief (20 sessions over 12–16 wks) structured treatment aimed at changing the dysfunctional beliefs and negative automatic thoughts that characterise depressive disorders.[22] Cognitive behavioural therapy requires a high level of training in the therapist, and has been adapted for children and adolescents suffering depression. A course of treatment is characterised by 8–12 weekly sessions, in which the therapist and the child collaborate to solve current difficulties. The treatment is structured and often directed by a manual. Treatment generally includes cognitive elements, such as the challenging of negativistic thoughts, and behavioural elements, such as structuring time to engage in pleasurable activity.

Interpersonal therapy A standardised form of brief psychotherapy (usually 12–16 weekly sessions) intended primarily for outpatients with unipolar non-psychotic depressive disorders. It focuses on improving the individual's interpersonal functioning and identifying the problems associated with the onset of the depressive episode.[23] In children and adolescents, interpersonal therapy has been adapted for adolescents to address common adolescent developmental issues, for example separation from parents, exploration of authority in relationship to parents, development of dyadic interpersonal relationships, initial experience with the death of a relative or friend, and peer pressure.

Pulsed intravenous clomipramine An intravenous loading procedure for clomipramine.

Systemic behavioural family therapy A combination of two treatment approaches that have been used effectively for dysfunctional families. In the first phase of treatment, the therapist clarifies the concerns that brought the family into treatment, and provides a series of reframing statements designed to optimise engagement in therapy and identification of dysfunctional behaviour patterns (systemic therapy). In the second phase, the family members focus on communication and problem solving skills and the alteration of family interactional patterns (family behaviour therapy).

REFERENCES

1. Costello EJ, Angold A, Burns BJ, et al. The Great Smoky Mountains Study of Youth. Goals, design, methods, and the prevalence of DSM-III-R disorders. *Arch Gen Psychiatry* 1996;53: 1129–1136.

2. Costello EJ. Developments in child psychiatric epidemiology. *J Am Acad Child Adolesc Psychiatry* 1989;28:836–841.

3. Lewinsohn PM, Rohde P, Seely JR. Major depressive disorder in older adolescents: prevalence, risk factors, and clinical implications. *Clin Psychol Rev* 1998;18:765–794.

4. Birmaher B, Ryan ND, Williamson DE, Brent DA. Childhood and adolescent depression: a review of the past 10 years, Part I. *J Am Acad Child Adolesc Psychiatry* 1996;35:1427–1439.

5. Geller B, Fox LW, Fletcher M. Effect of tricyclic antidepressants on switching to mania and on the onset of bipolarity in depressed 6- to 12-year-olds. *J Am Acad Child Adolesc Psychiatry* 1993; 32:43–50.

6. Hazell P, O'Connell D, Heathcote D, Henry D. Tricyclic drugs for depression in children and adolescents. In: The Cochrane Library, Issue 2, 2001. Oxford: Update Software. Search date 2000; primary sources Medline, Excerpta Medica, and Cochrane trials database.

7. Maneeton N, Srisurapanont M. Tricyclic antidepressants for depressive disorders in children and adolescents: A meta-analysis of randomized-controlled trials. *J Med Assoc Thai*

2000;83:1367–1374. Search date October 1999; primary sources Medline, Controlled Clinical Trials Register, and hand searches of the reference lists of identified papers and a previous meta-analyisis.

8. Sallee FR, Vrindavanam NS, Deas-Nesmith D, Carson SW, Sethuraman G. Pulse intravenous clomipramine for depressed adolescents: double-blind, controlled trial. *Am J Psychiatry* 1997;154: 668–673.

9. Avci A, Diler RS, Kibar M, Sezgin F. Comparison of moclobemide and placebo in young adolescents with major depressive disorder. *Ann Med Sci* 1999;8:31–40.

10. Williams JW, Mulrow CD, Chiquette E, Noel PH, Aguilar C, Cornell J. A systematic review of newer pharmacotherapies for depression in adults: evidence report summary. *Ann Intern Med* 2000; 132:743–756. Search date 1998; primary sources Medline, Embase, Psychlit, Lilacs, Psyindex, Sigle, Cinahl, Biological Abstracts, Cochrane Controlled Trials, hand searches, and personal contacts.

11. Geller B, Cooper TB, Zimerman B, et al. Lithium for prepubertal depressed children with family history predictors of future bipolarity: a double-blind, placebo-controlled study. *J Affect Disord* 1998;51:165–175.

12. Harrington R, Whittaker J, Shoebridge P, Campbell F. Systematic review of efficacy of cognitive behavioural therapies in childhood and adolescent

depressive disorder. *BMJ* 1998;316:1559–1563. Search date 1997; primary sources Medline, Psychlit, Cochrane, and hand searches of reference lists, book chapters, conference proceedings, and relevant journals in the field.

13. Lewinsohn PM, Clarke GN. Psychosocial treatments for adolescent depression. *Clin Psychol Rev* 1999;19:329–342.

14. Reinecke MA, Ryan NE, DuBois DL. Cognitive-behavioral therapy of depression and depressive symptoms during adolescence: a review and meta-analysis. *J Am Acad Child Adolesc Psychiatry* 1998;37:26–34.

15. Mendez Carrillo FX, Moreno PJ, Sanchez-Meca J, Olivares J, Espada JP. Effectiveness of psychological treatment for child and adolescent depression: a qualitative review of two decades of research. *Psicol Conductual* 2000;8:487–510.

16. Mufson L, Weissman MM, Moreau D, Garfinkel R. Efficacy of interpersonal psychotherapy for depressed adolescents. *Arch Gen Psychiatry* 1999;56:573–579.

17. Rossello J, Bernal G. The efficacy of cognitive-behavioral and interpersonal treatments for depression in Puerto Rican adolescents. *J Consult Clin Psychol* 1999;67:734–745.

18. Brent DA, Holder D, Kolko D, et al. A clinical psychotherapy trial for adolescent depression comparing cognitive, family, and supportive therapy. *Arch Gen Psychiatry* 1997;54:877–885.

19. Clarke GN, Rohde P, Lewinsohn PM, Hops H, Seeley JR. Cognitive-behavioral treatment of adolescent depression: efficacy of acute group treatment and booster sessions. *J Am Acad Child Adolesc Psychiatry* 1999;38:272–279.

20. Fine S, Forth A, Gilbert M, Haley G. Group therapy for adolescent depressive disorder: a comparison of social skills and therapeutic support. *J Am Acad Child Adolesc Psychiatry* 1991;30:79–85.

21. Birmaher B, Brent DA, Kolko D, et al. Clinical outcome after short-term psychotherapy for adolescents with major depressive disorder. *Arch Gen Psychiatry* 2000;57:29–36.

22. Haaga DAF, Beck AT. Cognitive therapy. In: Paykel ES, ed. *Handbook of affective disorders.* Edinburgh: Churchill Livingstone, 1992;511–523.

23. Klerman GL, Weissman H. Interpersonal psychotherapy. In: Paykel ES, ed. *Handbook of affective disorders.* Edinburgh: Churchill Livingstone, 1992;501–510.

Philip Hazell
Conjoint Professor of Child and Adolescent Psychiatry/Director Child and Youth Mental Health Service
University of Newcastle
New South Wales
Australia

Competing interests: The author has been paid a fee by Pfizer, the manufacturer of sertraline, for speaking to general practitioners about the evidence for the treatment of depression in young people. The author's service has been in receipt of funding from Eli Lilly to participate in a relapse prevention trial of tomoxetine for attention deficit hyperactivity disorder.

Search date July 2001

Peter Struijs and Gino Kerkhoffs

Musculoskeletal disorders

QUESTIONS

INTERVENTIONS

Key Messages

- One systematic review and one subsequent RCT have found limited evidence that functional treatment is better than a minimal treatment regimen. One systematic review and one subsequent RCT have found no clear difference between functional treatment and immobilisation. We found insufficient evidence comparing different functional treatment strategies.

- One systematic review has found no good evidence that surgery is superior to immobilisation. We found conflicting evidence comparing surgery versus functional treatment.

- One systematic review has found no significant benefit from ultrasound versus sham treatment.

- One systematic review has found no evidence of beneficial effects from cold pack placement compared with no treatment or with heat or contrast baths.

- One systematic review has found conflicting evidence on diathermy compared with placebo.

- One systematic review has found significant improvement in pain scores after 10 days with homeopathic ointment versus placebo treatment.

DEFINITION	Ankle sprain is an injury of the lateral ligament complex of the ankle joint. Such injury can range from mild to severe and is graded according to the following scale on the basis of severity.[1-5] Grade I is a mild stretching of the ligament complex without joint instability. Grade II is a partial rupture of the ligament complex with mild instability of the joint (such as isolated rupture of the anterior talofibular ligament). Grade III involves complete rupture of the ligament complex with instability of the joint.
INCIDENCE/ PREVALENCE	Ankle sprain is a common problem in acute medical care occurring at a rate of about one injury/10 000 population a day.[6] Injuries of the lateral ligament complex of the ankle form a quarter of all sports injuries.[6]
AETIOLOGY/ RISK FACTORS	The usual mechanism of injury is inversion and adduction (usually referred to as supination) of the plantar-flexed foot. Predisposing factors are a history of ankle sprains and specific malalignment, like crus varum and pes cavo-varus.
PROGNOSIS	Some sports (e.g. basketball, soccer, and volleyball) have a particularly high incidence of ankle injuries. Pain is the most frequent residual problem, often localised on the medial side of the ankle.[4] Other residual complaints include mechanical instability, intermittent swelling, and stiffness. People with more extensive cartilage damage have a higher incidence of residual complaints.[4] Long term cartilage damage can lead to degenerative changes and this is especially true if there is persistent or recurrent instability; every sprain has the potential to add new damage.
AIMS	Reduction of swelling and pain, and the restoration of the stability of the ankle joint.
OUTCOMES	Return to pre-injury level of sports; return to pre-injury level of work; pain; swelling; subjective instability; objective instability; recurrent injury; ankle mobility; complications; patient satisfaction.
METHODS	*Clinical Evidence* search and appraisal July 2001.

QUESTION   What are the effects of treatment strategies for acute ankle ligament ruptures?

OPTION   IMMOBILISATION

One systematic review and one subsequent RCT have found no clear difference between immobilisation versus functional treatment. One systematic review has found no good evidence that surgery is superior to immobilisation. Two other systematic reviews and five additional RCTs have found no clear differences between these treatment strategies.

Benefits: We found three systematic reviews (search dates 1993,[7] 1994,[8] and 1998[9]) describing 16 RCTs and five additional RCTs.[10-14] The most recent review included RCTs with a range of follow up from 6 months to 3.8 years.[9] It did not report the time spans from injury to treatment in the trials. **Immobilisation versus functional treatment:** We found three systematic reviews describing 13 RCTs

Musculoskeletal disorders

(1782 people), and three additional RCTs comparing immobilisation (see glossary, p 266) with a cast versus an early mobilisation programme with the use of an external support (e.g. tape, elastic bandage, orthotic support) and/or with physiotherapy (coordination training).[7-10,12-14] The most recent review found significantly less persistent subjective instability with functional treatment (see glossary, p 266) (5 RCTs; RR 0.6, 95% CI 0.4 to 0.8; absolute risks not provided; time of measuring outcome not provided), but no significant difference in pain (5 RCTs; RR 0.8, 95% CI 0.5 to 1.2; absolute risks not provided).[9] It included a variety of different forms of functional treatment, including strapping, bracing, use of an orthosis, elastic wrapping, special shoes for at least 5 weeks, and short term (up to 3 weeks) cast immobilisation. The first additional RCT is being translated.[12] The second RCT followed only 78 of the 149 people, making the results uninterpretable.[13] The third RCT (105 people with severe ankle sprains diagnosed by stress radiographs) compared three treatment options:[14] Schantz wrap (see glossary, p 267) plus advice to use ice, avoid heat, and start range of motion and isometric exercises immediately versus a short leg cast for 5–6 weeks followed by replacement cast plus maximum dorsiflexion versus a cast with the foot set immediately to maximum dorsiflexion. It found a significant reduction of functional instability at 1 year with Schantz wrap and cast versus the short leg cast, but the difference was not significant at 5 or 7 years. Follow up for other outcomes was too low to interpret results. **Immobilisation versus surgery:** We found one systematic review (search date 1998, 9 RCTs, 694 people) that compared operative treatment followed by 6 weeks of cast treatment versus 6 weeks of cast treatment alone.[9] It found no significant differences for either pain (5 RCTs; RR 1.1, 95% CI 0.6 to 2.1; absolute risks not provided) or subjective instability (5 RCTs; RR 1.0, 95% CI 0.7 to 1.4; absolute risks not provided). One of the RCTs (150 people) found immobilisation to be less effective than surgery at long term follow up (minimum 2 years' follow up; RR 3.6, 95% CI 1.1 to 11.5).[11] For recurrent sprains, return to sports, and objective instability, no significant differences were identified.

Harms: One RCT of immobilisation versus surgery reported two cases of deep venous thrombosis after cast immobilisation (4%) compared with three cases in the surgery group (9%).[11] Other RCTs did not specifically address harms. Other known harms of immobilisation include pain and impairment in activities of daily living.[11]

Comment: The most recent systematic review provided outcomes expressed only as relative risks; this makes assessing the absolute effect and balancing benefits and harms difficult.[7] The different treatment modalities included as functional treatment in the review makes interpretation of its results difficult. The review did not make clear at what time after injury the interventions were given in the various trials. A systematic review of immobilisation for acute lateral ankle ligament injuries in adults is under preparation.[15]

OPTION	FUNCTIONAL TREATMENT

One systematic review and one subsequent RCT have found limited evidence of improved outcomes with functional treatment compared with minimal treatment. One systematic review and one RCT have found no clear difference between functional treatment and immobilisation. We found conflicting evidence comparing surgical versus functional treatment.

Benefits: We found three systematic reviews (search dates 1993,[7] 1994,[8] and 1998,[9] 27 RCTs and 11 additional RCTs[12-14,16-23]) comparing functional treatment (see glossary, p 266) as a treatment strategy. **Versus minimal treatment:** We found two systematic reviews and one subsequent RCT.[8,9,16] The most recent systematic review (search date 1998, 3 RCTs, 214 people) compared functional treatment versus a minimal treatment policy.[9] It found that functional treatment significantly reduced the risk of giving way (RR 0.34, 95% CI 0.17 to 0.71). Although pain scores were better with functional treatment the difference was not significant (RR 0.53, 95% CI 0.27 to 1.02). The subsequent RCT (30 people with subacute or chronic ankle sprain without gross mechanical instability) compared the mortise separation adjustment (see glossary, p 267) versus detuned ultrasound.[16] It found mobilisation significantly reduced pain, increased ankle range of motion, and improved ankle function (results presented graphically) at 1 month. **Versus immobilisation:** See immobilisation option, p 261. **Versus surgery:** We found three systematic reviews (search dates 1993,[7] 1994,[8] and 1998[9]) including 15 RCTs and one additional RCT.[20] The most recent systematic review (7 RCTs, 914 people) included only people with rupture of the lateral ankle ligament.[9] It did not specify the kinds of surgery included within the RCTs. It found that surgery significantly reduced long term subjective instability (7 RCTs; RR 0.2, 95% CI 0.2 to 0.3; absolute risks not provided), but had no significant effect on long term pain (6 RCTs; RR 0.5, 95% CI 0.2 to 1.5; absolute risks not provided). One RCT in the review (116 people) found that surgery increased the proportion of people with impaired range of movement (ROM) over the short term compared to those treated with a semi-rigid device (RR 60, 95% CI 3.8 to 946).[18] No significant differences were found in the other reviews or RCTs. **Versus functional treatment:** We found five RCTs comparing different functional treatment strategies.[18,19,21-23] One RCT (61 people without previous fractures in the ankle joint or clinically demonstrable ankle instability; mean follow up of 230 days) found a reduced risk of recurrent sprains after elastic bandage plus propriocepsis training versus elastic bandage only (RR 0.46, 95% CI 0.2 to 1.0).[21] Thirteen people withdrew from the trial and were not included in the analysis. The second RCT (73 people with time from injury to treatment of < 24 h) identified a faster return to work for the semi-rigid device group compared with treatment with an elastic bandage (up to 10 weeks' follow up; 9.1 v 5.3 days; mean difference 3.8 days, 95% CI 1.1 to 6.5).[19] Fifteen people did not complete 10 weeks' follow up and it was not reported if results were intention to treat. The third RCT (41 people within 72 h of injury and requiring assisted ambulation but without previous injury, presence of severe vascular disease, or use of anticoagulant or anti-inflammatory medications) compared anteroposterior mobilisation plus rest, ice, compression, and elevation versus rest, ice, compression, and elevation alone.[23] People treated with anteroposterior mobilisation required fewer treatment sessions, had greater improvement in range of motion (after 2 treatment sessions 10.5° with added mobilisation v 5.8°: P < 0.05), and greater increases in stride speed. Three people withdrew from the mobilisation group and analysis was not intention to treat. The remaining 2 RCTs found no significant differences. One RCT (116 people with all grades of ankle sprain) compared a semi-rigid device with tape (recurrent sprains were found in 4% v 0%).[18] The other RCT (119 people not requiring surgery treated within 24 h of injury) compared two types of tape treatment with follow up of 5–7 days (short term pain 8% v 5%; swelling 58% v 47%; limited range of movement [ROM] 36% v 47%).[22]

Harms: Allergic reactions and skin problems have been reported with tape;[24] however, none of the RCTs reported this.

Comment: The more recent systematic review of functional treatment versus surgery presented results only as relative risks, which does not allow assessment of the number of people who benefited. It also categorised short term cast use as a functional treatment. The older systematic reviews did not perform meta-analysis and included people with different severities of ankle sprain.

OPTION   SURGERY

We found no good evidence in favour of surgery compared with immobilisation. We found conflicting evidence comparing functional treatment (see glossary, p 266) versus surgery.

Benefits: We found three systematic reviews (search dates 1993,[7] 1994,[8] and 1998[9]) describing 19 RCTs and three additional RCTs.[13,20,25] **Versus immobilisation:** See immobilisation option, p 261. **Versus functional treatment:** See functional treatment option, p 263.

Harms: Neurological injuries, infections, bleeding, osteoarthritis, and death are known harms of surgery.[11,25,26] One RCT of immobilisation (see glossary, p 266) versus surgery reported two cases of deep venous thrombosis after cast immobilisation (4%) compared with three cases in the surgery group (9%).[11] Another RCT found dysaesthesia (see glossary, p 266) in 6% after surgery.[27]

Comment: The RCT is being translated.[27]

OPTION   ULTRASOUND

One systematic review and one subsequent RCT have found no benefits with ultrasound versus sham ultrasound. Three RCTs found no clear difference between ultrasound and other treatments.

Benefits: We found one systematic review (search date 1997, 5 RCTs)[28] and one subsequent RCT.[29] The quality of the included RCTs was described as "modest". The review did not report the details of the trial populations. All trials followed participants for less than 4 weeks. The largest RCT (72 people in the smallest group) compared ultrasound plus placebo gel versus ultrasound plus felbinac gel versus sham ultrasound plus felbinac gel over an average of 7 days. It found 84% of people were assessed as moderate or better with ultrasound plus placebo gel versus 86% with ultrasound plus felbinac gel versus 85% with sham ultrasound plus felbinac gel. The differences were not significant. The second RCT (74 people in the smallest group) compared ultrasound versus sham ultrasound. It found no significant difference in overall clinical score. The third low quality RCT (40 people in the smallest group) compared ultrasound versus immobilisation (see glossary, p 266) over 2 weeks' follow up. It found a significant improvement in the number of people recovered with ultrasound (86%) versus immobilisation (59%; ARR 27%, 95% CI 8% to 46%). The fourth, small, short term RCT (20 people in the smallest group) found no significant difference between ultrasound versus sham ultrasound after 10 days in the ability to walk 20 metres without a limp. The fifth, small, short term RCT (20 people in the smallest group) found a significant difference between ultrasound versus electrotherapy after 10 days in the ability to walk 20 metres without a limp (AR 100% v 80%; ARR 20%, 95% CI 3% to 38%). One subsequent RCT (58 people with injury < 100 h before trial entry) found no significant effect of ultrasound compared with sham ultrasound for either pain, swelling, or range of motion.[29] Four people with sham ultrasound and three with ultrasound did not complete the trial. They all reported full recovery and their results were not included.

Harms: Harms were not specifically addressed in the review. The subsequent RCT found none.[29]

Comment: None.

OPTION   **COLD PACK COMPRESSION**

One systematic review found no beneficial effects with cold pack compression compared with no treatment or with heat or contrast baths.

Benefits: We found one systematic review (search date 1994, 3 RCTs, 203 people).[8] Two of the RCTs compared cold pack compression with no treatment.[30,31] In both RCTs, no significant differences were found compared with sham treatment. The grade of the injuries was not reported in the RCTs. The largest RCT (143 people, 50% unable to bear weight) found that by day 7, 88% of people had improved by two, three, or four scale points on a five-point linear analogue scale with cold pack compression versus 79% with dummy therapy (P = 0.15).[30] The third RCT (30 people) compared cold with heat and with a contrast bath. It found less oedema with cold pack placement after 3–5 days (P < 0.05).[32]

Harms: None of the RCTs addressed harms from cold pack placement.

Comment: None.

Musculoskeletal disorders

Ankle sprain

| OPTION | DIATHERMY |

One systematic review found conflicting evidence on diathermy. One large and one smaller RCT found that diathermy significantly reduces swelling compared with placebo treatment. Three RCTs found no significant difference.

Benefits: We found one systematic review (search date 1994, 5 RCTs, 490 people).[8] The review included a range of severity of ankle sprains but excluded the most severe injuries (avulsion and osteochondral fractures). The largest high quality RCT (300 people with time from injury to treatment of 4 days or less) compared two forms of pulsating shortwave treatment versus placebo.[33] The trial found that walking ability improved significantly more quickly with high frequency electromagnetic pulsing than with placebo (P < 0.01). The difference was not significant with low frequency electromagnetic pulsing. However, reduction of swelling was significantly better for the low frequency group versus placebo but not for high frequency versus placebo (change in circumference of ankle with high frequency 4.5 mm v low frequency 5.0 mm v placebo 2.6 mm; P < 0.01 for low frequency v placebo). A second RCT (50 people) found significantly reduced oedema compared with placebo.[34] The other RCTs (73, 37, and 30 people) found no significant differences for pain, oedema, or range of motion compared with placebo.[35–37] The first of these presented results only as graphs.[35] From these RCTs the grades of injuries were not clear. No other outcome measures were reported and no results were pooled.

Harms: No evidence of any harm was reported.

Comment: None.

| OPTION | HOMEOPATHIC OINTMENT |

One systematic review has found significant improvement in pain scores with homeopathic ointment after 10 days.

Benefits: We found one systematic review (search date 1990,[38] 1 RCT,[39] 69 people). The high quality RCT (69 people) found that people treated with a homeopathic ointment had significantly better pain scores after 10 days compared with placebo. The review did not provide specific numeric results or describe the type of ointment.

Harms: Harms were not addressed in the review.

Comment: The RCT is awaiting translation.

GLOSSARY

Dysaesthesia Decreased sensitivity of the skin for stimuli.

Functional treatment Diverse functional treatments have been used. The main differences are the type of external device applied for treatment. The supports can be divided according to rigidity into elastic bandage; tape; lace-up ankle support; and semi-rigid ankle support. Propriocepsis training (to enhance joint stability) has also been used.

Immobilisation Limiting the mobility of a joint complex to zero degrees.

Mortise separation adjustment An adjustment technique involving special manual manipulation of the foot and ankle.[16]
Schantz wrap The ankle is wrapped in a cast, padding, and gauze.

REFERENCES

1. Bernett P, Schirmann A. Sportverletzungen des sprunggelenkes. *Unfallheilkunde* 1979;82: 155–160.

2. Lassiter TE, Malone TR, Garret WE. Injuries to the lateral ligaments of the ankle. *Orthop Clin North Am* 1989;20:629–640.

3. Marti RK. Bagatelletsels van de voet. 56–61. 1982. Capita selecta, Reuma Wereldwijd.

4. Van Dijk CN, Bossuyt PM, Marti RK. Medial ankle pain after lateral ligament rupture. *J Bone Joint Surg (Br)* 1996;78:562–567.

5. Watson-Jones R. Fractures and joint injuries. London: Churchill, Livingstone, 1976.

6. Katcherian DA. Treatment of Freiberg's disease. *Orthop Clin North Am* 1994;25:69–81.

7. Shrier I. Treatment of lateral collateral ligament sprains of the ankle: A critical appraisal of the literature. *Clin J Sport Med* 1995;5:187–195. Search date 1993; primary sources hand searches of bibliographies and reference lists.

8. Ogilvie-Harris DJ, Gilbert M. Treatment modalities for soft tissue injuries of the ankle: A critical review. *Clin J Sport Med* 1995;5:175–186. Search date 1994; primary sources Medline, and Excerpta Medica.

9. Pijnenburg AC, Van Dijk CN, Bossuyt PM, Marti RK. Treatment of ruptures of the lateral ankle ligaments: a meta-analysis. *J Bone Joint Surg (Am)* 2000;82:761–773. Search date 1998; primary sources Cochrane, Medline, Embase, hand searches of references from the published reviews, and personal contact with authors.

10. Cetti R, Christensen SE, Corfitzen MT. Ruptured fibular ankle ligament: plaster or Pliton brace? *Br J Sports Med* 1984;18:104–109.

11. Korkala O, Rusanen M, Jokipii P, Kytomaa J, Avikainen V. A prospective study of the treatment of severe tears of the lateral ligament of the ankle. *Int Orthop* 1987;11:13–17.

12. Lind T. Conservative treatment of rupture of the lateral ligament of the ankle. Prospective comparison of 2 conservative therapeutic methods. *Ugeskr Laeger* 1984;146:4017–4019.

13. Munk B, Holm-Christensen K, Lind T. Treatment of acute lateral ankle ligament ruptures. A prospective 9–13-year follow-up study of three different therapies in 79 patients. *Ugeskr Laeger* 1996;158:6912–6914.

14. Vitellas KM, Mueller CF, Blau NA, Verner JJ, Zuelzer WA. The role of stress radiographs for the severe ankle sprain: A 7-year prospective study. *Em Radiol* 1995;2:339–344.

15. Kerkhoffs GMMJ, Rowe BH, Assendelft WJJ, Kelly K, Struijs PAA, van Dijk CN. Immobilisation for acute lateral ankle ligament injuries in adults (Protocol for a Cochrane Review). In: The Cochrane Library, Issue 2, 2001. Oxford: Update Software.

16. Pellow JE, Brantingham JW. The efficacy of adjusting the ankle in the treatment of subacute and chronic grade I and Grade II ankle inversion sprains. *J Manipulative Physiol Ther* 2001;24: 17–24.

17. Dettori JR, Basmania CJ. Early ankle mobilization, Part II: A one-year follow-up of acute, lateral ankle sprains (a randomized clinical trial). *Mil Med* 1994;159:20–24.

18. Johannes EJ, Sukul DM, Spruit PJ, Putters JL. Controlled trial of a semi-rigid bandage ('Scotchrap') in patients with ankle ligament lesions. *Curr Med Res Opin* 1993;13:154–162.

19. Leanderson J, Wredmark T. Treatment of acute ankle sprain. Comparison of a semi-rigid ankle brace and compression bandage in 73 patients. *Acta Orthop Scand* 1995;66:529–531.

20. Otto M, Novak L, Fekecs G. Functional conservative versus operative treatment of outer ankle ligament ruptures. *J Bone Joint Surg (Br)* 1997;(suppl II):250.

21. Wester JU, Jespersen SM, Nielsen KD, Neumann L. Wobble board training after partial sprains of the lateral ligaments of the ankle: a prospective randomized study. *J Orthop Sports Phys Ther* 1996;23:332–336.

22. Viljakka T, Rokkanen P. The treatment of ankle sprain by bandaging and antiphlogistic drugs. *Ann Chir Gynaecol* 1983;72:66–70.

23. Green T, Refshauge K, Crosbie J, Adams R. A randomized controlled trial of a passive accessory joint mobilization on acute ankle inversion sprains. *Phys Ther* 2001;81:984–994.

24. Zeegers AVCM. Supination injury of the ankle joint. University of Utrecht, the Netherlands, Thesis, 1995.

25. Biegler M, Lang A, Ritter J. Comparative study on the effectiveness of early functional treatment using special shoes following surgery of ruptures of fibular ligaments (German). *Unfallchirurg* 1985; 88:113–117.

26. Sommer HM, Schreiber H. Early functional conservative therapy of fresh fibular capsular ligament rupture from the socioeconomic viewpoint. *Sportverletz Sportschaden* 1993;7: 40–46.

27. Zwipp H, Hoffmann R, Thermann H, Wippermann BW. Rupture of the ankle ligaments. *Int Orthop* 1991;15:245–249.

28. Van der Windt DA, Van der Heyden GJ, Van den Berg SG, et al. Ultrasound therapy for musculoskeletal disorders: a systematic review. *Pain* 1999;81:257–271. Search date July 1997; primary sources Medline, Embase, Cochrane Database of Randomised Controlled Trials, the database of the Cochrane Rehabilitation and Related Therapies Field, and hand searches of references of relevant retrieved publications.

29. Nyanzi CS, Langridge J, Heyworth JR, Mani R. Randomized controlled study of ultrasound therapy in the management of acute lateral ligament sprains of the ankle joint. *Clin Rehabil* 1999;13: 16–22.

30. Sloan JP, Hain R, Pownall R. Clinical benefits of early cold therapy in accident and emergency following ankle sprain. *Arch Emerg Med* 1989;6: 1–6.

31. Laba E, Roestenburg M. Clinical evaluation of ice therapy for acute ankle sprain injuries. *New Zeal J Physiother* 1989;17:7–9.

32. Cote DJ, Prentice WEJ, Hooker DN, Shields EW. Comparison of three treatment procedures for minimizing ankle sprain swelling. *Physical Ther* 1988;68:1072–1076.

33. Pasila M, Visuri T, Sundholm A. Pulsating shortwave diathermy: value in treatment of recent ankle and foot sprains. *Arch Phys Med Rehabil* 1978;59:383–386.

34. Pennington GM, Danley DL, Sumko MH, Bucknell A, Nelson JH. Pulsed, non-thermal, high-frequency

electromagnetic energy (DIAPULSE) in the treatment of grade I and grade II ankle sprains. *Mil Med* 1993;158:101–404.

35. Barker AT, Barlow PS, Porter J, Smith ME, Clifton S. A double-blind clinical trial of low power pulsed shortwave therapy in the treatment of a soft tissue injury. *Physiotherapy* 1985;71:500–504.

36. McGill SN. The effects of pulsed shortwave therapy on lateral ligament sprain of the ankle. *New Zeal J Physiother* 1988;16:21–24.

37. Michlovitz S, Smith W, Watkins M. Ice and high voltage pulsed stimulation in treatment of acute lateral ankle sprains. *J Orthop Sports Phys Ther* 1988;9:301–304.

38. Kleijnen J, Knipschild P, ter Riet G. Clinical trials of homeopathy. *BMJ* 1991;301:316–323. Search date 1990; primary sources Medline, and hand searches of reference lists, journals, libraries, and conference proceedings, and personal communication with manufacturers and researchers.

39. Zell R, Connert WD, Mau J, Feuerstake G. Treatment of acute sprains of the ankle joint. Double-blind study assessing the effectiveness of a homeopathic ointment preparation. *Fortschr Med* 1988;106:96–100.

Peter Struijs
MSc

Gino Kerkhoffs
MD

Academic Medical Center
Amsterdam
The Netherlands

Competing interests: None declared.

Search date October 2001

Stephen Worrall

QUESTIONS

Effects of prophylactic removal of impacted wisdom teeth 270

INTERVENTIONS

Likely to be ineffective or harmful
Extraction of asymptomatic
    impacted wisdom teeth 270

Key Messages

- We found limited evidence that the harms of removing asymptomatic impacted wisdom teeth outweigh the benefits.

Impacted wisdom teeth

DEFINITION	Wisdom teeth are third molars that develop in almost all adults by about the age of 20 years. In some people, the teeth become partially or completely impacted below the gumline because of lack of space, obstruction, or abnormal position. Impacted wisdom teeth may be diagnosed because of pain and swelling or incidentally by routine dental radiography.
INCIDENCE/ PREVALENCE	Third molar impaction is common. Over 72% of Swedish people aged 20–30 years have at least one impacted lower third molar.[1] The surgical removal of impacted third molars (symptomatic and asymptomatic) is the most common procedure performed by oral and maxillofacial surgeons. It is performed on about 4/1000 people per year in England and Wales, making it one of the top 10 inpatient and day case procedures.[2–4] Up to 90% of people on oral and maxillofacial surgery hospital waiting lists are awaiting removal of wisdom teeth.[3]
AETIOLOGY/ RISK FACTORS	Impacted wisdom teeth are partly a by-product of improved oral hygiene and changes in diet. Less gum disease and dental caries, and less wear and tear on teeth because of a more refined diet, have increased the likelihood of retaining teeth into adult life, leaving less room for wisdom teeth.
PROGNOSIS	Impacted wisdom teeth can cause pain, swelling, and infection, as well as destroying adjacent teeth and bone. The removal of diseased and symptomatic wisdom teeth alleviates pain and suffering and improves oral health and function. We found no good evidence on what happens without treatment in people with asymptomatic impacted wisdom teeth.
AIMS	To prevent harms and maximise benefits of wisdom teeth removal.
OUTCOMES	Pain; rates of infection; oral health and function.
METHODS	*Clinical Evidence* search and appraisal October 2001.

QUESTION Should asymptomatic and disease-free impacted wisdom teeth be removed prophylactically?

One systematic review of two RCTs, one of which is still in progress, comparing prophylactic extraction of wisdom teeth versus no extraction found no evidence of benefit with prophylactic extraction. Removal of lower wisdom teeth causes permanent numbness of the lower lip or tongue in about 1/200 people. One systematic review of mainly observational studies found that the use of a lingual nerve retractor significantly increased the incidence of temporary lingual nerve damage, but that permanent damage was rare.

Benefits: We found one systematic review evaluating people with unerupted or impacted third molars (search date 1999, 2 RCTs, 34 reviews).[5] It addressed both clinical preventative and cost effectiveness issues. The first RCT in the review (164 people) investigated the effects of early third molar extraction on late crowding of the lower incisors and randomised people to extraction or to no extraction of third molars.[6] It found no clinically significant difference between the groups. However, the RCT had a low follow up rate (77 people [47%] at an average of 66 months). The second RCT in the review is still in progress, but preliminary results also suggest that no extraction could be the better option in terms of benefits such as functional health status and harms. However, more participants and longer follow up times are needed to establish this preliminary conclusion.

Harms: Pain and swelling are almost universal after removal of impacted wisdom teeth.[7,8] The removal of the lower wisdom teeth carries the risk of damage to the inferior alveolar nerve (injured in 1–8% of people[9,10] with permanent damage in up to 1% of people[11]) and to the lingual nerve (permanently injured in up to 1% of people).[12] The risks appear to be greater with greater depth of impaction. The risks are the same whether the wisdom tooth is symptomatic or asymptomatic. One systematic review (search date 1999, 7 prospective case series, 1 RCT) evaluated the effects of three different surgical techniques on the lingual nerve: buccal approach with lingual nerve retraction (3040 procedures), buccal approach without lingual nerve retraction (1336 procedures), and the lingual split technique with lingual nerve retraction (2077 procedures).[13] It found that, compared to the buccal approach without retraction, temporary lingual nerve injury (lasting < 6 months) was significantly more common with the buccal approach with lingual retraction (RR 8.8, 95% CI 4.3 to 17.8) and the lingual split technique with retraction (RR 13.3, 95% CI 6.6 to 26.9). Permanent lingual nerve injury (lasting > 6 months) occurred in 0.2% of people after the buccal approach without retraction versus 0.6% with the buccal approach with retraction versus 0.1% with lingual split with retraction. The significance of any difference between groups was not calculated because of the low event rates.[13]

Comment: The two RCTs identified by the systematic review were of poor quality. Surgical morbidity is operator and technique sensitive; estimates of the incidence of nerve damage vary widely between reports.[14,15]

REFERENCES

1. Hugoson A, Kugelberg CF. The prevalence of third molars in a Swedish population. An epidemiological study. *Community Dent Health* 1988;5:121–138.

2. Mercier P, Precious D. Risks and benefits of removal of impacted third molars. *Int J Oral Maxillofac Surg* 1992;21:17–27.

3. Shepherd JP, Brickley M. Surgical removal of third molars. *BMJ* 1994;309:620–621.

4. Worrall SF, Riden K, Corrigan AM. UK National Third Molar project: the initial report. *Br J Oral Maxillofac Surg* 1998;36:14–18.

5. Song F, O'Meara S, Wilson P, Golder S, Kleijnen J. The effectiveness and cost-effectiveness of prophylactic removal of wisdom teeth. *Health Technol Assess* 2000;4:15. Search date 1999; primary sources Medline, Embase, Science Citation Index, Cochrane Controlled Trials Register, National Research Register, Database of Reviews of Effectiveness, hand searches of paper sources, web-based resources, and contact with relevant organisations and professional bodies.

6. Harradine N, Pearson M, Toth B. The effect of extraction of third molars on late lower incisor crowding: a randomised controlled trial. *Br J Orthodont* 1998;25:117–122.

7. Bramley P. Sense about wisdoms? *J R Soc Med* 1981;74:867–868.

8. Capuzzi P, Montebugnoli L, Vaccaro MA. Extraction of impacted third molars. *Oral Surg Oral Med Oral Pathol Oral Radiol Endod* 1994;77:341–343.

9. Schultze-Mosgau S, Reich RH. Assessment of inferior alveolar and lingual nerve disturbances after dentoalveolar surgery, and recovery of sensitivity. *Int J Oral Maxillofac Surg* 1993;22: 214–217.

10. Rood JP. Permanent damage to inferior alveolar nerves during the removal of impacted mandibular third molars: comparison of two methods of bone removal. *Br Dent J* 1992;172:108–110.

11. Blackburn CW, Bramley PA. Lingual nerve damage associated with removal of lower third molars. *Br Dent J* 1989;167:103–107.

12. Robinson PP, Smith KG. Lingual nerve damage during lower third molar removal: a comparison of two surgical methods. *Br Dent J* 1996;180: 456–461.

13. Pichler JW, Beirne OR. Lingual flap retraction and prevention of lingual nerve damage associated with third molar surgery: a systematic review of the literature. *Oral Surg Oral Med Oral Pathol Oral Radiol Endod* 2001;91:395–401. Search date 1999; primary sources Medline, Healthstar, Current Contents, Allied and Alternative Medicine, Life Sciences, Web of Science, Nursing Allied Health, Cochrane Library, and hand searching of

references retrieved and the indexes of the journal Oral and Maxillofacial Surgery Clinics of North America 1989–1998.

14. Sisk AL, Hammer WB, Shelton DW, Joy ED Jr. Complications following removal of impacted third molars: the role of the experience of the surgeon. *J Oral Maxillofac Surg* 1986;44:855–859.

15. Moss CE, Wake MJC. Lingual access for third molar surgery: a 20-year retrospective audit. *Br J Oral Maxillofac Surg* 1999;37:255–258.

Stephen Worrall
Consultant Oral and
Maxillofacial Surgeon
St Luke's Hospital
Bradford
UK

Competing interests: None declared.

Search date July 2001

Nick Buckley and Michael Eddleston

INTERVENTIONS

Key Messages

- We found no good evidence on the effectiveness of ipecacuanha, gastric lavage, or activated charcoal in paracetamol poisoning.

- One small RCT found that acetylcysteine reduced mortality in people with established paracetamol-induced liver failure. One observational study found that people given early treatment with acetylcysteine were less likely to develop liver damage than untreated historical controls.

- One small RCT found that the risk of hepatotoxicity was lower with methionine than with supportive care.

Paracetamol (acetaminophen) poisoning

DEFINITION Paracetamol poisoning occurs as a result of either accidental or intentional overdose with paracetamol (acetaminophen).

INCIDENCE/ PREVALENCE Paracetamol is the most common drug used for self poisoning in the UK.[1] It is also a common means of self poisoning in the rest of Europe, North America, and Australasia. An estimated 41 200 cases of poisoning with products containing paracetamol occurred in 1989–1990 in England and Wales, with a mortality of 0.40% (95% CI 0.38% to 0.46%). Overdoses owing to paracetamol alone result in an estimated 150–200 deaths and 15–20 liver transplants each year in England and Wales.

AETIOLOGY/ RISK FACTORS Most cases in the UK are impulsive acts of self harm in young people.[1,2] In one study of 80 people who had overdosed with paracetamol, 42 had obtained the tablets for the specific purpose of taking an overdose and 33 had obtained them less than 1 hour before the act.[2]

PROGNOSIS People with blood paracetamol concentrations above the standard treatment line (defined in the UK as a line joining 200 mg/L at 4 h and 30 mg/L at 15 h on a semilogarithmic plot) have a poor prognosis without treatment (see figure 1, p 279).[4,5] In one study of 57 untreated people with blood concentrations above this line, 33 developed severe liver damage and three died.[4] People with a history of chronic alcohol misuse, use of enzyme inducing drugs, eating disorders, or multiple paracetamol overdoses may be at risk of liver damage with blood concentrations below this line.[6] In the USA, a lower line is used as an indication for treatment but we found no data relating this line to prognostic outcomes.[7] **Dose effect:** The dose ingested also indicates the risk of hepatotoxicity. People ingesting less than 125 mg/kg had no significant hepatotoxicity with a sharp dose dependent rise for higher doses.[8] The threshold for toxicity after acute ingestion may be higher in children, where a single dose of less than 200 mg/kg has not been reported to lead to death and rarely causes hepatotoxicity.[9]

AIMS To prevent liver failure, liver transplantation, or death, with minimal adverse effects.

OUTCOMES Hepatotoxicity (most commonly defined by the objective criterion of blood aspartate aminotransferase > 1000 U/L), liver failure, liver transplantation, or mortality.

METHODS *Clinical Evidence* search and appraisal July 2001. We also contacted experts in the field to identify unpublished studies. We evaluated only interventions that are currently in common use (not, for example, mercaptamine [cysteamine], cimetidine, or dimercaprol).

OPTION **ACETYLCYSTEINE**

One small RCT found that acetylcysteine reduced mortality in people with established paracetamol-induced liver failure. One observational study found that people given early treatment with acetylcysteine were less likely to develop liver damage than untreated historical controls.

Benefits: We found no systematic review. We found one RCT (50 people with established paracetamol-induced liver failure) that compared intravenous acetylcysteine (150 mg/kg over 15 min, 50 mg/kg over 4 h, and then 100 mg/kg over 16 h, continued until death or recovery) versus a placebo infusion of 5% dextrose.[10] It found a borderline significant effect in survival favouring acetylcysteine over dextrose (12/25 [48%] with acetylcysteine v 5/25 [20%] with 5% dextrose; ARR 28%, 95% CI 3% to 53%; RR 2.4, 95% CI 1.0 to 5.8; NNT 4, 95% CI 2 to 16).

Harms: The RCT did not specifically assess adverse outcomes and none were noted.[10] Four case series suggested that the incidence of adverse effects from intravenous acetylcysteine is 5–15%.[11–14] These were predominantly rash, urticaria, and occasionally more serious anaphylactoid reactions occurring with the initial "loading" dose. In most or all cases, adverse effects responded to temporary stopping of infusions and symptomatic treatment, and did not recur when treatment recommenced. Two deaths have been reported due to a tenfold miscalculation of the dose, although only half of the loading dose was given in one case.[15] Adverse reactions seem to be more common in people with asthma and those who have non-toxic paracetamol concentrations.[13] Vomiting is common after oral acetylcysteine and occurred in 63% of people in one series despite previous administration of metoclopramide.[14] Oral acetylcysteine can also cause hypersensitivity and anaphylactoid reactions.[16]

Comment: In the RCT, allocation was concealed but treatment was not blinded.[10] There were differences between the groups in prognostic variables (prothrombin time, coma grade) and other treatments, but a possible confounding effect could not be adequately assessed because of the small size of the study. One observational study evaluated the effects of intravenous acetylcysteine in people presenting early to hospital.[4] It found that people treated within 10 hours of ingestion were less likely to develop liver damage than untreated historical controls (2% in treated group v 58% in controls; ARR 56%, 95% CI 47% to 58%; RRR 97%, 95% CI 81% to 100%; NNT 2, 95% CI 2 to 3). As a result, subsequent RCTs were considered unethical. A systematic review of numerous case series found evidence that acetylcysteine is beneficial in paracetamol poisoning.[11] For both oral and intravenous acetylcysteine, overall hepatotoxicity was worse if treatment was delayed beyond 8–10 hours (1% in those treated within 8 h v 46% in those treated after 16 h).[4,11] We found no RCTs of different regimens and no evidence of a difference between oral and intravenous routes of administration.[11] The optimal dose, route, and duration of treatment is unknown. Two recent observational studies comparing different protocols for intravenous[17] and oral[18] acetylcysteine did not find marked differences in outcomes.

| OPTION | METHIONINE |

One RCT was too small to detect a clinically important effect of methionine on mortality in people with blood paracetamol concentrations above the UK standard treatment line. The RCT found a lower risk of hepatotoxicity with methionine than supportive care.

Benefits: We found no systematic review. One RCT (40 people) compared oral methionine (2.5 g 4 hourly for 4 doses), intravenous mercaptamine (3.6 g over 20 h), and supportive care in people with blood paracetamol concentrations above the UK standard treatment line.[19] There was no significant effect on death (0 deaths in the methionine group v 1 in the supportive care group). Only 27 people had a liver biopsy. Fewer people suffered grade III hepatic necrosis (0/9 with methionine v 6/10 with supportive care), or had peak aspartate aminotransferase greater than 1000 U (1/13 [7%] with methionine v 8/13 [62%] with supportive care; ARR 54%, 95% CI 16% to 61%; RR 0.13, 95% CI 0.02 to 0.86; NNT 2, 95% CI 2 to 6).

Harms: No serious adverse effects associated with treatment were reported in the RCT, but vomiting after administration of methionine occurred in 8/13 people (62%). The incidence of adverse effects in the control group was not reported.[19]

Comment: Interpretation of liver biopsy results from the RCT was difficult as not all people were tested and an intention to treat analysis was not possible. We found one case series in people treated with methionine in early and late paracetamol poisoning, but there was no untreated group for comparison.[20]

| OPTION | IPECACUANHA |

We found no evidence of the effectiveness of ipecacuanha in paracetamol poisoning.

Benefits: We found no systematic review and no RCTs that reported clinical end points.

Harms: We found no large study of complications in people poisoned with paracetamol receiving ipecacuanha. Specific complications of ipecacuanha may include aspiration, diarrhoea, ileus, arrhythmia during vomiting, dystonia from treatment for vomiting, and haematemesis from vomiting.[21]

Comment: Human simulated overdose studies suggest that ipecacuanha given within 1 hour could reduce paracetamol absorption but no studies have shown a change in clinical outcome.[22] One non-systematic review of ipecacuanha in all forms of poisoning found no evidence that ipecacuanha improved outcome in poisoned people.[22] Administration of ipecacuanha may delay the administration of activated charcoal and oral antidotes.

We found no evidence of the effectiveness of activated charcoal, whether in single or multiple dose regimens, in paracetamol poisoning.

Benefits: We found no systematic review and no RCTs that reported clinical outcomes.

Harms: We found no large study of complications in paracetamol poisoned people receiving single doses of activated charcoal. We found no large, high quality RCT comparing activated charcoal with placebo in any form of poisoning that might have allowed calculation of the incidence of complications. Harms may include aspiration pneumonia, vomiting, diarrhoea, constipation, ileus, and interference with regular medications.

Comment: **Single dose regimens:** Studies of simulated overdose in human volunteers suggest that activated charcoal given within 2 hours of paracetamol ingestion decreases absorption by a variable amount and that this amount diminishes with time.[23,24] One cohort study in 450 consecutive people who had taken 10 g or more of paracetamol found that those who had been given activated charcoal were significantly less likely to have high risk blood paracetamol concentrations (OR 0.36, 95% CI 0.23 to 0.58).[3] The effect was seen only in those treated within 2 hours, and the study was not large enough to assess the effect of numerous potential confounders.[3] One non-systematic review of activated charcoal in all forms of poisoning found no evidence that activated charcoal improved outcome in poisoned people.[23] **Multiple dose regimens:** We found no studies of simulated overdose that evaluated multiple dose regimens in paracetamol poisoning. One non-systematic review of multiple dose regimens in all forms of poisoning found no evidence that multiple dose regimens improve outcomes in poisoned people.[25] The rapid absorption and short half life of paracetamol suggest a beneficial effect is unlikely.

We found no evidence of the effectiveness of gastric lavage in paracetamol poisoning.

Benefits: We found no systematic review and no RCTs that reported clinical outcomes.

Harms: We found no large study of complications in paracetamol poisoned people receiving gastric lavage. Harms may include aspiration of stomach contents, hypoxia, and oesophageal perforation.[21]

Comment: Studies of simulated overdose in human volunteers suggest that gastric lavage carried out within 1 hour removes a variable number of paracetamol tablets and that the number diminishes with time.[26] One cohort study (450 consecutive people who took at least 10 g or more of paracetamol) found that those given activated charcoal were significantly less likely to have high risk blood paracetamol concentrations (OR 0.36, 95% CI 0.23 to 0.58).[3] The addition of gastric lavage did not decrease the risk further (OR 1.12, 95%

CI 0.57 to 2.20). One non-systematic review of gastric lavage in all forms of poisoning found no evidence that gastric lavage improved outcome in poisoned people.[26]

REFERENCES

1. Gunnell D, Hawton K, Murray V, et al. Use of paracetamol for suicide and non-fatal poisoning in the UK and France: are restrictions on availability justified? *J Epidemiol Community Health* 1997; 51:175–179.

2. Hawton K, Ware C, Mistry H, et al. Paracetamol self-poisoning. Characteristics, prevention and harm reduction. *Br J Psychiatry* 1996;168:43–48.

3. Buckley NA, Whyte IM, O'Connell DL, Dawson AH. Activated charcoal reduces the need for N-acetylcysteine treatment after acetaminophen (paracetamol) overdose. *J Toxicol Clin Toxicol* 1999;37:753–757.

4. Prescott LF, Illingworth RN, Critchley JAJH, Stewart MJ, Adam RD, Proudfoot AT. Intravenous N-acetylcysteine: the treatment of choice for paracetamol poisoning. *BMJ* 1979;2:1097–1100.

5. Rumack BH, Matthew H. Acetaminophen poisoning and toxicity. *Pediatrics* 1975;55:871–876.

6. Vale JA, Proudfoot AT. Paracetamol (acetaminophen) poisoning. *Lancet* 1995;346: 547–552.

7. Smilkstein MJ, Knapp GL, Kulig KW, Rumack B. Efficacy of oral N-acetylcysteine in the treatment of acetaminophen overdose. Analysis of the National Multicentre Study (1976–1985). *N Engl J Med* 1988;319:1557–1562.

8. Prescott LF. Paracetamol overdosage. Pharmacological considerations and clinical management. *Drugs* 1983;25:290–314.

9. Caravati EM. Unintentional acetaminophen ingestion in children and the potential for hepatotoxicity. *J Toxicol Clin Toxicol* 2000;38: 291–296.

10. Keays R, Harrison PM, Wendon JA, et al. Intravenous acetylcysteine in paracetamol induced fulminant hepatic failure: a prospective controlled trial. *BMJ* 1991;303:1026–1029.

11. Buckley NA, Whyte IM, O'Connell DL, Dawson AH. Oral or intravenous N-acetylcysteine: which is the treatment of choice for acetaminophen (paracetamol) poisoning? *J Toxicol Clin Toxicol* 1999;37:759–767.

12. Chan TY, Critchley JA. Adverse reactions to intravenous N-acetylcysteine in Chinese patients with paracetamol (acetaminophen) poisoning. *Hum Exp Toxicol* 1994;13:542–544.

13. Schmidt LE, Dalhoff K. Risk factors in the development of adverse reactions to N-acetylcysteine in patients with paracetamol poisoning. *Br J Clin Pharmacol* 2001;51:87–91.

14. Wright RO, Anderson AC, Lesko SL, Woolf AD, Linakis JG, Lewander WJ. Effect of metoclopramide dose on preventing emesis after oral administration of N-acetylcysteine for acetaminophen overdose. *J Toxicol Clin Toxicol* 1999;37:35–42.

15. Mant TG, Tempowski JH, Volans GN, Talbot JC. Adverse reactions to acetylcysteine and effects of overdose. *BMJ* 1984;289:217–219.

16. Perry HE, Shannon MW. Efficacy of oral versus intravenous N-acetylcysteine in acetaminophen overdose: results of an open-label, clinical trial. *J Pediatr* 1998;132:149–152.

17. Dougherty T, Greene T, Roberts JR. Acetaminophen overdose: comparison between continuous and intermittent intravenous N-acetylcysteine 48-hour protocols. *Ann Emerg Med* 2000;36:S83.

18. Woo OF, Mueller PD, Olson KR, Anderson IB, Kim SY. Shorter duration of oral N-acetylcysteine therapy for acute acetaminophen overdose. *Ann Emerg Med* 2000;35:363–368.

19. Hamlyn AN, Lesna M, Record CO, et al. Methionine and cysteamine in paracetamol (acetaminophen) overdose, prospective controlled trial of early therapy. *J Int Med Res* 1981;9: 226–231.

20. Vale JA, Meredith TJ, Goulding R. Treatment of acetaminophen poisoning. The use of oral methionine. *Arch Intern Med* 1981;141: 394–396.

21. Pond SM, Lewis-Driver DJ, Williams GM, Green AC, Stevenson NW. Gastric emptying in acute overdose: a prospective randomised controlled trial. *Med J Aust* 1995;163:345–349.

22. Krenzelok EP, McGuigan M, Lheur P. Position statement: ipecac syrup. American Academy of Clinical Toxicology and European Association of Poisons Centres and Clinical Toxicologists. *J Toxicol Clin Toxicol* 1997;35:699–709.

23. Chyka PA, Seger D. Position statement: single-dose activated charcoal. American Academy of Clinical Toxicology; European Association of Poisons Centres and Clinical Toxicologists. *J Toxicol Clin Toxicol* 1997;35:721–741.

24. Rose SR, Gorman RL, Oderda GM, Klein-Schwartz W, Watson WA. Simulated acetaminophen overdose: pharmacokinetics and effectiveness of activated charcoal. *Ann Emerg Med* 1991;20: 1064–1068.

25. American Academy of Clinical Toxicology, European Association of Poison Centres and Clinical Toxicologists. Position statement and practice guidelines on the use of multi-dose activated charcoal in the treatment of acute poisoning. *J Toxicol Clin Toxicol* 1999;37:731–751.

26. Vale JA. Position statement: gastric lavage. American Academy of Clinical Toxicology and European Association of Poisons Centres and Clinical Toxicologists. *J Toxicol Clin Toxicol* 1997; 35:711–719.

Nick Buckley
Consultant Clinical Pharmacologist
and Toxicologist
Canberra Hospital
Canberra
Australia

Michael Eddleston
Wellcome Trust Career Development
Fellow
Centre for Tropical Medicine
University of Oxford
Oxford
UK

Competing interests: None declared.

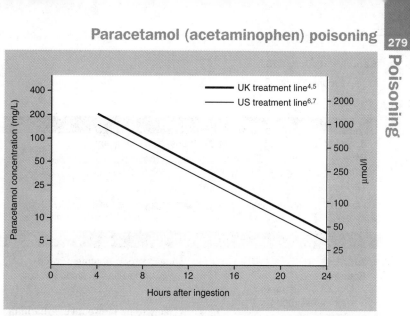

FIGURE 1 Nomograms used to determine acetylcysteine or methionine treatment, based on the blood concentrations between 4 and 24 hours after ingestion of paracetamol. Published with permission (see text, p 274).[3]

Bacterial vaginosis

Search date July 2001

M Joesoef and George Schmid

Key Messages

- Bacterial vaginosis can resolve spontaneously.

In non-pregnant women

- One systematic review found no significant difference in cure rates between oral and intravaginal antianaerobic drugs. Another systematic review has found that a 7 day course of twice daily oral metronidazole is more effective than a single 2 g dose. Limited evidence from RCTs found no significant difference in cure rates between oral clindamycin and oral metronidazole, and no difference between once and twice daily dosing with intravaginal metronidazole gel. One RCT found no difference between 3 day treatment with intravaginal ovules versus 7 day treatment with intravaginal clindamycin cream.

In pregnant women

- Limited evidence from a subgroup analysis in a systematic review found that in pregnant women who had a previous preterm birth, oral antianaerobic treatment (except clindamycin) for bacterial vaginosis reduced the risk of premature delivery. The systematic review and subsequent RCTs found no benefit from antianaerobic treatment for bacterial vaginosis in pregnant women without previous preterm delivery.

- Two RCTs found a higher risk of preterm delivery before 34 weeks in women without bacterial vaginosis who received intravaginal clindamycin cream or oral metronidazole and erythromycin.

- Four RCTs found a higher risk of preterm delivery and low birth weight in women with bacterial vaginosis who received intravaginal clindamycin cream. In all RCTs the increase was not statistically significant.

Preventing recurrence

- One systematic review has found that, in women with one steady male sexual partner, treating the partner with an oral antianaerobic agent does not reduce the woman's risk of recurrence.

Before procedures

- Two RCTs found that antianaerobic treatment for bacterial vaginosis in women about to undergo surgical abortion reduced the risk of pelvic inflammatory disease.

- We found no evidence on the effects of treatment of women with bacterial vaginosis about to undergo other gynaecological procedures, including abdominal hysterectomy, caesarean section, or insertion of an intrauterine contraceptive device.

DEFINITION Bacterial vaginosis is a microbial disease characterised by an alteration in the bacterial flora of the vagina from a predominance of *Lactobacillus* species to high concentrations of anaerobic bacteria. Diagnosis requires three out of four features: the presence of clue cells; a homogenous discharge adherent to the vaginal walls; pH of vaginal fluid > 4.5; and a "fishy" amine odour of the vaginal discharge before or after addition of 10% potassium hydroxide. The condition is asymptomatic in 50% of infected women. Women with symptoms have an excessive white to grey, or malodorous vaginal discharge, or both; the odour may be particularly noticeable during sexual intercourse.

INCIDENCE/ Bacterial vaginosis is the most common infectious cause of vagin-
PREVALENCE itis, being about twice as common as candidiasis.[1] Prevalences of 10–61% have been reported among unselected women from a range of settings.[2] Data on incidence are limited but one study found that, over a 2 year period, 50% of women using an intra-uterine contraceptive device had at least one episode, as did 20% of women using oral contraceptives.[3] Bacterial vaginosis is particularly prevalent in lesbians.[4]

AETIOLOGY/ The cause is not understood fully. Risk factors include new or
RISK FACTORS multiple sexual partners[1,3,5] and early age of sexual debut,[6] but no causative microorganism has been shown to be transmitted between partners. Use of an intrauterine contraceptive device[3] and douching[5] have also been reported as risk factors. Infection seems to be most common around the time of menstruation.[7]

PROGNOSIS The course of bacterial vaginosis varies and is poorly understood. Without treatment, symptoms may persist or resolve in both pregnant and non-pregnant women. Recurrence after treatment occurs in about a third of women. The condition is associated with complications of pregnancy: low birth weight; preterm birth (pooled OR from 10 cohort studies: 1.8, 95% CI 1.5 to 2.6);[8] preterm labour; premature rupture of membranes; late miscarriage; chorioamnionitis (48% v 22%, OR 2.6, 95% CI 1.0 to 6.6);[9] endometritis after normal delivery (8.2% v 1.5%, OR 5.6, 95% CI 1.8 to 17.2);[10] endometritis after caesarean section (55% v 17%, OR 5.8, 95% CI 3.0 to 10.9);[11] and surgery to the genital tract. Women who have had a previous premature delivery are especially at risk of complications in pregnancy, with a sevenfold increased risk of preterm birth (AR 24/428 [6%] in all women v 10/24 [42%] in women with a previous preterm birth).[12] Bacterial vaginosis can also enhance HIV acquisition and transmission.[13]

| AIMS | To alleviate symptoms and to prevent complications relating to childbirth, termination of pregnancy, and gynaecological surgery, with minimal adverse effects; to reduce adverse neonatal outcomes. |

| OUTCOMES | Preterm delivery; puerperal and neonatal morbidity and mortality; clinical or microbiological cure rates, usually at 1–2 weeks or 4 weeks after completing treatment. |

| METHODS | *Clinical Evidence* search and appraisal July 2001. In addition the authors searched Medline (keywords: bacterial vaginosis, non-specific vaginosis, clindamycin, metronidazole) from 1988 to September 1998, and also used information from drug manufacturers. |

QUESTION **What are the effects of different antianaerobic regimens in non-pregnant women with symptomatic bacterial vaginosis?**

One systematic review found no significant difference in cure rates between oral and intravaginal antianaerobic drugs. Another systematic review has found that a 7 day course of twice daily oral metronidazole is more effective than a single 2 g dose. Limited evidence from RCTs found no significant difference in cure rates between oral clindamycin and oral metronidazole, and no difference between once and twice daily dosing with intravaginal metronidazole gel. One RCT found no difference between 3 day treatment with intravaginal ovules versus 7 day treatment with intravaginal clindamycin cream.

Benefits: **Oral versus intravaginal antianaerobic treatment:** We found one systematic review (search date 1996, 5 RCTs) comparing oral and intravaginal formulations of metronidazole and clindamycin,[14] and one subsequent RCT.[15] Three RCTs were in symptomatic non-pregnant women and two were in symptomatic and asymptomatic non-pregnant women. There was no significant difference in cumulative cure rates 5–10 days after completing treatment (86% for oral metronidazole 500 mg twice daily for 7 days v 85% for clindamycin vaginal cream 5 g at bedtime for 7 days v 81% for metronidazole vaginal gel 5 g twice daily for 5 days). Four weeks after completing treatment, the cumulative cure rates were 78% for oral metronidazole versus 82% for clindamycin vaginal cream versus 71% for metronidazole vaginal gel. The subsequent RCT (233 women) of clindamycin vaginal cream versus oral metronidazole also found no significant difference in cure rates between clindamycin cream and oral metronidazole (68% v 67%).[15] **Different oral antianaerobic regimens:** We found one systematic review (search date 1996, 4 RCTs) comparing metronidazole 500 mg twice daily for 7 days versus a single 2 g dose of metronidazole.[14] It found significantly higher cumulative cure rates at 3–4 weeks after completing treatment with 7 day metronidazole (82% with 7 days of metronidazole v 62% with single dose metronidazole; P < 0.05). We found two additional RCTs comparing oral metronidazole 500 mg twice daily for 7 days versus oral clindamycin 300 mg twice daily for 7 days.[16] The first RCT (143 symptomatic non-pregnant women) found no significant difference in cure rates within 7–10 days of starting treatment (women cured: AR 46/49 [94%] with clindamycin v 48/50 [96%] with metronidazole; RR 0.98, 95% CI 0.89 to 1.07). A quarter of women were lost to follow up. The second RCT (96 non-pregnant women) found no significant difference in cure rates (AR 39/41 [95%] with clindamycin v 41/44 [93%] with metronidazole; ARI 2%; RR 1.0, 95% CI 0.92 to 1.14).[17] **Different intravaginal antianaerobic regimens:** We found two RCTs.[18,19] The first RCT (514 women) found no significant difference in effectiveness between once daily versus twice daily dosing of intravaginal metronidazole gel (AR 118/207 [57%] with once daily gel v 129/209 [62%] with twice daily gel; RR 0.92, 95% CI 0.79 to 1.08).[18] The second RCT (662 women) compared 3 day treatment with intravaginal clindamycin ovules versus 7 day treatment with intravaginal clindamycin cream. It found no significant difference in cure rates at 35 day assessment (AR 134/238 [56%] with 3 day regimen v 113/224 [50%] with 7 day regimen; ARI 5.9; RR 1.1, 95% CI 0.94 to 1.3).[19] **Recurrence:** One RCT (139 women) found that recurrence occurred in 30% of women after 12 weeks' treatment with clindamycin vaginal cream whose partner received placebo versus 32% of women whose partner received clindamycin capsules.[20] In another RCT (61 people, 19 withdrew), more than 50% of women taking clindamycin vaginal cream versus oral metronidazole had recurrent bacterial vaginosis 2 months after treatment.[21] We found no good studies of maintenance regimens for recurrent bacterial vaginosis.

Harms: The review of different oral antianaerobic regimens found that adverse effects occurred in a quarter to two thirds of women taking oral metronidazole, including mild to moderate nausea/dyspepsia, unpleasant metallic taste, headache, and dizziness.[14] Infrequent adverse effects from oral clindamycin included heartburn, nausea, vomiting, diarrhoea, constipation, headache, dizziness, and vertigo; the trials gave no data on frequency. Intravaginal clindamycin has been associated, rarely, with mild to severe colitis[22] and vaginal candidiasis. The RCT of once versus twice daily intravaginal metronidazole gel found no significant difference in frequency of adverse effects.[18] Yeast vulvovaginitis can be less common with intravaginal than with oral metronidazole (4% for intravaginal[23] v 8–22% for oral[24]).

Comment: Intravaginal administration reduces systemic absorption and systemic adverse effects. Some women may prefer oral medication because it is more convenient.

QUESTION **What are the effects of treatments in pregnant women with bacterial vaginosis?**

One systematic review of antianaerobic treatment of bacterial vaginosis during pregnancy has found that antibiotics versus placebo are associated with a lower incidence of preterm delivery, but the difference is not significant. Subgroup analysis in women with bacterial vaginosis who had a previous preterm delivery found that oral antianaerobic treatment significantly reduced the risk of preterm delivery. Subsequent RCTs found no significant difference between antianaerobic treatment versus placebo in the rate of preterm birth in women with bacterial vaginosis. Four RCTs found an increase in preterm birth and low birth weight in women with bacterial vaginosis treated with clindamycin cream.

Benefits: We found one systematic review (search date 1998, 5 RCTs, 1508 women)[25] and three subsequent RCTs comparing one or more antibiotic regimens versus placebo.[26–28] The review found that women taking antibiotics versus placebo had lower risk of preterm delivery, but the result did not quite reach significance (144/985 [14.6%] with antibiotics v 136/891 [15%] with placebo; RR 0.83, 95% CI 0.67 to 1.02). However, in the subgroup of women who had a previous preterm birth, the risk of preterm delivery was significantly less (57/187 [30%] with antibiotics v 58/116 [50%] with placebo; RR 0.55, 95% CI 0.41 to 0.74; NNT 4, 95% CI 3 to 8).[25] The first subsequent large RCT (1953 pregnant women with asymptomatic bacterial vaginosis) compared oral metronidazole versus placebo and found no significant difference in the risk of preterm birth (116/953 [12%] with metronidazole v 121/966 [12.5%] with placebo; RR 0.97, 95% CI 0.76 to 1.23).[26] In the subgroup of women who had a previous preterm birth, there was no significant difference in preterm birth (30/101 [30%] with metronidazole v 26/109 [24%] with placebo; RR 1.24, 95% CI 0.78 to 1.84).[26] The second RCT (129 evaluable pregnant women with bacterial vaginosis) comparing intravaginal clindamycin cream (5 g at bedtime for 7 days) versus placebo found no significant difference in preterm birth (9/60 [15%] with clindamycin v 5/69 [7%] with placebo; RR 2.1, 95% CI 0.7 to 5.0), or in low birth weight babies (8/59 [14%] with clindamycin v 3/69 [4%] with placebo; RR 3.1, 95% CI 0.9 to 11.2).[27] A small subgroup analysis of a third RCT (168 women) comparing clindamycin cream versus placebo found no significant difference in rates of preterm birth (before 34 weeks' gestation) in women with bacterial vaginosis (1/11 [9%] with clindamycin cream v 1/11 [9%] with placebo) and in women without bacterial vaginosis (9/72 [13%] with clindamycin cream v 3/74 [4%] with placebo; RR 3.1, 95% CI 0.9 to 10.9).[28]

Harms: The review found adverse effects occurred in 4% of women receiving antibiotics for bacterial vaginosis.[25] **In women without bacterial vaginosis:** Two RCTs of antibiotic administration[28,29] found an increase in preterm birth (before 34 weeks' gestation) in a subgroup of women without bacterial vaginosis who received intravaginal clindamycin cream[28] or oral metronidazole and erythromycin.[29] For the first RCT, differences between groups did not reach statistical significance (AR 9/72 [12.5%] with clindamycin v 3/74 [4%] with placebo; recalculation by *Clinical Evidence*: ARI 8.4%;

RR 3.1, 95% CI 0.9 to 10.9).[28] A subgroup analysis of the second RCT found no significant difference for preterm birth before 37 weeks' gestation (AR 56/254 [22%] with metronidazole and erythromycin v 26/104 [25%] with placebo; RR 0.88, 95% CI 0.57 to 1.3), but found a significant difference for preterm birth before 34 weeks' gestation (AR 34/254 [13%] with metronidazole and erythromycin v 5/104 [5%] with placebo; RR 2.8, 95% CI 1.2 to 6.0; NNH 12, 95% CI 4 to 136).[29] **In women with bacterial vaginosis:** Four RCTs[27,30-32] found an increase in preterm birth and low birth weight of women with bacterial vaginosis who received intravaginal clindamycin cream. In all RCTs, the increase was not significant. In the second trial, the rate of preterm birth (< 32 weeks' gestation) was higher with clindamycin cream than with placebo (AR 16/340 [5%] with clindamycin v 9/341 [3%] with placebo; ARI 2.1%, 95% CI –0.8% to 5.1%; RR 1.78, 95% CI 0.80 to 3.98). The rate of low birth weight was higher with clindamycin (AR 30/334 [9%] with clindamycin cream v 23/338 [7%] with placebo; RR 1.32, 95% CI 0.78 to 2.22).[30] In the third RCT the rate of preterm birth (< 37 weeks' gestation) was higher with clindamycin cream than placebo (AR 7/51 [14%] with clindamycin cream v 3/50 with placebo; RR 2.3, 95% CI 0.6 to 8.4).[31] In the fourth RCT the rate of preterm birth (< 37 weeks' gestation) was slightly higher with clindamycin cream than placebo (AR 9/187 [5%] with clindamycin cream v 7/188 [4%] with placebo; RR 1.29, 95% CI 0.49 to 3.40).[32] One large RCT (1953 women) found significantly more adverse effects with metronidazole versus placebo, particularly gastrointestinal symptoms (20% with metronidazole v 7.5% with placebo; CI not provided).[26]

Comment: The average quality of the trials in the systematic review was good. All trials reported loss to follow up between 1% and 17% for the various treatment groups.[25] Results from the two subsequent RCTs conflict with those of the systematic review.[26,27] The subgroup analysis for the third trial had a small sample size.[28]

QUESTION   **Does treating male partners prevent recurrence?**

One systematic review has found that, in women with one steady male sexual partner, treating the partner with an oral antianaerobic agent does not reduce the woman's risk of recurrence.

Benefits: We found one systematic review (search date not stated, 5 RCTs) with a variety of treatment regimens and populations.[33] It found that treatment of a sexual partner with metronidazole or clindamycin had no significant effect on recurrence rates.

Harms: No harmful effects were reported.

Comment: The lack of evidence of effectiveness of both metronidazole and clindamycin suggests that anaerobes are unlikely to be the sole pathogenic agents linking bacterial vaginosis with sexual intercourse.

Bacterial vaginosis

QUESTION   What are the effects of treatment before gynaecological procedures?

In women with bacterial vaginosis who are about to undergo surgical abortion, three RCTs found that oral or intravaginal antianaerobic treatment reduced the risk of pelvic inflammatory disease. We found no RCTs on the effects of treatment before other gynaecological procedures, including abdominal hysterectomy, caesarean section, or insertion of an intrauterine contraceptive device.

Benefits: We found no systematic review. **Before surgical abortion:** We found three RCTs. The first RCT (174 women with bacterial vaginosis) compared oral metronidazole 500 mg three times daily for 10 days versus placebo in women about to undergo surgical abortion.[34] Fewer women taking metronidazole developed pelvic inflammatory disease than those taking placebo, although the result did not quite reach significance (AR 3/84 [4%] with metronidazole v 11/90 [12%] with placebo; RR 0.29, 95% CI 0.08 to 1.01; NNT 12, 95% CI 6 to 279). The second RCT (1655 women) compared intravaginal clindamycin cream versus placebo in women about to undergo surgical abortion. It found that clindamycin significantly reduced the risk of post-abortion infection (recalculation by *Clinical Evidence*: post-abortion infection AR 3/181 [2%] with clindamycin cream v 12/181 [7%] with placebo; RR 0.25, 95% CI 0.07 to 0.87; NNT 20, 95% CI 10 to 125).[35] The third RCT compared a single dose metronidazole suppository 2 mg versus placebo.[36] It found that metronidazole suppository was associated with a lower risk of postoperative upper genital tract infection (AR 12/142 [8%] with metronidazole v 21/131 [16%] with placebo; RR 0.53, 95% CI 0.27 to 1.03). **Before gynaecological surgery:** Bacterial vaginosis is associated with an increased risk of endometritis after caesarean section and vaginal cuff cellulitis after abdominal hysterectomy,[11,37] but we found no RCTs of antianaerobic treatment in women before such surgery. **Before insertion of an intrauterine contraceptive device:** Bacterial vaginosis has been associated with pelvic inflammatory disease (see pelvic inflammatory disease, p 324) in women using intrauterine contraceptive devices,[3] but we found no RCTs of antianaerobic treatment in women with bacterial vaginosis before insertion of these devices.

Harms: The RCTs provided no information on adverse effects.[34]

Comment: None.

REFERENCES

1. Barbone F, Austin H, Louv WC, Alexander WJ. A follow-up study of methods of contraception, sexual activity, and rates of trichomoniasis, candidiasis, and bacterial vaginosis. Am J Obstet Gynecol 1990;163:510–514.

2. Mead PB. Epidemiology of bacterial vaginosis. Am J Obstet Gynecol 1993;169:446–449.

3. Avonts D, Sercu M, Heyerick P, et al. Incidence of uncomplicated genital infections in women using oral contraception or an intrauterine device: a prospective study. Sex Transm Dis 1990;17:23–29.

4. Berger BJ, Kolton S, Zenilman JM, et al. Bacterial vaginosis in lesbians: a sexually transmitted disease. Clin Infect Dis 1995;21:1402–1405.

5. Hawes SE, Hillier SL, Benedetti J, et al. Hydrogen peroxide-producing lactobacilli and acquisition of vaginal infections. J Infect Dis 1996;174:1058–1063.

6. Hillier SL, Nugent RP, Eschenbach DA, et al. Association between bacterial vaginosis and preterm delivery of a low-birth-weight infant. N Engl J Med 1995;333:1737–1742.

7. Schwebke JR, Morgan SC, Weiss HL. The use of sequential self-obtained vaginal smears for detecting changes in the vaginal flora. Sex Transm Dis 1997;24:236–239.

8. Flynn CA, Helwig AL, Meurer LN. Bacterial vaginosis in pregnancy and the risk of prematurity: a meta-analysis. J Fam Pract 1999;48:885–892.

9. Hillier SL, Martius J, Krohn MA, et al. Case-control study of chorioamnionic infection and

chorioamnionitis in prematurity. *N Engl J Med* 1988;319:972–975.

10. Newton ER, Prihoda TJ, Gibbs RS. A clinical and microbiologic analysis of risk factors for puerperal endometritis. *Obstet Gynecol* 1990;75:403–406.

11. Watts D, Krohn M, Hillier S, Eschenbach DA. Bacterial vaginosis as a risk factor for postcesarean endometritis. *Obstet Gynecol* 1990; 75:52–58.

12. McDonald HM, O'Loughlin JA, Vigneswaran R, et al. Impact of metronidazole therapy on preterm birth in women with bacterial vaginosis flora (*Gardnerella vaginalis*): a randomised, placebo controlled trial. *Br J Obstet Gynaecol* 1997;104:1391–1397.

13. Schmid G, Markowitz L, Joesoef R, Koumans E. Bacterial vaginosis and HIV infection [editorial]. *Sex Transm Infect* 2000;76:3–4.

14. Joesoef MR, Schmid GP. Bacterial vaginosis: review of treatment options and potential clinical indications for therapy. *Clin Infect Dis* 1999; 28(suppl 1):72–79. Search date 1996; primary sources Medline, hand searches of text books about sexually transmitted diseases, meeting abstracts, and contact with drug manufacturers.

15. Paavonen J, Mangioni C, Martin MA, Wajszczuk CP. Vaginal clindamycin and oral metronidazole for bacterial vaginosis: a randomized trial. *Obstet Gynecol* 2000;96:256–260.

16. Greaves WL, Chungafung J, Morris B, Haile A, Townsend JL. Clindamycin versus metronidazole in the treatment of bacterial vaginosis. *Obstet Gynecol* 1988;72:799–802.

17. Aubert JM, Oliete S, Leira J. Treatment of bacterial vaginosis: clindamycin versus metronidazol. *Prog Obst Gin* 1994;37:287–292.

18. Livengood CH, Soper DE, Sheehan KL, et al. Comparison of once daily and twice daily dosing of 0.75% metronidazole gel in the treatment of bacterial vaginosis. *Sex Transm Dis* 1999;26:137–142.

19. Sobel J, Peipert JF, McGregor JA, et al. Efficacy of clindamycin vaginal ovule (3-day treatment) versus clindamycin vaginal cream (7-day treatment) in bacterial vaginosis. *Infect Dis Obstet Gynecol* 2001;9:9–15.

20. Colli E, Landoni M, Parazzini F. Treatment of male partners and recurrence of bacterial vaginosis: a randomised trial. *Genitourin Med* 1997;73:267–270.

21. Sobel JD, Schmitt C, Meriwether C. Long-term follow-up of patients with bacterial vaginosis treated with oral metronidazole and topical clindamycin. *J Infect Dis* 1993;167:783–784.

22. Trexler MF, Fraser TG, Jones MP. Fulminant pseudomembranous colitis caused by clindamycin phosphate vaginal cream. *Am J Gastroenterol* 1997;92:2112–2113.

23. Hillier SL, Lipinski C, Briselden AM, Eschenbach DA. Efficacy of intravaginal 0.75% metronidazole gel for the treatment of bacterial vaginosis. *Obstet Gynecol* 1993;81:963–967.

24. Schmitt C, Sobel JD, Meriwether C. Bacterial vaginosis: treatment with clindamycin cream versus oral metronidazole. *Obstet Gynecol* 1992; 79:1020–1023.

25. Brocklehurst P, Hannah M, McDonald H. The management of bacterial vaginosis in pregnancy. In: The Cochrane Library, Issue 2, 2001. Oxford: Update Software. Most recent substantive amendment/search date July 1998; primary sources Cochrane Pregnancy and Childbirth Group Trials Register.

26. Carey JC, Klebanoff MA, Hauth JC, et al. Metronidazole to prevent preterm delivery in pregnant women with asymptomatic bacterial vaginosis. *N Engl J Med* 2000;342:534–540.

27. McGregor JA, French JI, Jones W, et al. Bacterial vaginosis is associated with prematurity and vaginal fluid mucinase and sialidase: results of a controlled trial of topical clindamycin cream. *Am J Obstet Gynecol* 1994;170:1048–1059.

28. Vermeulen GM, Bruinse HW. Prophylactic administration of clindamycin 2% vaginal cream to reduce the incidence of spontaneous preterm birth in women with an increased recurrence risk: a randomized placebo-controlled double-blind trial. *Br J Obstet Gynaecol* 1999;106:652–657.

29. Hauth JC, Goldenberg RL, Andrews WW, DuBard MB, Copper RL. Reduced incidence of preterm delivery with metronidazole and erythromycin in women with bacterial vaginosis. *N Engl J Med* 1995;333:1732–1736.

30. Joesoef MR, Hillier SL, Wiknjosastro G, et al. Intravaginal clindamycin treatment for bacterial vaginosis: effect on preterm delivery and low birth weight. *Am J Obstet Gynecol* 1995;173:1527–1531.

31. Kurkinen-Raty M, Vuopala S, Koskela M, et al. A randomised controlled trial of vaginal clindamycin for early pregnancy bacterial vaginosis. *BJOG* 2000;107:1427–1432.

32. Kekki M, Kurki T, Pelkonen J, Kurkinen-Raty M, Cacciatore B, Paavonen J. Vaginal clindamycin in preventing preterm birth and periparital infections in asymptomatic women with bacterial vaginosis: a randomized, controlled trial. *Obstet Gynecol* 2001; 97:643–648.

33. Hamrick M, Chambliss ML. Bacterial vaginosis and treatment of sexual partners. *Arch Fam Med* 2000; 9:647–648. Search date not stated; primary sources Medline and The Cochrane Library.

34. Larsson PG, Platz-Christensen JJ, Thejls H, Forsum U, Pahlson C. Incidence of pelvic inflammatory disease after first-trimester legal abortion in women with bacterial vaginosis after treatment with metronidazole: a double-blind, randomized study. *Am J Obstet Gynecol* 1992;166:100–103.

35. Larsson PG, Platz-Christensen JJ, Dalaker K, et al. Treatment with 2% clindamycin vaginal cream prior to first trimester surgical abortion to reduce signs of postoperative infection: a prospective, double-blinded, placebo-controlled, multicenter study. *Acta Obstet Gynecol Scand* 2000;79:390–396.

36. Crowley T, Low N, Turner A, Harvey I, Bidgood K, Horner P. Antibiotic prophylaxis to prevent post-abortal upper genital tract infection in women with bacterial vaginosis: randomised controlled trial. *BJOG* 2001;108:396–402.

37. Soper DE, Bump RC, Hurt WG. Bacterial vaginosis and trichomoniasis vaginitis are risk factors for cuff cellulitis after abdominal hysterectomy. *Am J Obstet Gynecol* 1990;163:1016–1021.

M Joesoef
Medical Epidemiologist
National Center for HIV STD and TB
Prevention
Atlanta
USA

George Schmid
Medical Epidemiologist
World Health Organization
Geneva
Switzerland

Competing interests: None declared.

Genital chlamydial infection

Search date May 2001

Nicola Low and Frances Cowan

INTERVENTIONS

Key Messages

- Short term microbiological cure is the outcome used in most trials, but this may not mean eradication of *Chlamydia trachomatis*. Long term cure rates have not been studied extensively because of high default rates and difficulty in distinguishing persistent infection from reinfection due to re-exposure.

In men and non-pregnant women

- Small RCTs with short term follow up and high withdrawal rates have found that multiple dose regimens of tetracyclines (doxycycline, tetracycline) and mac-rolides (rosaramicin) achieve microbiological cure in at least 95% of people with genital chlamydia. Erythromycin (2 g/day) is likely to be beneficial. Cipro-floxacin is unlikely to be beneficial. We found limited evidence on the effec-tiveness of other antibiotics. We found no differences in microbiological cure rates between men and women or between those with proven or presumed infection.

- A meta-analysis of short term RCTs has found that a single dose of azithromycin may be as effective in achieving microbiological cure of *C trachomatis* as a 7 day course of doxycycline. Rates of adverse effects were similar.

In pregnant women

- Two systematic reviews have found that both amoxicillin (amoxycillin) and erythromycin are likely to be effective in achieving microbiological cure.

- One small RCT has found that clindamycin and erythromycin have a similar effect on cure rates.

- One systematic review has found that a single dose of azithromycin is more effective in achieving microbiological cure of C trachomatis than a 7 day course of erythromycin.

DEFINITION   Uncomplicated genital chlamydia is a sexually transmitted infection of the urethra in men and of the endocervix, urethra, or both, in women that has not ascended to the upper genital tract. Infection is asymptomatic in up to 80% of women, but may cause non-specific symptoms, including vaginal discharge and intermenstrual bleeding. Infection in men causes urethral discharge and urethral irritation or dysuria, but may also be asymptomatic in up to half of cases.[1]

INCIDENCE/   Genital chlamydia is the commonest bacterial sexually transmitted
PREVALENCE infection in developed countries. In the USA, over 642 000 cases of chlamydia were reported in the year 2000.[2] The prevalence of uncomplicated genital chlamydia in women attending general practice surgeries in the UK is reported to be 3–5%.[3] Prevalence is highest in young adults. Reported rates in 15–19 year old women are about 800/100 000 in the UK,[4] 1000/100 000 in Sweden,[1] and 2500/100 000 in the USA.[5]

AETIOLOGY/   Infection is caused by the bacterium C trachomatis serotypes D–K.
RISK FACTORS It is transmitted primarily through sexual intercourse.

PROGNOSIS   Untreated chlamydial infection may persist asymptomatically in women for at least 15 months[6] and for an unknown period in men. In women, untreated chlamydial infection that ascends to the upper genital tract causes pelvic inflammatory disease in an estimated 30–40% of women[7] (see pelvic inflammatory disease, p 324). Tubal infertility has been found to occur in about 11% of women after a single episode of pelvic inflammatory disease, and the risk of ectopic pregnancy is increased six to sevenfold.[8] Ascending infection in men causes epididymitis, but evidence that this causes male infertility is limited.[9] Maternal to infant transmission can lead to neonatal conjunctivitis and pneumonitis in 30–40% of cases.[1] Chlamydia may coexist with other genital infections and may facilitate transmission and acquisition of HIV infection.[1]

AIMS   To eradicate C trachomatis; to prevent the development of upper genital tract infection; and to prevent further sexual transmission, with minimal adverse effects of treatment.

OUTCOMES   Microbiological cure rate (calculated as the percentage of people attending a follow up visit at least 1 week after the end of antibiotic treatment who had a negative test for C trachomatis); adverse effects of treatment, including effects on the fetus; short term microbiological cure may not mean eradication of C trachomatis but long term cure rates have not been studied extensively because of high default rates and difficulty in distinguishing persistent infection from reinfection due to re-exposure; pelvic inflammatory disease; infertility.

METHODS   *Clinical Evidence* search and appraisal May 2001. All relevant systematic reviews and masked clinical trials were included. We present the range of cure rates (with exact binomial CIs) or, if there was no evidence of statistical heterogeneity between trials, the summary cure rate (95% CIs) weighted by the standard error. Summary rates do not include cure rates of 100% because the standard error cannot be computed if there are no treatment failures. Where two or more trials compared the same regimens with no evidence of statistical heterogeneity, we used a fixed effects meta-analysis to calculate the summary odds ratio with 95% confidence intervals. Trial quality was assessed in terms of randomisation, blinding, and numbers of withdrawals from analysis.[10] Trials with methodological limitations have been included but relevant problems are mentioned in the text. **Categorising interventions:** We considered a regimen beneficial if the summary cure rate from two or more RCTs was 95% or greater, as previously suggested,[11] and if the lower confidence limit was also above 90%. There were insufficient data to differentiate reinfections from persistent infections. We considered regimens to be likely (or unlikely) to be beneficial on the basis of positive (or negative) results from two or more RCTs, and of unknown effectiveness if there was only one RCT or if results were conflicting.

QUESTION   **What are the effects of antibiotic treatment for men and non-pregnant women with uncomplicated genital chlamydial infection?**

OPTION   MULTIPLE DOSE REGIMENS

Small RCTs, with short term follow up and high withdrawal rates, have found that tetracyclines (doxycycline, tetracycline) and macrolides (rosaramicin) achieve microbiological cure in 95% or more cases of genital chlamydia. We found no differences in microbiological cure rates between men and women or between those with proven or presumed infection. We found limited evidence on the effectiveness of other macrolides, quinolones, and penicillins.

Benefits: We found no systematic review. We found 22 RCTs reported to be double blind or with blinded outcome assessment comparing 19 different antibiotic regimens (see web extra table A at www.clinicalevidence.com).[12–33] Results were similar in men and women and in populations with proven and presumed infection, so data were combined. **Doxycycline:** We found 11 RCTs (1434 men and women) comparing doxycycline with another antibiotic.[12-14,16-23] The cure rate was 100% in six RCTs and the weighted average 98% (95% CI 96% to 99%) in the other five. We found no trials comparing different regimens for doxycycline, but the most frequent schedule (in 6 trials) was 100 mg twice daily for 7 days. **Tetracycline:** The summary cure rate in four trials (201 men and women) comparing tetracycline hydrochloride (500 mg 4 times daily for 7 days) versus another antibiotic was 97% (95% CI 94% to

99%).[24–27] Our own meta-analysis of three trials[25–27] found that rates of treatment failure with rosaramicin compared with tetracycline were similar (OR 1.55, 95% CI 0.54 to 4.43; see web extra figure A at www.clinicalevidence.com). **Erythromycin:** Cure rates with erythromycin stearate 1 g daily for 7 days (3 trials, 191 people) ranged from 77–95%,[30–32] and with erythromycin 2 g daily for 7 days (2 trials, 40 people) from 94–100%.[29,32] **Ciprofloxacin:** In two trials (190 men and women), the cure rate for ciprofloxacin ranged from 63–92%.[20,21] Our meta-analysis found that failure of microbiological cure was more frequent with ciprofloxacin than doxycycline (OR 5.0, 95% CI 1.2 to 10.0). A variety of other antibiotics were studied in single trials (see web extra table A at www.clinicalevidence.com). No trial measured the effect of antibiotics on pelvic inflammatory disease or infertility.

Harms: Reported adverse effects varied widely between trials but were mostly gastrointestinal (see web extra table A at www.clinicalevidence.com).

Comment: Most trials were conducted in sexually transmitted diseases clinics where follow up is difficult; in seven of 14 trials with available data, more than 15% of randomised participants were not included in the analysis.[15,22,29–33] Most trials were small (three had fewer than 40 people with chlamydia)[16,24,29] and many antibiotic regimens were compared so it is difficult to draw conclusions about relative efficacy. Only five trials reported that sexual partners of participants were offered treatment. Amoxicillin and ampicillin have not been adequately assessed in the treatment of genital chlamydia infection (see web extra table A at www.clinicalevidence.com) because *in vitro* studies suggest that amoxicillin does not eradicate *C trachomatis*,[34] raising the concern that infection may persist and recrudesce *in vivo*.

| OPTION | SINGLE DOSE VERSUS MULTIPLE DOSE REGIMENS |

A meta-analysis of short term RCTs has found that a single dose of azithromycin may be as effective in achieving microbiological cure of *C trachomatis* as a 7 day course of doxycycline. Rates of adverse effects were similar.

Benefits: We found one systematic review (search date 1996, 9 blinded and unblinded RCTs, 1800 people) comparing azithromycin 1 g as a single dose versus doxycycline 100 mg twice daily for 7 days in people with proven or presumed genital chlamydia.[35] Data about laboratory diagnosed infection were available for five RCTs (554 men and women). Cure rates for azithromycin ranged from 90–100% and for doxycycline from 93–100%. Microbiological failure tended to be more frequent with azithromycin than with doxycycline, but this did not reach statistical significance (AR 22/301 v 10/253; OR recalculated from data in the paper 1.8, 95% CI 0.9 to 3.9; P = 0.11).

Harms: Short term adverse effects of both azithromycin and doxycycline were reported to be mild.

Genital chlamydial infection

Comment: Azithromycin can be given in a single dose as directly observed therapy. More comparisons of azithromycin and doxycycline are needed to rule out a clinically important difference between them.

QUESTION **What are the effects of treatment for pregnant women with uncomplicated genital chlamydial infection?**

OPTION **MULTIPLE DOSE REGIMENS**

Two systematic reviews have found that both amoxicillin (amoxycillin) and erythromycin are likely to be effective in achieving microbiological cure of genital chlamydia in pregnant women. One small RCT has found that clindamycin and erythromycin have a similar effect on cure rates.

Benefits: We found two systematic reviews, (search date 1998[36] and search date not stated[37]), the most recent of which (11 blinded and unblinded trials, 1449 people)[36] included all studies in the earlier review. **Erythromycin and amoxicillin:** Both achieved high rates of microbiological cure (cure rates 182/199 [91%] with amoxicillin 500 mg 3 times daily for 7 days v 163/191 [85%] with erythromycin 500 mg 4 times daily for 7 days; OR for failure of cure with amoxicillin compared with erythromycin 0.54, 95% CI 0.28 to 1.02; P = 0.059), and treatment with any antibiotic was better than placebo (OR for failure of cure 0.06, 95% CI 0.03 to 0.12). **Clindamycin:** One small RCT found no significant difference in cure rates between clindamycin and erythromycin (38/41 [93%] v 31/37 [84%]).

Harms: Rates of adverse effects were similar for clindamycin and erythromycin, but adverse effects sufficient to stop treatment were less frequent with amoxicillin than erythromycin (OR 0.16, 95% CI 0.09 to 0.30). None of the trials gave information on adverse clinical outcomes in the offspring.

Comment: We found no long term follow up data.

OPTION **SINGLE VERSUS MULTIPLE DOSE REGIMENS**

One systematic review has found that, in pregnant women, a single dose of azithromycin is as effective in achieving microbiological cure of C trachomatis as a 7 day course of erythromycin.

Benefits: We found one systematic review (search date 1998, 4 non-blinded RCTs, 290 pregnant women) comparing a single dose of azithromycin 1 g versus erythromycin 500 mg four times daily for 7 days.[36] Failure of microbiological cure was less frequent with azithromycin than erythromycin (11/145 [8%] v 27/145 [19%]; OR 0.38, 95% CI 0.19 to 0.74).[36] There was no significant difference in the rate of premature delivery (OR 0.73, 95% CI 0.24 to 2.20).

Harms: The RCTs found that azithromycin was associated with fewer adverse effects. Fetal anomaly was reported in one infant in each group.[36] Effects of azithromycin in pregnancy have not been extensively studied.

Comment: None.

REFERENCES

1. Holmes KK, Sparling PF, Mårdh PA, et al, eds. *Sexually transmitted diseases*. 3rd edition. New York: McGraw Hill Inc, 1999.
2. Anonymous. Notifiable diseases/deaths in selected cities weekly information. *MMR Morb Mortal Wkly Rep* 2001;49:1168.
3. Stokes T. Screening for chlamydia in general practice: a literature review and summary of the evidence (review). *J Public Health Med* 1997;19: 222–232.
4. http://www.phls.co.uk/facts/STI/sti.htm Last accessed 13 March 2001.
5. *Sexually Transmitted Disease Surveillance, 1999*. US Department of Health and Human Services, Public Health Service. Atlanta. Centers for Disease Control and Prevention (CDC), September 2000.
6. McCormack WM, Alpert S, McComb DE, Nichols RL, Semine DZ, Zinner SH. Fifteen-month follow-up study of women infected with *Chlamydia trachomatis*. *N Engl J Med* 1979;300:123–125.
7. Cates W Jr, Rolfs RT Jr, Aral SO. Sexually transmitted diseases, pelvic inflammatory disease, and infertility: an epidemiologic update. *Epidemiol Rev* 1990;12:199–220.
8. Weström L, Bengtsson LP, Mårdh PA. Incidence, trends, and risks of ectopic pregnancy in a population of women. *BMJ* 1981;282:15–18.
9. Ness RB, Markovic N, Carlson CL, Coughlin MT. Do men become infertile after having sexually transmitted urethritis? An epidemiologic examination [review]. *Fertil Steril* 1997;68: 205–213.
10. Chalmers I, Adams M, Dickersin K, et al. A cohort study of summary reports of controlled trials. *JAMA* 1990;263:1401–1405.
11. Clinical Effectiveness Group. National guideline for the management of *Chlamydia trachomatis* genital tract infection. *Sex Transm Infect* 1999;75(suppl 1):4–8.
12. Nilsen A, Halsos A, Johansen A, et al. A double blind study of single dose azithromycin and doxycycline in the treatment of chlamydial urethritis in males. *Genitourin Med* 1992;68: 325–327.
13. Steingrímsson Ó, Ólafsson JH, Thórarinsson H, Ryan RW, Johnson RB, Tilton RC. Single dose azithromycin treatment of gonorrhea and infections caused by *C trachomatis* and *U urealyticum* in men. *Sex Transm Dis* 1994;21: 43–46.
14. Stamm WE, Hicks CB, Martin DH, et al. Azithromycin for empirical treatment of the nongonococcal urethritis syndrome in men. A randomized double-blind study. *JAMA* 1995;274: 545–549.
15. Brihmer C, Mårdh PA, Kallings I, et al. Efficacy and safety of azithromycin versus lymecycline in the treatment of genital chlamydial infections in women. *Scand J Infect Dis* 1996;28:451–454.
16. Stein GE, Mummaw NL, Havlichek DH. A preliminary study of clarithromycin versus doxycycline in the treatment of nongonococcal urethritis and mucopurulent cervicitis. *Pharmacotherapy* 1995;15:727–731.
17. Romanowski B, Talbot H, Stadnyk M, Kowalchuk P, Bowie WR. Minocycline compared with doxycycline in the treatment of nongonococcal urethritis and mucopurulent cervicitis. *Ann Intern Med* 1993; 119:16–22.
18. Boslego JW, Hicks CB, Greenup R, et al. A prospective randomized trial of ofloxacin vs. doxycycline in the treatment of uncomplicated male urethritis. *Sex Transm Dis* 1988;15: 186–191.
19. Phillips I, Dimian C, Barlow D, et al. A comparative study of two different regimens of sparfloxacin versus doxycycline in the treatment of non-gonococcal urethritis in men. *J Antimicrob Chemother* 1996;37(suppl A):123–134.
20. Hooton TM, Rogers ME, Medina TG, et al. Ciprofloxacin compared with doxycycline for nongonococcal urethritis. Ineffectiveness against *Chlamydia trachomatis* due to relapsing infection. *JAMA* 1990;264:1418–1421.
21. Jeskanen L, Karppinen L, Ingervo L, Reitamo S, Happonen HP, Lassus A. Ciprofloxacin versus doxycycline in the treatment of uncomplicated urogenital *Chlamydia trachomatis* infections. A double-blind comparative study. *Scand J Infect Dis Suppl* 1989;60:62–65.
22. McCormack WM, Dalu ZA, Martin DH, et al. Double-blind comparison of trovafloxacin and doxycycline in the treatment of uncomplicated Chlamydial urethritis and cervicitis. Trovafloxacin Chlamydial Urethritis/Cervicitis Study Group. *Sex Transm Dis* 1999;26:531–536.
23. Lassus AB, Virrankoski T, Reitamo SJ, et al. Pivampicillin versus doxycycline in the treatment of chlamydial urethritis in men. *Sex Transm Dis* 1990;17:20–22.
24. Lassus A, Juvakoski T, Kanerva L. Comparison between rifampicin and tetracycline in the treatment of nongonococcal urethritis in males with special reference to *Chlamydia trachomatis*. *Eur J Sex Transm Dis* 1984;2:15–17.
25. Lassus A, Allgulander C, Juvakoski T. Efficacy of rosaramicin and tetracycline in chlamydia-positive and -negative nongonococcal urethritis. *Eur J Sex Transm Dis* 1982;1:29–31.
26. Juvakoski T, Allgulander C, Lassus A. Rosaramicin and tetracycline treatment in *Chlamydia trachomatis*-positive and -negative nongonococcal urethritis. *Sex Transm Dis* 1981;8:12–15.
27. Brunham RC, Kuo CC, Stevens CE, Holmes KK. Therapy of cervical chlamydial infection. *Ann Intern Med* 1982;97:216–219.
28. Batteiger BE, Zwickl BE, French ML, Jones RB. Women at risk for gonorrhea: comparison of rosaramicin and ampicillin plus probenecid in the eradication of *Neisseria gonorrhoeae*, *Chlamydia trachomatis* and genital mycoplasmas. *Sex Transm Dis* 1985;12:1–4.
29. Robson HG, Shah PP, Lalonde RG, Hayes L, Senikas VM. Comparison of rosaramicin and erythromycin stearate for treatment of cervical infection with *Chlamydia trachomatis*. *Sex Transm Dis* 1983;10:130–134.
30. Worm AM, Hoff G, Kroon S, Petersen CS, Christensen JJ. Roxithromycin compared with erythromycin against genitourinary chlamydial infections. *Genitourin Med* 1989;65: 35–38.
31. Worm AM, Avnstorp C, Petersen CS. Erythromycin against *Chlamydia trachomatis* infections. A double blind study comparing 4- and 7-day treatment in men and women. *Dan Med Bull* 1985;32:269–271.
32. Linnemann CCJ, Heaton CL, Ritchey M. Treatment of *Chlamydia trachomatis* infections: comparison of 1- and 2-g doses of erythromycin daily for seven days. *Sex Transm Dis* 1987;14:102–106.
33. Paavonen J, Kousa M, Saikku P, Vartiainen E, Kanerva L, Lassus A. Treatment of nongonococcal urethritis with trimethoprim-sulphadiazine and with placebo. A double-blind partner-controlled study. *Br J Venereal Dis* 1980;56: 101–104.

34. Kuo CC, Wang SP, Grayston JT. Antimicrobial activity of several antibiotics and a sulfonamide against *Chlamydia trachomatis* organisms in cell culture. *Antimicrob Agents Chemother* 1977;12:80–83.

35. Chlamydial STD treatment. *Bandolier* 1996;28: 4–6. Search date 1996; primary source Medline. http://www.jr2.ox.ac.uk/bandolier/band28/b28–4. html. Last accessed 13 March 2001.

36. Brocklehurst P, Rooney G. Interventions for treating genital *Chlamydia trachomatis* infection in pregnancy. In: The Cochrane Library, Issue 4, 1999. Oxford: Update Software. Search date 1998; primary sources Cochrane Pregnancy and Childbirth Review Group Specialised Register of Controlled Trials, and Cochrane Controlled Trials Register.

37. Turrentine MA, Newton ER. Amoxicillin or erythromycin for the treatment of antenatal chlamydial infection: a meta-analysis. *Obstet Gynecol* 1995;86:1021–1025. Search date not stated; primary sources Medline, and Cochrane Pregnancy and Childbirth Database.

Nicola Low
Department of Social Medicine University of Bristol
Bristol
UK

Frances Cowan
Department of Sexually
Transmitted Diseases
Royal Free and
University College Medical School
London
UK

Competing interests: FC has received research and symposium funding from Glaxo Wellcome in relation to HSV research. NL, none declared.

Search date July 2001

Anna Wald

INTERVENTIONS

Key Messages

Treating first and recurrent episodes of genital herpes

- RCTs have found that oral antiviral treatment in people with first episode genital herpes reduces the duration of symptoms, lesions, and viral shedding in first and recurrent episodes of genital herpes.

- RCTs found no evidence of significant differences in effectiveness or adverse events between aciclovir, valaciclovir, and famciclovir.

- One systematic review has found that oral antiviral treatment taken at the start of a recurrence reduces the duration of lesions, symptoms, and viral shedding in people with recurrent genital herpes. RCTs found no significant differences between different antivirals.

- One systematic review has found that daily maintenance treatment with oral antiviral agents reduces the frequency of recurrences and viral shedding.

- One systematic review found that the effects of psychotherapy on genital herpes recurrence have not yet been adequately studied.

- We found limited evidence of an effect of antiviral treatment versus placebo for genital herpes in people with HIV infection.

Genital herpes

Preventing transmission of herpes simplex virus

- Limited evidence from a prospective cohort study suggested that male condom use reduced the risk of sexual transmission of herpes simplex virus type 2 in women who had disconcordant sexual partners. The study found no evidence of a benefit in men who had disconcordant sexual partners. Other interventions aimed at preventing transmission (antiviral treatment and immunisation) have not been adequately studied.

- We found that the effect of abdominal delivery on mother to baby transmission has not been adequately evaluated. The procedure carries the risk of increased maternal morbidity and mortality.

- The highest risk of mother to baby transmission is in women newly infected with genital herpes in late pregnancy. We found that interventions to prevent infection in late pregnancy (such as serological screening and counselling) have not been adequately studied.

- Limited evidence from RCTs suggests that antiviral treatment may reduce the number of pregnant women with genital lesions at term. Because women with genital lesions at term are usually offered abdominal deliveries, antiviral treatment may reduce the rate of abdominal delivery.

DEFINITION	Genital herpes is an infection with herpes simplex virus type 1 or type 2, causing ulceration in the genital area. Herpes simplex virus infections can be defined on the basis of virological and serological findings. Types of infection include first episode primary infection, which is herpes simplex virus in a person without prior herpes simplex virus type 1 or type 2 antibodies; first episode non-primary infection, which is herpes simplex virus type 2 in a person with prior herpes simplex virus type 1 antibodies or vice versa; first recognised recurrence, which is herpes simplex virus type 2 (or type 1) in a person with prior herpes simplex virus type 2 (or type 1) antibodies; and recurrent genital herpes, which is caused by reactivation of latent herpes simplex virus.
INCIDENCE/ PREVALENCE	Genital herpes infections are among the most common sexually transmitted diseases. Seroprevalence studies show that 22% of adults in the USA have herpes simplex virus type 2 antibodies.[1] A UK study found that 23% of adults attending sexual medicine clinics and 7.6% of blood donors in London had antibodies to herpes simplex virus type 2.[2]
AETIOLOGY/ RISK FACTORS	Both herpes simplex virus type 1 and 2 can cause a first episode of genital infection, but herpes simplex virus type 2 is more likely to cause recurrent disease.[3] Most people with herpes simplex virus type 2 infection are not aware that they have genital herpes, as their symptoms are mild. However, these people can pass on the infection to sexual partners and newborns.[4,5]
PROGNOSIS	Sequelae of herpes simplex virus infection include neonatal herpes simplex virus infection, opportunistic infections in immuno-compromised people, recurrent genital ulceration, and psychosocial morbidity. Herpes simplex virus type 2 infection is associated with an increased risk of HIV transmission and acquisition. The most common neurological complications are aseptic meningitis (reported in about a quarter of women during primary infection) and urinary retention. The absolute risk of neonatal infection is high (41%, 95% CI 26% to 56%) in babies born to women who acquire

infection near the time of labour[6,7] and low (< 3%) in women with established infection, even in those who have a recurrence at term. About 15% of neonatal infections result from postnatal transmission from oral lesions.

AIMS
To reduce the morbidity of the first episode; to reduce the risk of recurrent disease after a first episode; to prevent further transmission, with minimal adverse effects of treatment.

OUTCOMES
Severity and duration of symptoms; healing time; duration of viral shedding; recurrence rates; psychosocial morbidity; rates of transmission; adverse effects of treatment.

METHODS
Clinical Evidence search and appraisal July 2001, using the terms herpes simplex virus, aciclovir, valaciclovir, famciclovir, cidofovir, trifluridine, and neonatal herpes. We also included preliminary results of clinical trials published in the abstracts of the Interscience Conference on Antimicrobial Agents and Chemotherapy and International Society for STD Research. We also contacted experts in the field and makers of antiviral drugs to identify completed studies that were undergoing peer review, but which had not yet been published.

QUESTION **What are the effects of antiviral treatment in people with a first episode of genital herpes?**

RCTs have found that oral antiviral treatment decreases the duration of lesions, symptoms, and viral shedding, and reduces neurological complications in people with first episode genital herpes. Limited data provide no evidence that oral antiviral treatment reduced the rate of recurrence compared with placebo. RCTs have found no evidence of a significant difference in terms of clinical or biological variables of a first episode of genital herpes between aciclovir, valaciclovir, and famciclovir treatments.

Benefits:
We found no systematic review. **Immediate effects:** We found five RCTs (350 men and women) of oral aciclovir for the treatment of first episode genital herpes.[8–12] In the largest RCT (150 people), aciclovir (200 mg 5 times daily) versus placebo decreased the duration of viral shedding (median 2 days with aciclovir *v* 9 days with placebo), pain (5 days with aciclovir *v* 7 days with placebo), time to healing of lesions (12 days with aciclovir *v* 14 days with placebo), and reduced formation of new lesions (18% with aciclovir *v* 62% with placebo).[10] The other RCTs found similar results.[8,9,11,12] Neurological complications (aseptic meningitis and urinary retention) were also reduced. Numbers were small so no firm estimates of effectiveness were available. **Different regimens:** We found two RCTs.[13,14] The first international RCT (643 otherwise healthy adults with first episode genital herpes) compared oral valaciclovir (1000 mg twice daily) versus oral aciclovir (200 mg 5 times daily) for 10 days.[13] It found no significant differences between the two medications in any clinical or virological variables. The second RCT (951 adults with first episode genital herpes) compared three different doses of oral famciclovir (125, 250, or 500 mg 3 times daily) versus oral aciclovir (200 mg 5 times daily).[14] It found no significant differences. **Recurrence rates:** A meta-analysis of two small placebo controlled RCTs (61 people with first episode genital

herpes) found no significant difference in time to recurrence or frequency of recurrence between people given oral aciclovir and those given placebo.[15] **Systemic versus topical treatment:** We found no direct randomised comparisons of oral, intravenous, or topical antiviral treatment.

Harms: Adverse effects (mostly headache and nausea) were rare and frequency was similar for aciclovir, valaciclovir, famciclovir, and placebo.

Comment: Oral aciclovir has the advantage of convenience over intravenous aciclovir.[16] A non-randomised comparison of results from different trials performed at one institution suggests that systemic treatment is more effective than topical.[16]

QUESTION   **What interventions reduce the impact of recurrence?**

OPTION   **ANTIVIRAL TREATMENT AT THE START OF RECURRENCE**

One systematic review has found that oral antiviral treatment taken at the start of a recurrence reduces the duration of lesions, symptoms, and viral shedding in people with recurrent genital herpes. RCTs found no significant differences between different antivirals.

Benefits: We found one systematic review (search date 1997, 4 RCTs, 3393 people).[17] **Famciclovir versus placebo:** The review found one RCT (467 people with recurrent genital herpes) of famciclovir versus placebo.[17] It found that oral famciclovir (125–500 mg twice daily) significantly reduced the duration of lesions (5 days with famciclovir v 4 days with placebo) and viral shedding (3 days with famciclovir v 2 days with placebo). **Valaciclovir versus placebo:** The review found one RCT of valaciclovir versus placebo.[17] The RCT (987 people with recurrent genital herpes) found that self initiated oral valaciclovir (500 or 1000 mg twice daily) for 5 days versus placebo decreased the episode duration (4 days with valaciclovir v 6 days with placebo) and viral shedding (2 days with valciclovir v 4 days with placebo), and increased the rate of aborted recurrences (31% with valciclovir v 21% with placebo). **Valaciclovir versus aciclovir:** The review found two RCTs (1939 people), which found no significant difference between oral valaciclovir and aciclovir. **Aciclovir versus placebo:** We found one non-systematic review of several RCTs (more than 650 healthy adults with recurrent genital herpes).[18] These evaluated 5 days of oral aciclovir (200 mg 5 times daily or 800 mg twice daily), started at the first sign of recurrence. Aciclovir versus placebo reduced the period of viral shedding (1 with aciclovir v 2 days with placebo) and duration of lesions (5 with aciclovir v 6 days with placebo). **Famciclovir versus aciclovir:** We found one RCT (204 people with recurrent genital herpes), which found no significant difference in time to heal between oral famciclovir versus aciclovir (mean lesion healing time 5.1 days with famciclovir v 5.4 days with aciclovir, mean difference 0.3 days, 95% CI –0.3 to +0.8 days).[19]

Harms: Adverse effects (mostly headache and nausea) were rare, and frequency was similar for aciclovir, valaciclovir, famciclovir, and placebo.

Comment: The benefit was found to be greater if the person with recurrent herpes initiated treatment at the first symptom or sign of a recurrence.[20] People can learn to recognise recurrences early on and should have an adequate supply of medication at home.

OPTION   **DAILY MAINTENANCE ANTIVIRAL TREATMENT**

One systematic review has found that daily maintenance treatment with oral antiviral agents reduces the frequency of recurrences and viral shedding in people with genital herpes.

Benefits: **Recurrence rates:** We found one systematic review (search date 1997, 4 placebo controlled RCTs).[17] Two RCTs evaluated treatment for 1 year. In the first RCT (1479 people), freedom from recurrence was reported in 40–50% of people who received valaciclovir (500 or 1000 mg once daily), valaciclovir (250 mg twice daily), or aciclovir (400 mg twice daily) as compared with 5% who received placebo.[21] In the other RCT (455 people), the median time to first recurrence was 11 months with famciclovir (250 mg twice daily) and 1.5 months with placebo.[22] One non-systematic review (published in 1990) identified several placebo controlled RCTs of aciclovir.[18] Most participants had a history of frequent recurrence ($\geq$ 6/year). Daily aciclovir was associated with reduced recurrence rate (74–93%) and duration of recurrences (3.5 v 5 days). One double blind, placebo controlled RCT (1146 adults) found significantly fewer recurrences during the first year with aciclovir (1.7 with aciclovir v 12.5 with placebo; P < 0.0001).[23] Of 210 adults in the trial who completed 5 years of continuous treatment with aciclovir (400 mg twice daily), 53–70% were free of recurrence each year. **Viral shedding:** We found one RCT (34 women with recently acquired genital herpes simplex virus type 2 infection) of daily maintenance treatment versus placebo that assessed viral shedding in women.[24] Women obtained swabs for viral cultures daily for 70 days while receiving aciclovir (400 mg twice daily) or placebo. Viral shedding was reduced by 95% with aciclovir on days with reported lesions and by 94% on days without lesions. **Psychosocial morbidity:** We found one RCT (1479 people) that evaluated the effect of daily oral antiviral treatment on a genital herpes quality of life scale.[25] People receiving daily aciclovir or valaciclovir had significantly greater mean improvements from baseline than those receiving placebo.[26]

Harms: Daily treatment with aciclovir, famciclovir, and valaciclovir was well tolerated.[27] People taking aciclovir were followed for up to 7 years, and those taking famciclovir and valaciclovir for up to 1 year. Nausea and headache were infrequent, and participants rarely discontinued treatment because of adverse effects. We found no studies evaluating whether daily maintenance treatment increases high risk sexual behaviour. We found no evidence that daily treatment with aciclovir results in emergence of aciclovir resistant herpes simplex virus during or after stopping treatment in healthy adults.[27]

Comment: Viral shedding is an intermediate outcome, but may be important to people with herpes as it reflects the risk of transmitting infection.

Genital herpes

OPTION **PSYCHOTHERAPY**

One systematic review found that the effects of psychotherapy on the rate of genital herpes recurrence have not yet been adequately studied.

Benefits: We found one systematic review (search date 1991), which identified six poor quality studies of psychotherapeutic interventions in 69 participants (4 studies had < 10 participants).[28] Interventions varied from hypnotherapy and progressive muscle relaxation to cognitive therapy and multifaceted intervention. The largest RCT (31 people with > 4 recurrences a year) compared psychosocial intervention, versus social support, versus waiting list. Participants receiving psychosocial intervention had significantly lower recurrence rates (6 recurrences/year) as compared with the pretreatment frequency (11/year) and with the other groups (11/year).

Harms: No adverse effects were noted.

Comment: Small numbers of people, inadequate controls, and subjective and retrospective assessment of recurrence frequency at baseline limit the usefulness of these studies. Controlled studies that include prospective clinical evaluation of disease activity are needed.

QUESTION **What interventions prevent transmission of herpes simplex virus?**

OPTION **CONDOMS, ANTIVIRAL TREATMENT, IMMUNISATION**

Limited evidence from one prospective cohort study suggested that male condom use may decrease the risk of sexual transmission of herpes simplex virus 2 among women who have a sexual partner disconcordant for herpes simplex virus 2. However, no benefit was found among men. We found no good evidence on the effects of antiviral treatments. One RCT found no evidence of effectiveness of glycoprotein vaccine.

Benefits: **Condoms:** We found no RCTs. In a prospective cohort study (528 couples discordant for herpes simplex virus [HSV] type 2 infection and followed for 18 months), the male use of condoms in more than 25% of sexual acts was associated with a lower risk of HSV-2 acquisition among women (adjusted HR 0.09, 95% CI 0.01 to 0.67) but not among men (adjusted HR 2.02, 95% CI 0.32 to 12.5).[29] Only 61% of couples ever used condoms during the study and only 8% used them consistently. One person acquired HSV-2 despite consistent condom use. **Antiviral treatment:** We found no direct evidence that treatment reduces HSV transmission in serologically discordant couples. However, RCTs have shown that daily antiviral treatment decreases the frequency of clinical and subclinical viral shedding (see text, p 298). **Immunisation:** We found one RCT (2393 HSV-2 and HIV seronegative people) of recombinant glycoprotein vaccine (gB2 and gD2) versus placebo.[30] It found no significant difference in vaccine efficacy (4.6 cases per 100 person years with placebo v 4.2 cases per 100 person years with glycoprotein vaccine; P = 0.58). It found no significant difference in the duration of initial genital herpes, or the frequency of subsequent recurrences in people who acquired genital HSV infection.

Harms: As for individual interventions (see harms of daily maintenance antiviral treatment, p 299).

Comment: Controlled trials of condoms for prevention of HSV-2 transmission are impractical. Even with routine counselling, many couples do not regularly use condoms. Trials of different methods of advising people to use condoms or providing condoms could be performed.

OPTION   ABDOMINAL DELIVERY TO PREVENT NEONATAL HERPES

We found insufficient evidence for the effect of abdominal delivery on the risk of neonatal herpes. The procedure carries a risk of increased maternal morbidity and mortality.

Benefits: We found no systematic review and no RCTs that assessed the effects of abdominal delivery on the risk of mother to child transmission of herpes simplex virus. In the Netherlands, women with recurrent genital herpes at delivery have been allowed vaginal birth since 1987. This policy has not resulted in an increase in neonatal herpes: 26 cases from 1981–1986 and 19 cases from 1987–1991.[7]

Harms: Abdominal delivery is associated with significant maternal morbidity and mortality. A study pooling data from different studies estimated that, for every two neonatal deaths from herpes simplex virus infection prevented by abdominal delivery, one maternal death may be caused.[31]

Comment: Countries vary in their approach to obstetric management of women with recurrent genital herpes at term. In the USA and the UK, these women are advised to undergo abdominal delivery, with its attendant risks to the mother. The absolute risk of neonatal infection is high (AR 41%, 95% CI 26% to 56%) in babies born to women who acquired infection near the time of labour[6,7] and low (AR < 3%) in women with established infection, even in those who have recurrence at term. Most women who acquired infection toward the end of pregnancy are undiagnosed, and most cases of neonatal herpes simplex virus infection are acquired from women without a history of genital herpes. The available evidence suggests that efforts to prevent neonatal herpes simplex virus infection should focus on preventing the acquisition of infection in late pregnancy.

OPTION   ANTIVIRAL TREATMENT DURING PREGNANCY

We found limited evidence from one systematic review suggesting that aciclovir reduces the rate of genital lesions at term in women with first or recurrent episodes of genital herpes simplex virus during pregnancy. We found that adverse effects have not been adequately studied.

Benefits: We found one systematic review (search date 1996),[7] which identified two RCTs,[32,33] and one controlled study,[34] of daily aciclovir versus placebo in 210 pregnant women near term with genital herpes. The studies differed in terms of the dose and duration of aciclovir and the populations enrolled. Abdominal delivery was performed in women with genital lesions at term. All three studies found lower rates of abdominal delivery in women treated with aciclovir, although in two studies the effect was not significant (AR of abdominal delivery 4/21 [19%] in women receiving aciclovir v 10/25 [40%] in women receiving placebo, RR 0.48, 95% CI 0.17 to 1.30;[32] AR of abdominal delivery 6/46 [13%] in women receiving aciclovir v 15/46 [33%] in women receiving no treatment, RR 0.4, 95% CI 0.17 to 0.94, NTT 6, 95% CI 3 to 43;[34] and AR of abdominal delivery 7/31 [23%] in women receiving aciclovir v 10/32 [31%] in women receiving placebo, RR 0.72, 95% CI 0.32 to 1.66).[33]

Harms: No adverse effects for women or newborns were reported, but the number of women was small. Rare adverse events, such as an increase in asymptomatic viral shedding or aciclovir related obstructive uropathy in the newborns, would be difficult to detect.

Comment: None.

OPTION   **SEROLOGICAL SCREENING AND COUNSELLING TO PREVENT ACQUISITION OF HERPES SIMPLEX VIRUS DURING PREGNANCY**

We found insufficient evidence on the effects of serological screening and counselling during pregnancy on infection rates.

Benefits: We found no systematic review or RCTs that assessed either serological screening with type specific assays to identify women at risk for acquisition of herpes simplex virus infection in late pregnancy, or counselling to avoid genital–genital and oral–genital contact in late pregnancy.

Harms: We found insufficient evidence.

Comment: None.

QUESTION   **What are the effects of treatments in people with genital herpes and HIV infection?**

OPTION   **ANTIVIRAL TREATMENTS**

We found limited evidence of the effect of antiviral treatment for genital herpes in people with HIV infection. However, evidence from other settings suggests that antivirals may be effective treatment of genital herpes in immunocompromised people.

Benefits: We found no systematic review and no RCTs on the treatment of first episode genital herpes in people with HIV infection. **Treatment of recurrence:** We found two RCTs.[35,36] One RCT (193 people on stable antiretroviral treatment) compared famciclovir (500 mg twice daily) versus aciclovir (400 mg 5 times daily) for 1 week.[35] It found no difference between the two drugs in mucocutaneous recurrence of herpes simplex virus. The other RCT (467 people) compared valaciclovir (1 g twice daily) versus aciclovir (200 mg 5 times daily) for 5 days.[36] It found no significant differences between the two drugs. **Prevention of recurrence:** We found two RCTs.[37,38] One crossover RCT (48 people with antibodies to HIV and herpes simplex virus; 38 with a history of genital herpes) compared famciclovir versus placebo over 8 weeks.[37] The conclusions of that study are difficult to interpret (see comment below). The other RCT (1062 people with a median CD4 count of $320/mm^3$) compared valaciclovir (500 mg twice daily) versus valaciclovir (1000 mg once daily) versus aciclovir (400 mg twice daily) over 1 year.[38] It found no significant difference between either dose of valaciclovir versus aciclovir, although recurrence was less likely with valaciclovir (500 mg twice daily) than with the valaciclovir (1000 mg once daily; 82% v 71% recurrence free at 48 weeks; $P < 0.05$).

Harms: Adverse effects (mostly headache and nausea) occurred with similar frequencies with aciclovir, valaciclovir, and famciclovir. Thrombotic microangiopathy, which has been reported in people receiving valaciclovir (8 g daily), has not been reported among 713 HIV infected persons who received oral valaciclovir in daily doses ranging from 250–1000 mg for up to 1 year (A Wald, personal communication, 2000).

Comment: Three of the four RCTs did not have a placebo control. Most studies compared new treatments with aciclovir rather than placebo. The crossover trial of famciclovir versus placebo was difficult to interpret because the withdrawal rate was high.[37] Although we found only limited evidence of an effect of antivirals for treatment of genital herpes in people with HIV infection, there was a consensus that antiviral treatment may be helpful, based on evidence from immunocompromised people who do not have HIV. Aciclovir has been found effective in immunocompromised populations. With the availability of effective treatments for HIV, trials of antiviral (anti-herpes simplex virus) versus placebo may now be conducted. A trial of valaciclovir versus placebo is now in progress (A Wald, personal communication, 2000). In HIV infected people, there is a markedly increased rate of herpes simplex virus shedding.[39] HIV has been recovered from genital herpes lesions.[40] We found no evidence on the effect of daily antiviral treatment on transmission of HIV to sexual partners.

REFERENCES

1. Fleming DT, McQuillan GM, Johnson RE, et al. Herpes simplex virus type 2 in the United States, 1976 to 1994. *N Engl J Med* 1997;337:1105–1111.

2. Cowan FM, Johnson AM, Ashley R, et al. Antibody to herpes simplex virus type 2 as serological marker of sexual lifestyle in populations. *BMJ* 1994;309:1325–1329.

3. Benedetti J, Corey L, Ashley R. Recurrence rates in genital herpes after symptomatic first-episode infection. *Ann Intern Med* 1994;121:847–854.

4. Mertz GJ, Schmidt O, Jourden JL, et al. Frequency of acquisition of first-episode genital infection with herpes simplex virus from symptomatic and asymptomatic source contacts. *Sex Transm Dis* 1985;12:33–39.

5. Whitley RJ, Kimberlin DW, Roizman B. Herpes simplex viruses. *Clin Infect Dis* 1998;26:541–553.

6. Brown ZA, Selke SA, Zeh J, et al. Acquisition of herpes simplex virus during pregnancy. *N Engl J Med* 1997;337:509–515.

7. Smith J, Cowan FM, Munday P. The management of herpes simplex virus infection in pregnancy. *Br J Obstet Gynaecol* 1998;105:255–268. Search date 1996; primary source Medline.

8. Nilsen AE, Aasen T, Halsos AM, et al. Efficacy of oral acyclovir in treatment of initial and recurrent genital herpes. *Lancet* 1982;2:571–573.

9. Corey L, Fife K, Benedetti JK, et al. Intravenous acyclovir for the treatment of primary genital herpes. *Ann Intern Med* 1983;98:914–921.

10. Mertz G, Critchlow C, Benedetti J, et al. Double-blind placebo-controlled trial of oral acyclovir in the first episode genital herpes simplex virus infection. *JAMA* 1984;252:1147–1151.

11. Mindel A, Adler MW, Sutherland S, et al. Intravenous acyclovir treatment for primary genital herpes. *Lancet* 1982;2:697–700.

12. Bryson YJ, Dillon M, Lovett M, et al. Treatment of first episodes of genital herpes simplex virus infections with oral acyclovir: a randomized double-blind controlled trial in normal subjects. *N Engl J Med* 1983;308:916–1920.

13. Fife KH, Barbarash RA, Rudolph T, et al. Valaciclovir versus acyclovir in the treatment of first-episode genital herpes infection: results of an international, multicenter, double-blind randomized clinical trial. *Sex Transm Dis* 1997;24: 481–486.

14. Loveless M, Harris W, Sacks S. *Treatment of first episode genital herpes with famciclovir. Programs and abstracts of the 35th Interscience Conference on Antimicrobial Agents and Chemotherapy.* San Francisco, California, 1995.

Genital herpes

15. Corey L, Mindel A, Fife KH, et al. Risk of recurrence after treatment of first episode genital herpes with intravenous acyclovir. *Sex Transm Dis* 1985;12:215–218.

16. Corey L, Benedetti J, Critchlow C, et al. Treatment of primary first-episode genital herpes simplex virus infections with acyclovir: results of topical, intravenous and oral therapy. *J Antimicrob Chemother* 1983;12(suppl B):79–88.

17. Wald A. New therapies and prevention strategies for genital herpes. *Clin Infect Dis* 1999;28:S4–13. Search date 1997; primary source Medline.

18. Stone K, Whittington W. Treatment of genital herpes. *Rev Infect Dis* 1990;12(suppl 6):610–619.

19. Chosidow O, Drouault Y, Leconte-Veyriac F, et al. Famciclovir versus aciclovir in immunocompetent patients with recurrent genital herpes infections: a parallel-groups, randomised, double-blind clinical trial. *Br J Dermatol* 2001;144:818–824.

20. Reichman RC, Badger GJ, Mertz GJ, et al. Treatment of recurrent genital herpes simplex infections with oral acyclovir: a controlled trial. *JAMA* 1984;251:2103–2107.

21. Reitano M, Tyring S, Lang W, et al. Valaciclovir for the suppression of recurrent genital herpes simplex virus infection: a large-scale dose range finding study. *J Infect Dis* 1998;178:603–610.

22. Diaz-Mitoma F, Sibbald RG, Shafran SD. Oral famciclovir for the suppression of recurrent genital herpes: a randomized controlled trial. *JAMA* 1998; 280:887–892.

23. Goldberg L, Kaufman R, Kurtz T, et al. Continuous five-year treatment of patients with frequently recurring genital herpes with acyclovir. *J Med Virol* 1993(suppl 1):45–50.

24. Wald A, Zeh J, Barnum G, et al. Suppression of subclinical shedding of herpes simplex virus type 2 with acyclovir. *Ann Intern Med* 1996;124:8–15.

25. Doward LC, McKenna SP, Kohlmann T, et al. The international development of the RGHQoL: a quality of life measure for recurrent genital herpes. *Qual Life Res* 1998;7:143–153.

26. Patel R, Tyring S, Strand A, et al. Impact of suppressive antiviral therapy on the health related quality of life of patients with recurrent genital herpes infection. *Sex Transm Infect* 1999;75: 398–402.

27. Fife KH, Crumpacker CS, Mertz GJ. Recurrence and resistance patterns of herpes simplex virus following stop of ≥ 6 years of chronic suppression with acyclovir. *J Infect Dis* 1994;169:1338–1341.

28. Longo D, Koehn K. Psychosocial factors and recurrent genital herpes: a review of prediction and psychiatric treatment studies. *Int J Psychiatry*

29. Wald A, Langenberg A, Link K, et al. Effect of condoms on reducing the transmission of herpes simplex virus type 2 from men to women. *Dermatol* 2001;285:3100–3106.

30. Corey L, Langenberg AG, Ashley R, et al. Recombinant glycoprotein vaccine for the prevention of genital HSV-2 infection: two randomised controlled trials. *JAMA* 1999;282: 331–340.

31. Randolph A, Washington A, Prober C. Cesarean delivery for women presenting with genital herpes lesions. *JAMA* 1993;270:77–82.

32. Scott LL, Sanchez PJ, Jackson GL, Zeray F, Wendel Jr GD. Acyclovir suppression to prevent cesarean delivery after first-episode genital herpes. *Obstet Gynecol* 1996;87:69–73.

33. Brocklehurst P, Kinghorn G, Carney O, et al. A randomised placebo controlled trial of suppressive acyclovir in late pregnancy in women with recurrent genital herpes infection. *Br J Obstet Gynaecol* 1998;105:275–280.

34. Stray-Pedersen B. Acyclovir in late pregnancy to prevent neonatal herpes simplex [Letter] [see comments]. *Lancet* 1990;336:756.

35. Romanowski B, Aoki FY, Martel AY, Lavender EA, Parsons JE, Saltzman RL. Efficacy and safety of famciclovir for treating mucocutaneous herpes simplex infection in HIV-infected individuals. Collaborative Famciclovir HIV Study Group. *AIDS* 2000;14:1211–1217.

36. Schacker T, International Valaciclovir Study Group. *Valaciclovir as acute treatment for recurrent ano-genital herpes in immunocompromised (HIV positive) individuals*. 13th International Society for STD Research. Denver, Colorado, 1999.

37. Schacker T, Hu HL, Koelle DM, et al. Famciclovir for the suppression of symptomatic and asymptomatic herpes simplex virus reactivation in HIV-infected persons. A double-blind, placebo-controlled trial. *Ann Intern Med* 1998;128:21–28.

38. Gold J, Bell A, Valaciclovir International HSV Study Group. *Valaciclovir prevents herpes simplex virus recurrences in HIV-infected individuals – a double-blind controlled trial*. Programs and abstracts of the 20th International Congress of Chemotherapy. Sydney, Australia, 1997.

39. Schacker T, Zeh J, Hu HL, et al. Frequency of symptomatic and asymptomatic HSV-2 reactivations among HIV-infected men. *J Infect Dis* 1998;178:1616–1622.

40. Schacker T, Ryncarz A, Goddard J, et al. Frequent recovery of HIV from genital herpes simplex virus lesions in HIV infected persons. *JAMA* 1998;280: 61–66.

Med 1993;23:99–117. Search date 1991; primary sources Psychological Abstracts, Medline, and hand searches of reference lists.

Anna Wald

Assistant Professor of Medicine and Epidemiology

University of Washington

Seattle

USA

Competing interests: The author has received research support from GlaxoSmithKline, Wyeth Lederly Vacccines and Pediatrics, and 3M. The author is a consultant to GlaxoSmithKline.

INTERVENTIONS

Key Messages

- We found five treatments that were compared with placebo. Podophyllotoxin, imiquimod, and intralesional interferon have been found to be significantly more effective in the clearance of warts compared with placebo, but data on recurrence are lacking. Placebo controlled RCTs of topical interferon give conflicting results, and those of systemic interferon show no evidence of benefits.

- We found no RCTs comparing placebo with cryotherapy, electrosurgery, surgical excision, or laser surgery.

- We found no clear evidence that one treatment is superior to another.

- Topical 5-fluorouracil and bi- and trichloroacetic acid have not been adequately evaluated.

- We found no evidence that treatment of external genital warts decreased infectivity, and the preventive effects of condoms have not been adequately evaluated.

DEFINITION External genital warts are benign epidermal growths on the external perianal and perigenital region. There are four morphological types: condylomatous, keratotic, papular, and flat warts.

INCIDENCE/ PREVALENCE In 1996, external and internal genital warts accounted for over 180 000 initial visits to private physicians' offices in the USA: about 60 000 fewer than were reported for 1995.[1] In the USA, 1% of sexually active men and women aged 18–49 years are estimated to have external genital warts.[2]

AETIOLOGY/ RISK FACTORS External genital warts are caused by the human papillomavirus (HPV). Although more than 70 types of HPV have been identified, most external genital warts in immunocompetent people are caused by HPV types 6 and 11.[3,4] HPV infections and, more specifically, external genital warts are sexually transmissible.

PROGNOSIS Clinical trials have found that recurrences are frequent and may necessitate repeated treatment. Without treatment, external genital warts may remain unchanged, may increase in size or number, or may completely resolve. They rarely, if ever, progress to cancer.[5] Juvenile laryngeal papillomatosis, a rare and sometimes life threatening condition, occurs in children of women with a history of genital warts. Its rarity makes it hard to design studies that can evaluate whether treatment in pregnant women alters the risk.[6,7]

AIMS To eliminate symptomatic warts from the external genitalia; to prevent recurrence; and to avoid sequelae, with minimal adverse effects.

OUTCOMES Wart clearance (generally accepted as complete eradication of warts from the treated area); recurrence; sequelae; adverse effects of treatment; quality of life; transmission.

METHODS *Clinical Evidence* search and appraisal from 1985 to May 2001. We also performed selected Medline searches for papers published before 1985. Other data came from abstract booklets, conference proceedings, references identified from bibliographies of pertinent articles and books, and manufacturers of therapeutic agents. This review is limited to systematic reviews and subsequent RCTs, unless no RCTs were found for a particular treatment. This limitation may have biased the review in favour of newer and heavily marketed treatments.

QUESTION **What are the effects of non-surgical treatments?**

OPTION **PODOPHYLLOTOXIN**

RCTs have found that podophyllotoxin is more effective than placebo.

Benefits: We found no systematic review. **Versus placebo:** Data from eight placebo controlled RCTs (1035 people) found that, within 16 weeks of treatment, podophyllotoxin was more effective than placebo (wart clearance occurred in 45–77% of people on treatment; RR of clearance v placebo between 2.0, 95% CI 0.9 to 4.3[8] and 48, 95% CI 3.0 to 773[9–15]). **Recurrence rates:** RCTs of 0.5% cream or solution found recurrence rates ranging from 4%[15] to 33%.[9] One RCT (57 people) of 0.5% podophyllotoxin solution as prophylaxis against recurrence of external genital warts (initially treated in an open label study) found fewer recurrences among people taking placebo.[16] **Versus podophyllin:** Five RCTs compared podophyllotoxin versus podophyllin.[17–21] They found no significant difference in wart clearance (RRs for podophyllin v podophyllotoxin between 0.7, 95% CI 0.4 to 1.12 and 1.7, 95% CI 0.9 to 3.2).[20] One RCT used a 2% solution in a limited study of self treatment for penile warts and found no significant difference with podophyllotoxin versus podophyllin (RR for podophyllin v podophyllotoxin 0.6, 95% CI 0.3 to 1.3).[21]

Harms: Safety during pregnancy is unknown. Podophyllotoxin does not contain the mutagenic flavonoid compounds, quercetin and kaempherol, which are contained in podophyllin resin preparations.[22] Local inflammation or irritation, erosion, burning, pain, and itching are reported in most trials. Balanoposthitis,[23,24] dyspareunia, bleeding, scarring, and insomnia are reported rarely.[8] One large RCT reported burning and inflammation in 75% and bleeding in 25% of treated people.[12] Although rare, preputial tightening has been reported.[17]

Comment: RCTs examined the efficacy of podophyllotoxin solutions more often than cream preparations, but cream or gel preparations may be easier to apply than solutions. This and other differences may cause variable efficacy.

OPTION   **IMIQUIMOD**

RCTs have found that imiquimod is more effective at clearing warts than placebo.

Benefits: We found no systematic review. **Versus placebo:** We found two RCTs in a total of 968 people. Wart clearance within 3 months occurred twice as often with 1% cream as placebo (clearance rate 37–56% with imiquimod v 0–56% with placebo; RR 1.9, 95% CI 1.1 to 3.3).[25,26] For 5% cream, clearance was 13 times greater than with placebo (RR 13, 95% CI 4.2 to 40.2).[26] **Recurrence:** No recurrences were reported in people using 1% cream, but recurrences were reported in 13–19% of people treated with 5% cream.[25,26] This compared to 10% among placebo treated people in one study.[25]

Harms: One RCT reported local itching, erythema, and burning in more than 15% of people, and irritation, tenderness, ulceration, and pain in less than 10%.[26]

Comment: We found one other small RCT[27] of imiquimod versus placebo, but excluded it pending review of its methods (it used 2% imiquimod cream versus placebo in only 60 men and found cure rates consistent with the studies included above).[25,26]

OPTION   **CRYOTHERAPY**

We found no trials comparing cryotherapy with placebo. RCTs have found similar wart clearance rates with cryotherapy compared with podophyllin, trichloroacetic acid, or electrosurgery. One RCT found that recurrence rates were similar after cryotherapy and electrosurgery. Cryotherapy has been used successfully in pregnancy.

Benefits: We found no systematic review. **Versus placebo:** We found no RCTs. **Versus other treatments:** We found six comparative RCTs: two compared cryotherapy plus interferon versus cryotherapy alone;[28,29] the other four compared cryotherapy versus podophyllin,[30] trichloroacetic acid,[31,32] or electrosurgery.[30,33] **Clearance:** Four RCTs reported 63–88% clearance 3 months or more after cryotherapy.[30–33] Although one RCT found cryotherapy was more effective than podophyllin after six treatments (RR of wart clearance compared with podophyllin 1.9, 95% CI 1.4 to 2.6), there was no significant difference in wart clearance 3 months after treatment (RR 1.4, 95% CI 0.9 to 2.2) suggesting merely a difference in speed of effect.[30] Two of the trials found no significant difference between cryotherapy and trichloroacetic acid at the end of treatment or 3 months later (RRs 1.1, 95% CI 0.8 to 1.5,[31] and 0.9, 95% CI 0.8 to 1.1[32]). Two trials found that electrosurgery was slightly more effective than cryotherapy (RRs of wart clearance with electrosurgery v cryotherapy at the end of treatment: 1.2, 95% CI 1.1 to 1.3; and after 3 months 1.4, 95% CI 1.0 to 2.0).[30,33] **Recurrence:** One trial found no significant difference in recurrence rates between cryotherapy and electrosurgery (21% v 22%).[30]

Harms: Discomfort, ulceration, and scabbing were reported in nearly a fifth of people after cryotherapy.[30,33] One RCT reported local infection in one of 86 people taking cryotherapy versus none of 149 people taking podophyllin resin or electrosurgery.[30]

Comment: One case series of 34 pregnant women who received three or fewer treatments of cryotherapy found no subsequent infection or premature rupture of membranes.[34]

OPTION PODOPHYLLIN

RCTs have found that podophyllin resin is as effective as most other treatments, but is less effective than surgical excision. We found no trials comparing podophyllin with placebo.

Benefits: We found no systematic review. **Versus placebo:** We found no RCTs. **Versus other treatments:** We found 13 RCTs: four compared podophyllin versus podophyllotoxin,[17–20] one versus cryotherapy,[29] one versus electrosurgery,[30] three with and without interferon,[35–37] one with and without trichloroacetic acid,[38] two versus surgical excision,[38,39] and one compared alternative doses of podophyllin.[40] **Clearance:** None of the four RCTs comparing podophyllin with podophyllotoxin found a significant difference in wart clearance (RRs ranging between 0.7, 95% CI 0.4 to 1.1[18] and 1.7, 95% CI 0.9 to 3.2[20]). The trials comparing cryotherapy or electrosurgery versus podophyllin found no significant difference 3 months after treatment (RR for both comparison treatments 1.4, 95% CI 0.9 to 2.1).[30] One RCT found that podophyllin and intralesional interferon together were more effective than podophyllin alone for clearance 3 weeks after treatment (RR 2.0, 95% CI 1.1 to 3.6); however, it found no significant difference at 11 weeks (RR 2.3, 95% CI 0.9 to 5.8).[36] Two RCTs found that podophyllin was less effective than surgical excision (RRs 0.3, 95% CI 0.2 to 0.7 and

0.5, 95% CI 0.2 to 0.9).[38,39] **Recurrence:** Two RCTs found that recurrence was more frequent with podophyllin versus surgical excision (60–65% v 19–29% after surgery).[38,39]

Harms: Eight RCTs reported pain, erythema, irritation, and tenderness in 3–17% of people treated with podophyllin.[17,18,20,30,35,36,38,39] Skin burns (1–3%),[37,38] bleeding (4%),[39] and erosion or ulcerations (1%[18]–11%[34]) were also reported. Faecal incontinence (4%)[39] and preputial tightening (1%)[17] were reported rarely.

Comment: Safety during pregnancy is unknown. Podophyllin may contain the mutagenic flavonoid compounds, quercetin and kaempherol.[22]

OPTION   BI- AND TRICHLOROACETIC ACID

We found inadequate evidence to evaluate the efficacy of bi- and trichloroacetic acid.

Benefits: We found no systematic review. **Versus placebo:** We found no RCTs. **Versus other treatments:** We found two RCTs (192 people) comparing trichloroacetic acid versus cryotherapy. These found no significant difference in wart clearance (RRs of trichloroacetic acid v cryotherapy 1.1, 95% CI 0.8 to 1.5 and 0.9, 95% CI 0.8 to 1.1).[31,32] We also reviewed one RCT (73 people) comparing trichloroacetic acid plus podophyllin versus podophyllin alone.[41] Participants were followed for 3 months. The RCT found no significant difference in wart clearance between the two groups.

Harms: Insufficient data are available to comment on possible harms.

Comment: Small numbers of participants and inadequate study designs make it difficult to evaluate effectiveness. In pregnant women, only case series are available: 31 of 32 pregnant women treated with trichloroacetic acid showed wart clearance, and two of 31 showed recurrence.[42] The evidence is inadequate to evaluate adverse effects of trichloroacetic acid in pregnancy.

OPTION   TOPICAL INTERFERON

Three RCTs have found increased wart clearance with topical interferon versus placebo.

Benefits: We found no systematic review. **Versus placebo:** We found three RCTs (223 men and women). Complete wart clearance 4 weeks after treatment occurred in more people using interferon versus placebo (6% v 3%, P value not provided;[43] 73% v 10%, P < 0.0001;[44] 90% v 20%, P value not provided[11]). About a third of each group in the first study had cleared their warts by 16 weeks.[43] Recurrence rates were not evaluated. **Versus podophyllotoxin:** One of the RCTs also compared topical interferon versus podophyllotoxin and found that interferon was significantly more effective than podophyllotoxin about 4 weeks after treatment (RR compared with podophyllotoxin 1.5, 95% CI 1.03 to 1.63).[11] **As adjuvant to other treatment:** One RCT compared recombinant β interferon at two doses plus CO_2 laser versus CO_2 laser alone, electrotherapy, and liquid nitrogen. Recurrences occurred in 62% of people (21/36) treated with 1 million IU interferon, in 54% (19/35) treated with 150 000 IU interferon, and 75% (27/36) treated with placebo.[45]

Harms: One placebo controlled study reported local burning and itching in 39% of treated people.[43] Another RCT reported fever, headache, and itching in 18% of people treated with interferon.[11]

Comment: Differences in the RCTs' findings may be attributable to the preparations used; one preparation was incorporated into a methyl cellulose aqueous base[43] and the other was instilled into a cream base.[11]

OPTION   INTRALESIONAL INJECTION OF INTERFERON

RCTs have found that intralesional injection of interferon is more effective than placebo.

Benefits: We found no systematic review. We found eight placebo controlled trials,[46–54] and one RCT (1000 people) comparing interferon plus podophyllin versus podophyllin alone.[36] Doses and follow up intervals varied. Two of the placebo controlled RCTs randomised treatment to lesions rather than to people.[49,51] Complete wart clearance was reported in 17–63% of people on intralesional interferon within 8–20 weeks of treatment. **Versus placebo:** In studies using 1 MU/ml, intralesional interferon was between twofold (95% CI 0.8 to 4.6)[50] and 3.5-fold (95% CI 1.4 to 8.8)[47] more likely to achieve complete wart clearance than placebo. One RCT found no significant difference for complete wart clearance between 1 MU/ml intralesional interferon and placebo. However, it found a twofold improvement if complete and partial responders were grouped together for analysis (RR of clearance 2.3, 95% CI 1.2 to 4.3).[54] **Added to podophyllin:** One RCT found that podophyllin and intralesional interferon together were more effective than podophyllin alone 3 weeks after treatment (RR 2.0, 95% CI 1.1 to 3.6); however, no significant difference was observed at 11 weeks (RR 2.3, 95% CI 0.9 to 5.8).[36]

Harms: Flu like symptoms (dizziness, fever, malaise, myalgia, nausea and vomiting, headache, and pain) were reported in 0–100% of people. Eight of nine studies reported local irritation and one reported hypopigmentation among treated individuals.[54] Several studies reported a fall in white cell counts,[36,46-48,50-53] thrombocytopenia (1%),[46] and raised serum aspartate transaminase concentrations (6%)[36] in people on interferon.

Comment: None.

OPTION   SYSTEMIC INTERFERON

RCTs have found no evidence that systemic interferon is more effective than placebo, and it is associated with a range of adverse effects.

Benefits: We found no systematic review. We found 16 RCTs (1992 men and women): six placebo controlled trials; two trials that compared systemic interferon versus podophyllin or diathermocoagulation; and eight trials that evaluated its use with one or more adjunct therapies.[28,29,55-68] **Clearance:** Fourteen of the RCTs reported wart clearance within 3 months of treatment in 17–67% of people. However, four RCTs comparing systemic interferon with placebo found no significant difference in rates of wart clearance.[56-61] One study found that people taking systemic interferon showed greater wart clearance than people treated with placebo, which was significant at 8 weeks' follow up (51% v 29%; P < 0.05), but no difference was detected 12 months after treatment.[59] **Recurrence:** Recurrence rates varied from 9–69%.[28,56,58,68]

Harms: Flu like symptoms were reported at variable frequencies. Headache, fatigue and malaise, myalgia, nausea and vomiting, fever, chills, and dizziness were reported in 0.5–100% of people on interferon.[28,29,55-63,65,66,68-70] Anaphylactic reaction occurred in 2% of people in one RCT,[63] leukopenia in 6–28%,[58,65,66] thrombocytopenia in 3–4%,[58,66] and raised liver enzymes in 3%.[58,69] Bronchospasm and depression were rarely reported (1/97 people for each symptom in 1 trial).[28]

Comment: None.

OPTION   **TOPICAL 5-FLUOROURACIL**

Topical 5-fluorouracil has not yet been adequately evaluated in the treatment of external genital warts.

Benefits: We found no systematic review or RCTs.

Harms: One case series of 1% solution reported minor local erosions (48%), urinary meatus erosions (5%), vulvar irritation (10%), burning (10%), and dysuria (4%).[71]

Comment: We found three case series in 224 men and women treated with 1% and 5% cream and solution preparations in various doses.[71-73] Wart clearance was reported in 10–50% of people within 3 months of treatment. Only one study reported recurrence rates based on data from only 20 of its 49 participants; recurrences were noted in 10.[72] 5-Fluorouracil has teratogenic and mutagenic properties. Safety in pregnancy is not known. Exposure to 5-fluorouracil during pregnancy has been reported rarely, with no untoward outcomes.[74,75]

QUESTION   **What are the effects of surgical treatments?**

OPTION   **ELECTROSURGERY**

Limited evidence from RCTs suggests that electrosurgery is more effective than intramuscular and subcutaneous interferon. We found no trials comparing electrosurgery with no treatment.

Benefits: We found no systematic review. **Clearance:** We found no RCTs versus no or sham treatment and found three RCTs (482 men and women) comparing electrosurgery versus interferon, cryotherapy, or podophyllin resin.[30,33,63] Complete wart clearance was reported in 61–94% of people 3–6 weeks after treatment. Electrosurgery was more effective than intramuscular interferon (RR v im 3.3, 95% CI 1.8 to 5.9) or subcutaneous interferon (RR v sc 6.9, 95% CI 2.8 to 17.1).[63] One RCT found that electrosurgery was more effective than podophyllin resin 4 weeks after treatment (RR 2.3, 95% CI 1.7 to 3.0), but this difference ceased to be significant after 3 months (RR 1.4, 95% CI 0.9 to 2.1).[30] Two studies found that electrosurgery was slightly more effective than cryotherapy within 3–4 weeks of treatment (RRs 1.2, 95% CI 1.1 to 1.3[30] and 1.4, 95% CI 1.0 to 2.0[33]). One of these trials followed people for 3 months, after which time this difference ceased to be significant (RR 1.0, 95% CI 0.8 to 1.2).[30] **Recurrence:** One trial found recurrence in 22% of people after electrosurgery versus 21% after cryotherapy and 44% using podophyllin resin.[30]

Harms: Pain and local irritation were reported in 17% of treated people.[30]

Comment: None.

OPTION   SURGICAL EXCISION

RCTs have found that surgical (scissor) excision is as effective as laser surgery and more effective than podophyllin. We found no trials comparing surgical excision with no treatment.

Benefits: We found no systematic review. **Clearance:** We found no RCTs versus no treatment or sham treatment, but found three RCTs comparing surgical excision versus CO_2 laser[76] or podophyllin.[38,39] Within 1 year of treatment, complete wart clearance occurred in 35–72% of people treated with surgical excision. Two studies found that podophyllin was less effective than surgery for clearance (RRs of clearance 0.3, 95% CI 0.2 to 0.7[38,39] and 0.5, 95% CI 0.2 to 0.9[37]). One trial found no significant difference in clearance between laser and conventional surgery (RR 1.2, 95% CI 0.6 to 2.4).[76] **Recurrence:** Recurrence occurred in 19–29% of excision treated people versus 60–65% of those treated with podophyllin.[38,39] The trial comparing conventional and laser surgery found no significant difference in recurrence rates between the two treatments.[76]

Harms: All surgically treated participants experienced pain. Scar formation (9%)[76] and bleeding (37%)[39] were less frequent.

Comment: None.

OPTION   LASER SURGERY

One RCT found limited evidence of a difference in wart clearance or recurrence rates between laser and conventional surgery. We found no trials comparing laser surgery with no treatment.

Benefits: We found no systematic review. We found no RCT versus no or sham treatment, three RCTs (285 people) evaluating laser surgery plus interferon versus laser alone,[65–67] and one RCT (50 people) comparing laser surgery versus conventional surgical excision.[76] **Clearance:** Complete wart clearance was reported in 23–52% of people within 36 months of laser surgery. This was not significantly different from clearance after conventional surgery (RR for laser v

conventional surgery 1.2, 95% CI 0.6 to 2.4).[76] **Recurrence:** Recurrence was reported in 60–77% of people after laser surgery.[65,67,76] This did not differ significantly from recurrence rates with conventional surgery.[76]

Harms: The RCT comparing laser with conventional surgery found no significant difference in the rate of local scar formation (28% after laser surgery v 9% after conventional surgery; P > 0.2).[76] Postoperative pain was reported equally in both groups.

Comment: We found two case series of laser surgery, which included 47 pregnant women.[42,77] These reported premature rupture of membranes (2/32 women), prolonged rupture of membranes (1/32), the need for postoperative suprapubic catheterisation (7/32), pyelonephritis (1/32), prolonged healing time (1/52), and rectal perforation with secondary abscess (1/52).

QUESTION **Does treatment of external genital warts or the use of barrier contraceptives prevent transmission of human papillomavirus (HPV)?**

We found insufficient evidence about barrier contraceptives or treatment of external genital warts to prevent transmission of HPV.

Benefits: We found no controlled studies about the effects of barrier contraceptives or treatment of external genital warts on the rate of transmitting HPV.

Harms: None reported.

Comment: Penetrative intercourse may not be required for transmission of HPV infection, and it is unclear whether sexual contact with any infected and uninfected perigenital tissues is sufficient to cause external genital warts.

REFERENCES

1. US Department of Health and Human Services, Public Health Service. Division of STD Prevention. *Sexually transmitted disease surveillance*. Atlanta: Centers for Disease Control and Prevention, 1996.

2. Koutsky LA, Galloway DA, Holmes KK. Epidemiology of genital human papillomavirus infection. *Epidemiol Rev* 1988;10:122–163.

3. Gissmann L, zur Hausen H. Partial characterization of viral DNA from human genital warts (condylomata acuminata). *Int J Cancer* 1980;25:605–609.

4. Gissmann L, Boshart M, Durst M, Ikenberg H, Wagner D, zur Hausen H. Presence of human papillomavirus in genital tumors. *J Invest Dermatol* 1984;83(suppl 1):26–28.

5. IARC Working Group on Evaluation of Carcinogenic Risks to Humans. *IARC monographs on the evaluation of carcinogenic risks to humans: human papillomaviruses*. Lyon, France: World Health Organization, International Agency for Research on Cancer, 1995.

6. Bonnez W, Kashima HK, Leventhal B, et al. Antibody response to human papillomavirus (HPV) type 11 in children with juvenile-onset recurrent respiratory papillomatosis (RRP). *Virology* 1992;188:384–387.

7. Hallden C, Majmudar B. The relationship between juvenile laryngeal papillomatosis and maternal condylomata acuminata. *J Reprod Med* 1986;31:804–807.

8. Greenberg MD, Rutledge LH, Reid R, Berman NR, Precop SL, Elswick RK Jr. A double-blind, randomized trial of 0.5% podofilox and placebo for the treatment of genital warts in women. *Obstet Gynecol* 1991;77:735–739.

9. Beutner KR, Conant MA, Friedman-Kien AE, et al. Patient-applied podofilox for treatment of genital warts. *Lancet* 1989;i:831–834.

10. Kirby P, Dunne King D, Corey L. Double-blind randomized clinical trial of self-administered podofilox solution versus vehicle in the treatment of genital warts. *Am J Med* 1990;88:465–469.

11. Syed TA, Khayyami M, Kriz D, et al. Management of genital warts in women with human leukocyte interferon-α vs podophyllotoxin in cream: a placebo-controlled, double-blind, comparative study. *J Mol Med* 1995;73:255–258.

12. Tyring S, Edwards L, Cherry LK, et al. Safety and efficacy of 0.5% podofilox gel in the treatment of anogenital warts. *Arch Dermatol* 1998;134:33–38.

13. Von Krogh G, Hellberg D. Self-treatment using a 0.5% podophyllotoxin cream of external genital condylomata acuminata in women. A placebo-controlled, double-blind study. *Sex Transm Dis* 1992;19:170–174.

14. Von Krogh G, Szpak E, Andersson M, Bergelin I. Self-treatment using 0.25%–0.50% podophyllotoxin-ethanol solutions against penile

condylomata acuminata: a placebo-controlled comparative study. *Genitourin Med* 1994;70: 105–109.

15. Syed TA, Lundin S, Ahmad SA. Topical 0.3% and 0.5% podophyllotoxin cream for self-treatment of condylomata acuminata in women: a placebo-controlled, double-blind study. *Dermatology* 1994; 189:142–145.

16. Bonnez W, Elswick RK Jr, Bailey-Farchione A, et al. Efficacy and safety of 0.5% podofilox solution in the treatment and suppression of anogenital warts. *Am J Med* 1994;96:420–425.Edwards A, Atma-Ram A, Thin RN. Podophyllotoxin 0.5% v podophyllin 20% to treat penile warts. *Genitourin Med* 1988;64:263–265.

18. Hellberg D, Svarrer T, Nilsson S, Valentin J. Self-treatment of female external genital warts with 0.5% podophyllotoxin cream (Condyline) vs weekly applications of 20% podophyllin solution. *Int J STD AIDS* 1995;6:257–261.

19. Kinghorn GR, McMillan A, Mulcahy F, Drake S, Lacey C, Bingham JS. An open, comparative, study of the efficacy of 0.5% podophyllotoxin lotion and 25% podophyllotoxin solution in the treatment of condylomata acuminata in males and females. *Int J STD AIDS* 1993;4:194–199.

20. Lassus A, Haukka K, Forsstrom S. Podophyllotoxin for treatment of genital warts in males: a comparison with conventional podophyllin therapy. *Eur J Sex Transm Dis* 1984;2:31–33.

21. White, DJ, Billingham C, Chapman S, et al. Podophyllin 0.5% or 2.0% v podophyllotoxin 0.5% for self treatment of penile warts: a double blind randomised study. *Genitourin Med* 1997;73: 184–187.

22. Petersen CS, Weismann K. Quercetin and kaempherol: an argument against the use of podophyllin? *Genitourin Med* 1995;71:92–93.

23. Von Krogh G. Topical self-treatment of penile warts with 0.5% podophyllotoxin in ethanol for four or five days. *Sex Transm Dis* 1987;14:135–140.

24. Von Krogh G. Penile condylomata acuminata: an experimental model for evaluation of topical self-treatment with 0.5–1.0% ethanolic preparations of podophyllotoxin for three days. *Sex Transm Dis* 1981;8:179–186.

25. Edwards L, Ferenczy A, Eron L, et al. Self-administered topical 5% imiquimod cream for external anogenital warts. *Arch Dermatol* 1998; 134:25–30.

26. Beutner KR, Spruance SL, Hougham AJ, Fox TL, Owens ML, Douglas JM Jr. Treatment of genital warts with an immune-response modifier (imiquimod). *J Am Acad Dermatol* 1998;38(2 pt 1):230–239.

27. Syed TA, Hadi SM, Qureshi ZA, Ali SM, Kwah MS. Treatment of external genital warts in men with imiquimod 2% in cream. A placebo-controlled, double-blind study. *J Infect* 2000;41:148–51

28. Eron LJ, Alder MB, O'Rourke JM, Rittweger K, DePamphilis J, Pizzuti DJ. Recurrence of condylomata acuminata following cryotherapy is not prevented by systemically administered interferon. *Genitourin Med* 1993;69:91–93.

29. Handley JM, Horner T, Maw RD, Lawther H, Dinsmore WW. Subcutaneous interferon α 2a combined with cryotherapy vs cryotherapy alone in the treatment of primary anogenital warts: a randomised observer blind placebo controlled study. *Genitourin Med* 1991;67:297–302.

30. Stone KM, Becker TM, Hadgu A, Kraus SJ. Treatment of external genital warts: a randomised clinical trial comparing podophyllin, cryotherapy, and electrodesiccation. *Genitourin Med* 1990;66: 16–19.

31. Abdullah AN, Walzman M, Wade A. Treatment of external genital warts comparing cryotherapy (liquid nitrogen) and trichloroacetic acid. *Sex Transm Dis* 1993;20:344–345.

32. Godley MJ, Bradbeer CS, Gellan M, Thin RN. Cryotherapy compared with trichloroacetic acid in treating genital warts. *Genitourin Med* 1987;63: 390–392.

33. Simmons PD, Langlet F, Thin RN. Cryotherapy versus electrocautery in the treatment of genital warts. *Br J Venereal Dis* 1981;57:273–274.

34. Bergman A, Bhatia NN, Broen EM. Cryotherapy for treatment of genital condylomata during pregnancy. *J Reprod Med* 1984;29:432–435.

35. Condyloma International Collaborative Study Group. A comparison of interferon alfa-2a and podophyllin in the treatment of primary condylomata acuminata. *Genitourin Med* 1991;67:394–399.

36. Douglas JM Jr, Eron LJ, Judson FN, et al. A randomized trial of combination therapy with intralesional interferon α 2b and podophyllin versus podophyllin alone for the therapy of anogenital warts. *J Infect Dis* 1990;162:52–59.

37. Potkul RK, Lancaster WD, Kurman RJ, Lewandowski G, Weck PK, Delgado G. Vulvar condylomas and squamous vestibular micropapilloma. Differences in appearance and response to treatment. *J Reprod Med* 1990;35: 1019–1022.

38. Khawaja HT. Podophyllin versus scissor excision in the treatment of perianal condylomata acuminata: a prospective study. *Br J Surg* 1989;76: 1067–1068.

39. Jensen SL. Comparison of podophyllin application with simple surgical excision in clearance and recurrence of perianal condylomata acuminata. *Lancet* 1985;2:1146–1148.

40. Simmons PD. Podophyllin 10% and 25% in the treatment of ano-genital warts: a comparative double-blind study. *Br J Venereal Dis* 1981;57: 208–209.

41. Gabriel G, Thin RN. Treatment of anogenital warts. Comparison of trichloroacetic acid and podophyllin versus podophyllin alone. *Br J Venereal Dis* 1983; 59:124–126.

42. Schwartz DB, Greenberg MD, Daoud Y, Reid R. Genital condylomas in pregnancy: use of trichloroacetic acid and laser therapy. *Am J Obstet Gynecol* 1988;158(6 pt 1):1407–1416.

43. Keay S, Teng N, Eisenberg M, Story B, Sellers PW, Merigan TC. Topical interferon for treating condyloma acuminata in women. *J Infect Dis* 1988;158:934–939.

44. Syed TA, Ahmadpour OA: Human leukocyte derived interferon-α in a hydrophilic gel for the treatment of intravaginal warts in women: a placebo-controlled, double-blind study. *Int J STD AIDS* 1998;9:769–772.

45. Gross G, Rogozinski T, Schofer H, et al. Recombinant interferon β gel as an adjuvant in the treatment of recurrent genital warts: results of a placebo-controlled double blind study of 120 patients. *Dermatology* 1998;196:330–334.

46. Eron LJ, Judson F, Tucker S, et al. Interferon therapy for condylomata acuminata. *N Engl J Med* 1986;315:1059–1064.

47. Friedman-Kien AE, Eron LJ, Conant M, et al. Natural interferon alfa for treatment of condylomata acuminata. *JAMA* 1988;259:533–538.

48. Friedman-Kien A. Management of condylomata acuminata with Alferon N injection, interferon alfa-n3 (human leukocyte derived). *Am J Obstet Gynecol* 1995;172(4 pt 2):1359–1368.

49. Monsonego J, Cessot G, Ince SE, Galazka AR, Abdul-Ahad AK. Randomised double-blind trial of recombinant interferon-β for condyloma acuminatum. *Genitourin Med* 1996;72:111–114.

50. Reichman RC, Oakes D, Bonnez W, et al. Treatment of condyloma acuminatum with three different interferons administered intralesionally: a double-blind, placebo-controlled trial. *Ann Intern Med* 1988;108:675–679.

51. Scott GM, Csonka GW. Effect of injections of small doses of human fibroblast interferon into genital warts: a pilot study. *Br J Venereal Dis* 1979;55: 442–445.

52. Vance JC, Bart BJ, Hansen RC, et al. Intralesional recombinant α-2 interferon for the treatment of patients with condyloma acuminatum or verruca plantaris. *Arch Dermatol* 1986;122:272–277.

53. Welander CE, Homesley HD, Smiles KA, Peets EA. Intralesional interferon alfa-2b for the treatment of genital warts. *Am J Obstet Gynecol* 1990;162: 348–354.

54. Bornstein J, Pascal B, Zarfati D, et al. Recombinant human interferon-β for condylomata acuminata: a randomized, double-blind, placebo controlled study of intralesional therapy. *Int J STD AIDS* 1997;8:614–621.

55. Armstrong DK, Maw RD, Dinsmore WW, et al. A randomised, double-blind, parallel group study to compare subcutaneous interferon α-2a plus podophyllin with placebo plus podophyllin in the treatment of primary condylomata acuminata. *Genitourin Med* 1994;70:389–393.

56. Armstrong DK, Maw RD, Dinsmore WW, et al. Combined therapy trial with interferon α-2a and ablative therapy in the treatment of anogenital warts. *Genitourin Med* 1996;72:103–107.

57. Condylomata International Collaborative Study Group. Recurrent condylomata acuminata treated with recombinant interferon alfa-2a: a multicenter double-blind placebo-controlled clinical trial. *JAMA* 1991;265:2684–2687.

58. Condylomata International Collaborative Study Group. Recurrent condylomata acuminata treated with recombinant interferon α-2a: a multicenter double-blind placebo-controlled clinical trial. *Acta Derm Venereol* 1993;73:223–226.

59. Gall SA, Constantine L, Koukol D. Therapy of persistent human papillomavirus disease with two different interferon species. *Am J Obstet Gynecol* 1991;164(1 pt 1):130–134.

60. Olmos L, Vilata J, Rodriguez Pichardo A, Lloret A, Ojeda A, Calderon MD. Double-blind, randomized clinical trial on the effect of interferon-β in the treatment of condylomata acuminata. *Int J STD AIDS* 1994;5:182–185.

61. Reichman RC, Oakes D, Bonnez W, et al. Treatment of condyloma acuminatum with three different interferon-α preparations administered parenterally: a double-blind, placebo-controlled trial. *J Infect Dis* 1990;162:1270–1276.

62. Condylomata International Collaborative Study Group. A comparison of interferon alfa-2a and podophyllin in the treatment of primary condylomata acuminata. *Genitourin Med* 1991;67:394–399.

63. Benedetti Panici P, Scambia G, Baiocchi G, Perrone L, Pintus C, Mancuso S. Randomized clinical trial comparing systemic interferon with diathermocoagulation in primary multiple and widespread anogenital condyloma. *Obstet Gynecol* 1989;74(3 pt 1):393–397.

64. Bonnez W, Oakes D, Bailey-Farchione A, et al. A randomized, double-blind, placebo-controlled trial of systemically administered interferon-α, -β, or -γ in combination with cryotherapy for the treatment of condyloma acuminatum. *J Infect Dis* 1995; 171:1081–1089.

65. Condylomata International Collaborative Study Group. Randomized placebo-controlled double-blind combined therapy with laser surgery and systemic interferon-α 2a in the treatment of anogenital condylomata acuminatum. *J Infect Dis* 1993;167:824–829.

66. Petersen C, Bjerring P, Larson J, et al. Systemic interferon α-2b increases the cure rate in laser treated patients with multiple persistent genital warts: a placebo-controlled study. *Genitourin Med* 1991;67:99–102.

67. Reid R, Greenberg MD, Pizzuti DJ, Omoto KH, Rutledge LH, Soo W. Superficial laser vulvectomy. V. Surgical debulking is enhanced by adjuvant systemic interferon. *Am J Obstet Gynecol* 1992; 166:815–820.

68. Bonnez W, Oakes D, Bailey-Farchione A, et al. A randomized, double blind trial of parenteral low dose versus high dose interferon β in combination with cryotherapy for treatment of condyloma acuminatum. *Antiviral Res* 1997;35:41–52.

69. Kirby PK, Kiviat N, Beckman A, Wells D, Sherwin S, Corey L. Tolerance and efficacy of recombinant human interferon γ in the treatment of refractory genital warts. *Am J Med* 1988;85:183–188.

70. Reichman RC, Micha JP, Weck PK, et al. Interferon α-n1 (Wellferon) for refractory genital warts: efficacy and tolerance of low dose systemic therapy. *Antiviral Res* 1988;10(1–3):41–57.

71. Von Krogh G. The beneficial effect of 1% 5-fluorouracil in 70% ethanol on therapeutically refractory condylomas in the preputial cavity. *Sex Transm Dis* 1978;5:137–140.

72. Krebs H. Treatment of extensive vulvar condylomata acuminata with topical 5-fluorouracil. *South Med J* 1990;83:761–764.

73. Haye KR. Treatment of condyloma acuminata with 5 per cent 5-fluorouracil (5-FU) cream [letter]. *Br J Vener Dis* 1974;50:466.

74. Dreicer R, Love RR. High total dose 5-fluorouracil treatment during pregnancy. *Wis Med J* 1991;90: 582–583.

75. Van Le L, Pizzuti DJ, Greenberg M, Reid R. Accidental use of low-dose 5-fluorouracil in pregnancy. *J Reprod Med* 1991;36:872–874.

76. Duus BR, Philipsen T, Christensen JD, Lundvall F, Sondergaard J. Refractory condyloma acuminata: a controlled clinical trial of carbon dioxide laser versus conventional surgical treatment. *Genitourin Med* 1985;61:59–61.

77. Kryger-Baggesen N, Falck Larsen J, Hjortkjaer Pedersen P. CO_2 laser treatment of condylomata acuminata. *Acta Obstet Gynecol Scand* 1984;63: 341–343.

DJ Wiley

Assistant Professor in Residence
School of Nursing Primary Care
University of California
Los Angeles, CA
USA

Competing interests: DJW has been a consultant to 3M Pharmaceuticals and has received research funding from Merck and Co.

Sexual health

Gonorrhoea

Search date August 2001

John Moran

INTERVENTIONS

Beneficial
Single dose regimens using selected fluoroquinolones, selected cephalosporins, or spectinomycin in uncomplicated infection* . . .318
Single dose regimens using selected cephalosporins or spectinomycin in uncomplicated infection in pregnant women 319

Likely to be beneficial
Selected injectable fluoroquinolones or selected injectable cephalosporins in disseminated infection** . . .320

Unknown effectiveness
Dual treatment for gonorrhoea and chlamydia infections in all people diagnosed with gonorrhoea 320

*Based on comparisons of results across arms of different trials.
**Based only on non-RCT evidence and consensus.

Key Messages

- One systematic review and other clinical trials have found that many anti-microbial agents other than penicillin and tetracycline achieve cure rates of 97% or higher. Cure rates were lower (≤ 80%) for pharyngeal infection. Most regimens cause few adverse effects. Resistance is now widespread to penicillins, tetracyclines, and sulphonamides.

- We found little evidence on treatment in pregnant women. Two RCTs found that antibiotics were effective in pregnant women. We found no reports of serious adverse effects.

- We found no recent trials evaluating treatments for disseminated gonococcal infection, but found no reports of treatment failures.

- Dual treatment for gonorrhoea and chlamydia infections is based on theory and expert opinion rather than on evidence from clinical trials. The balance between benefits and harms will vary with the prevalence of co-infection in each population.

DEFINITION Gonorrhoea is caused by infection with *Neisseria gonorrhoeae*. In men, uncomplicated urethritis is the most common manifestation, with dysuria and urethral discharge. Less typically, signs and symptoms are mild and indistinguishable from chlamydial urethritis. In women the most common manifestation is cervicitis, which produces symptoms (e.g. vaginal discharge, lower abdominal discomfort, and dyspareunia) in only half of the women. Co-infection with chlamydia is reported in 20–40% of people.[1]

INCIDENCE/ Between 1975 and 1996, the incidence of reported gonorrhoea in
PREVALENCE the USA fell by 74%, reaching a level in 1996 of 122/100 000 people. Since 1996, between 123 and 133 cases have been reported per 100 000 people each year.[2] In the UK, diagnoses of gonorrhoea have increased since 1994, reaching 39/100 000 males and 17/100 000 females in 1999.[3] In poor communities, rates may be higher: the estimated incidence in people aged 15–59 years living in three inner London boroughs in 1994–1995 was 138/100 000 women and 292/100 000 men.[4] Rates are highest in younger people. In the USA in 1999, incidence was highest in women aged 15–19 years (716/100 000) and men aged 20–24 years (590/100 000).[2]

AETIOLOGY/ Most infections result from penile-vaginal, penile-rectal, or penile-
RISK FACTORS pharyngeal contact. An important minority of infections are transmitted from mother to child during birth, which can cause ophthalmia neonatorum. Less common are ocular infections in older children and adults as a result of sexual exposure, poor hygiene, or the medicinal use of urine.

PROGNOSIS The natural history of untreated gonococcal infection is spontaneous resolution after weeks or months of unpleasant symptoms. During this time, there is a substantial likelihood of transmission to others and of complications developing in the infected individual.[5] Symptoms in most men are severe enough to cause them to seek treatment, but an estimated 1–3% of infected men remain asymptomatic. These men, and men who are infectious but not yet symptomatic, are largely responsible for the spread of the disease. In many women, the lack of readily discernible signs or symptoms of cervicitis means that infections go unrecognised and untreated. An unknown proportion of untreated infections causes local complications, including lymphangitis, periurethral abscess, bartholinitis, and urethral stricture; epididymitis in men; and in women involvement of the uterus, fallopian tubes, or ovaries causing pelvic inflammatory disease (see pelvic inflammatory disease, p 324). It is the association of gonorrhoea with pelvic inflammatory disease — a major cause of secondary infertility, ectopic pregnancy, and chronic pelvic pain — that makes gonorrhoea an important public health issue. Manifestations of disseminated infection are petechial or pustular skin lesions; asymmetrical arthropathies, tenosynovitis or septic arthritis; and, rarely, meningitis or endocarditis.

AIMS To relieve symptoms; avoid complications; and prevent further transmission, with minimal adverse effects of treatment.

OUTCOMES   Microbiological cure rates (number of infected people or infected sites culture-negative 1–14 days after treatment, divided by number of infected people or infected sites cultured 1–14 days after treatment).

METHODS   *Clinical Evidence* search and appraisal August 2001. Additional author PubMed search October 2001. Key words: gonorrhoea and *N gonorrhoeae* infections, plus a search of references of key articles and books. Studies were excluded if they defined possible treatment failures as "re-infections", if they did not use end points based on microbiological cure, or if they were based on drug regimens unlikely to be of general use (e.g. those using antibiotic regimens that are toxic or to which resistance is now widespread).[6]

QUESTION   **What are the effects of treatments for uncomplicated infections in men and non-pregnant women?**

One systematic review and other clinical trials have found that many antimicrobial agents other than penicillin and tetracycline achieve cure rates of 97% or higher (see table 1, p 323). Cure rates are lower (≤ 80%) for pharyngeal infection. Most regimens cause few adverse effects. Resistance is now widespread to penicillins, tetracyclines, and sulphonamides.

Benefits: **Uncomplicated urogenital, rectal, and pharyngeal infections:** We found one systematic review (search date 1993).[6] The results were updated to 2001 by the author of the review using the original methods and are tabulated (see table 1, p 323) (JS Moran, personal communication, 2001). The original review identified studies (both RCTs and other clinical trials) published from 1981–1993 that used a single dose regimen based on an antimicrobial other than a β lactamase sensitive penicillin or a tetracycline.[6] The search retrieved studies with a total of 24 383 evaluable people or infections. Combining results across arms of trials, 96% were cured on the basis of culture results. Sites of infection, when specified, included the cervix, urethra, rectum, and pharynx. Comparison of cure rates by site of infection found that cure rates were over 95% for all sites except the pharynx, for which they were about 80% (see table 1, p 323).[9] **Eye infections:** We found no systematic review or RCTs. In the only recent published study of the treatment of gonococcal conjunctivitis, all 12 participants responded well to a single 1 g dose of ceftriaxone.[10]

Harms: Single dose regimens using fluoroquinolones, third generation and extended spectrum cephalosporins, or spectinomycin are generally safe and well tolerated. The most important adverse effects are rare hypersensitivity reactions. Minor adverse effects are most troublesome for the 800 mg cefixime regimen,[11,12] and the 2 g azithromycin regimen;[13] both cause frequent gastrointestinal upset. All the other doses found effective are associated with a low incidence of adverse outcomes. One large observational cohort study of azithromycin, cefixime, ciprofloxacin, and ofloxacin "in everyday use" found few serious adverse effects.[14] Quinolones may cause arthropathy in animals. No evidence of joint toxicity has been observed in clinical use, even with prolonged, multiple dose regimens used for the management of children with cystic fibrosis.[15-19]

Comment: There is good agreement between antigonococcal activity of antimicrobials *in vitro* and their efficacy in clinical trials. A large number of people were evaluated in a range of settings, suggesting that the results can be generalised. However, comparative results from different settings were not provided. Single dose regimens may make adherence more likely. The ceftriaxone and spectinomycin regimens require intramuscular injection. Resistance is now widespread for all penicillins, sulphonamides, and tetracyclines, and is common for fluroquinolones in Asia and the Pacific but not elsewhere. Resistance to third generation and extended spectrum cephalosporins or spectinomycin is rarely reported (see table 2, p 323).

QUESTION What are the effects of treatments for uncomplicated infections in pregnant women?

One systematic review and one subsequent RCT have found that antibiotic treatment in pregnancy is effective. We found no reports of serious adverse effects.

Benefits: We found one systematic review (search date 1998; 2 RCTs)[25] of treatments of gonococcal infection during pregnancy. One of the RCTs (267 pregnant women with positive cultures for gonorrhoea) compared amoxicillin versus probenecid, spectinomycin, and ceftriaxone regimens. Eradication rates ranged from 89–97%. Single dose ceftriaxone 250 mg cured 95% (95% CI 89.2% to 98.5%) of rectal and cervical infections and 100% (95% CI 54.1% to 100%) of pharyngeal infections; spectinomycin 2 g cured 97% (95% CI 91.5% to 99.4%) of rectal and cervical infections and 83% (95% CI 35.9% to 99.6%) of pharyngeal infections. The second RCT (95 women with positive cultures for gonorrhoea) was only included in the review in abstract form. The subsequent full publication compared a single dose of ceftriaxone intramuscularly versus a single dose of cefixime orally.[26] It found that eradication rates were similar in the two groups: ceftriaxone 125 mg eradicated 96.8% (95% CI 89.0% to 99.6%) of cervical and rectal infections and 100% (95% CI 47.8% to 100%) of pharyngeal infections versus cefixime 400 mg that eradicated 96% (95% CI 88.8% to 99.6%) of cervical and rectal infections and 100% (95% CI 54.1% to 100%) of pharyngeal infections.

Harms: The systematic review reported vomiting after treatment in 1/267 women included in one trial.[25] The second RCT reported soreness at the injection site among women receiving ceftriaxone and some "minor" malformations among their children, generally cosmetic (e.g. nevus, café au lait spots, skin tag; 10/60 [16.7%] with ceftriaxone *v* 7/62 [11.3%] with cefixime).[26] Because quinolones cause arthropathy in animals, their use is not recommended in pregnancy, although we found no reports of adverse effects of quinolones on pregnancy outcome in humans. A single, multicentre, prospective, controlled study of 200 exposed women found no evidence of adverse effects.[27] We found no evidence that the non-quinolone regimens listed above are less safe or less well tolerated by pregnant women than by men or non-pregnant women.

Comment: None.

QUESTION **What are the effects of treatments for disseminated gonococcal infection?**

We found no recent trials evaluating treatment for disseminated gonococcal infection. We found no reports of treatment failures with multidose regimens using injectable cephalosporins or quinolones.

Benefits: We found no systematic review and no studies of the treatment of disseminated gonococcal infection published in the last 20 years.

Harms: We found no reports of adverse effects of multidose regimens using injectable cephalosporins or quinolones in this context.

Comment: More than a hundred clinical trials involving over 20 000 people have found that many single dose antimicrobial regimens cure uncomplicated infections more than 90% of the time.[6] Given the protracted natural history without treatment, this evidence suggests that treatment with these antimicrobial regimens is beneficial. Which regimens are most beneficial cannot be determined precisely because direct randomised comparisons of the best different regimens have not been performed. However, analysis of available trials supports the consensus that the most effective regimens are those using selected third generation or expanded spectrum cephalosporins and, except where resistance is common, those using selected fluoroquinolones or spectinomycin. We found no RCTs of antibiotic treatment in complicated gonorrhoea, but there is a strong consensus supporting the view that the most effective treatments for these conditions are multidose regimens using injectable cephalosporins or quinolones. Although we found no published data establishing the efficacy of this treatment, we found no reports of treatment failures.

QUESTION **What are the effects of dual treatment for gonorrhoea and chlamydia infection?**

Dual treatment with an antimicrobial effective against *Chlamydia trachomatis* is based on theory and expert opinion rather than evidence. The balance between benefits and harms from controlled trials will vary with the prevalence of co-infection in each population.

Benefits: We found no systematic review or RCTs.

Harms: We found no good evidence on the harms of dual treatment. Treatment for chlamydia can cause mild gastrointestinal distress, and there is the possibility that using a second drug could stimulate the emergence or spread of resistance in *N gonorrhoeae* or other bacteria.

Comment: Routine dual treatment has been advocated and implemented for the last 10 years, and is believed to have two potential benefits. First, it is believed by some to have contributed to the decline in the prevalence of chlamydia infection observed in some populations.

We found no evidence for any direct effect of dual treatment on chlamydia prevalence. Other factors may have contributed to reduced chlamydia prevalence (including widespread screening for asymptomatic chlamydia infection and changes in sexual behaviour), making it difficult to attribute decreases in the prevalence of chlamydia infection to any specific cause. Secondly, routine dual treatment may retard the spread of resistant gonococcal strains. Limited data from case reports support this belief. In the past, chlamydia testing was often unavailable, expensive, time consuming, and not highly sensitive, whereas dual treatment with a tetracycline, such as doxycycline, was safe and inexpensive. Chlamydia testing has now become more widely available, more affordable, quicker, and more sensitive, and the prevalence of chlamydia has fallen in some populations. Nevertheless, chlamydia is still found in 20–40% of people with gonorrhoea in many clinics.[1]

REFERENCES

1. Centers for Disease Control and Prevention. 1998 Guidelines for the treatment of sexually transmitted diseases. *Morb Mortal Wkly Rep* 1998;47(RR-1):60.

2. Division of STD Prevention, Centers for Disease Control and Prevention, Sexually transmitted diseases surveillance, 2000. Atlanta, GA: US Department of Health and Human Services, Centers for Disease Control and Prevention, September 2001. http://www.cdc.gov/std/stats

3. PHLS, DHSS and PS, Scottish ISD(D)5 Collaborative Group. Trends in sexually transmitted infections in the United Kingdom, 1990 to 1999. London: Public Health Laboratory Service, 2000. http://www.phls.co.uk/facts/STI/sti.htm

4. Low N, Daker-White G, Barlow D, Pozniak AI. Gonorrhoea in inner London: results of a cross-sectional study. *BMJ* 1997;314:1719–1723.

5. Hook EW, Handsfield HH. Gonococcal infections in the adult. In: Holmes KK, Mardh P-A, Sparling PF, et al, eds. *Sexually Transmitted Diseases* 3rd ed. New York: McGraw-Hill, 1999.

6. Moran JS, Levine WC. Drugs of choice for the treatment of uncomplicated gonococcal infections. *Clin Infect Dis* 1995;20(suppl 1):47–65. Search date 1993; primary sources Medline, reference lists from retrieved articles, abstracts from the annual Interscience Conference on Antimicrobial Agents and Chemotherapy, and meetings of the International Society for Sexually Transmitted Disease Research 1990–1993.

7. Aplasca de los Reyes MR, Pato-Mesola V et al. A randomized trial of ciprofloxacin versus cefixime for treatment of gonorrhea after rapid emergence of gonococcal ciprofloxacin resistance in the Philippines. *Clin Infect Dis* 2001;32:1313–1318.

8. Rahman M, Alam A, Nessa K, et al. Treatment failure with the use of ciprofloxacin for gonorrhea correlates with the prevalence of fluoroquinolone-resistant *Neisseria gonorrhoeae* strains in Bangladesh. *Clin Infect Dis* 2001;32:884–889.

9. Moran JS. Treating uncomplicated *Neisseria gonorrhoeae* infections: is the anatomic site of infection important? *Sex Transm Dis* 1995;22:39–47.

10. Haimovici R, Roussel TJ. Treatment of gonococcal conjunctivitis with single-dose intramuscular ceftriaxone. *Am J Ophthalmol* 1989;107:511–514.

11. Handsfield HH, McCormack WM, Hook EW III, et al. The Gonorrhea Treatment Study Group. A comparison of single-dose cefixime with

ceftriaxone as treatment for uncomplicated gonorrhea. *N Engl J Med* 1991;325:1337–1341.

12. Megran DW, LeFebvre K, Willets V, Bowie WR. Single-dose oral cefixime versus amoxicillin plus probenecid for the treatment of uncomplicated gonorrhea in men. *Antimicrob Agents Chemother* 1990;34:355–357.

13. Handsfield HH, Dalu ZA, Martin DH, et al. Azithromycin Gonorrhea Study Group. Multicenter trial of single-dose azithromycin vs. ceftriaxone in the treatment of uncomplicated gonorrhea. *Sex Transm Dis* 1994;21:107–111.

14. Wilton LV, Pearce GL, Mann RD. A comparison of ciprofloxacin, norfloxacin, ofloxacin, azithromycin and cefixime examined by observational cohort studies. *Br J Clin Pharmacol* 1996;41:277–284.

15. Green SD. Indications and restrictions of fluoroquinolone use in children. *Br J Hosp Med* 1996;56:420–423.Grenier B. Use of fluoroquinolones in children. An overview. *Adv Antimicrob Antineoplastic Chemother* 1992; 11–12:135–140.

16. Schaad UB. Use of quinolones in children and articular risk. *Arch Pediatr* 1996;3:183–184.

17. Hampel B, Hullmann R, Schmidt H. Ciprofloxacin in pediatrics: worldwide clinical experience based on compassionate use. Safety report. *Pediatr Infect Dis J* 1997;16:127–129.

18. Warren RW. Rheumatologic aspects of pediatric cystic fibrosis patients treated with fluoroquinolones. *Pediatr Infect Dis J* 1997;16:118–122.

19. Ye SZ. Survey on antibiotic sensitivity of Neisseria gonorrhoeae strains isolated in China, 1987–1992. *Sex Transm Dis* 1994;21:237–240.

20. Guoming L, Qun C, Shengchun W. Resistance of Neisseria gonorrhoeae epidemic strains to antibiotics: report of resistant isolates and surveillance in Zhanjiang, China: 1998–1999. *Sex Transm Dis* 2000;27:115–118.

21. The WHO Western Pacific Region Gonococcal Antimicrobial Surveillance Programme. Surveillance of antibiotic resistance in *Neisseria gonorrhoeae* in the WHO Western Pacific Region, 2000. *Commun Dis Intell* 2001;25:274–276.

22. Public Health Laboratory Service. The Gonococcal Resistance to Antimicrobials Surveillance Programme Annual Report, Year 2000 Collection. http://www.phls.co.uk/facts/STI/files/grasp_report.pdf

23. Fiorito S, Galarza P, Pagano I, et al. Emergence of high level ciprofloxacin resistant Neisseria gonorrhoeae strain in Buenos Aires, Argentina. *Sex Transm Infect* 2001;77:77.

25. Brocklehurst P. Interventions for treating gonorrhoea in pregnancy (Cochrane Review). In: The Cochrane Library, Issue 2, 2001. Oxford: Update Software. Search date 1998; primary sources Cochrane Pregnancy and Childbirth Group Register, and The Cochrane Controlled Trials Register.
26. Ramus RM, Sheffield JS, Mayfield JA, Wendel GD Jr. A randomized trial that compared oral cefixime and intramuscular ceftriaxone for the treatment of gonorrhea in pregnancy. *Am J Obstet Gynecol* 2001;185:629–632.
27. Loebstein R, Addis A, Ho E, et al. Pregnancy outcome following gestational exposure to fluoroquinolones: a multicenter prospective controlled study. *Antimicrob Agents Chemother* 1998;42:1336–1339.

John Moran
Medical Epidemiologist
Centers for Disease Control and
Prevention
Atlanta
USA

Competing interests: None declared.

TABLE 1	Effectiveness of selected single dose regimens in published clinical trials[6] and updated to 2001 (see text, p 318).

Drug and dose	Pharyngeal infections		Urogenital and rectal infections	
	% cured	95% CI	% cured	95% CI
Ceftriaxone 250 mg	98.9	94.0 to 100	99.2	98.8 to 99.5
Ciprofloxacin 500 mg*	97.2	85.5 to 99.9	99.8	98.7 to 100
Ciprofloxacin 250 mg	88.5	81.8 to 95.2	98.7	98.0 to 99.4
Ceftriaxone 125 mg	94.1	85.6 to 98.4	98.8	97.9 to 99.8
Gatifloxacin 600 mg	100	82.3 to 100	99.6	97.7 to 100
Spectinomycin 2 g	51.8	38.7 to 64.9	98.2	97.6 to 98.9
Azithromycin 2 g	100	82.3 to 100	99.2	97.2 to 99.9
Ofloxacin 400 mg	89.7	71.6 to 97.8	98.6	97.8 to 99.4
Gatifloxacin 400 mg	100	63.1 to 100	99.2	97.1 to 99.9
Cefixime 800 mg	80.0	51.9 to 95.7	98.4	95.9 to 99.6
Cefixime 400 mg	92.3	74.9 to 99.1	97.3	95.9 to 98.6

Data have been updated to include those from eligible studies published between 1993 and 2001. Only those regimens that are available in the USA, and have been shown in published studies to cure more than 95% of uncomplicated urogenital and rectal infections (with a lower 95% confidence limit > 95%), have been selected.
* Excludes two published clinical trials among people known to be at high risk of harbouring fluoroquinolone resistant strains; ciprofloxacin 500 mg cured only 48/72 [67%] of cervical infections in one trial [7] and 41/66 [62%] in the other.[8]

TABLE 2	Reported resistance of N gonorrhoeae to antimicrobials (see text, p 319).

Drug	Resistance
Sulphonamides	Widespread
Penicillins	Widespread
Tetracyclines	Widespread
Third generation cephalosporins (e.g. ceftriaxone, cefixime)	Two reports from China[20,21]
Spectinomycin	Rare
Quinolones	Parts of Asia: common[22]
	USA: in 2000, resistance to ciprofloxacin was reported in 0.2% of isolates from the mainland and in 14% of isolates from Hawaii[2]
	UK: among 3166 gonorrhoeae isolates tested in 2000, 1.8% were flouroquinolone resistant and a further 2.4% showed decreased susceptibility[23]
	Australia, New Zealand, and Pacific Islands: 0–14%[22]
	South America: One fluoroquinolone resistant isolate reported[24]

Pelvic inflammatory disease

Search date August 2001

Jonathan Ross

INTERVENTIONS

Key Messages

- We found no good evidence comparing empirical treatment with antibiotics (before receiving results of microbiological tests) versus delaying treatment until test results are available.

- One systematic review has found that several regimens of antibiotic treatment are effective in relieving the symptoms of pelvic inflammatory disease and achieving high rates of microbiological cure.

- We found no good evidence on the optimal duration of treatment. Two RCTs found no significant difference between different oral and parenteral regimens.

- One systematic review found that routine prophylaxis with doxycycline prior to intrauterine contraceptive device insertion did not reduce the risk of pelvic inflammatory disease. The absolute risk of pelvic inflammatory disease following intrauterine contraceptive device insertion was low. However, the systematic review may have insufficient power to rule out a clinically important difference.

DEFINITION	Pelvic inflammatory disease is inflammation and infection of the upper genital tract in women, typically involving the fallopian tubes, ovaries, and surrounding structures.
INCIDENCE/ PREVALENCE	The exact incidence of pelvic inflammatory disease is unknown because the disease cannot be diagnosed reliably from clinical symptoms and signs.[1–3] Direct visualisation of the fallopian tubes by laparoscopy is the best single diagnostic test, but it is invasive and not used routinely in clinical practice. Pelvic inflammatory disease is the most common gynaecological reason for admission to hospital in the USA, accounting for 49/10 000 recorded hospital discharges. However, because most pelvic inflammatory diseases are asymptomatic, this figure underestimates the true prevalence.[1,4] A crude marker of pelvic inflammatory disease in developing countries can be obtained from reported hospital admission rates, where it accounts for 17–40% of gynaecological admissions in sub-Saharan Africa, 15–37% in Southeast Asia, and 3–10% in India.[5]
AETIOLOGY/ RISK FACTORS	Factors associated with pelvic inflammatory disease mirror those for sexually transmitted infections: young age, reduced socioeconomic circumstances, African/Afro-Caribbean ethnicity, lower educational attainment, and recent new sexual partner.[2,6,7] Most cases seem to result from ascending infection from the cervix. Initial epithelial damage caused by bacteria (especially *Chlamydia trachomatis* and *Neisseria gonorrhoeae*) allows the opportunistic entry of other organisms. Isolates from the upper genital tract are polymicrobial, including *Mycoplasma hominis* and anaerobes.[8] The spread of infection to the upper genital tract may be increased by vaginal douching and instrumentation of the cervix, but reduced by the barrier method and oral contraceptives compared with other forms of contraception.[9–12]
PROGNOSIS	Pelvic inflammatory disease has high morbidity; about 20% of affected women become infertile, 20% develop chronic pelvic pain, and 10% of those who conceive have an ectopic pregnancy.[2] We found no placebo controlled trials of antibiotic treatment. Uncontrolled observations suggest that clinical symptoms and signs resolve in a significant number of untreated women.[13] Repeated episodes of pelvic inflammatory disease are associated with a four to six times increase in the risk of permanent tubal damage.[14]
AIMS	To alleviate the pain and systemic malaise associated with infection; to achieve microbiological cure; to prevent development of permanent tubal damage with associated sequelae, such as chronic pelvic pain, ectopic pregnancy, and infertility; and to prevent the spread of infection to others.
OUTCOMES	Incidence and severity of acute symptoms and signs; microbiological cure of the upper genital tract; incidence of chronic pelvic pain, ectopic pregnancy, and infertility; rate of transmission to others.
METHODS	*Clinical Evidence* search and appraisal August 2001.

| QUESTION | What are the effects of empirical treatment versus treatment delayed until the results of microbiological investigations are known? |

| OPTION | EMPIRICAL ANTIBIOTIC TREATMENT |

We found no good evidence on the effects of empirical treatment versus delayed treatment for suspected pelvic inflammatory disease.

Benefits: We found no systematic review or RCTs comparing empirical versus delayed treatment.

Harms: We found no reliable evidence on harms.

Comment: Because there are no reliable clinical diagnostic criteria for pelvic inflammatory disease, early empirical treatment is common.[3] The positive predictive value of a clinical diagnosis is 65–90% compared with laparoscopy.[1–3] The absence of infection from the lower genital tract, where samples are usually taken, does not exclude pelvic inflammatory disease[2] and so may not influence the decision to treat. One case control study (76 cases and 367 controls) found that delaying treatment is associated with impaired fertility (OR 2.6, 95% CI 1.2 to 5.9).[15]

| QUESTION | How do different antimicrobial regimens compare? |

One systematic review of observational trials and RCTs has found that several regimens of parenteral followed by oral antibiotic treatment are effective in resolving the acute symptoms and signs associated with pelvic inflammatory disease (see table 1, p 329). We found no good evidence on the optimal duration of treatment. Two RCTs found no significant difference between different oral and parenteral regimens.

Benefits: We found one systematic review (search date 1997, 26 studies, 1925 women),[16] which was subsequently updated (search date 1997, 26 studies, 1925 women).[17] These reviews answer different questions and cover different aspects. They evaluated 16 different antimicrobial regimens. The identified studies included case series, and it is not possible from the aggregated data published in the reviews to ascertain how many studies were RCTs. Inclusion criteria were a diagnosis of pelvic inflammatory disease (clinical, microbiological, laparoscopic, or by endometrial biopsy) and microbiological testing for *C trachomatis* and *N gonorrhoeae*. The reviews found antibiotics were effective in relieving the symptoms associated with pelvic inflammatory disease, with clinical and microbiological cure rates of 90–100% (see table 1, p 329). **Duration of treatment:** The duration of treatment was not addressed, although the most common treatment period was 14 days. **Oral versus parenteral treatment:** The reviews did not analyse outcomes by oral or parenteral route of administration. Most regimens started with parenteral treatment and continued with oral treatment at different points. Two RCTs (249 and 72 women) compared oral ofloxacin versus parenteral cefoxitin and doxycycline. The trials found no significant difference in cure rates among groups (clinical cure rates about 95% for all treatments).[18,19]

Harms: The harms associated with treatment were not specifically addressed by the systematic reviews.[16,17] In two RCTs reporting adverse effects, withdrawal from treatment was uncommon (2/20 for doxycycline/metronidazole; 0/20 for perfloxacin/metronidazole; 0/16 for ciprofloxacin).[20,21]

Comment: We found little evidence about long term sequelae of pelvic inflammatory disease, adverse effects of treatment, treatment of pelvic inflammatory disease of differing severity, the effect of ethnicity, or the relevance of tracing sexual contacts. The risks of tubal occlusion and subsequent infertility relate to the severity of pelvic inflammatory disease prior to starting treatment,[22] and clinical improvement may not translate into preserved fertility.[23,24] The inclusion of observational studies in the systematic review without a sensitivity analysis may compromise the validity of the conclusions. Two papers are awaiting translation.[25,26]

QUESTION **What are the effects of routine antibiotic prophylaxis to prevent pelvic inflammatory disease prior to intrauterine contraceptive device insertion?**

One systematic review found that routine prophylaxis with doxycycline prior to intrauterine contraceptive device insertion did not reduce the risk of pelvic inflammatory disease. The absolute risk of pelvic inflammatory disease following intrauterine contraceptive device insertion was low.

Benefits: We found one systematic review (search date 2000, 4 RCTs, 3598 women requesting intrauterine contraceptive device insertion).[27] The trials compared a single dose of doxycycline (200 mg) 1 hour prior to intrauterine device insertion. Meta-analysis found no significant difference in the incidence of pelvic inflammatory disease (doxycycline v placebo OR 0.89, 95% CI 0.53 to 1.51). The rate of pelvic inflammatory disease in all women was low (0.5–1.6%).

Harms: The harms associated with treatment were not specifically addressed by the systematic review.[27] Nausea and vomiting has been reported with 17–28% of healthy volunteers on doxycycline, depending on the formulation administered.[28]

Comment: In the populations included in the systematic review the risk of pelvic inflammatory disease following intrauterine device insertion was low.[27] The occurrence of pelvic inflammatory disease in this group usually reflects the introduction of infection into the uterus during intrauterine device insertion and will therefore vary with the prevalence of sexually transmitted infections in the population. The confidence intervals are wide, suggesting that the study may have insufficient power to rule out a clinical important difference.

REFERENCES

1. Morcos R, Frost N, Hnat M, Petrunak A, Caldito G. Laparoscopic versus clinical diagnosis of acute pelvic inflammatory disease. *J Reprod Med* 1993; 38:53–56.
2. Metters JS, Catchpole M, Smith C, et al. *Chlamydia trachomatis: summary and conclusions of CMO's expert advisory group.* London: Department of Health, 1998.
3. Centers for Disease Control. *1998 guidelines for treatment of sexually transmitted diseases.* Bethesda, Maryland: CDC, 1998. http://www.cdc.gov/epo/mmwr/preview/mmwrhtml/00050909.htm.
4. Velebil P, Wingo PA, Xia Z, Wilcox LS, Peterson HB. Rate of hospitalization for gynecologic disorders among reproductive-age women in the United States. *Obstet Gynecol* 1995;86:764–769.
5. Kani J, Adler MW. Epidemiology of pelvic inflammatory disease. In: Berger GS, Weström L, eds. *Inflammatory disease.* New York: Raven Press, 1992.
6. Simms I, Catchpole M, Brugha R, Rogers P, Mallinson H, Nicoll A. Epidemiology of genital *Chlamydia trachomatis* in England and Wales. *Genitourin Med* 1997;73:122–126.

7. Grodstein F, Rothman KJ. Epidemiology of pelvic inflammatory disease. *Epidemiology* 1994;5: 234–242.

8. Bevan CD, Johal BJ, Mumtaz G, Ridgway GL, Siddle NC. Clinical, laparoscopic and microbiological findings in acute salpingitis: report on a United Kingdom cohort. *Br J Obstet Gynaecol* 1995;102:407–414.

9. Wolner-Hanssen P, Eschenbach DA, Paavonen J, et al. Association between vaginal douching and acute pelvic inflammatory disease. *JAMA* 1990; 263:1936–1941.

10. Jacobson L, Westrom L. Objectivized diagnosis of acute pelvic inflammatory disease. Diagnostic and prognostic value of routine laparoscopy. *Am J Obstet Gynecol* 1969;105:1088–1098.

11. Kelaghan J, Rubin GL, Ory HW, Layde PM. Barrier-method contraceptives and pelvic inflammatory disease. *JAMA* 1982;248:184–187.

12. Wolner-Hanssen P, Eschenbach DA, Paavonen J, et al. Decreased risk of symptomatic chlamydial pelvic inflammatory disease associated with oral contraceptive use. *JAMA* 1990;263:54–59.

13. Curtis AH. Bacteriology and pathology of fallopian tubes removed at operation. *Surg Gynecol Obstet* 1921;33:621.

14. Hillis SD, Owens LM, Marchbanks PA, Amsterdam LF, MacKenzie WR. Recurrent chlamydial infections increase the risks of hospitalization for ectopic pregnancy and pelvic inflammatory disease. *Am J Obstet Gynecol* 1997;176: 103–107.

15. Hillis SD, Joesoef R, Marchbanks PA, et al. Delayed care of pelvic inflammatory disease as a risk factor for impaired fertility. *Am J Obstet Gynecol* 1993;168:1503–1509.

16. Walker CK, Kahn JG, Washington AE, Peterson HB, Sweet RL. Pelvic inflammatory disease: metaanalysis of antimicrobial regimen efficacy. *J Infect Dis* 1993;168:969–978. Search date 1997; primary sources Medline, and bibliographies from reviews, textbooks, and references.

17. Walker CK, Workowski KA, Washington AE, Soper DE, Sweet RL. Anaerobes in pelvic inflammatory disease: implications for the Centers for Disease Control and Prevention's guidelines for treatment of sexually transmitted diseases. *Clin Infect Dis* 1999;28(suppl):29–36. Search date 1997; primary sources Medline, and bibliographies from reviews, textbooks, and references.

18. Martens MG, Gordon S, Yarborough DR, Faro S, Binder D, Berkeley A. Multicenter randomized trial of ofloxacin versus cefoxitin and doxycycline in outpatient treatment of pelvic inflammatory disease. Ambulatory PID Research Group. *South Med J* 1993;86:604–610.

19. Wendel GD, Cox SM, Bawdon RE, Theriot SK, Heard MC, Nobles BJ. A randomized trial of ofloxacin versus cefoxitin and doxycycline in the outpatient treatment of acute salpingitis. *Am J Obstet Gynecol* 1991;164:1390–1396.

20. Witte EH, Peters AA, Smit IB, et al. A comparison of pefloxacin/metronidazole and doxycycline/ metronidazole in the treatment of laparoscopically confirmed acute pelvic inflammatory disease. *Eur J Obstet Gynecol Reprod Biol* 1993;50:153–158.

21. Heinonen PK, Teisala K, Miettinen A, Aine R, Punnonen R, Gronroos P. A comparison of ciprofloxacin with doxycycline plus metronidazole in the treatment of acute pelvic inflammatory disease. *Scand J Infect Dis* 1989;60(suppl): 66–73.

22. Soper DE, Brockwell NJ, Dalton HP. Microbial etiology of urban emergency department acute salpingitis: treatment with ofloxacin. *Am J Obstet Gynecol* 1992;167:653–660.

23. Buchan H, Vessey M, Goldacre M, Fairweather J. Morbidity following pelvic inflammatory disease. *Br J Obstet Gynaecol* 1993;100:558–562.

24. Brunham RC, Binns B, Guijon F, et al. Etiology and outcome of acute pelvic inflammatory disease. *J Infect Dis* 1988;158:510–517.

25. Fischbach F, Deckardt R, Graeff H. Ciprofloxacin/ Metronidazol vs. Cefoxitin/Doxycyclin: Vergleich zweier Therapieschemata zur Behandlung der akuten pelvinen Infektion. *Geburtsh u. Frauenheilk* 1994;54:337–340.

26. Ciraru-Vigneron N, Bergcau G, Sauvanet E, et al. Amoxicillin-clavulanic acid combination versus triple drug therapy for the treatment of severe pelvic inflammatory disease. *Path Biol* 1986;34: 665–668.

27. Grimes DA, Schulz KF. Antibiotic prophylaxis for intrauterine contraceptive device insertion. In: The Cochrane Library, Issue 2, 2001. Oxford: Update Software. Search date December 2000; primary sources Medline, Embase, hand search of journals through CENTRAL, lists of references, and contact with experts in the field.

28. Story MJ, McCloud PI, Boehm G. Doxycycline tolerance study. Incidence of nausea after doxycycline administration to healthy volunteers: a comparison of 2 formulations (Doryx' vs Vibramycin'). *Eur J Clin Pharmacol* 1991;40: 419–421.

Jonathan Ross
Honorary Senior Lecturer
University of Birmingham
Birmingham
UK

Competing interests: None declared.

TABLE 1	Cure rates for the antibiotic treatment of acute pelvic inflammatory disease: aggregated data from systematic reviews of RCTs and case series (see text, p 326).[16,17]

Drug regimen	Number of studies	Number of women	Cure rate (%) clinical/ microbiological*
Inpatient treatment (initially parenteral switching to oral)			
Clindamycin + aminoglycoside	11	470	91/97
Cefoxitin + doxycycline	8	427	91/98
Cefotetan + doxycycline	3	174	95/100
Ceftizoxime + tetracycline	1	18	88/100
Cefotaxime + tetracycline	1	19	94/100
Ciprofloxacin	4	90	94/96
Ofloxacin	1	36	100/97
Sulbactam/ ampicillin + doxycycline	1	37	95/100
Co-amoxiclav	1	32	93/–
Metronidazole + doxycycline	2	36	75/71
Outpatient treatment (oral unless indicated otherwise)			
Cefoxitin (im) + probenecid + doxycycline	3	219	89/93
Ofloxacin	2	165	95/100
Co-amoxiclav	1	35	100/100
Sulbactam/ampicillin	1	36	70/70
Ceftriaxone (im) + doxycycline	1	64	95/100
Ciprofloxacin + clindamycin	1	67	97/94

im, intramuscular; *N gonorrhoeae, C trachomatis, or both, when detected in lower genital tract.

Skin disorders

Search date October 2001

Fay Crawford

INTERVENTIONS

Key Messages

- Systematic reviews have found strong evidence that topical treatments (including allylamines, azoles, undecenoic acid, and tolnaftate) versus placebo increase mycological cure rates in fungal skin infections of the foot.

- One systematic review has found that topical allylamines produce a faster response than azoles but the cure rates are similar. We found no evidence of significant differences in efficacy between individual allylamines or individual azoles, or between allylamines and butenafine.

- One systematic review has found that both oral allylamines and azoles improve cure rates of tinea pedis compared with placebo. We found no evidence of significant differences in cure rate among different oral allylamines, different oral azoles, or between oral allylamines and oral azoles.

- Single RCTs found that topical ciclopiroxolamine, griseofulvin, or acidified nitrite cream were more effective than placebo, but griseofulvin was less effective than terbinafine for curing athlete's foot.

- We found limited evidence from small RCTs that topical butenafine combined with urea or tea tree oil may cure fungal nail infections more frequently than placebo.

- Two RCTs found that topical ciclopiroxolamine improved cure rate compared with placebo in people with fungally infected toenails.

- We found little evidence about long term recurrence rates after different treatments.

DEFINITION	Athlete's foot is a cutaneous fungal infection that causes the skin to itch, flake, and fissure. Nail involvement is characterised by ungual thickening and discolouration.
INCIDENCE/ PREVALENCE	In the UK, athlete's foot is present in about 15% of the general population,[1] and 1.2 million people have fungally infected toe nails.[2]
AETIOLOGY/ RISK FACTORS	Swimming pool users and industrial workers may have increased risk of fungal foot infection. However, one survey found fungal foot infection in only 9% of swimmers, with the highest incidence (20%) in men aged 16 years and over.[1]
PROGNOSIS	Fungal infections of the foot are not life threatening in people with normal immunity, but in some people they cause persistent symptoms. Others are apparently oblivious of persistent infection. The infection can spread to other parts of the body and to other individuals.
AIMS	To control symptoms and prevent recurrence, with minimal adverse effects.
OUTCOMES	Rates of fungal eradication, shown by negative microscopy and culture, and resolution of clinical signs and symptoms at follow up.
METHODS	*Clinical Evidence* search and appraisal October 2001. We initially searched Medline, Embase, and the Cochrane Controlled Trials Register to May 2000 for systematic reviews and subsequent RCTs (all languages). Studies were excluded if foot specific data could not be extracted. We excluded studies that did not use microscopy and culture (skin infections) or culture (nail infections) for diagnosis and as an outcome measure. The evidence is presented for classes of treatment (allylamines, azoles, etc); individual members of each class are described in the text and listed in table 1, see p 338.

QUESTION   **What are the effects of topical antifungals for athlete's foot?**

OPTION   **TOPICAL ALLYLAMINES (NAFTIFINE, TERBINAFINE)**

One systematic review and two subsequent RCTs have found that allylamines are more effective than placebo for curing fungal skin infections. It found insufficient evidence comparing different allylamines with one another. Allylamines produce a faster response than azoles but the cure rates are similar.

Benefits: **Versus placebo:** We found one systematic review,[3,4] and three subsequent RCTs.[5-7] The systematic review (search date 1997, 12 RCTs, 1433 people with fungal infections of the foot) found that topical allylamines versus placebo for 1–4 weeks significantly reduced the risk of treatment failure assessed by culture or microscopy after 6–8 weeks (192/724 [27%] v 570/709 [80%] for placebo; ARR 55%, 95% CI 41% to 70%; RR 0.30, 95% CI 0.24 to 0.38; NNT 2 at 6 wks). The first subsequent RCT (70 people with interdigital tinea pedis and positive fungal culture) found a significant increase in the cure rate after 7 weeks with 7 days of 1%

terbinafine cream versus placebo (mycological cure: 91% with terbinafine v 37% with placebo; CI not provided; P < 0.001).[5] The second subsequent RCT (60 people with moccasin type tinea pedis) compared 1% terbinafine cream versus 1% butenafine (a benzylamine derivative) cream versus placebo.[6] People receiving butenafine applied the cream for 1 week. Placebo and terbinafine were applied for 2 weeks. The RCT found significantly more people cured after 16 weeks with both terbinafine versus placebo and with butenafine versus placebo. The third subsequent RCT (153 people with interdigital tinea pedis) found significantly increased clinical cure after 8 weeks with terbinafine (1% solution) versus placebo (35/56 [65%] terbinafine v 1/23 [4%] with placebo; ARR 60%, 95% CI 45% to 75%). **Different allylamines:** The systematic review identified one small RCT (60 people), which found no significant difference in treatment failure with naftifine versus terbinafine (75% with naftifine v 81% with terbinafine; ARR 5%, 95% CI −17% to +21%). **Versus topical azoles:** See topical azoles, p 332. **Versus butenafine:** We found one RCT (60 people with moccasin type tinea pedis), which compared 1% terbinafine cream versus 1% butenafine cream versus placebo.[6] The RCT found no significant difference in cure rate with terbinafine versus butenafine after 16 weeks (ARR 10%, 95% CI −12% to +32%).

Harms: The systematic review[3,4] did not report frequency of adverse effects. We found few reports of local irritation in any of the trials.

Comment: The systematic review assessed the quality of reporting in the trials. Out of a possible 12 points, the mean quality score for all 72 included studies was 6.3. Few demographic details of participants were reported.[3]

OPTION	TOPICAL AZOLES

One systematic review has found that azole creams administered for 4–6 weeks increase cure rate compared with placebo. We found no evidence of differences in efficacy between individual azoles. Allylamines produce a faster response than azoles but the cure rates are similar.

Benefits: **Versus placebo:** We found one systematic review (search date 1997, 17 RCTs, 1259 people with fungal skin infections of the foot).[3,4] Interventions lasted for 4–6 weeks. The review found a significant reduction of the risk of treatment failure (determined by culture or microscopy after 6–10 wks) with azoles versus placebo (126/664 [19%] with azoles v 362/595 [61%] with placebo; ARR 42%, 95% CI 38% to 48%; RR 0.31, 95% CI 0.25 to 0.38; NNT 2, 95% CI 2 to 3). **Different azoles:** The systematic review (12 RCTs, 584 people) found no consistent difference over 3–10 weeks with one azole for 3–4 weeks versus another.[3,4] **Versus topical allylamines:** We found one systematic review (search date 1997, 12 RCTs, 1487 people with fungal infections of the foot)[3,4] and two additional RCTs.[8,9] The systematic review found a significant reduction after 3–12 weeks in the risk of treatment failure with 1–6 weeks of topical allylamine versus at least 4 weeks of topical azole (146/773 [19%] with topical allylamine v 224/714 [31%] for topical azole; ARR 13%, 95% CI 9% to 16%; RR 0.60, 95% CI 0.49 to

0.73; NNT 8, 95% CI 6 to 12). Four included RCTs found that a 1 week course of allylamine had similar failure rates as a 4 week course of azoles (53/464 [11%] with 1 wk of allylamine v 71/448 [16%] with 4 weeks of azole; ARR 4.4%, 95% CI 0% to 8%).[3,4] The first additional RCT (429 people with interdigital athlete's foot) found no significant difference in mycological cure after 8 weeks with 1% terbinafine solution (twice daily for 1 wk followed by 3 wks of placebo) versus 4 weeks of 1% clotrimazole solution (83% with terbinafine v 82% with clotrimazole; ARR +1%, 95% CI −5% to +8%).[8] The second RCT (48 people) also found no significant difference for mycological cure with 1% terbinafine cream (for 1 wk) versus 4 weeks of 2% clotrimazole cream after 10 weeks (ARR −2%, 95% CI −33% to +28%).[9]

Harms: One subsequent RCT found similar adverse events with 1% terbinafine solution and 1% clotrimazole solution.[8] About 5% of the people experienced mild to moderate local skin reactions, such as itching, erythema, or scaling.

Comment: See table 1 for a list of compounds categorised as topical azoles, p 338.

OPTION   OTHER TOPICAL AGENTS

One systematic review has found that topical undecenoic acid and tolnaftate are more effective than placebo. Single RCTs found that topical ciclopiroxolamine, griseofulvin, or nitrite cream improved cure rates compared with placebo.

Benefits: **Topical ciclopiroxolamine versus placebo:** We found one systematic review (search date 1997, 1 RCT, 144 people with fungal skin infection of the foot).[3,4] The RCT found a significant reduction of treatment failure after 6 weeks with topical ciclopiroxolamine versus placebo for 4 weeks (31/71 [44%] with ciclopiroxolamine v 67/73 [92%] with placebo; ARR 48%, 95% CI 25% to 69%; RRR 0.48, 95% CI 0.25 to 0.73; NNT 2, 95% CI 1 to 4). **Topical griseofulvin versus placebo:** The review identified one RCT (94 people), which found a significant reduction of treatment failure with griseofulvin versus placebo (9/47 [19%] with griseofulvin v 31/47 [66%] with placebo; ARR 47%, 95% CI 28% to 58%; RR 0.29, 95% CI 0.13 to 0.57; NNT 2, 95% CI 2 to 4). **Topical undecenoic acid versus placebo:** The review identified four RCTs (223 people), which found a significant reduction of treatment failure with undecenoic acid versus placebo (40/123 [33%] with undecenoic acid v 81/103 [79%] with placebo; ARR 46%, 95% CI 32% to 58%; RRR 0.41, 95% CI 0.27 to 0.60; NNT 2, 95% CI 2 to 3). **Topical tolnaftate versus placebo:** The review identified three RCTs (148 people), which found a significant reduction after 5–8 weeks in treatment failure with tolnaftate for 4 weeks versus placebo (20/78 [26%] with tolnaftate v 49/70 [70%] with placebo; ARR 44%, 95% CI 29% to 56%; RR 0.37, 95% CI 0.21 to 0.59; NNT 2, 95% CI 2 to 4). **Topical acidified nitrite cream and salicylate versus salicylate:** The review identified one RCT (60 people with interdigital athlete's foot), which found a significant improvement in cure rate with 3% nitrite plus 3% salicylic acid cream for 4 weeks versus 3% salicylic acid alone (completer analysis: 18/19 [95%] with nitrite plus salicylate v 11/16 [69%] with salicylate; ARR 26%, 95% CI 1% to 51%).[10]

Harms: The systematic review did not report frequency of adverse effects. The RCT comparing nitrite plus salicylate found no drug associated adverse events in active or salicylate only groups.[10]

Comment: In the RCT of nitrite plus salicylate versus salicylate alone, only 58% [36/60] of those randomised completed the RCT.

QUESTION **What are the effects of oral antifungal treatments for athlete's foot?**

OPTION **ORAL AZOLES**

We found one systematic review. One included RCT found that oral azoles improved cure rate compared with placebo. The review found no evidence of significant differences in cure rates between individual azoles, between oral azoles and oral allylamines, or between oral azoles and oral griseofulvin.

Benefits: **Versus placebo**: We found one systematic review (search date 2000, 1 RCT, 72 people with tinea pedis).[11] The RCT found a significantly improved cure rate with 1 week of oral itraconazole (200 mg) versus placebo (mycological cure after 8 wks: 20/36 [56%] v 3/36 [8%]; ARR 47%, 95% CI 28% to 65%).[12] **Versus oral allylamines:** See benefits of oral allylamines, p 335. **Versus other azoles:** We found one systematic review (search date 2000, 2 RCTs) of oral fluconazole (50 mg daily for 4 wks) versus another azole.[11] Results were not pooled. The first RCT (35 people with tinea pedis) found no significant difference in cure rate with fluconazole versus itraconazole (100 mg daily) (ARR −5%, 95% CI −24% to +13%).[13] The second RCT (42 people) also found no significant differences in cure rate with fluconazole versus ketoconazole (200 mg daily) (ARR 4%, 95% CI −4% to +12%).[14] **Versus griseofulvin:** We found one systematic review (search date 2000, 1 RCT, 29 people with tinea pedis).[11] The RCT found no significant difference in cure rate with ketoconazole (200 mg daily for 4 wks) versus griseofulvin (1000 mg daily) (ARR −4%, 95% CI −40% to +32%).[15]

Harms: The systematic review[11] found that all RCTs of oral antifungal drugs reported adverse events, mainly gastrointestinal effects. Fluconazole had a lower frequency of adverse events (11%), but the rate was not significantly lower than the rates for griseofulvin or oral allylamines (18%).

Comment: None.

OPTION	ORAL ALLYLAMINES

One RCT found that 2 weeks of oral terbinafine versus 2 weeks of oral itraconazole significantly increased the chance of cure. No differences were detected in the cure rates in RCTs comparing 2 weeks of oral terbinafine versus 4 weeks of oral itraconazole. One systematic review found limited evidence that oral allylamines improved cure rates compared with oral griseofulvin or placebo.

Benefits:
Versus placebo: We found one systematic review (search date 2000, 1 RCT, 41 people with athlete's foot).[11] It found significantly improved cure rates after 8 weeks with terbinafine (250 mg daily for 6 wks) versus placebo (15/23 [65%] with terbinafine v 0/18 [0%] with placebo; ARR 65%, 95% CI 46% to 85%; RR 23.5, 95% CI 2.8 to 226; NNT 2).[16] **Versus azoles:** We found one systematic review (search date 2000, 4 RCTs, 339 people with cutaneous fungal infections of the foot).[11] One of the included RCTs found a significant difference between 2 wks of terbinafine (250 mg daily) and 2 weeks of itraconazole (100mg daily) (ARR 32%, 95% CI 16% to 47%), but the other 3 RCTs (comparing 2 wks of terbinafine versus 4 wks of itraconazole) found no significant difference. Overall, the review found no significant difference in cure rate with oral allylamines (terbinafine 250 mg for 2 wks) versus oral azoles (itraconazole 100 mg for 2 or 4 wks) after 4–16 weeks (128/161 [80%] with terbinafine v 116/178 [65%] with itraconazole; ARR 5%, 95% CI −6% to +17%). **Versus griseofulvin:** We found one systematic review (search date 2000, 2 RCTs, 81 people with tinea pedis).[11] One RCT included only people with interdigital infection; the other included only those with plantar tinea pedis. Pooled analysis found a significantly improved cure rate with terbinafine (250 mg daily) versus griseofulvin (500 mg daily) after 4–6 weeks (35/38 [92%] with terbinafine v 13/33 [39%] with griseofulvin; ARR 52%, 95% CI 33% to 70%).

Harms:
The systematic review found all oral antifungal drugs were associated with adverse events (mainly gastrointestinal).[11] Terbinafine was associated with a greater risk of adverse events (18%), but the rate was not significantly different from that for griseofulvin or oral azoles.

Comment:
None.

QUESTION	What are the effects of topical antifungals for nail infections?

OPTION	FUNGAL NAILS: TOPICAL AGENTS

We found limited evidence from single RCTs that butenafine cream in combination with urea or tea tree oil may improve cure rates compared with placebo in people with fungally infected toe nails. Two RCTs found that ciclopiroxolamine lacquer produced improved cure rates compared with placebo.

Athlete's foot and fungally infected toe nails

Benefits: We found one systematic review (search date 1997, 2 RCTs, 153 people),[3,4] and four subsequent RCTs.[17–19] The systematic review found insufficient evidence to draw conclusions. **Butenafine plus urea:** One subsequent RCT[17] (60 people with fungally infected toenails) found significantly improved cure rate (based on microscopy and culture after 36 wks) with 2% butenafine plus 20% urea cream (twice daily for 1 wk) versus placebo (44/50 [88%] with butenafine plus urea cream v 0/10 [0%] with placebo; ARR 88%, 95% CI 79% to 97%; NNT 2).[17] **Butenafine plus tea tree oil:** One subsequent RCT (60 people, mean age 30 years, mean duration of disease 15 months) found significantly improved cure rates at 16 weeks with 2% butenafine plus 5% tea tree oil versus 5% tea tree oil alone (placebo) (32/40 [80%] with active cream v 0/20 [0%] with placebo; ARR 80%, 95% CI 54% to 90%).[18] **Ciclopiroxolamine versus placebo:** Two subsequent RCTs were reported together.[19] Both found significantly improved mycological cure rates at 48 weeks with 8% ciclopiroxolamine nail lacquer versus placebo (intention to treat analysis, first trial: 211 people, 29% with ciclopiroxolamine v 11% with placebo; ARR 17%, 95% CI 7% to 27%; second trial: 229 people, 36% with ciclopiroxolamine v 9% with placebo; ARR 26% 95% CI 16% to 37%).

Harms: In the RCT of butenafine plus tea tree oil versus tea tree oils alone (placebo), four people reported mild inflammation in the active arm, although adherence to treatment was not affected.[18] The RCTs of ciclopiroxolamine versus placebo found no significant difference in the frequency of adverse events between intervention and control groups except for rash (10% with ciclopiroxolamine v 2% with placebo).[19] Butenafine plus urea cream was associated with mild inflammation in 10% of people.[17]

Comment: Ciclopiroxolamine nail lacquer (8%) is not currently available in the UK. The article describing the RCTs of ciclopiroxolamine referred to 13 other trials of ciclopiroxolamine nail lacquer in people with fungally infected toenails or fingernails, but details were not stated. Reported mycological cure rates with ciclopiroxolamine ranged from about 30% to about 80%.

REFERENCES

1. Gentles JC, Evans EGV. Foot infections in swimming baths. *BMJ* 1973;3:260–262.

2. Roberts DT. Prevalence of dermatophyte onychomycosis in the UK: results of an omnibus survey. *Br J Dermatol* 1992;126(suppl 39): 23–27.

3. Crawford F, Hart R, Bell-Syer S, Torgerson D, Young P, Russell I. Topical treatments for fungal infections of the skin and nails of the foot. In: The Cochrane Library, Issue 3, 2001. Oxford: Update Software. Search date 1997; primary sources Medline, Embase, Cinahl, Cochrane Controlled Trials Register, Science Citation Index, Biosis, CAB-Health, Healthstar, DARE, the NHS Economic Evaluation Database, Econlit, hand searched references and key journals, and pharmaceutical companies contacted.

4. Hart R, Bell-Syer EM, Crawford F, Torgerson DJ, Young P, Russell I. Systematic review of topical treatments for fungal infections of the skin and nails of the feet. *BMJ* 1999;319:79–82. Search date 1997; primary sources Medline, Embase,

Cinahl, Cochrane Controlled Trials Register, Science Citation Index, Biosis, CAB-Health, Healthstar, DARE, the NHS Economic Evaluation Database, Econlit, hand searched references and key journals, and pharmaceutical companies contacted.

5. Korting HC, Tietz HJ, Brautigam M, Mayser P, Rapatz G, Pauls C, for the LAS-INT-06 study group. *Med Mycology* 2000;39:335–340.

6. Syed TA, Hadi SM, Quereshi ZA, Ali SA, Ahamed SA. Butenafine 1% versus terbinafine 1% in cream for the treatment of Tinea Pedis. A placebo controlled double-blind comparative study. *Clin Drug Invest* 2000;19:393–397.

7. Lebwohl M, Elewski B, Eisen D, Savin RC. Efficacy and safety of terbinafine 1% solution in the treatment of interdigital tinea pedis and tinea corporis or tinea cruris. *Cutis* 2001;67:261–266.

8. Schopf R, Hettler O, Brautigam M, et al. Efficacy and tolerability of terbinafine 1% topical solution used for 1 week compared with 4 weeks clotrimazole 1% topical solution in the treatment

of interdigital tinea pedis: a randomised controlled clinical trial. *Mycoses* 1999;42:415–420.

9. Leenutaphong V, Tangwiwat S, Muanprasat C, Niumpradit N, Spitaveesuawan R. Double-blind study of the efficacy of 1 week topical terbinafine cream compared to 4 weeks miconazole cream in patients with tinea pedis. *J Med Assoc Thailand* 1999;82:1006–1009.

10. Weller R, Omerod AD, Hobson RP, Benjamin NJ. A randomised trial of acidified nitrite cream in the treatment of tinea pedis. *J Am Acad Dermatol* 1998;38:559–563.

11. Bell-Syer SEM, Hart R, Crawford F, et al. A systematic review of oral treatments for fungal infections of the skin of the feet. *J Dermatol* 2001;12:69–74. Search date 2000; primary sources DARE, Ecolit, Embase, Healthstar, NHS Economic Evaluation Database, BIDS, Cinahl, Cochrane Controlled Trials Register, Embase, Medline, hand searching of *Brit Podiatr Med*, *The Foot*, *Foot Ankle Int*, and *J Am Podiatr Med Assoc*. Pharmaceutical companies and UK podiatry schools were contacted for unpublished material.

12. Svejgaard E, Avnstorp C, Wanscher B, et al. Efficacy and safety of short-term itraconazole in tinea pedis: a double blind, randomised, placebo controlled trial. *Dermatology* 1998;197:368–372.

13. Difonzo EM, Papini M, Cilli P, et al. A double-blind study comparison of itraconazole and fluconazole in tinea pedis and tinea manuum. *J Eur Acad Dermatol Venereol* 1995;4:148–152.

14. Fischbein A, Haneke E, Lacner K. Comparative evaluation of oral fluconazole and oral ketoconazole in the treatment of fungal infections of the skin. *Int J Dermatol* 1992;31(suppl 2):12–16.

15. Roberts DT, Cox NH, Gentles JC, et al. Comparison of ketoconazole and griseofulvin in the treatment of tinea pedis. *J Med Vet Mycology* 1987;25: 347–350.

16. Savin RC, Zaias N. Treatment of chronic moccasin-type tinea pedis with terbinafine: a double-blind placebo-controlled trial. *J Am Acad Dermatol* 1990;23:804–807.

17. Syed TA, Ahamadpour OA, Ahamad SA, et al. Management of toenail onychomycosis with 2% butenafine and 20% urea cream: a placebo controlled trial. *J Dermatol* 1998;25:648–652.

18. Syed TA, Qureshi ZA, Ali SM, Ahmad SA. Treatment of toenail onychomycosis with 2% butenafine and 5% melaleuca (tea tree) oil in cream. *Trop Med Internat Health* 1999;4: 284–287.

19. Gupta AK, Fleckman P, Baran R. Ciclopirox nail lacquer topical solution 8% in the treatment of toenail onychomycosis. *J Am Acad Dermatol* 2000;43;S70–S80.

Fay Crawford
Senior Research Fellow
University of York
York
UK

Competing interests: None declared.

TABLE 1 Antifungal drugs and antifungal drug classes cited in this topic (See text, p 331).

Antifungal drug classes	Topical compounds	Oral drugs
Azoles	Bifonazole	Fluconazole
	Clotrimazole	Itraconazole
	Econazole	Ketoconazole
	Fenticonazole	
	Ketoconazole	
	Miconazole	
	Oxiconazole	
	Sulconazole	
	Tioconazole	
Allylamines	Naftifine	Terbinafine
	Terbinafine	
Polyenes	Nystatin	Amphotericin B
		Nystatin
Benzylamine derivative	Butenafine	
Morpholines	Amorolfine	
Miscellaneous	Ciclopiroxolamine	Griseofulvin
	Tea Tree Oil	
	Tolnaftate	
	Undecanoates	

Search date September 2001

Dominic Smethurst

INTERVENTIONS

Key Messages

Treatments

- One systematic review has found that topical corticosteroids versus placebo provide symptomatic relief of atopic eczema and are safe in the short term. We found little good information on their long term adverse effects. One RCT found insufficient evidence of the effects of topical steroids in preventing relapse.

- One systematic review has found no significant difference between topical antimicrobial agents plus steroids versus topical steroids alone in improving the clinical signs and symptoms of atopic eczema.

- Limited evidence from one systematic review suggests that emollient plus topical corticosteroid versus topical corticosteroid alone significantly improves clinical signs and symptoms of atopic eczema.

- One systematic review identified no RCTs on the effects of wet wrap or other forms of bandaging.

- RCTs found limited evidence suggesting that controlling house dust mite reduces severity of symptoms, especially in people with positive mite radioallergosorbent test scores and in children, but only if very low levels of mites are achieved.

Atopic eczema

- One systematic review in children and adults with atopic eczema has found inconclusive evidence of the effects of dietary manipulation, such as exclusion of egg and cow's milk.

Prevention in predisposed infants

- Limited observational evidence suggests that exclusive breast feeding for at least 5 months reduces the risk of eczema in infants with a family history of atopy.
- Limited evidence from one systematic review suggests that maternal dietary restriction during lactation may protect against the development of eczema in infants with a family history of atopy. One systematic review has found no significant difference between maternal diet restriction during pregnancy versus no restriction in development of atopic eczema in the infant at 12–18 months.

Avoidance of provoking factors

- RCTs found limited evidence that, in people with atopic eczema, the roughness of clothing textiles is a more important factor for skin irritation than the type of textile fibre (synthetic or natural). One RCT in infants with atopic eczema comparing cotton nappy/diaper versus cellulose core nappy/diaper versus cellulose core nappy/diaper containing absorbent gelling found no significant difference in eczema scores.
- One systematic review has found no significant difference between washing detergents that contain enzymes versus washing detergents without enzymes in eczema severity at 1 month. We found no RCTs of the effect of avoidance of all contact with washing detergents.
- We found no evidence on the effects of vaccination or avoiding animal contact on the severity of atopic eczema.

DEFINITION Atopic eczema (atopic dermatitis) is an inflammatory skin disease characterised by an itchy erythematous poorly demarcated skin eruption with a predilection for skin creases.[1]

INCIDENCE/ PREVALENCE Atopic eczema affects 15–20% of school children in the UK and 2–3% of adults.[2] Prevalence has increased substantially over the past 30 years,[3] possibly because of environmental and lifestyle changes.

AETIOLOGY/ RISK FACTORS Aetiology is believed to be multifactorial. Recent interest has focused on airborne allergens (house dust mites, pollen, animal dander), outdoor pollution, climate, diet, and prenatal/early life factors such as infections.

PROGNOSIS Although there is currently no cure, several interventions can help to control symptoms. Atopic eczema clears in 60–70% of children by their early teens, although relapses may occur.

AIMS To prevent atopic eczema in predisposed infants and children; to minimise the impact of atopic eczema on quality of life in children and adults.

OUTCOMES Severity of symptoms (itching, sleep disturbance) and signs (erythema, oozing/crusting, lichenification, cracking, oedema/papulation, excoriation, and dryness); quality of life; area of skin involvement. Trials used a range of atopic eczema scoring systems, including scoring of atopic dermatitis (SCORAD), six area six sign atopic dermatitis severity score (SASSAD), Rajka and Langeland scoring system, and the dermatology life quality index.

METHODS   *Clinical Evidence* search and appraisal September 2001 and personal contact with experts. Because of the limited studies available for many questions, we included some with shortcomings in methods, which we mention in the text.

QUESTION   **What are the effects of treatments in adults and children with atopic eczema?**

OPTION   **TOPICAL STEROIDS**

One systematic review has found that topical corticosteroids versus placebo improve atopic eczema after 1–4 weeks. Another systematic review comparing a variety of topical steroids versus each other found significant improvement in 22–100% of people after 1–6 weeks. Short term RCTs and one longer term cohort study found no serious systemic adverse effects or skin atrophy associated with topical steroids. Small volunteer studies have found that potent topical steroid preparations cause skin thinning after twice daily application for up to 6 weeks, although skin thickness returns to normal within 4 weeks of stopping treatment. One RCT found insufficient evidence of the effects of topical steroids in preventing relapse.

Benefits: **Versus placebo:** We found one systematic review (search date 1999, 11 RCTs[4–14] in children and adults with atopic eczema) comparing topical steroids versus placebo cream.[15] All of the RCTs found that topical steroid versus placebo significantly improved clinical signs and symptoms of eczema (see table 1, p 353). **Versus each other:** One systematic review (search date 1999, 40 RCTs in children and adults with atopic eczema) comparing a wide variety of topical steroids versus each other found significant improvements in 22–100% of people after 1–6 weeks of treatment.[15] Many of the RCTs identified by the review were of poor quality and the review was unable to draw conclusions about differences in effectiveness between different corticosteroids. **Prevention of relapse:** We found one systematic review (search date 1999),[15] which identified one RCT.[16] The RCT (56 adults with atopic eczema that had "completely healed" with a 4 wk course of fluticasone propionate) compared fluticasone propionate (2 consecutive days a wk for 16 wks) versus placebo.[16] It found that fluticasone propionate versus placebo significantly maintained improvement of scoring of atopic dermatitis scores at 16 weeks (P = 0.018; no further data provided).[16]

Harms: The short term RCTs identified by the review[4–13] and one longer term cohort study (14 pre-pubertal children, median treatment 6.5 years taking mild to moderate dose topical steroids) found no serious systemic effects or cases of skin atrophy.[17] Minor adverse effects, such as burning, stinging, irritation, folliculitis, hypertrichosis, contact dermatitis, and pigmentary disturbances, occurred in less than 10% of people. **Skin thinning:** The RCT examining prevention of relapse in people with atopic eczema found no significant difference between corticosteroids twice weekly to healed lesions versus placebo in histological evidence of skin atrophy after 16 weeks.[16] We found no further RCTs looking at skin thinning in people with atopic eczema. Four very small RCTs in healthy volunteers (12 people) used ultrasound to evaluate skin thickness.[18–21] The RCTs found that clobetasol 17-propionate 0.05% twice daily versus placebo significantly increased skin thinning after 1 week , and that triamcinolone acetate 0.1% or betamethasone 17-valerate 0.1% twice daily versus placebo significantly increased skin thinning after 3 weeks. They found no significant difference between hydrocortisone prednicarbate twice daily or mometasone furoate once daily versus placebo in skin thinning after 6 weeks. All preparations were used for up to 6 weeks, and skin thinning reversed within 4 weeks of stopping treatment.

Comment: Studies that did not specify the type of eczema, or those that included other dermatoses in the overall analysis, were excluded. The RCTs identified by the review used different clinical scoring systems, making it difficult to compare results.[15] In the RCT (56 adults) comparing fluticasone propionate versus placebo to prevent relapse, participants using fluticasone propionate were advised to apply cream to both known "healed" sites and any newly occurring sites of eczema and improvement in scoring of atopic dermatitis scores was measured overall;[16] therefore, it is uncertain whether improvements in scoring of atopic dermatitis scores were because of prevention of relapse or improvement in newly occurring sites of eczema.

OPTION   **TOPICAL ANTIMICROBIAL PLUS STEROID COMBINATIONS**

One systematic review has found no significant difference between topical antimicrobial agents plus steroids versus topical steroids alone in improving the clinical signs and symptoms of atopic eczema. One systematic review and three additional RCTs have found no significant difference between different antimicrobial agents plus steroids in improving the clinical signs and symptoms of atopic eczema.

Benefits: **Versus topical steroid alone:** We found one systematic review (search date 1999, 3 RCTs, 329 people) with atopic dermatitis, comparing topical antimicrobial plus steroid combinations versus topical steroid alone.[15] It found no significant difference between betamethasone valerate plus fusidic acid, hydrocortisone acetate plus fusidic acid, or betamethasone valerate plus gentamicin versus topical steroid alone in clinical signs and symptoms of eczema (no further data provided). **Versus each other:** We found one systematic review (search date 1999, 4 RCTs, 322 people)[15] and three additional RCTs in people with clinically infected eczema (atopic eczema not specified) comparing different topical antimicrobial plus steroid combinations with each other.[22–24] The systematic review and subsequent RCTs found clinical improvement in 54–95% of participants, with no significant difference between the various preparations with respect to improvement in clinical signs and symptoms. People treated with fusidic acid plus hydrocortisone showed a more rapid clinical response than those treated with miconazole plus hydrocortisone.[15,22-24]

Harms: Overall, the RCTs identified by the review reported minor adverse effects comprising itching, stinging, burning, and irritation in fewer than 2% of people.[15]

Comment: Only two of the RCTs identified by the review specified a degree of infection in most participants at recruitment.[15] One of these also included people with contact dermatitis in the overall analysis, and the use of left/right comparisons within individual participants may have reduced the difference between groups because of systemic absorption of the antimicrobial agent.

OPTION EMOLLIENTS

One systematic review has found that emollient plus topical corticosteroid versus topical corticosteroid alone significantly improves clinical signs and symptoms of atopic eczema.

Benefits: **As adjunct to topical steroids:** We found one systematic review (search date 1999, 2 RCTs,[25,26] 130 people)[15] and one additional controlled clinical trial[27] comparing topical corticosteroid plus moisturising cream versus topical corticosteroid alone. The first RCT identified by the review (80 people with mild to moderate atopic eczema) compared moisturising cream three times daily plus a topical corticosteroid (desonide 0.05%) twice daily versus topical corticosteroid alone.[25] It found that the combined regimen significantly improved clinical signs and symptoms of eczema at 3 weeks (70% v 55%; P < 0.01). The second RCT identified by the review (50 people with atopic eczema) compared emollient cream once daily plus hydrocortisone 2.5% cream once daily versus emollient lotion once daily plus hydrocortisone 2.5% cream once daily.[26] It found significant improvement in signs and symptoms with both treatment regimens after 3 weeks. One additional controlled clinical trial (25 children, randomisation not mentioned) found no significant difference between emollient cream once daily plus hydrocortisone 2.5% cream once daily versus hydrocortisone 2.5% cream twice daily in signs and symptoms after 3 weeks (P > 0.545).[27]

Harms: Minor adverse effects, such as a burning sensation, were reported in fewer than 2% of people in the RCTs identified by the review.[15]

Comment: We excluded many of the studies located in our search as they did not specify the type of eczema, or they included people with other forms of eczema. We have not included studies looking at bath additives.

| OPTION | WET WRAP DRESSINGS AND BANDAGING |

We found no RCTs on the effects of wet wrap or other forms of bandaging in people with atopic eczema.

Benefits:
We found one systematic review (search date 1999), which identified no RCTs on the effects of wet wrap or other forms of bandaging in people with atopic eczema.[15]

Harms:
Uncontrolled studies have found enhanced topical steroid absorption and adverse effects have been found with earlier forms of wet wrap dressings (see glossary, p 351).[28]

Comment:
We found three uncontrolled studies.[28–30] The first study used wet wrap dressings in 30 children with acute erythrodermic eczema.[28] All children responded well to treatment after 2–5 days, with no relapses 2 weeks later (no quantitative results provided). The second study (21 children with chronic severe atopic eczema treated with wet wrap dressings ≤ 2/wk for 3 months) found that in all children the eczema improved after starting treatment and sleep disturbance was reduced. Most parents reported a reduction in topical steroid requirements (no quantitative results provided).[29] As both studies were uncontrolled, the improvement may have been attributable to the additional medical or nursing input during the study rather than to the effect of the wet wraps. The third uncontrolled study (40 children) compared topical mometasone furoate for 2 weeks followed by an additional 2 weeks of mometasone furoate applied with or without wet wraps versus fluticasone proprionate for 2 weeks followed by an additional 2 weeks of fluticasone proprionate applied with or without wet wraps.[30] It found that wet wraps versus no wet wraps improved eczema severity but as most of the improvement occurred in the first 2 weeks, prior to application of wet wraps, it is impossible to isolate the effects of wet wraps.

| OPTION | CONTROL OF HOUSE DUST MITE |

Three RCTs in people with atopic eczema found that extreme reduction in dust levels (achieved by measures such as synthetic mattress covers, acaricidal spraying, and high filtration vacuuming) versus placebo significantly reduced eczema severity score, but one controlled clinical trial found no significant difference between polyurethane coated cotton covers versus placebo in eczema severity scores. The clinical relevance of the reduction in severity score in the RCTs is uncertain. One small RCT comparing natamycin spray plus vacuuming versus placebo found no correlation between improvement in eczema severity score and reduction in mite levels, but the reduction in mite numbers was only 68%. One RCT and one controlled clinical trial in people with atopic eczema or dermatitis and positive mite radioallergosorbent test scores found conflicting evidence of the effects of reducing the number of dust mites in improving eczema severity.

Benefits:
We found one systematic review (search date 1999,[15] 5 RCTs[31–35]) and two additional controlled clinical trials that were excluded from the review because of lack of explicit randomisation.[36,37] The first RCT identified by the review (24 atopic adults and 24 atopic children > 7 years old, skin prick and radioallergosorbent [RAST]

status not specified) compared extreme reduction in dust levels (achieved by a trained nurse visiting to apply bed covers made of a breathable synthetic material plus benzyltannate spray and high filtration vacuuming) versus placebo (nurse visit to apply cotton bedcovers plus placebo spray and standard vacuum cleaners).[31] It found that extreme reduction in dust levels versus placebo significantly reduced eczema severity scores at 6 months ([maximum score 108 units], mean difference in severity score 4.3 units, 95% CI 1.3 to 7.3). This was associated with a 98% reduction in mean mattress dust load versus 16% in the placebo group (P = 0.002) and a 91% reduction in the concentration of mite allergen Der p1 on bedroom carpet and 76% reduction on living room carpet versus 89% reduction (P = 0.94) and 38% reduction (P = 0.27) in the placebo group.[31] The second RCT identified by the review (28 people with atopic dermatitis) compared extreme reduction in dust levels (achieved by nurse visits to apply bed covers made of a breathable synthetic material plus mitocidal spray plus high filtration vacuuming) versus placebo (nurse visits to apply cotton bed covers plus water spraying plus low filtration vacuuming).[35] It found that extreme reduction in dust levels versus placebo significantly reduced eczema surface area (mean difference in area 10%, 95% CI 3 to 17; P = 0.0006) and significantly improved eczema severity score after 6 months (mean improvement in score 4.2 v 12.6; P = 0.006; results presented graphically).[35] The third RCT identified by the review (20 atopic dermatitis patients, aged 12–47 years with positive skin prick and RAST tests to house dust mite) compared 4 groups: natamycin spray alone; natamycin spray plus vacuuming; placebo spray alone; and placebo spray plus vacuuming.[32] It found no correlation between improvement in clinical score and lowered mite numbers. However, the maximum reduction in mite numbers in mattresses was only 68%. The fourth RCT identified by the review (57 infants with atopic dermatitis, unblinded) compared reduction in house mite levels (achieved by special pillows, washing of bedding, removal of pets and soft toys and intensive vacuuming) plus mite blocking bedding versus reduction in house mite levels plus regular bedding.[33] The RCT did not assess the effects on atopic eczema severity. It found that mite reduction bedding versus regular bedding significantly reduced serum and skin prick responses to dust mite allergens after 1 year (17/27 [63%] v 8/26 [31%]; P < 0.02).[33] The fifth RCT identified by the review (30 children aged 3–12 years with stable eczema, unblinded) compared intensive versus gentle cleaning of mattresses, quilts, and floors every 3 weeks by a team of dust mite specialists. Both groups also received advice to clean either intensively or gently. It found that intensive versus gentle cleaning significantly improved clinically scored eczema after 1 year (P < 0.01; results presented graphically).[34] The first controlled clinical trial (51 people with atopic eczema, randomisation not mentioned) compared three groups: 3 weeks in a "clean room" with reduced dust levels in people with positive mite RAST scores; 3 weeks in an ordinary hospital room in people with positive mite RAST scores; and 3 weeks in a "clean room" in people with negative RAST scores. It found that "clean room" treatment in people with high RAST scores resulted in induction of an itch free period and prolonged remission but found no itch free period in people with positive RAST scores treated in an ordinary hospital room or in people with negative RAST scores treated in a "clean room".[36] The second controlled clinical trial (40 people with atopic dermatitis, randomisation not mentioned) compared polyurethane coated cotton bed covers plus monthly vacuuming of mattresses and bedroom carpets versus placebo (cotton covers without monthly vacuuming).[37] It found no significant difference between polyurethane coated cotton covers versus placebo in eczema severity SCORAD scores at 12 months (no further data provided).

Harms: The RCTs identified by the review and the additional controlled clinical trials gave no information on adverse effects.[31–37]

Comment: In the first RCT of extreme reduction of dust levels, the clinical relevance of the reduction in eczema severity score is uncertain.[31] The extreme dust control measures in the RCTs, such as home visits for intensive cleaning and removal of all pets and toys, may not be applicable to the general population.[31,33–35] In the first controlled clinical trial, where people spent 3 weeks in a "clean room" with reduced dust levels, participants were only allowed out of the room for toilet and shower breaks.[36] The use of bedding covers seems to be the simplest and most effective measure to reduce house dust mite levels in the home (see table 2, p 354).

<hr>

OPTION   **DIETARY MANIPULATION**

One systematic review in children or adults with atopic eczema found inconclusive evidence of the effects of dietary manipulation, such as exclusion of egg and cow's milk.

Benefits: **In children:** We found one systematic review (search date 1999,[15] 4 RCTs[38–41]) of the effects of an egg and milk exclusion diet in unselected children with eczema. The review could not perform a meta-analysis because of trial heterogeneity. The first RCT identified by the review (20 children aged 2–8 years) compared an egg and cow's milk exclusion diet with soya milk substitution versus a control diet with egg and cow's milk.[38] It found that an egg and cow's milk exclusion diet versus control diet significantly improved eczema severity (14/20 [70%] treated children improved v 1/20 [5%] controls; RR 7.5, 95% CI 4.85 to 9.73).[38] The second RCT identified by the review (40 children and young adults) found no significant difference between an egg and cow's milk exclusion diet with soya milk substitution versus a control diet with egg and cow's milk in mean eczema area score, itch score, or use of topical corticosteroids (no further data provided).[39] The third RCT identified by the review (55 children with proven sensitivity to eggs; positive mite radioallergosorbent) comparing an egg exclusion diet versus general dietary advice found that an egg free diet significantly reduced the surface area affected by eczema (from 19.6% to 10.9% v from 21.9% to 18.9%; P = 0.02). It also found that an egg exclusion diet versus general dietary advice significantly improved mean severity score (from 33.9 to 24 v from 36.7 to 33.5; P = 0.04).[40] The fourth RCT identified by the review (85 children, 46 evaluable) comparing a "few foods diet"(in which all but a handful of foods were excluded) versus usual diet found no significant difference in eczema severity.[41] **In adults:** We found one systematic review (search date 1999,[15] 2 RCTs[39,42]). The first RCT identified by the review (18 adults aged 16–23 years) found no significant difference between an egg and cow's milk exclusion diet with soya milk substitution versus a control diet with egg and cow's milk in mean eczema area score, itch score, or use of topical corticosteroids (no further data provided).[39] The second RCT identified by the review (33 adults) found no significant difference between a liquid elemental diet (containing amino acids, essential fatty acids, glucose, trace elements, sorbic acid, and vitamins) versus placebo diet in the number of people with an improvement eczema severity score (5/16 [31%] with elemental diet v 4/9 [44%] with placebo; RR 1.02., 95% CI 0.34 to 3.03).[43]

Harms: The RCTs gave no information on adverse effects.[38–41]

Comment: Calcium, protein, and calorie deficiency are risks of dairy free diets in children. The clinical relevance of changes in severity scores obtained in many studies is unknown. We have not included studies looking at the role of food additives, fatty acid supplementation, or trace elements in eczema. Two of the RCTs identified by the review used potentially allergenic soya based milk substitute during the trial period.[38,39] One of the RCTs identified by the review included both children and adults but assessed them separately.[39] Double blind placebo controlled food challenges have been used to identify people with food allergy, but the clinical relevance of positive reactions (which may include gastrointestinal, respiratory, or cutaneous symptoms) to subsequent eczema control is unclear. One retrospective diagnostic study examined hypersensitivity reactions up to 48 hours after double blind, placebo controlled food challenges in 107 children aged 5 months to 12 years with moderate to severe atopic dermatitis and a history suggestive of food allergy.[44] This study found positive reactions in 81% of children, with 70% of reactions occurring within 2 hours. Egg and cow's milk accounted for 83% of the positive reactions.[44] In three further studies, double blind, placebo controlled food challenges caused hypersensitivity reactions (all within 2 h of the challenge) in 63% of children with moderate to severe atopic eczema (320 children), and in 33–39% of children with mild to severe atopic eczema (211 children). Egg, milk, and peanut accounted for 67–78% of the reactions. The effect of subsequent dietary elimination was studied in only 27 of these children. This showed a greater improvement in children on exclusion diets than in non-randomly selected controls, using a crude scoring system.[42]

QUESTION **What are the effects of preventive interventions in predisposed infants?**

OPTION **PROLONGED BREAST FEEDING IN PREDISPOSED INFANTS**

We found limited observational evidence suggesting that exclusive breast feeding for at least 5 months reduced the risk of eczema in infants with a family history of atopy.

Benefits: We found no systematic review or RCTs (see comment below). One 17 year prospective cohort study (236 healthy infants) found that infants breast fed exclusively for more than 6 months versus breast fed for less than 1 month and weaned onto cow's milk formula had a significantly lower prevalence of eczema at 1 year (all infants) and 3 years (infants with a family history of atopy).[45] It found no reduction in the prevalence of eczema in infants who were intermittently breast fed for 2–6 months. Two prospective studies compared prevalence of eczema in exclusively breast fed infants and in non-breast fed infants (non-breast fed infants were randomised to different formulae).[46,47] The studies found that in infants with a family history of atopy, breast feeding for an average of 5 months versus feeding with soya or cow's milk significantly reduced the incidence of eczema at 18 months, but found no significant difference between breast feeding for an average of 5 months versus whey hydrolysate or casein hydrolysate. One further prospective study found that breast feeding for 6–13 months versus conventional formula significantly reduced the incidence of eczema at 3 years (8% v 24%), but found no significant difference between breast feeding versus hydrolysed milk formula (8% v 10%).[48] All infants were given a hypoantigenic weaning diet.

Harms: We found no evidence of harms associated with prolonged breast feeding.

Comment: It is unlikely that an RCT would be conducted in this area. Much of the available evidence was limited by what would be formally considered as poor methodology, for example selection and information bias, short duration of breast feeding, and inadequate control for confounding factors such as introducing supplemental milk or solid foods. Prolonged self selected breast feeding may be associated with unknown protective factors, leading to bias.

OPTION   **MATERNAL DIETARY RESTRICTION**

We found limited evidence from one systematic review that maternal dietary restriction during lactation may protect against the development of eczema in infants with a family history of atopy. One systematic review found no significant difference between maternal diet restriction during pregnancy versus no restriction in development of atopic eczema in the infant at 12–18 months.

Benefits: We found one systematic review (search date 1999;[15] 2 earlier systematic reviews[49,50]). **During lactation:** The review[15] did not fully describe the earlier review it identified.[49] The earlier review (search date not stated, 3 RCTs, 194 women) found that maternal antigen avoidance diet versus normal diet during lactation (range 36 weeks gestation to 6 months lactation) significantly reduced the number of breast fed infants who developed atopic eczema at 12–18 months.[49] **During pregnancy:** The review[15] did not fully describe the earlier systematic review it identified.[50] The earlier review (search date not stated, 3 RCTs, 504 women at high risk of giving birth to an atopic child) compared a maternal antigen avoidance diet during pregnancy versus no restricted diet.[50] It found no significant difference between maternal diet restriction versus no restriction in development of atopic eczema in the infant at 12–18 months (47/77 [26%] v 52/195 [27%]; RR 0.97, 95% CI 0.71 to 1.34).

Harms: **During lactation:** The systematic review gave no information on adverse effects.[49] **During pregnancy:** One RCT (212 women) identified by the review found that mean birth weight was lower with a restricted diet versus no restricted diet (mean 3% lower; no further data provided), but the difference may not be clinically significant.[50]

Comment: All of the RCTs identified by the review of antigen diets during lactation were limited by poor methods; therefore, the results should be interpreted with caution.[49]

QUESTION **What are the effects of avoidance of provoking factors in adults and children with atopic eczema?**

OPTION **CLOTHING TEXTILES**

RCTs found limited evidence that, in people with atopic eczema, the roughness of clothing textiles is a more important factor for skin irritation than the type of textile fibre (synthetic or natural). It found that polyester and cotton of similar textile fineness seemed to be equally well tolerated. One RCT in infants with atopic eczema comparing cotton nappy/diaper versus cellulose core nappy/diaper versus cellulose core nappy/diaper containing absorbent gelling found no significant difference in eczema scores. We found no RCTs on the long term effects of different textiles on the severity of atopic eczema.

Benefits: We found one systematic review (search date 1999,[15] 3 RCTs[51–53]) and one additional RCT.[54] The first RCT identified by the review (20 people with atopic eczema and 20 healthy controls; mean age 25 years, double blind) compared cotton and polyester shirts of different fabric structure and coarseness at rest and after exercise to induce sweating.[51] It found no significant difference between fabrics in comfort ratings. Knitted fabrics (polyester or cotton) were better tolerated than woven fabrics (all polyester). Of the knitted fabrics, polyester was as well tolerated by people with eczema as the comparable cotton shirt of similar textile fineness. At rest, people with eczema tolerated the less coarse knitted polyester better than the other polyester knitted fabrics, although there was no significant difference during exercise. Of the woven fabrics, the finer polyester was better tolerated by people with eczema than the coarser fabrics, both at rest and during exercise, although controls showed no significant difference. The second RCT identified by the review (55 people with atopic dermatitis) compared four different shirts: one cotton and three synthetic with differing fibre structure.[52] It found that cotton shirts versus synthetic shirts that were rougher or heavier in fibre composition significantly improved comfort as measured by a comfort score (P < 0.0001).[52] The third RCT identified by the review (85 infants) comparing cotton nappy/diaper versus cellulose core nappy/diaper (conventional disposable nappy/diaper) versus cellulose core nappy/diaper containing absorbent gelling found no significant difference in eczema scores after

26 weeks (no further data provided).[53] One additional RCT (25 women with atopic eczema, aged 15–20 years, with a history of wool irritation) compared the effects of two different wool fibres on itching.[54] It found that coarser 36 μm wool fibre versus thin 20 μm wool fibre increased the frequency of wool induced itching after 12 hours. Visible skin changes, disappearing within 24 hours in all cases, were seen in more women wearing thick versus thin fibre wool but the difference was not significant (6/9 [67%] v 11/16 [69%]; RR 0.97, 95% CI 0.55 to 1.71).[54]

Harms:
With the exception of short term skin irritation, no harmful effects were reported in the RCTs.[51–54]

Comment:
The RCT comparing cotton nappy/diaper versus cellulose core nappy/diaper (conventional disposable nappy/diaper) versus cellulose core nappy diaper containing absorbent gelling stratified randomisation by severity of nappy rash and atopic eczema (assessed by a grading scale) and by age, weight, and maturity.[53]

| OPTION | WASHING DETERGENTS |

One systematic review found no significant difference between washing detergents that contain enzymes versus washing detergents without enzymes in eczema severity at 1 month. We found no RCTs of the effect of avoidance of all contact with washing detergents.

Benefits:
Biological versus non-biological detergents: One systematic review (search date 1999, 1 RCT, 25 people with atopic eczema, aged 17–59 years) comparing washing detergents with enzymes versus detergents without enzymes found no significant difference in clinical disease severity (using scoring of atopic dermatitis [SCORAD] scale), subjective symptoms, or corticosteroid use after detergent use for 1 month.[15] **Avoidance of all washing detergents:** We found no RCTs.

Harms:
No harmful effects were reported in this trial.

Comment:
None.

| OPTION | VACCINATION/IMMUNISATION |

We found no evidence about the effects of vaccination on atopic eczema severity.

Benefits:
We found no systematic review, RCTs, or cohort studies.

Harms:
One observational study in 134 allergic children (with atopic eczema, asthma, or cows milk allergy) reported transient mild generalised urticaria and fever in two children with atopic eczema within 24 hours of vaccination.[55]

Comment:
The study found that the lowest rate of positive skin prick tests to measles, mumps, and rubella vaccine was in the 68 children with atopic eczema (4% positive), compared with the 47 children with asthma (9% positive), and the 11 children with cow's milk allergy (18% positive).[55] The 64 children with atopic eczema who were subsequently vaccinated had no serious reactions, although the long term effect on eczema severity was not studied.

We found no evidence on the effects of avoiding animal contact on the severity of atopic eczema.

Benefits: We found no systematic review, RCTs, or cohort studies of the effects of avoiding animals or removing the family pet on the severity of atopic eczema.

Harms: We found no evidence.

Comment: Observational studies have suggested that keeping pets is associated with an increased prevalence of atopic eczema. Following removal of animals from the home it may take many months for the allergen load to decrease because of widespread distribution in carpets and soft furnishings.

GLOSSARY

Wet wrap dressings Wet occlusive tubifast dressings that are applied over topical steroid or emollient.

REFERENCES

1. Williams HC, Burney PGJ, Pembroke AC, Hay RH. The UK working party's diagnostic criteria for atopic dermatitis. III Independent hospital validation. *Br J Dermatol* 1994;131:406–417.

2. Kay J, Gawkrodger DJ, Mortimer MJ, Jaron AG. The prevalence of childhood atopic eczema in a general population. *J Am Acad Dermatol* 1994;30:35–39.

3. Williams HC. Is the prevalence of atopic dermatitis increasing? *Clin Exp Dermatol* 1992;17:385–391.

4. Lawlor F, Black AK, Greaves M. Prednicarbate 0.25% ointment in the treatment of atopic dermatitis: A vehicle-controlled double-blind study. *J Dermatol Treat* 1995;6:233–235.

5. Roth HL, Brown EP. Hydrocortisone valerate. Double-blind comparison with two other topical steroids. *Cutis* 1978;21:695–698.

6. Maloney JM, Morman MR, Stewart DM, et al. Clobetasol propionate emollient 0.05% in the treatment of atopic dermatitis. *Int J Dermatol* 1998;37:128–144.

7. Sears HW, Bailer JW, Yeadon A. Efficacy and safety of hydrocortisone buteprate 0.1% cream in patients with atopic dermatitis. *Clin Ther* 1997; 19:710–719.

8. Vanderploeg DE. Betamethasone dipropionate ointment in the treatment of psoriasis and atopic dermatitis: a double-blind study. *South Med J* 1976;69:862–863.

9. Lupton ES, Abbrecht MM, Brandon ML. Short-term topical corticosteroid therapy (halcinonide ointment) in the management of atopic dermatitis. *Cutis* 1982;30:671–675.

10. Stalder JF, Fleury M, Sourisse M, et al. Local steroid therapy and bacterial skin flora in atopic dermatitis. *Br J Dermatol* 1994;131:536–540.

11. Sefton J, Loder JS, Kyriakopoulos AA. Clinical evaluation of hydrocortisone valerate 0.2% ointment. *Clin Ther* 1984;6:282–293.

12. Wahlgren CF, Hägermark O, Bergström R, Hedin B. Evaluation of a new method of assessing pruritus and antipruritic drugs. *Skin Pharmacol* 1988;1: 3–13.

13. Sudilovsky A, Muir JG, Bocobo FC. A comparison of single and multiple applications of Halcinonide cream. *Int J Dermatol* 1981;20:609–613.

14. Lebwohl M. Efficacy and safety of fluticasone propionate ointment, 0.005%, in the treatment of eczema. *Cutis* 1996;57(2 suppl):62–68.

15. Hoare C, Li Wan PA, Williams HC. A systematic review of treatments for atopic eczema. *Health Technol Assess* 2000;4:1–203. Search date 1999; primary sources Medline, Embase, Cochrane Library, and Cochrane Skin Group Specialised Trials Register.

16. Van der Meer JB, Glazenburg EJ, Mulder PGH, et al. The management of moderate to severe atopic dermatitis in adults with topical fluticasone propionate. *Br J Dermatol* 1999;140:1114–1121.

17. Patel L, Clayton PE, Addison GM, Price DA, David TJ. Adrenal function following topical steroid treatment in children with atopic dermatitis. *Br J Dermatol* 1995;132:950–955.

18. Kerscher MJ, Hart H, Korting HC, Stalleicken D. In vivo assessment of the atrophogenic potency of mometasone furoate, a newly developed chlorinated potent topical glucocorticoid as compared to other topical glucocorticoids old and new. *Int J Clin Pharmacol Ther* 1995;33:187–189.

19. Kerscher MJ, Korting HC. Comparative atrophogenicity potential of medium and highly potent topical glucocorticoids in cream and ointment according to ultrasound analysis. *Skin Pharmacol* 1992;5:77–80.

20. Kerscher MJ, Korting HC. Topical glucocorticoids of the non-fluorinated double-ester type. *Acta Derm Venereol* 1992;72:214–216.

21. Korting HC, Vieluf D, Kerscher M. 0.25% prednicarbate cream and the corresponding vehicle induce less skin atrophy than 0.1% betamethasone-17-valerate cream and 0.05% clobetasol-17-propionate cream. *Eur J Clin Pharmacol* 1992;42:159–161.

22. Hill VA, Wong E, Corbett MF, Menday AP. Comparative efficacy of betamethasone/clioquinol (Betnovate-C) cream and betamethasone/fusidic acid (Fucibet) cream in the treatment of infected hand eczema. *J Dermatol Treat* 1998;9:15–19.

23. Poyner TF, Dass BK. Comparative efficacy and tolerability of fusidic acid/hydrocortisone cream (Fucidin H cream) and miconazole/hydrocortisone cream (Daktacort cream) in infected eczema. *J Eur Acad Dermatol Venereol* 1996;7(suppl 1):23–30.

24. Jaffe GV, Grimshaw JJ. A clinical trial of hydrocortisone/potassium hydroxyquinolone

Atopic eczema

sulphate (Quinocort) in the treatment of infected eczema and impetigo in general practice. *Pharmatherapeutica* 1986;4:628–636.

25. Hanifin JM, Hebert AA, Mays SR, et al. Effects of a low-potency corticosteroid lotion plus a moisturizing regimen in the treatment of atopic dermatitis. *Curr Ther Res* 1998;59:227–233.

26. Kantor I, Milbauer J, Posner M, et al. Efficacy and safety of emollients as adjunctive agents in topical corticosteroid therapy for atopic dermatitis. *Today Ther Trend* 1993;11:157–166.

27. Lucky AW, Leach AD, Laskarzewski P, Wenck H. Use of an emollient as a steroid-sparing agent in the treatment of mild to moderate atopic dermatitis in children. *Pediatr Dermatol* 1997;14:321–324.

28. Goodyear HM, Spowart K, Harper JI. "Wet wrap" dressings for the treatment of atopic eczema in children. *Br J Dermatol* 1991;125:604.

29. Mallon E, Powell S, Bridgman A. "Wet-wrap" dressings for the treatment of atopic eczema in the community. *J Dermatol Treat* 1994;5:97–98.

30. Pei AYS, Chan HL, Ho KM. The effectiveness of wet wrap dressings using 0.1% mometasone furoate and 0.005% fluticasone proprionate ointments in the treatment of moderate to severe atopic dermatitis in children. *Pedriatr Dermatol* 2001;18:343–348.

31. Tan B, Weald D, Strickland I, Frieman PS. Double-blind controlled trial of effect of house dust-mite allergen avoidance on atopic dermatitis. *Lancet* 1996;347:15–18.

32. Colloff MJ, Lever RS, McSharry C. A controlled trial of house dust mite eradication using natamycin in homes of patients with atopic dermatitis: effect on clinical status and mite populations. *Br J Dermatol* 1989;121:199–208.

33. Nishioka K, Yasueda H, Saito H. Preventative effect of bedding encasement with microfine fibres on mite sensitisation. *J Allergy Clin Immunol* 1998; 101; 28–32.

34. Endo K, Fukuzumi T, Adachi J, et al. Effect of vacuum cleaning of floors and bed clothes of patients on house dust mite counts and clinical scores of atopic dermatitis. A double blind control trial. [Japanese]. *Aerrerugi* 1997;46:1013–1024.

35. Friedmann PS, Tan BB. Mite elimination – clinical effect on eczema. *Allergy* 1998; 53 Suppl 48:97–100.

36. Sanda T, Yasue T, Oohashi M, Yasue A. Effectiveness of house dust-mite allergen avoidance through clean room therapy in patients with atopic dermatitis. *J Allergy Clin Immunol* 1992;89:653–657.

37. Holm L, Ohman S, Bengtsson A, et al. Effectiveness of occlusive bedding in the treatment of atopic dermatitis–a placebo-controlled trial of 12 months' duration *Allergy* 2001;56:152–158.

38. Atherton DJ, Sewell M, Soothill JF, Wells RS, Chilvers CE. A double-blind controlled crossover trial of an antigen avoidance diet in atopic eczema. *Lancet* 1978;1:401–403.

39. Neild VS, Marsden RA, Bailes JA, Bland JM. Egg and milk exclusion diets in atopic eczema. *Br J Dermatol* 1986;114:117–123.

40. Lever R, MacDonald C, Waugh P, Aitchison T. Randomised controlled trial of advice on an egg

exclusion diet in young children with atopic eczema and sensitivity to eggs. *Pediatr Allergy* 1998;9:13–19.

41. Mabin DC, Sykes AE, David TJ. Controlled trial of a few foods diet in severe atopic dermatitis. *Arch Dis Child* 1995;73:202–207.

42. Sampson HA, McCaskill CM. Food hypersensitivity and atopic dermatitis: evaluation of 113 patients. *J Pediatr* 1985;107:669–675.

43. Munkvad M, Danielsen L, Høj L, et al. Antigen-free diet in adult patients with atopic eczema. *Acta Derm Venereol* 1984;64:524–528.

44. Niggemann B, Sielaff B, Beyer K, Binder C, Wahn U. Outcome of double-blind, placebo-controlled food challenge tests in 107 children with atopic dermatitis. *Clin Exp Allergy* 1999;29: 91–96.

45. Saarinen UM, Kajosaari M. Breast-feeding as prophylaxis against atopic disease: prospective follow-up study until 17 years old. *Lancet* 1995; 346:1065–1069.

46. Chandra RK. Five year follow up of high risk infants with a family history of allergy. *J Pediatr Gastroenterol Nutr* 1997;24:380–388.

47. Chandra RK, Shakuntla P, Hamed A. Influence of maternal diet during lactation and use of formula feeds on development of atopic eczema in high risk infants. *BMJ* 1989;299:228–230.

48. Marini A, Agostoi M, Motta G, Mosca F. Effects of a dietary and environmental prevention programme on the incidence of allergic symptoms in high atopic risk infants: three years follow-up. *Acta Paediatr* 1996; 414(suppl): 1–22.

49. Kramer MS. Maternal antigen avoidance during lactation for preventing atopic disease in infants of women at high risk. In: The Cochrane Library, Issue 4, 2000. Oxford: Update Software. Search date not stated; primary sources The Cochrane Pregnancy and Childbirth Group Trials Register and contact with authors of studies.

50. Kramer MS. Maternal antigen avoidance during pregnancy for preventing atopic disease in infants of women at high risk. In: The Cochrane Library, Issue 3, 2001. Oxford: Update Software. Search date not stated; primary sources The Cochrane Pregnancy and Childbirth Group Trials Register.

51. Diepgen TL, Salzer B, Tepe A, Hornstein OP. A study of skin irritations caused by textiles under standardized sweating conditions in patients with atopic eczema [German]. *Melliand Deutsch/ English* 1995;12:E268–E269.

52. Diepgen TL, Stabler A, Tepe A, Hornsein OP. A study of skin irritation by textiles under standardised sweating conditions in patients with atopic eczema. [German] *Z Hautkrankheiten* 1990;65:907–910.

53. Seymour JL, Keswick BH, Hanifin JM, Jordan WP, Milligan MC. Clinical effects of diaper types on the skin of normal infants and infants with atopic dermatitis. *J Am Acad Dermatol* 1987;17: 988–997.

54. Bendsöe N, Björnberg A, Åsnes H. Itching from wool fibres in atopic eczema. *Contact Dermatitis* 1987;17:21–22.

55. Juntunen-Backman K, Peltola H, Backman A, Salo OP. Safe immunisation of allergic children against measles, mumps and rubella. *Am J Dis Child* 1987;141:1103–1105.

Dominic Smethurst

Dr

Department of Evidence-based Dermatology

Nottingham

UK

Competing interests: None declared.

TABLE 1	Topical steroids versus placebo in atopic eczema: results of RCTs* (see text, p 341).[4-13]

Methods	Results*
Mattress, pillow and duvet covers (micro-porous or polyurethane coated)	Very effective (3 RCTs). Dust mite allergen levels 1–25% of control levels after 3–12 months; 44–98% reduction in dust load after 3 months.
Washing bedding at 55°C	Effective (2 RCTs). Reduces levels of dust mite allergen by > 95% and kills 100% of mites.
Removal of carpets and curtains	Unknown.
Acaricides (e.g. benzyl benzoate)	Conflicting results from RCTs — better when used on carpets than on mattresses. Effect may be short lived.
Intensive vacuuming	Small effect on mite levels in mattresses (1 RCT, 1 crossover trial) but not correlated with improvement in symptoms, possibly because conventional rather than high filtration cleaners may increase levels of airborne mite allergens, which may aggravate atopic disease (1 RCT in 16 rooms).
Air filters and dehumidifiers	Conflicting results from RCTs.

*Trials have tended to use a combination of control measures, making it difficult to see which measures were responsible for beneficial effects.

TABLE 2 Methods for reducing house dust mite levels: results of controlled trials (see text, p 346).

	Number of participants (age in years)	Outcome
Prednicarbate ointment, 0.25% twice daily for 4 weeks.[4]	51 (18–60)	Reduced dermatitis: 87% active treatment, 8% controls. Significantly reduced patient-assessed pruritis on active treatment.
Hydrocortisone valerate cream, 0.2% three times daily for 2 weeks.[5]	20 (2–75)	Excellent or better: 75% active treatment, 20% controls.
Clobetasol propionate cream, 0.05% twice daily for 4 weeks.[6]	81 (≥ 12)	Good, excellent, or clear: 82% active treatment, 29% controls.
Hydrocortisone buteprate cream, 0.1% once daily for 2 weeks.[9]	194 (17–76)	Excellent or good: 69% active treatment, 26% controls.
Betamethasone dipropionate ointment, 0.05% twice daily for 3 weeks.[8]	36 (2–63)	Good or excellent: 94% active treatment, 13% controls.
Halcinonide ointment, 0.1% three times daily for 2 weeks.[7]	233 (2–67)	Good or excellent: 85% active treatment, 44% controls.
Desonide cream once daily for 1 week.[10]	40 (0.4–15)	Improvement or resolution: 67% active treatment, 16% controls.
Hydrocortisone valerate 0.2% ointment twice daily for 2 weeks.[11]	64 (> 12)	Disease severity score: 70% reduction with active treatment, 15% controls.
Betamethasone dipropionate twice daily for 4 days.[12]	30 (19–57)	Itch free on days 3–4: 36% active treatment, 22% controls.
Halcinonide cream, 0.1% twice daily for 3 weeks.[13]	58 (0.8–86)	57% of people achieved a better response with active treatment than control treatment ("better response" was not defined).

*Confidence intervals not reported.

Key Messages

- We found limited evidence from two systematic reviews that chemical insecticides are effective.

- We found limited evidence that insecticide treatment is more effective than combing with conditioner.

- We found no good evidence on combing, herbal medicines, or repellents.

Head lice

DEFINITION	Head lice are obligate ectoparasites of socially active humans. They infest the scalp and attach their eggs to the hair shafts. Itching, resulting from multiple bites, is not diagnostic but may increase the index of suspicion. Infestation can be diagnosed only by finding living lice. Eggs glued to hairs, whether hatched (nits) or unhatched, are not proof of active infection, because eggs may retain a viable appearance for weeks after death.
INCIDENCE/ PREVALENCE	We found no studies on incidence and no recent published prevalence results from any developed country. Anecdotal reports suggest that prevalence has increased in the past few years in most communities in the UK and USA.
AETIOLOGY/ RISK FACTORS	Observational studies indicate that infections occur most frequently in school children, although there is no proof of a link with school attendance.[1,2] We found no evidence that lice prefer clean hair to dirty hair.
PROGNOSIS	The infection is almost harmless. Sensitisation reactions to louse saliva and faeces may result in localised irritation and erythema. Secondary infection of scratches may occur. Lice have been identified as primary mechanical vectors of scalp pyoderma caused by streptococci and staphylococci usually found on the skin.[3]
AIMS	To eliminate infestation by killing or removing all head lice and their eggs.
OUTCOMES	Treatment success is given as the percentage of people completely cleared of head lice. There are no standard criteria for judging treatment success. Trials used different methods, and in many cases the method was not stated. Few studies are pragmatic (see glossary, p 359).
METHODS	The initial search was performed by the Cochrane Infectious Diseases Group at the Liverpool School of Tropical Medicine for a systematic review compiled in July 1998.[4] *Clinical Evidence* search and appraisal October 2001.

QUESTION **What are the effects of treatment for head lice?**

OPTION **INSECTICIDE BASED PHARMACEUTICAL PRODUCTS**

We found two systematic reviews of small, poor quality RCTs of insecticide based pharmaceutical products. One systematic review has found that permethrin and malathion were more effective than placebo, and synergised pyrethrins and permethrin were of similar effectiveness. An earlier systematic review has found that permethrin is more effective than lindane. All RCTs had flawed methods. The most recently added RCT compared malathion with combing and is discussed under mechanical removal of lice or viable eggs by combing, p 358.

Benefits: We found two systematic reviews.[4,5] The first systematic review (search date 1995, 7 RCTs, 1808 people) was of 11 insecticide products, including lindane, carbaryl, malathion, permethrin, and other pyrethroids in various vehicles.[4] Two RCTs found that only permethrin produced clinically significant differences in the rate of treatment success; both compared lindane (1% shampoo) versus permethrin (1% cream rinse). Permethrin was found to be more effective (lindane v permethrin; OR for not clearing head lice 15.2, 95% CI 8.0 to 28.8). The subsequent systematic review (search date 2001) set stricter criteria for RCTs and rejected all but four RCTs.[5] It excluded both studies on which the earlier review was based. One RCT (63 people) found that, after 7 days, permethrin (1% cream rinse) versus placebo was more effective against head lice (head lice cleared: 29/29 [100%] with permethrin v 3/34 [9%] with placebo; RR 11.3, 95% CI 3.9 to 33.4). Two weeks after permethrin treatment, more people had no head lice compared with placebo (head lice cleared: 28/29 [97%] with permethrin v 2/24 [8%] with placebo; RR 11.6, 95% CI 3.1 to 43.8). One RCT (115 people) compared malathion (0.5% alcoholic lotion) with the vehicle base as placebo. At 1 week, more people treated with malathion versus placebo had no head lice (head lice cleared: 62/65 [95%] with malathion v 21/47 [45%] with placebo; RR 2.1, 95% CI 1.5 to 2.9; NNT 2, 95% CI 1 to 3). One efficacy trial (22 people) of synergised pyrethrin (0.16% mousse) versus permethrin (1% cream rinse) found a non-significant reduction of head lice with permethrin at 6 days (17/19 [89%] with pyrethrin v 3/3 [100%] with permethrin; RR 0.89, 95% CI 0.8 to 1.0). These later data were obtained from an efficacy analysis instead of an intention to treat analysis.

Harms: Only minor adverse effects have been reported for most insecticides. The exception is lindane, where there are extensive reports of effects related to overdosing (treatment of scabies) and absorption (treatment of head lice). Transdermal passage of lindane occurs during treatment of head lice,[6] but we found no reports of adverse effects in this setting. We found no confirmed reports of adverse effects from the organophosphate malathion when used therapeutically. One observational study (32 people) found that 0.2–3.2% of the applied dose of 0.1–0.2 g of malathion, given in the form of head louse products, was excreted in urine as metabolites, suggesting limited transdermal absorption. No effect was observed on plasma or erythrocyte cholinesterase activity.[7]

Comment: Follow up for 6 days is inadequate, as the eggs take 7 days to hatch. Most investigators agree that a final examination after 14 days is appropriate for primary end point determination of cure. The three trials included in the most recent systematic review were conducted in developing countries where insecticide treatments were not regularly available.[4] This may have resulted in greater efficacy, because the insects have not been subjected to any kind of selection pressure. No RCT has yet tested the effect of a pediculicide's formulation on its activity. Studies in vitro suggest that other components of products (e.g. terpenoids and solvents) may be more effective pediculicides than the insecticide itself.[8] Resistance to one or more insecticides is now common.[9–11] One RCT (193 people) investigating resistance compared malathion (0.5% lotion with terpenoids) with phenothrin (0.3% lotion) in a community where lice were identified in vitro as being tolerant of phenothrin.[12] One day after treatment more people treated with malathion versus phenothrin were louse free (87/95 [92%] with malathion v 39/98 [40%] with phenothrin; RR 2.3, 95% CI 1.7 to 2.9) and this difference had increased by day 7 (90/95 [95%] with malathion v 38/98

[39%] with phenothrin; RR 2.4, 95% CI 1.8 to 3.2). However, some children not free from lice on day 1 had become louse free by day 7 in both groups, suggesting some parental intervention had influenced the results. Nevertheless, this study indicates that resistance to pyrethroid insecticide may have influenced about 60% of the treatments.

OPTION **MECHANICAL REMOVAL OF LICE OR VIABLE EGGS BY COMBING**

We found one RCT comparing an insecticide treatment with combing. It found that malathion was more effective than wet combing with conditioner.

Benefits: We found one RCT (72 people) comparing "bug busting" (wet combing with conditioner) with two applications of 0.5% malathion, 7 days apart.[13] Seven days after treatment, more people treated with malathion had no lice compared with "bug busting" (31/40 [78%] with malathion v 12/32 [38%] with "bug busting"; RR 2.1, 95% CI 1.3 to 3.3; NNT 3, 95% CI 2 to 5).[13] We found three RCTs comparing different pediculicides in combination with nit combing, but none included a non-combing control group.[14–16]

Harms: Apart from discomfort, we found no evidence of harms due to combing. Wet combing with conditioner may risk adverse reactions, which have been observed during normal cosmetic use, to hair conditioning agents.[17–21]

Comment: The systematic review comparing insecticide with wet combing and conditioner was designed to be a pragmatic RCT (see glossary, p 359) with results that are applicable to normal practice.[13]

OPTION **HERBAL TREATMENTS**

We found no good evidence on the effects of herbal treatments.

Benefits: We found no systematic review, RCTs, or cohort studies evaluating herbal treatments.

Harms: We found no evidence (see above).

Comment: None.

OPTION **ESSENTIAL OILS AND OTHER CHEMICALS USED AS REPELLENTS**

We found no good evidence on the effects of essential oils or other compounds, such as piperonal, as repellents.

Benefits: We found no systematic review, RCTs, or cohort studies evaluating repellents.

Harms: We found no evidence of harms, although a potential for toxic effects has been recognised for several essential oils.[22]

Comment: None.

GLOSSARY

Pragmatic RCT An RCT designed to provide results that are directly applicable to normal practice (compared to explanatory trials that are intended to clarify efficacy under ideal conditions). Pragmatic RCTs recruit a population that is representative of those who are normally treated, allow normal compliance with instructions (by avoiding incentives and by using oral instructions with advice to follow manufacturers instructions), and analyse results by "intention to treat" rather than by "on treatment" methods.[9]

REFERENCES

1. Burgess IF. Human lice and their management. *Adv Parasitol* 1995;36:271–342.
2. Gratz NG. *Human lice. Their prevalence, control and resistance to insecticides.* Geneva: World Health Organization, 1997.
3. Taplin D, Meinking TL. Infestations. In: Schachner LA, Hansen RC, eds. *Pediatric dermatology*, vol 2. New York: Churchill Livingstone, 1988:1465–1493.
4. Vander Stichele RH, Dezeure EM, Bogaert MG. Systematic review of clinical efficacy of topical treatments for head lice. *BMJ* 1995;311: 604–608. Search date 1995; primary sources Medline, International Pharmaceutical Abstracts, and Science Citation Index.
5. Dodd CS. Interventions for treating head lice (Cochrane Review). In: The Cochrane Library, Issue 3, 2001. Oxford: Update Software. Search date 2001; primary sources CCTR, Medline, Embase, BIDS SC, BIOSIS, and Toxline.
6. Ginsburg CM, Lowry W. Absorption of gamma benzene hexachloride following application of Kwell shampoo. *Pediatr Dermatol* 1983;1:74–76.
7. Dennis GA, Lee PN. A phase I volunteer study to establish the degree of absorption and effect on cholinesterase activity of four head lice preparations containing malathion. *Clin Drug Invest* 1999;18:105–115.
8. Burgess I. Malathion lotions for head lice: a less reliable treatment than commonly believed. *Pharm J* 1991;247:630–632.
9. Burgess IF, Brown CM, Peock S, et al. Head lice resistant to pyrethroid insecticides in Britain [letter]. *BMJ* 1995;311:752.
10. Pollack RJ, Kiszewski A, Armstrong P, et al. Differential permethrin susceptibility of head lice sampled in the United States and Borneo. *Arch Pediatr Adolesc Med* 1999;153:969–973.
11. Lee SH, Yoon KS, Williamson M, et al. Molecular analyses of *kdr*-like resistance in permethrin-resistant strains of head lice, *Pediculus capitis*. *Pestic Biochem Physiol* 2000;66:130–143.
12. Chosidow O, Chastang C, Brue C, et al. Controlled study of malathion and *d*-phenothrin lotions for *Pediculus humanus* var *capitis*-infested schoolchildren. *Lancet* 1994;334:1724–1727.
13. Roberts RJ, Casey D, Morgan DA, et al. Comparison of wet combing with malathion for treatment of head lice in the UK: a pragmatic randomised controlled trial. *Lancet* 2000;356:540–544.
14. Bainbridge CV, Klein GI, Neibart SI, et al. Comparative study of the clinical effectiveness of a pyrethrin-based pediculicide with combing versus a permethrin-based pediculicide with combing. *Clin Pediatr (Phila)* 1998;37:17–22.
15. Clore ER, Longyear LA. A comparative study of seven pediculicides and their packaged nit combs. *J Pediatr Health Care* 1993;7:55–60.
16. Hipolito RB, Mallorca FG, Zuniga-Macaraig ZO, et al. Head lice infestation: single drug versus combination therapy with one percent permethrin and trimethoprim/sulfamethoxazole. *Pediatrics* 2001;107:E30.
17. Korting JC, Pursch EM, Enders F, et al. Allergic contact dermatitis to cocamidopropyl betaine in shampoo. *J Am Acad Dermatol* 1992;27:1013–1015.
18. Niinimaki A, Niinimaki M, Makinen-Kiljunen S, et al. Contact urticaria from protein hydrolysates in hair conditioners. *Allergy* 1998;53:1070–1082.
19. Schalock PC, Storrs FJ, Morrison L. Contact urticaria from panthenol in hair conditioner. *Contact Dermatitis* 2000;43:223.
20. Pasche-Koo F, Claeys M, Hauser C. Contact urticaria with systemic symptoms caused by bovine collagen in hair conditioner. *Am J Contact Dermatol* 1996;7:56–57.
21. Stadtmauer G, Chandler M. Hair conditioner causes angioedema. *Ann Allergy Asthma Immunol* 1997;78:602.
22. Veal L. The potential effectiveness of essential oils as a treatment for headlice, *Pediculus humanus capitis*. *Complement Ther Nurs Midwifery* 1996;2: 97–101.

Ian Burgess
Director
Insect Research and Development Limited
Cambridge
UK

Competing interests: The author has been a consultant to several companies involved in development and marketing of pediculicides and has received payment for professional services, including development of educational materials.

Scabies

Search date September 2001

Godfrey Walker and Paul Johnstone

QUESTIONS

INTERVENTIONS

Beneficial

Likely to be beneficial

Trade off between benefits and harms

Unknown effectiveness

Key Messages

- One systematic review has found that permethrin versus crotamiton significantly increases clinical and parasitic cure after 28 days. The review suggests that permethrin is as effective as lindane in cure, with fewer adverse effects.

- One systematic review found limited evidence that lindane was as effective as crotamiton, permethrin, or oral ivermectin in clinical cure, but found rare reports of convulsions and other severe adverse effects.

- One systematic review has found no significant difference between crotamiton and lindane in clinical cure, but has found crotamiton to be less effective than permethrin.

- We found insufficient evidence on the effects of other topical agents (malathion, benzyl benzoate, and sulphur compounds).

- One systematic review found limited evidence that oral ivermectin versus placebo significantly increased clinical cure, and found no significant difference between oral ivermectin versus lindane in clinical cure. Experience of the use of oral ivermectin in onchocerciasis suggests that it is safe in younger adults, but no such experience exists for children, and there have been reports of increased risk of death in elderly people.

DEFINITION	Scabies is an infestation of the skin by the mite *Sarcoptes scabiei*.[1] Typical sites of infestation are skin folds and flexor surfaces. In adults, the most common sites are between the fingers and on the wrists, although infection may manifest in elderly people as a diffuse truncal eruption. In infants and children the face, scalp, palms, and soles are also often affected.
INCIDENCE/ PREVALENCE	Scabies is a common public health problem with an estimated prevalence of 300 million cases worldwide, mostly affecting people in developing countries where prevalence can exceed 50%.[2] In industrialised countries it is most common in institutionalised communities. Case studies suggest that epidemic cycles occur every 7–15 years and that these partly reflect the population's immune status.
AETIOLOGY/ RISK FACTORS	Scabies is particularly common where there is social disruption, overcrowding with close body contact, and limited access to water.[3] Young children, immobilised elderly people, people with HIV/AIDS, and other medically and immunologically compromised people are predisposed to infestation and have particularly high mite counts.[4]
PROGNOSIS	Scabies is not life threatening, but the severe, persistent itch and secondary infections may be debilitating. Occasionally, crusted scabies develops. This form of the disease is resistant to routine treatment and can be a source of continued reinfestation and spread to others.
AIMS	To eliminate the scabies mites and ova from the skin; to cure pruritus (itching); to prevent reinfestation; to prevent spread to other people.
OUTCOMES	**Clinical cure:** number of visible burrows and papular and vesicular eruptions; pruritus. **Parasitic cure:** presence of mites, ova, or faecal pellets in skin scrapings under a magnifying lens or microscope. Outcomes should be assessed 28–30 days after start of treatment, which is the time it takes for lesions to heal and for any eggs and mites to reach maturity if treatment fails.
METHODS	*Clinical Evidence* search and appraisal September 2001.

QUESTION What are the effects of topical treatments?

OPTION PERMETHRIN

One systematic review has found that permethrin versus crotamiton significantly increases clinical and parasitic cure after 28 days. The review suggests that permethrin is as effective as lindane in cure, with fewer adverse effects.

Benefits:	We found no RCTs comparing permethrin versus placebo. We found one systematic review (search date 1999, 6 RCTs)[5] and one subsequent RCT[6] comparing permethrin versus other topical and oral agents. **Versus crotamiton:** The review (2 RCTs, 194 people) found that permethrin versus crotamiton significantly increased clinical cure rates after 28 days (2 RCTs; OR for failed clinical cure with permethrin *v* crotamiton 0.21, 95% CI 0.10 to 0.47) and significantly increased parasitic cure after 28 days (1 RCT; 94 people; OR for failed parasitic cure with permethrin *v* crotamiton 0.21, 95% CI 0.08 to 0.53). It found no significant difference between permethrin and crotamiton in self reported pruritus (1 RCT: OR for itch persistence with permethrin

Skin disorders

v with crotamiton 0.38, 95% CI 0.12 to 1.19).[5] **Versus lindane:** The systematic review identified four RCTs comparing permethrin versus lindane.[5] Overall the review found that permethrin versus lindane appeared to be more effective in clinical cure after 28 days. However, it found significant trial heterogeneity (P < 0.005). Two RCTs, including the largest one (467 people), found no significant difference between permethrin and lindane.[5] **Versus oral ivermectin:** We found one subsequent RCT that compared topical permethrin versus oral ivermectin.[7] The RCT will be reported at a later date.

Harms: One RCT identified by the review reported five adverse effects: two in the permethrin group (rash and possible diarrhoea) and three in the lindane group (pruritic rash, papules, and diarrhoea).[8] During 1990–1995 six adverse events were reported per 100 000 units distributed in the USA (1 central nervous system adverse effect reported per 500 000 units of permethrin distributed).[9] Resistance to permethrin seems to be rare.[9]

Comment: None.

| OPTION | LINDANE |

One systematic review found limited evidence that lindane was as effective as crotamiton, permethrin, or oral ivermectin in clinical cure, but found rare reports of convulsions and other severe adverse effects.

Benefits: We found no RCTs comparing lindane versus placebo. We found one systematic review (search date 1999, 6 RCTs),[5] comparing lindane versus other topical and oral agents. **Versus crotamiton:** One RCT (100 adults and children) identified by the review found no significant difference in clinical cure rates (OR for failed clinical cure with crotamiton *v* lindane 0.41, 95% CI 0.15 to 1.10).[5] However, confidence intervals are broad and a clinically important difference cannot be ruled out. **Versus permethrin:** See benefits of permethrin, p 361. **Versus oral ivermectin:** One RCT (53 adults referred to hospital with scabies) identified by the review found no significant difference between lindane versus ivermection in clinical cure rates at 15 days (failed clinical cure 14/27 [52%] with gamma benzene hydrochloride *v* 12/26 [46%] with oral ivermectin; RR 0.89, 95% CI 0.51 to 1.55).[5]

Harms: The RCTs identified by the review reported no severe adverse effects.[5] Case reports and evidence from the World Health Organization Collaborating Centre for International Drug Monitoring included reports of rare severe adverse effects (e.g. convulsions and aplastic anaemia), particularly when lindane was applied to people with extensive skin disease and to children.[7,10,11] Summary reports from 47 countries suggest that lindane is more toxic than other preparations.[11] Four convulsions were reported in people on benzyl benzoate, one in people on crotamiton, 38 in people on lindane, two in people on malathion, and six in people on permethrin. Deaths reported on benzyl benzoate were none, crotamiton one, lindane one, malathion none, and permethrin five.[11] Resistance has been reported in many countries.[12]

Comment: Lindane was withdrawn from the market in the UK in 1995 because of concern about possible adverse effects. The evidence linking lindane with convulsions is suggestive but not conclusive.[9–11] Summary reports are influenced by how much the products are used for the treatment of scabies and other infestations, and the quality of reporting. Safety results from trials and observational studies need to be summarised, particularly regarding additional risks in infants and pregnant women.

OPTION   CROTAMITON

One systematic review has found no significant difference between crotamiton and lindane in clinical cure, but found crotamiton to be less effective than permethrin.

Benefits: We found no RCTs comparing crotamiton versus placebo. We found one systematic review (search date 1999, 3 RCTs) comparing crotamiton versus other topical agents.[5] **Crotamiton versus permethrin:** See benefits of permethrin, p 361. **Crotamiton versus lindane:** See benefits of lindane, p 362.

Harms: We found limited evidence on the toxicity of crotamiton, but reports of serious adverse effects are rare.[10] There have been a few reports of deaths, convulsions, and resistance (see harms of lindane, p 362).[10]

Comment: None.

OPTION   MALATHION

One systematic review found no RCTs of malathion. Cure rates of over 80% have been reported in case series.

Benefits: We found one systematic review (search date 1999) that identified no RCTs.[5] Case series suggest that malathion is effective in curing infestation with scabies, with a cure rate of over 80% at 4 weeks.[13,14]

Harms: No important adverse events have been reported (see harms of lindane, p 362).

Comment: The safety results from trials and observational studies need to be summarised, particularly with regard to additional risks in infants and pregnant women.

OPTION   BENZYL BENZOATE

One systematic review found insufficient evidence of the effects of benzyl benzoate in clinical cure. Cure rates of about 50% have been reported in non-randomised trials.

Benefits: We found no RCTs comparing benzyl benzoate versus placebo. We found one systematic review (search date 1999, 2 RCTs, 202 people) comparing benzyl benzoate versus other agents.[5] **Versus oral ivermectin:** One small RCT (44 adults and children) identified by the review found no significant difference between benzyl benzoate versus oral ivermectin (see benefits of oral ivermectin, p 364). **Versus sulphur ointment:** One RCT identified by the review compared benzyl benzoate versus sulphur ointment (158 adults and children identified in a house to house survey of a semi-urban area of India).[15] It found no significant difference in the number of people with apparently cured lesions by 8 days (AR 68/89 [76%] with benzyl benzoate *v* 45/69 [65%] with sulphur ointment; RR 1.17, 95% CI 0.95 to 1.33) or by 14 days (AR 81/89 [91%] with benzyl benzoate *v* 67/69 [97%] with sulphur ointment; RR 0.94, 95% CI 0.86 to 1.01).

Harms: The RCT comparing benzyl benzoate versus oral ivermectin found that about a quarter of people treated with benzyl benzoate reported a transient increase in pruritus and dermatitis.[16] No other important adverse events have been reported (see harms of lindane, p 362).

Comment: Non-randomised trials suggest benzyl benzoate has variable effectiveness (as low as 50%).[17–19] The low cure rate may be related to the concentration of the preparation and resistance of the mite to benzyl benzoate.

OPTION SULPHUR COMPOUNDS

We found insufficient evidence of the effects of sulphur compounds.

Benefits: We found no RCTs comparing sulphur compounds versus placebo. **Versus benzyl benzoate:** We found one RCT (see benefits of benzyl benzoate, p 363).[15]

Harms: Use of sulphur was associated with increased local irritation in about a quarter of cases.[9]

Comment: None.

QUESTION What are the effects of systemic treatments?

OPTION ORAL IVERMECTIN

One systematic review found limited evidence that oral ivermectin versus placebo significantly increased clinical cure, and found no significant difference between oral ivermectin versus lindane in clinical cure. Experience of the use of oral ivermectin in onchocerciasis suggests that it is safe in younger adults, but no such experience exists for children, and there have been reports of increased risk of death in elderly people.

Benefits: We found one systematic review (search date 1999, 3 RCTs)[5] and one subsequent RCT[6] comparing oral ivermectin versus placebo or other agents. **Versus placebo:** One RCT (55 young adults and children aged > 5 years) identified by the review found that oral ivermectin versus placebo significantly increased clinical cure rates after 7 days (23/29 [79%] with oral ivermectin *v* 4/26 [15%] with placebo; RR 5.2, 95% CI 2.1 to 12.9; NNT 2, 95% CI 1 to 3).[5] **Versus benzyl benzoate:** One small RCT (44 adults and children) identified by the review found no significant difference in clinical cure rates at 30 days (16/23 [70%] with oral ivermectin *v* 10/21 [48%] with benzyl benzoate; RR 1.5, 95% CI 0.9 to 2.5).[16] **Versus lindane:** See benefits of lindane, p 362. **Versus permethrin:** See benefits of permethrin, p 361.

Harms: The RCTs identified by the review were too small to give adequate data on harms.[5] Oral ivermectin has been used widely in adults with onchocerciasis and even with repeated doses serious adverse effects have been rare.[20,21] We found no good evidence about its safety in children. An increased risk of death has been reported among elderly people taking oral ivermectin for scabies in a long term care facility.[22] It is not clear whether this was caused by oral ivermectin, interactions with other scabicides (including lindane and permethrin), or other treatments such as psychoactive drugs. Other studies reported no such complications from its use in elderly people.[23]

Comment: Case series suggest that oral ivermectin may be effective when included in the treatment of hyperkeratotic crusted scabies (also known as Norwegian scabies)[24,25] and in people with concomitant HIV disease.[4] The RCT comparing oral ivermection versus placebo assessed outcomes 7 days after the intervention was administered, which may be insufficient time to achieve cure.[5]

REFERENCES

1. Meinking TL, Taplin D. Infestations. In: Schachner LA, Hansen RC, eds. *Pediatric dermatology.* New York: Churchill Livingston, 1995.
2. Stein DH. Scabies and pediculosis. *Curr Opin Pediatr* 1991;3:660–666.
3. Green M. Epidemiology of scabies. *Epidemiol Rev* 1989;11:126–150.
4. Meinking TL, Taplin D, Hermida JL, Pardo R, Kerddel FA. The treatment of scabies with ivermectin. *N Engl J Med* 1995;333:26–30.
5. Walker GJA, Johnstone PW. Interventions for treating scabies. In: The Cochrane Library, Issue 3, 2001. Oxford: Update Software. Search date 1999; primary sources Medline, Embase, records of military trials from UK, USA, and Russia, and specialist register of the Cochrane Diseases Group.
6. Usha V, Gopalakrishnan Nair TV. A comparative study of oral ivermectin and topical permethrin cream in the treatment of scabies. *J Am Acad Dermatol* 2000;42:236–240.
7. McLeod WA. Acute lindane poisoning [letter]. *Can Med Assoc J* 1978;118:123–125.
8. Schultz MW, Gomez M, Hansen RC, et al. Comparative study of 5% permethrin cream and 1% lindane lotion for the treatment of scabies. *Arch Dermatol* 1990;126:167–170.
9. Meinking TL, Taplin D. Safety of permethrin vs lindane for the treatment of scabies. *Arch Dermatol* 1996;132:959–962.
10. Elgart ML. A risk-benefit assessment of agents used in the treatment of scabies. *Drug Saf* 1996; 14:386–393.
11. WHO Collaborating Centre for International Drug Monitoring. Reported adverse reactions to ectoparasiticodes, including scabicides, insecticides and repellents. Uppsala, Sweden, 1998.
12. Brown S, Belcher J, Brady W. Treatment of ectoparasitic infections: review of the English-language literature. *Clin Infect Dis* 1995;20(suppl 1):104–109.
13. Hanna NF, Clay JC, Harris JRW. *Sarcoptes scabiei* infestation treated with malathion liquid. *Br J Vener Dis* 1978;54:354.
14. Thianprasit M, Schuetzenberger R. Prioderm lotion in the treatment of scabies. *Southeast Asian J Trop Med Public Health* 1984;15:119–120.
15. Gulati PV, Singh KP. A family based study on the treatment of scabies with benzyl benzoate and sulphur ointment. *Indian J Dermatol Venereol Lepr* 1978;44:269–273.
16. Glaziou P, Cartel JL, Alzieu P, Moulia-Pelat JP, Martin PMV. Comparison of ivermectin and benzyl benzoate for treatment of scabies. *Trop Med Parasitol* 1993;44:331–332.
17. Burgess I, Robinson RJF, Robinson J, Maunder JW, Hassan Z. Aqueous malathion 0.5% as a scabicide: clinical trial. *BMJ* 1986;292:1172.
18. Kaur GA, Nadeswary K. Field trials on the management of scabies in Jengka Triangle, Pahang. *Med J Malaysia* 1980;35:14–21.
19. Haustein UF, Hlawa B. Treatment of scabies with permethrin versus lindane and benzyl benzoate. *Acta Derm Venereol* 1989;69:348–351.
20. Pacque M, Munoz B, Greene BM, et al. Safety of and compliance with community-based ivermectin therapy. *Lancet* 1990;335:1377–1380.
21. De Sole G, Remme J, Awadzi K, et al. Adverse reactions after large-scale treatment of onchocerciasis with ivermectin: combined results from eight community trials. *Bull World Health Organ* 1989;67:707–719.
22. Barkwell R, Shields S. Deaths associated with ivermectin treatment of scabies. *Lancet* 1997; 349:1144–1145.
23. Diazgranados JA, Costa JL. Deaths after ivermectin treatment. *Lancet* 1997;349:1698.
24. Sullivan JR, Watt G, Barker B. Successful use of ivermectin in the treatment of endemic scabies in a nursing home. *Australas J Dermatol* 1997;38:137–140.
25. Aubin F, Humbert P. Ivermectin for crusted (Norwegian) scabies. *N Engl J Med* 1995;332:612.

Godfrey Walker
Specialist in Reproductive Health
UNFPA Country Technical Services
Team for Eastern Europe and Central
Asia
Bratislava
Slovak Republic

Paul Johnstone
Director of Public Health Visiting
Professor in Public Health
University of Teesside
Middlesbrough
UK

Competing interests: None declared.

Dysmenorrhoea

Search date October 2001

Cynthia Farquhar and Michelle Proctor

INTERVENTIONS

Key Messages

- One systematic review has found that aspirin is significantly more effective for pain relief than placebo, but less effective than naproxen or ibuprofen. The review found no significant difference between paracetamol versus placebo, aspirin, or ibuprofen in pain relief. It found limited evidence that co-proxamol versus placebo significantly reduced pain, but reduced pain significantly less and was associated with significantly more adverse effects than naproxen. It also found that co-proxamol reduced dysmenorrhoea-related symptoms significantly less than mefenamic acid.

- One systematic review has found that naproxen, ibuprofen, and mefenamic acid are significantly more effective than placebo for pain relief. The review found some evidence of increased adverse effects with naproxen.

- One systematic review found insufficient evidence of the effects of oral contraceptives in pain relief.

- One small RCT found limited evidence suggesting that laparoscopic uterine nerve ablation versus diagnostic laparoscopy significantly increased pain relief. Another RCT comparing laparoscopic uterine nerve ablation versus laparoscopic presacral neurectomy found no significant difference in pain relief in the short term, but found that laparoscopic presacral neurectomy significantly reduced pain in the long term.

- Two small RCTs found that high frequency transcutaneous electrical nerve stimulation versus placebo significantly increased pain relief. One RCT found no significant difference between low frequency transcutaneous electrical nerve stimulation versus placebo in pain relief. Two RCTs found conflicting evidence of the effects of transcutaneous electrical nerve stimulation versus non-steroidal anti-inflammatory drugs in pain relief.

- One small RCT found limited evidence that acupuncture versus placebo acupuncture or no treatment significantly reduced pain.

- Two RCTs found insufficient evidence of the effects of behavioural interventions.

- RCTs found conflicting evidence of the effects of spinal manipulation versus placebo or no treatment in pain relief.

- One systematic review found insufficient evidence of the effects of herbal remedies.

- Two RCTs found limited evidence that magnesium versus placebo significantly reduced pain, but one RCT found no significant difference between magnesium versus placebo in pain relief. One large RCT found that thiamine versus placebo significantly reduced pain. RCTs have found insufficient evidence of the effects of fish oil, dietary change, or vitamin E.

DEFINITION Dysmenorrhoea comprises painful menstrual cramps of uterine origin. It is commonly divided into primary dysmenorrhoea (pain without organic pathology) and secondary dysmenorrhoea (pelvic pain associated with an identifiable pathological condition, such as endometriosis or ovarian cysts). The initial onset of primary dysmenorrhoea is usually shortly after menarche (6–12 months) when ovulatory cycles are established. The pain duration is commonly 8–72 hours and is usually associated with the onset of the menstrual flow. Secondary dysmenorrhoea may arise as a new symptom during a woman's fourth and fifth decade.[1]

INCIDENCE/ PREVALENCE Variations in the definition of dysmenorrhoea make it difficult to determine the precise prevalence. However, various types of study have found a consistently high prevalence in women of different ages and nationalities. A systematic review (search date 1996) of the prevalence of chronic pelvic pain, summarising both community and hospital surveys, estimated the prevalence at 45–95%.[2] Reports focus on adolescent girls and generally include only primary dysmenorrhoea, although this is not always specified. Studies of prevalence are summarised in table 1, p 379.

AETIOLOGY/ RISK FACTORS A longitudinal study of a representative sample of women born in 1962 found that severity of dysmenorrhoea was significantly associated with duration of menstrual flow (average duration of menstrual flow was 5 days for women with no dysmenorrhoea and 5.8 days for women with severe dysmenorrhoea; $P < 0.001$; WMD −0.8, 95% CI −1.36 to −0.24); younger average menarcheal age (13.1 years in women without dysmenorrhoea v 12.6 years in women with severe dysmenorrhoea; $P < 0.01$; WMD 0.5, 95% CI 0.09 to 0.91); and cigarette smoking (41% of smokers and 26% of non-smokers experienced moderate or severe dysmenorrhoea).[9] There is also some evidence of a dose-response relationship between exposure to environmental tobacco smoke and increased incidence of dysmenorrhoea.[10]

PROGNOSIS　Primary dysmenorrhoea is a chronic recurring condition that affects most young women. Studies of the natural history of this condition are sparse. One longitudinal study in Scandinavia found that primary dysmenorrhoea often improves in the third decade of a woman's reproductive life, and is also reduced following childbirth.[9]

AIMS　To relieve pain from dysmenorrhoea, with minimal adverse effects.

OUTCOMES　Pain relief, measured either by a visual analogue scale (see glossary, p 378), other pain scales, or as a dichotomous outcome (pain relief achieved yes/no); overall improvement in dysmenorrhoea measured by change in dysmenorrhoeic symptoms either self reported or observed, quality of life scales, or other similar measures such as the Menstrual Distress or Menstrual Symptom Questionnaires; adverse effects of treatment (incidence and type of adverse effects); proportion of women requiring analgesics in addition to their assigned treatment; proportion of women reporting activity restriction or absences from work or school and hours or days of absence as a more selective measure.

METHODS　*Clinical Evidence* search and appraisal October 2001.

QUESTION　What are the effects of drug treatments?

OPTION　ASPIRIN, PARACETAMOL, AND COMPOUND ANALGESICS

One systematic review has found that aspirin is significantly more effective for pain relief than placebo, but less effective than naproxen or ibuprofen. The review found no significant difference between paracetamol versus placebo, aspirin, or ibuprofen in pain relief. It found limited evidence that co-proxamol versus placebo significantly reduced pain, but reduced pain significantly less and was associated with significantly more adverse effects than naproxen. It also found that co-proxamol reduced dysmenorrhoea-related symptoms significantly less than mefenamic acid.

Benefits:　We found one systematic review (search date 1997, 13 RCTs) of the effects of analgesics in primary dysmenorrhoea (see table 2, p 380), which compared analgesics versus placebo, versus each other, or versus non-steroidal anti-inflammatory drugs.[11] **Aspirin versus placebo:** The review identified eight RCTs comparing aspirin versus placebo (486 women, 650 mg 4 times daily). Aspirin was significantly more effective than placebo for pain relief (5 RCTs; RR 1.60, 95% CI 1.12 to 2.29; NNT 10, 95% CI 5 to 50). There was no significant difference between aspirin versus placebo in the need for additional medication (3 RCTs; RR 0.79, 95% CI 0.58 to 1.08), or restriction of daily activity and absence from work (3 RCTs: RR 0.82, 95% CI 0.64 to 1.04; 1 RCT: RR 1.28, 95% CI 0.24 to 6.76). **Paracetamol versus placebo:** One RCT identified by the review found no significant difference between paracetamol 500 mg four times daily versus placebo in pain relief (35 women; RR 1.0, 95% CI 0.3 to 3.6). **Co-proxamol versus placebo:** The review identified one RCT, which found that co-proxamol (see glossary, p 377) versus placebo significantly increased marked or moderate pain relief (72 women; 650 mg/65 mg 4 times daily; RR 3.72, 95% CI 2.13 to 6.52). **Paracetamol versus aspirin:** One RCT (35 volunteer medical, pharmacy, and dental students) identified by the review compared aspirin (500 mg 4 times daily) versus paracetamol (500 mg 4 times daily). It found no significant difference in pain relief (10 cm visual analogue scale [see glossary, p 378]: median change from baseline 1.6 cm, 95% CI 0.4 to 3.3 with paracetamol v 1.2 cm, 95% CI 0 to 2.7 with aspirin). **Aspirin or paracetamol versus non-steroidal anti-inflammatory drugs:** The review identified six RCTs comparing aspirin or paracetamol versus non-steroidal anti-inflammatory drugs (313 women). Aspirin (650 mg 4 times daily) reduced pain significantly less than both naproxen (275 mg 4 times daily) (1 RCT; RR 2.29, 95% CI 1.16 to 4.29) and ibuprofen (400 mg 4 times daily) (1 RCT; RR 1.9, 95% CI 1.13 to 2.78). One RCT found no significant difference between paracetamol (1000 mg 3 times daily) versus ibuprofen (400 mg 3 times daily) in pain relief (defined as at least moderate relief) (1 RCT; RR 0.86, 95% CI 0.68 to 1.10). **Co-proxamol versus non-steroidal anti-inflammatory drugs:** The review identified three RCTs. One RCT compared co-proxamol (650 mg/65 mg 3 times daily) versus mefenamic acid (500 mg 3 times daily). The RCT found that co-proxamol versus mefenamic acid was significantly less effective in reducing dysmenorrhoea related symptoms (P < 0.01). Co-proxamol versus mefenamic acid also increased the need for additional medication (mean number of tablets of additional medication 2.6 with mefenamic acid v 6.8 with co-proxamol; no P value provided). The RCT found no significant difference between treatments in absence from work or school. Two RCTs (98 women) compared co-proxamol (650 mg/65 mg 3 times daily) versus naproxen (275 mg 3 times daily). Neither RCT found a significant difference in pain severity (P > 0.05), but naproxen achieved more effective pain control on some of the days measured (P < 0.05).

Harms: The most common adverse effects described by the review were nausea or abdominal discomfort, headaches, and dizziness.[11] Adverse effects occurred in 7–17% of women taking aspirin versus 3–17% of women taking placebo. The review found no significant difference between aspirin or paracetamol versus placebo in the frequency of adverse effects (any adverse effect for aspirin v placebo: RR 1.31, 95% CI 0.79 to 2.17; any adverse effect for paracetamol v placebo: RR 1.00, 95% CI 0.36 to 2.75). It found that co-proxamol versus naproxen significantly increased the number of women experiencing adverse effects (23–58% v 15–25%; RR 1.94, 95% CI 1.11 to 3.41).[11]

Comment: Most RCTs included in the systematic review were short (usually only 1 menstrual cycle on each treatment), small, and used a crossover design without a washout period. All of the RCTs (except one of co-proxamol versus naproxen) used double blinding. All the RCTs used oral administration of treatment in the form of tablets or capsules.

OPTION	NON-STEROIDAL ANTI-INFLAMMATORY DRUGS (OTHER THAN ASPIRIN)

One systematic review has found that naproxen, ibuprofen, and mefenamic acid are all significantly more effective than placebo for pain relief. The review found some evidence of increased adverse effects with naproxen.

Benefits: We found one systematic review (search date 1997) of the effects of non-steroidal anti-inflammatory drugs (NSAIDs) in primary dysmenorrhoea, which included 23 RCTs of naproxen (1728 women), 18 of ibuprofen (748 women), and five of mefenamic acid (257 women).[11] **NSAIDs versus placebo:** The systematic review found that all three NSAIDs versus placebo significantly increased pain relief (naproxen: 13 RCTs; RR 3.17, 95% CI 2.72 to 3.67, NNT 2.6, 95% CI 2 to 3.4; ibuprofen: 9 RCTs; RR 2.41, 95% CI 1.58 to 3.68, NNT 2.4, 95% CI 1.7 to 3.8; mefenamic acid: 3 RCTs; RR 2.03, 95% CI 1.65 to 2.48, NNT 2.4, 95% CI 1.6 to 4.5). The use of additional analgesics was significantly reduced for all NSAIDs versus placebo. Women taking naproxen were 60% less likely to use additional analgesics (10 RCTs; RR 0.4, 95% CI 0.3 to 0.4); those taking ibuprofen were 70% less likely (2 RCTs; RR 0.23, 95% CI 0.13 to 0.41); and those on mefenamic acid were 35% less likely (1 RCT; RR 0.65, 95% CI 0.52 to 0.80). Restriction of daily life was significantly less for naproxen (7 RCTs; RR 0.71, 95% CI 0.60 to 0.85) and ibuprofen (3 RCTs; RR 0.82, 95% CI 0.64 to 1.04). Absence from work or school was significantly reduced with naproxen (7 RCTs; RR 0.29, 95% CI 0.13 to 0.66) but not with ibuprofen (1 RCT; RR 0.14, 95% CI 0.02 to 1.10). **Comparison of NSAIDs:** The review identified five comparative RCTs. Three RCTs found no significant difference in pain relief between naproxen (550 mg loading dose followed by 275 mg) versus ibuprofen (400 mg) (RR 1.1, 95% CI 0.8 to 1.5). One RCT found that naproxen (550 mg loading dose followed by 275 mg) versus mefenamic acid (500 mg followed by 250 mg) significantly increased pain relief (RR 2.4, 95% CI 1.4 to 4.1), and another RCT found no significant difference between ibuprofen 400 mg versus mefenamic acid 250 mg (no RR or P values provided).

Harms: The most commonly reported adverse effects in the RCTs identified by the review were nausea, dizziness, and headaches.[11] Naproxen versus placebo significantly increased the number of adverse effects (number of RCTs not specified; RR 1.45, 95% CI 1.03 to 2.04). The review found no significant difference between ibuprofen versus placebo in the number of adverse effects (RR 1.12, 95% CI 0.85 to 1.47) or between mefenamic acid versus placebo (RR 0.59, 95% CI 0.28 to 1.23).[11]

Comment: All the RCTs identified by the review used oral treatment.[11] NSAIDs can be administered as suppositories, which seem to have a similar effect on overall pain relief but less effect than oral treatment for spasmodic pain.[12] Most RCTs in this systematic review used a crossover design without a washout period and were brief (usually only 1 menstrual cycle per treatment). Nine of the included RCTs did not blind the researchers to treatment allocation. Many of the trials on NSAIDs were sponsored by the pharmaceutical industry. The pain relief figures used above refer to RCTs that include women with primary dysmenorrhoea only. However, some of the figures regarding use of additional medication included data from women with undefined dysmenorrhoea. A systematic review with stricter inclusion criteria and methodological quality assessment is underway.[13]

OPTION   COMBINED ORAL CONTRACEPTIVES

One systematic review found insufficient evidence of the effects of oral contraceptives in pain relief.

Benefits: We found one systematic review (search date 1999, 5 RCTs, 379 women).[14] It found no significant difference between medium dose oestrogen (> 35 µg) plus first or second generation progestogens versus placebo in pain relief at 1–3 months (4 RCTs, 320 women; 112/216 [52%] v 32/104 [31%]; RR 1.40, 95% CI 0.58 to 3.42). It found that oral contraceptives versus placebo reduced the number of women absent from work or school, but the difference did not quite reach significance (1 RCT; 19/49 [39%] v 24/40 [60%]; RR 0.65, 95% CI 0.42 to 1.00).

Harms: The review found no significant difference between combined oral contraceptives versus placebo in the number of women experiencing adverse effects, such as nausea, vomiting, depression, and abdominal pain (1 RCT, 89 women; 15/49 [31%] v 8/40 [20%]; RR 1.53, 95% CI 0.72 to 3.24).[14] The results of two RCTs are difficult to interpret and could not be included in the meta-analysis of adverse effects performed by the review because the RCTs randomised menstrual cycles and not women.[15,16] One small RCT (18 women) identified by the review comparing combined oral contraceptives versus placebo found that more women receiving the contraceptive pill experienced breakthrough bleeding (2/12 [17%] v 0/6 [0%]).[15] Another RCT (59 women) identified by the review found that combined oral contraceptives versus placebo increased weight gain, nausea, and vomiting (no further data provided).[16]

Comment: Most of the RCTs identified by the review had weak methods.[14] Because of the small number of included trials and participants, the results of the systematic review are sensitive to the statistical methods of calculation used. One of the RCTs identified by the review could not be included in the meta-analysis because of poor reporting of data.[16] All of the RCTs identified by the review used oral contraceptives that are no longer commonly prescribed, so the results may not be applicable to women today who take different preparations.[14]

QUESTION   What are the effects of surgical treatments?

One small RCT found limited evidence suggesting that laparoscopic uterine nerve ablation versus diagnostic laparoscopy significantly increased pain relief. Another RCT comparing laparoscopic uterine nerve

Women's health

ablation versus laparoscopic presacral neurectomy found no significant difference in pain relief in the short term, but found that laparoscopic presacral neurectomy significantly reduced pain in the long term.

Benefits: We found one systematic review (search date 1998, 6 RCTs) of surgical pelvic nerve interruption for primary and secondary dysmenorrhoea.[17] Only two of the six RCTs included women with primary dysmenorrhoea. Meta-analysis was not performed because of RCT heterogeneity. One RCT identified by the review (21 women) comparing laparoscopic uterine nerve ablation (LUNA) (see glossary, p 377) versus diagnostic laparoscopy found that LUNA significantly increased pain relief at 3 months (OR 15.5, 95% CI 2.9 to 83) and at 12 months (OR 10.9, 95% CI 1.5 to 77). The other RCT (68 women) found no significant difference between LUNA versus laparoscopic presacral neurectomy (LPSN) (see glossary, p 377) in pain relief at 3 months' follow up (OR 0.7, 95% CI 0.2 to 2.7). However, at 12 months' follow up, the LPSN group had significantly better pain relief scores (OR 0.26, 95% CI 0.10 to 0.71).

Harms: One RCT identified by the review found that LPSN versus LUNA significantly increased constipation (31/33 [94%] with LPSN v 0/35 [0%] with LUNA; RR 0.01, 95% CI 0.00 to 0.24).[17]

Comment: Two larger RCTs of LUNA are underway (M Proctor, personal communication, 2001). We found a second relevant systematic review but we have not included it because it includes lower levels of evidence, such as case studies.[18]

QUESTION   What are the effects of complementary treatments?

OPTION   TRANSCUTANEOUS ELECTRICAL NERVE STIMULATION

Two small RCTs found that high frequency transcutaneous electrical nerve stimulation versus placebo significantly increased pain relief. One RCT found no significant difference between low frequency transcutaneous electrical nerve stimulation versus placebo in pain relief. Two RCTs found conflicting evidence of the effects of transcutaneous electrical nerve stimulation versus non-steroidal anti-inflammatory drugs in pain relief.

Benefits: We found no systematic review but found three RCTs [19–21] **High frequency transcutaneous electrical nerve stimulation (TENS) versus placebo:** We found two RCTs.[19,20] The first RCT (32 women, double blind, crossover) compared three groups: high frequency TENS (see glossary, p 377); placebo; and ibuprofen.[19] It found that TENS versus placebo significantly increased the number of women who experienced at least moderate pain relief (14/32 [44%] with TENS v 1/32 [3%] with placebo; OR 24, 95% CI 2.9 to 199). The second RCT (27 women, single blind) compared high frequency TENS versus low frequency TENS versus placebo.[20] It found that high frequency TENS versus placebo significantly reduced pain (18 women: mean decrease 72% with TENS v 26% with placebo; WMD using fixed effects model 45, 95% CI 23 to 67). **Low frequency TENS versus placebo:** The RCT (27 women, single blind) comparing high frequency TENS versus low frequency TENS versus placebo found no significant difference between low frequency TENS versus placebo (18 women; WMD 24, 95% CI −2.9 to +51).[20] **High frequency TENS versus low frequency TENS:** One RCT found no significant difference between high frequency and low frequency TENS for pain relief (WMD 21, 95% CI −4.4 to +46).[20] **High frequency TENS versus non-steroidal anti-inflammatory drugs:** The RCT (32 women) comparing high frequency TENS, ibuprofen, and placebo found that high frequency TENS was significantly less effective than ibuprofen in achieving pain relief (14/32 [44%] with TENS v 24/32 [75%] using ibuprofen; OR 0.26, 95% CI 0.09 to 0.75).[19] Another unblinded RCT (12 women, crossover) found no significant difference between naproxen versus high frequency/high intensity TENS in pain relief (data were presented in graphic form but no OR or P values provided) but both significantly reduced pain from baseline (P < 0.001).[21]

Harms: Adverse effects of muscle vibrations, tightness, headaches, and slight burning or redness after use were experienced by four women on treatment and none on placebo (OR 10, 95% CI 0.5 to 199; P = 0.12).[19] In the unblinded crossover RCT, 10/12 women considered TENS to be temporarily painful but were prepared to accept this effect for the pain relief achieved.[21] None of the 12 women reported any adverse effects during treatment with naproxen.

Comment: A systematic review is underway.[22]

OPTION   ACUPUNCTURE

One small RCT found limited evidence that acupuncture versus placebo acupuncture or versus no treatment significantly reduced pain.

Benefits: We found no systematic review. We found one RCT (48 women) comparing acupuncture versus placebo acupuncture (see glossary, p 377) versus two no-treatment control groups, one of which had extra visits from a physician.[23] Treatment was for 30–40 minutes once a week for 3 weeks a month, for a total of 3 months. It found that acupuncture versus placebo acupuncture or no treatment significantly increased the proportion of women experiencing pain relief (chi^2 = 13.6; P < 0.001). Acupuncture versus placebo acupuncture was significantly more effective in achieving pain relief (OR 17.5, 95% CI 1.6 to 192).

Harms: The RCT gave no information on adverse effects.

Comment: A systematic review is underway.[23]

OPTION   BEHAVIOURAL INTERVENTIONS

Two RCTs found insufficient evidence of the effects of behavioural interventions.

Benefits: We found no systematic review. We found two small RCTs on behavioural interventions (see glossary, p 377). One involved relaxation and imagery,[24] and the other involved aerobic exercise.[25] **Relaxation treatment:** The first RCT (69 women) compared muscle relaxation plus positive imagery regarding menstruation versus self directed group discussion about menstruation versus waiting list control. The groups were divided into women with spasmodic or congestive dysmenorrhoea using the Menstrual Symptom Questionnaire. Spasmodic dysmenorrhoea was defined as spasms of pain mainly around the abdomen, and congestive dysmenorrhoea was defined as a dull aching pain in the lower abdomen and other areas of the body. It found that, in women with spasmodic or congestive dysmenorrhoea, muscle relaxation versus waiting list control significantly improved symptoms (P < 0.01). However, it found that only the women with spasmodic dysmenorrhoea experienced significantly less pain with relaxation versus group discussion or versus waiting list control (P < 0.001).[24] **Aerobic exercise:** The second RCT (36 women) comparing a training group that participated in 30 minutes of exercise 3 days a week versus a sedentary control group found that aerobic exercise significantly lowered Menstrual Distress Questionnaire scores (P < 0.05; results presented graphically).[25]

Harms: The RCTs gave no information on adverse effects.

Comment: Both RCTs were small and of poor methodological quality.[24,25] The classification of dysmenorrhoea into spasmodic and congestive categories is no longer commonly used and has little meaning.[25] The RCT (36 women) comparing aerobic exercise versus a sedentary control analysed results for the 26 women (72%) who completed the trial (11 in the exercise group and 15 in the control group).[25] A systematic review is underway.[26]

OPTION   SPINAL MANIPULATION

RCTs found conflicting evidence of the effects of spinal manipulation versus placebo or no treatment in pain relief.

Benefits: We found one systematic review (search date 2000, 5 RCTs) comparing spinal manipulation versus placebo or no treatment.[27] There was significant trial heterogeneity and the outcome of pain intensity or pain relief was reported differently by each of the trials; therefore a meta-analysis could not be performed. The first RCT (11 women) identified by the review compared high velocity, low amplitude rotation manipulation (HVLA) (see glossary, p 377) versus no treatment versus placebo manipulation (see glossary, p 377). It found no significant difference between HVLA versus no treatment in pain relief after 1 month (7/8 [87%] with HVLA v 0/2 [0%] with no treatment; RR 5.00, 95% CI 0.39 to 63.85), or HVLA versus placebo treatment (7/8 [87%] with HVLA v 0/1 [0%] with placebo treatment; RR 3.33, 95% CI 0.30 to 37.42). The second RCT identified by the review (44 women) comparing HVLA versus placebo manipulation found that HVLA significantly reduced pain intensity as measured by a 10 cm visual analogue scale (see glossary, p 378) pain score after one treatment and one menstrual cycle (WMD −1.41, 95% CI −2.55 to −0.27). The third RCT (138 women) identified by the review found no significant difference between HVLA versus placebo manipulation in pain as measured by mean change in visual analogue scale pain score after one menstrual cycle (WMD +2.08, 95% CI −3.20 to +7.36). The fourth RCT (12 women) identified by the review found that HVLA versus placebo manipulation improved pain after one treatment during one menstrual cycle (no further data provided). The fifth RCT (26 women) identified by the review comparing 3 months of Toftness manipulation (see glossary, p 377) versus placebo manipulation found that manipulation versus placebo did not significantly reduce pain intensity as measured by 10 cm visual analogue scale pain scores after 3 months (WMD 2.20, 95% CI 1.38 to 3.02), but manipulation did significantly reduce pain intensity after 6 months (WMD −1.40, 95% CI −2.21 to −0.59).[27]

Harms: One RCT identified by the review (138 women) found no significant difference between HVLA versus placebo manipulation in the number of women experiencing soreness in the lower back region within 48 hours of the intervention (3/69 [4%] v 2/69 [3%]; RR 1.50, 95% CI 0.26 to 8.70).[27] Soreness resolved within 24 hours. No other adverse effects were reported. The other RCTs identified by the review gave no information on adverse effects.

Comment: The overall methodological quality of the RCTs identified by the review was good: low withdrawal rate (2%), adequate randomisation method, blinding of the outcome assessor, and potential blinding of the participants as the control procedure was very similar to the treatment.

OPTION   HERBAL REMEDIES

One systematic review found insufficient evidence of the effects of herbal remedies.

Benefits: We found one systematic review (search date 2000), which identified one RCT comparing a herbal remedy versus placebo.[28] It found that the Japanese herbal remedy toki-shakuyaku-san (taken 3 times daily) versus placebo remedy significantly reduced pain as measured by a visual analogue scale (see glossary, p 378) after 6 months (P < 0.005), and significantly reduced the need for additional medication (diclofenac sodium) (P < 0.01; results presented graphically).

Harms: The RCT gave no information on adverse effects.

Comment: Toki-shakuyaku-san is a mixture of six herbs, including angelica and peony root.

OPTION   DIETARY SUPPLEMENTS

Two RCTs found limited evidence that magnesium versus placebo significantly reduced pain, but one RCT found no significant difference between magnesium versus placebo in pain relief. One large RCT found that thiamine versus placebo significantly reduced pain. RCTs found insufficient evidence of the effects of fish oil, dietary change, or vitamin E.

Benefits: We found one systematic review (search date 2000, 6 RCTs)[28] and two additional RCTs.[29,30] **Fish oils versus placebo:** One RCT (42 women) identified by the review compared fish oil capsules twice daily for 1 month versus placebo. Menstrual symptom scores were significantly lower with fish oil than placebo (44 v 70; P < 0.001).[28] Less additional medication (ibuprofen 200 mg) was used in the fish oil group (mean 4.7 tablets with treatment v 10.1 with placebo; P = 0.015). One additional RCT (78 women) compared four interventions: fish oil (0.5–1 g 5 times daily); fish oil with vitamin B_{12} (0.015 mg); seal oil (higher in saturated fat than fish oil); and placebo for a minimum of 3 months.[29] It found that pain measured on a visual analogue scale (see glossary, p 378) significantly decreased only in the fish oil with vitamin B_{12} group (reduction in mean scores: placebo –0.19; seal oil –0.2; fish oil –0.15; fish oil with vitamin B_{12} –0.73; P = 0.015). However, all three active treatment groups experienced significant change in the number of other menstrual symptoms and the amount of interference with daily activities (P < 0.05). **Magnesium versus placebo:** Three RCTs identified by the review compared magnesium versus placebo.[28] The first RCT (50 women) identified by the review compared magnesium aspartate three times daily versus placebo. It found that magnesium aspartate versus placebo significantly increased the number of women without pain after 6 months (21/25 [84%] with magnesium v 7/25 [28%] with placebo; RR 3.0, 95% CI 1.6 to 5.8). The second RCT (27 women) identified by the review found no significant difference between magnesium (5 mmol 3 times daily) versus placebo in reducing pain as measured by visual analogue scale pain scores, or in the number of ibuprofen tablets taken (P = 0.07; no further data provided). The third RCT (21 women) identified by the review found that magnesium (500 mg daily during menses) versus placebo significantly reduced pain after 5 months (P < 0.01).[28] **Thiamine versus placebo:** The review identified one crossover RCT (556 Indian adolescents attending school) comparing thiamine (100 mg daily for 3 months) versus placebo, which found that thiamine significantly increased the number of people with no pain before crossover after 60 days (142/277 [51%] with thiamine v 0/279 [0%] with placebo).[28] After completion of the RCT, 87% of all women experienced no pain. **Dietary change versus vitamin B_{12}:** One additional RCT (33 women) comparing a low fat, vegetarian diet versus a supplement placebo tablet containing vitamin B_{12} (0.02 mg) found no significant difference in the number of days with menstrual pain (WMD –0.9, 95% CI –1.8 to 0.0).[30] **Vitamin E plus ibuprofen versus ibuprofen alone:** One crossover RCT identified by the review (50 women) compared vitamin E (100 mg daily for 20 days before menses) plus ibuprofen (400 mg at the outset of painful menstruation) versus ibuprofen alone (400 mg at the onset of pain).[28] It found no significant difference between vitamin E plus ibuprofen versus ibuprofen alone in pain relief (23/26 [88%] v 17/24 [71%]; RR 1.25, 95% CI 0.93 to 1.67).

Harms: **Fish oils versus placebo:** One RCT identified by the review found that two women taking fish oils reported nausea and one women reported acne.[28] No adverse effects were reported in the group of women receiving placebo. **Magnesium versus placebo:** One RCT identified by the review found that magnesium versus placebo significantly increased the number of women who experienced intestinal discomfort and other minor adverse effects (5/25 [20%] with magnesium v 0/25 [0%] with placebo; NNH 5, 95% CI 2 to 38), although relief of these symptoms occurred when the dose was reduced from three to two tablets daily.[28] **Dietary change versus vitamin B$_{12}$:** One additional RCT comparing a low fat, vegetarian diet versus a supplement placebo tablet found that stomach upset, slight nausea, burping, and a bad taste in the mouth were reported by eight women across the different treatment groups.[30] No additional information was reported in the trial.

Comment: None.

GLOSSARY

Behavioural interventions Treatments that attempt modification of thought and beliefs (cognition) about symptoms and pain and/or modification of behavioural or physiological responses to symptoms and pain.

Co-proxamol Non-proprietary label for a dextropropoxyphene hydrochloride and paracetamol combination. The most common presentation is tablets containing dextropropoxyphene hydrochloride 32.5 mg and paracetamol 325 mg.

High velocity, low amplitude manipulation A technique of spinal manipulation that uses high velocity, low amplitude thrusts to manipulate vertebral joints. The technique is designed to restore motion to a restricted joint and improve function. The physician positions the patient at the barrier of restricted motion and then gives a rapid, accurate thrust in the direction of the restricted barrier to resolve the restriction and improve motion.

Laparoscopic presacral neurectomy Involves the total removal of the presacral nerves lying within the boundaries of the interiliac triangle. This procedure interrupts the majority of the cervical sensory nerve fibres and is used to diminish uterine pain.

Laparoscopic uterine nerve ablation Involves laparoscopic surgery to transect (usually they are cut and then electrocauterised) the uterosacral ligaments at their insertion into the cervix. This procedure interrupts the majority of the cervical sensory nerve fibres and is used to diminish uterine pain.

Placebo acupuncture Also known as sham acupuncture, a commonly used control intervention involving the use of acupuncture needles to stimulate non-acupuncture points in areas outside of Chinese meridians. These points can be identified by a point detector as areas of the skin that do not have skin electrical activity similar to acupuncture points. There is some disagreement over correct needle placement, as placement of a needle in any position may elicit some biological response that can complicate interpretation of results.

Placebo manipulation Also known as sham manipulation, it is a control intervention. The main principle is to use a non-therapeutic level of torque. There are two common techniques for placebo manipulation. In one, thrust is administered but the posture of the participant is such that the mechanical torque of the manipulation is substantially reduced. In the other, an activator adjusting tool is used, which can make spinal adjustments using spring recoil, where the spring is set so no force is exerted.

Toftness technique A low force technique of chiropractic adjusting that uses a sensometer to detect sites of abnormal electromagnetic radiation, and to determine which sites to adjust. Adjustment is then delivered using a metered, hand-held pressure applicator.

Transcutaneous electrical nerve stimulation (TENS) Electrodes are placed on the skin and different electrical pulse rates and intensities are used to stimulate the area. Low frequency TENS (also referred to as acupuncture-like TENS) usually consists of pulses delivered at 1–4 Hz at high intensity so they evoke visible muscle fibre contractions. High frequency TENS (conventional TENS) usually consists of pulses delivered at 50–120 Hz at a low intensity, so there are no muscle contractions.

Visual analogue scale A commonly used scale in pain assessment. It is a 10 cm horizontal or vertical line with word anchors at each end, such as "no pain" and "pain as bad as it could be". The woman is asked to make a mark on the line to represent pain intensity. This mark is converted to distance in millimetres from the "no pain" anchor to give a pain score that can range from 0–100.

REFERENCES

1. Fraser I. Prostaglandins, prostaglandin inhibitors and their roles in gynaecological disorders. *Bailliere's Clinical Obstet Gynaecol* 1992;6: 829–857.

2. Zondervan KT, Yudkin PL, Vessey MP, et al. The prevalence of chronic pelvic pain in the United Kingdom: a systematic review. *Br J Obstet Gynaecol* 1998;105:93–99. Search date 1996; primary sources Medline, Embase, and Psychlit.

3. Harlow SD, Park M. A longitudinal study of risk factors for the occurrence, duration and severity of menstrual cramps in a cohort of college women. *Br J Obstet Gynaecol* 1996;103:1134–1142.

4. Campbell MA, McGrath PJ. Use of medication by adolescents for the management of menstrual discomfort. *Arch Pediatr Adolesc Med* 1997;151: 905–913.

5. Robinson JC, Plichta S, Weisman CS, et al. Dysmenorrhoea and the use of oral contraceptives in adolescent women attending a family planning clinic. *Am J Obstet Gynecol* 1992;166:578–583.

6. Andersch B, Milsom I. An epidemiologic study of young women with dysmenorrhea. *Am J Obstet Gynecol* 1982;144:655–660.

7. Pedron Neuvo N, Gonzalez-Unzaga LN, De Celis-Carrillo R, et al. Incidence of dysmenorrhoea and associated symptoms in women aged 12–24 years. *Ginecologia y Obstetrica de Mexico* 1998; 66:492–494.

8. Klein JR, Litt IF. Epidemiology of adolescent dysmenorrhea. *Pediatrics* 1981;68:661–664.

9. Sundell G, Milsom I, Andersch B. Factors influencing the prevalence and severity of dysmenorrhoea in young women. *Br J Obstet Gynecol* 1990;97:588–594.

10. Chen C, Cho SI, Damokosh AI, et al. Prospective study of exposure to environmental tobacco smoke and dysmenorrhea. *Environ Health Perspect* 2000;108:1019–1022.

11. Zhang WY, Li Wan Po A. Efficacy of minor analgesics in primary dysmenorrhoea: a systematic review. *Br J Obstet Gynaecol* 1998; 105:780–789. Search date 1997; primary sources Medline, Embase, and Science Citation Index.

12. Ylikorkala O, Puolakka J, Kauppila A. Comparison between naproxen tablets and suppositories in primary dysmenorrhea. *Prostaglandins* 1980;20: 463–468.

13. Proctor ML, Sinclair OJ, Farquhar CM, Ivanova I, Stones W. Non-steroidal anti-inflammatory drugs for primary dysmenorrhoea (Protocol for a Cochrane Review). In: The Cochrane Library, Issue 4, 2001. Oxford: Update Software.

14. Proctor ML, Roberts H, Farquhar C. Combined oral contraceptives for primary dysmenorrhoea. In: The Cochrane Library, Issue 4, 2001. Oxford, Update Software. Search date 1999; primary sources Medline, Embase, Cinahl, Cochrane Controlled Trials Register, and hand searched citation lists.

15. Nakano R, Takemura H. Treatment of function dysmenorrhoea: a double-blind study. *Acta Obstet Gynaecol Jpn* 1971;18:41–44.

16. Matthews AE, Clarke JE. Double-blind trial of a sequential oral contraceptive (Sequens) in the treatment of dysmenorrhoea. *J Obstet Gynaecol Br Commonw* 1968;75:1117–1122.

17. Proctor ML, Farquhar CM, Sinclair OJ, et al. Surgical interruption of pelvic nerve pathways for primary and secondary dysmenorrhoea. In: The Cochrane Library, Issue 4, 2001. Oxford: Update Software. Search date 1998; primary sources Medline, Embase, Cochrane Controlled Trials Register, hand searched citation lists, and conference proceedings.

18. Khan KS, Khan SF, Nwosu CR, et al. Laparoscopic uterosacral nerve ablation in chronic pelvic pain: an overview. *Gynaecol Endosc* 1999;8:257–265. Search date 1997; primary sources Medline, Embase, and Science Citation Index.

19. Dawood MY, Ramos J. Transcutaneous electrical nerve stimulation (TENS) for the treatment of primary dysmenorrhoea: a randomized crossover comparison with placebo TENS and ibuprofen. *Obstet Gynecol* 1990;75:656–660.

20. Mannheimer JS, Whalen EC. The efficacy of transcutaneous electrical nerve stimulation in dysmenorrhea. *Clin J Pain* 1985;1: 75–83.

21. Hedner N, Milsom I, Eliasson T, et al. Tens bra vid smatsam mens. [TENS is effective in painful menstruation.] *Lakartidningen* 1996;93: 1219–1222 [in Swedish].

22. Proctor ML, Farquhar C, Kennedy S, Jin X. Transcutaneous electrical nerve stimulation and acupuncture for the treatment of primary dysmenorrhoea (Protocol for a Cochrane Review). In: The Cochrane Library, Issue 4, 2001. Oxford: Update Software.

23. Helms JM. Acupuncture for the management of primary dysmenorrhea. *Obstet Gynecol* 1987;69: 51–56.

24. Chesney MA, Tasto DL. The effectiveness of behavior modification with spasmodic and congestive dysmenorrhea. *Behav Res Ther* 1975; 13:245–253.

25. Israel RG, Sutton M, O'Brien KF. Effects of aerobic training on primary dysmenorrhea symptomatology in college females. *J Am Coll Health* 1985;33: 241–244.

26. Proctor ML, Murphy PA, Pattison HM, Farquhar CM. Behavioural interventions for primary and secondary dysmenorrhoea (Protocol for a Cochrane Review). In: The Cochrane Library, Issue 4, 2001. Oxford: Update Software.

27. Proctor ML, Hing W, Johnson TC, Murphy PA. Spinal manipulation for primary and secondary dysmenorrhoea. In: The Cochrane Library, Issue 4, 2001. Oxford: Update Software. Search date 2000; primary sources Medline, Embase, Cinahl, Psychlit, Bioabstracts, SPORTDiscus, Cochrane Controlled Trials Register, and hand searched citation lists.

28. Proctor ML, Murphy PA. Herbal and dietary therapies for primary and secondary

dysmenorrhoea. In: The Cochrane Library, Issue 4, 2001. Oxford: Update Software. Search date 2000; Medline, Embase, Cinahl, Psychlit, Bioabstracts, Cochrane Controlled Trials Register, and hand searched citation lists.

29. Deutch B, Jorgensen EB, Hansen JC. Menstrual discomfort in Danish women reduced by dietary supplements of omega-3 PUFA and B12 (fish oil or seal oil capsules). *Nutrition Research* 2000;20: 621–631.

30. Barnard ND, Scialli AR, Hurlock D, Bertron P. Diet and sex-hormone binding globulin, dysmenorrhea, and premenstrual symptoms. *Obstet Gynecol* 2000;95:245–250.

Michelle Proctor
Cochrane Review Group Co-ordinator

Cynthia Farquhar
Associate Professor
School of Medicine
University of Auckland
Auckland
New Zealand

Competing interests: None declared.

TABLE 1	**Prevalence of dysmenorrhoea: results of community and hospital surveys (see text, p 367).[3–8]**

Study population	Population size	Location	Year	Prevalence
College students aged 17–19 years[3]	165	USA	1996	72% (13% severe)
High school students aged 14–21 years[4]	291	Canada	1997	93% (5% severe)
Adolescents attending an inner city family planning clinic[5]	308	USA	1992	80% (18% severe)
Women from an urban population aged 19 years[6]	596	Sweden	1982	73% (15% severe)
Students aged 12–24 years[7]	1066	Mexico	1998	52–64%
Adolescents aged 12–17 years[8]	2699	USA	1981	60% (14% severe)

TABLE 2 Effects of aspirin, paracetamol, and compound analgesics for dysmenorrhoea: results of a systematic review (see text, p 368).[11]

Comparison	Usual dosage	Number of RCTs	Number of women	Pain relief	Adverse effects	Conclusion
Aspirin v placebo	650 mg four times daily	8	486	RR 1.60 (95% CI 1.12 to 2.29)	More frequent on aspirin (7–17% v 3–17% on placebo; RR 1.3, 95% CI 0.79 to 2.17)	Aspirin more effective than placebo (NNT 10, 95% CI 5 to 50)
Aspirin v paracetamol	650 mg v 500 mg four times daily	1	35	Median pain relief: paracetamol 1.6 (95% CI 0.4 to 3.3); aspirin 1.2 (95% CI 0 to 2.7)	NA	No significant difference
Aspirin v naproxen	650 mg v 275 mg four times daily	1	32	RR 2.29 (95% CI 1.16 to 4.29)	NA	Naproxen more effective than aspirin
Aspirin v ibuprofen	650 mg v 400 mg four times daily	1	56	RR 1.9 (95% CI 1.13 to 2.78)	NA	Ibuprofen more effective than placebo
Paracetamol v placebo	500 mg four times daily	1	35	RR 1.00 (95% CI 0.28 to 3.63)	No significant difference (RR 1.00, 95% CI 0.36 to 2.75)	No significant difference
Paracetamol v ibuprofen	1000 mg v 400 mg three times daily	1	67	RR 0.86 (95% CI 0.68 to 1.10)	NA	No significant difference
Co-proxamol v placebo	650 mg/65 mg four times daily	1	72	RR 3.72 (95% CI 2.13 to 6.52)	NA	Co-proxamol more effective than placebo
Co-proxamol v naproxen	650 mg/65 mg v 275 mg three times daily	2	98	P > 0.05 (no other data could be obtained from the report)	More frequent on co-proxamol (23–58% v 15–25% on naproxen; RR 1.94, 95% CI 1.11 to 3.41)	No significant difference
Co-proxamo v mefenamic acid	650 mg/65 mg v 500 mg three times daily	1	30	P < 0.01 (no other evidence can be obtained from the trial)	NA	Mefenamic acid more effective than co-proxamol

NA, not available.

INTERVENTIONS

Key Messages

- One RCT found that intravaginal nystatin versus placebo significantly reduced the proportion of women with a poor symptomatic response (NNT 3 after 1 week).

- Six RCTs have found that intravaginal imidazoles (e.g. clotrimazole) versus placebo reduce persistent symptoms of vulvovaginal candidiasis (NNT 3 after 1 month). Numerous RCTs have found no clear evidence that effects differ significantly among the various intravaginal imidazoles. RCTs have found no clear evidence of any difference between shorter and longer durations of treatment (1–14 days). RCTs have found an increased frequency of mild vulvar irritation with intravaginal imidazoles compared with oral treatments.

- We found no RCTs of oral fluconazole versus placebo or no treatment. A systematic review has found no significant reduction of symptoms of vulvovaginal candidiasis with oral fluconazole versus intravaginal imidazoles. RCTs have found that fluconazole is associated with increased frequency of mild nausea, headache, and abdominal pain.

- One RCT found that oral itraconazole versus placebo significantly reduced persistent symptoms. No significant difference in the reduction of persistent symptoms was found between oral itraconazole and intravaginal imidazoles. An RCT found increased mild gastrointestinal adverse effects with itraconazole versus intravaginal imidazole.

Vulvovaginal candidiasis

- We found no RCT of oral ketoconazole versus placebo or no treatment. Four RCTs have found no significant difference in the reduction of persistent symptoms between oral ketoconazole and intravaginal imidazoles, but ketoconazole significantly increased the frequency of minor adverse events (mainly nausea). Case reports have associated ketoconazole with a low risk of serious fulminant hepatitis.

- Two RCTs found no clear evidence that treating a woman's male sexual partner significantly improved resolution of the woman's acute vulvovaginal candidiasis symptoms, or reduced the rate of symptomatic relapse.

- Two RCTs of regular prophylaxis with intravaginal imidazole versus placebo found inconsistent effects on the proportion of women with symptomatic relapse. One RCT found that regular prophylactic intravaginal imidazole versus treatment only at the onset of symptoms reduced the frequency of episodes of symptomatic vaginitis, but the difference was not significant. The RCTs were too small to exclude a clinically important benefit.

- One RCT found a significantly reduced recurrence of vulvovaginal candidiasis with oral itraconazole versus placebo. We found no good evidence about oral itraconazole versus intravaginal imidazoles.

- One RCT found that oral ketoconazole, given either intermittently or continuously at a lower dose, significantly reduced symptomatic recurrences compared with placebo.

DEFINITION Vulvovaginal candidiasis is symptomatic vaginitis (inflammation of the vagina), which often involves the vulva, caused by infection with a *Candida* yeast. Predominant symptoms are vulvar itching and abnormal vaginal discharge (which may be minimal, a "cheese like" material, or a watery secretion). Differentiation from other forms of vaginitis requires the presence of yeast on microscopy of vaginal fluid. The definition of recurrent vulvovaginal candidiasis varies among RCTs, but is commonly defined as four or more symptomatic episodes a year.[1] This summary excludes studies of asymptomatic women with vaginal colonisation by *Candida* species.

INCIDENCE/ PREVALENCE Vulvovaginal candidiasis is the second most common cause of vaginitis (after bacterial vaginosis). Estimates of its incidence are limited, and often derived from women attending hospital clinics. At least one episode of vulvovaginal candidiasis occurs during the lifetime of 50–75% of all women. About half of the women who have an episode develop recurrent vulvovaginal candidiasis.[2] Vulvovaginal candidiasis is diagnosed in 5–15% of women attending sexually transmitted disease and family planning clinics.[1]

AETIOLOGY/ RISK FACTORS *Candida albicans* accounts for 85–90% of vulvovaginal candidiasis infections. Development of symptomatic vulvovaginal candidiasis probably represents increased growth of yeast that previously colonised the vagina without causing symptoms. Risk factors for vulvovaginal candidiasis include pregnancy (RR 2–10), diabetes mellitus, and systemic antibiotics. The evidence that different types of contraceptives are risk factors is contradictory. The incidence of vulvovaginal candidiasis rises with initiation of sexual activity, but we found no direct evidence that vulvovaginal candidiasis is sexually transmitted.[3–5]

PROGNOSIS We found few descriptions of the natural history of untreated vulvovaginal candidiasis. Discomfort is the main complication, and can include pain while passing urine, or during sexual intercourse. Balanitis (see glossary, p 391) in male partners of women with vulvovaginal candidiasis can occur, but it is rare.

AIMS To alleviate symptoms with minimal adverse effects from treatment.

OUTCOMES Clinical cure rates, either measured in the short term (5–15 days) or medium term (3–6 wks) after treatment. The definition of clinical cure varies among RCTs but often includes both complete resolution of symptoms and negative culture of *Candida*.

METHODS *Clinical Evidence* search and appraisal November 2001. We included only those studies in which most recruits were from the target population (e.g. to answer the question for non-pregnant women we sought RCTs that excluded pregnant women or RCTs in which pregnant women represented < 20% of the recruits). Studies of women with HIV infection were excluded. Many RCTs excluded women with diabetes mellitus. Studies were included only if recruitment included only women with both symptoms of vaginal candidiasis and laboratory confirmation of candidal infection.

QUESTION **What are the effects of treatments for symptomatic vulvovaginal candidiasis in non-pregnant women**

OPTION **INTRAVAGINAL NYSTATIN**

One RCT found that intravaginal nystatin versus placebo significantly reduced the proportion of women with a poor symptomatic response (NNT 3 after 1 wk). One RCT found that intravaginal boric acid may reduce persistent symptoms more than intravaginal nystatin, but old case reports have described systemic toxicity from the use of intravaginal boric acid. We found limited evidence that intravaginal nystatin was less effective than intravaginal imidazoles at reducing persistent symptoms (NNH 4). We found no comparison of intravaginal nystatin versus oral fluconazole, itraconazole, or ketoconazole.

Benefits: **Versus placebo or no treatment:** We found no systematic review but found one RCT of nystatin versus placebo.[6] The RCT (double blind, 50 women) found that intravaginal nystatin (500 000 IU twice daily for 14 days) versus placebo significantly reduced the proportion of women with a symptomatic response categorised as "poor" (2/25 [8%] with nystatin v 10/25 [40%] with placebo; ARR 32%, 95% CI 8% to 56%; OR 0.18, 95% CI 0.05 to 0.65; NNT 3). **Versus antiseptics:** We found one systematic review (search date 1993, 1 RCT).[7] The RCT[8] identified by the review found that intravaginal nystatin (100 000 IU capsule once daily) versus intravaginal boric acid (600 mg capsule once daily) for 14 days significantly reduced the proportion of women with persistent symptoms or a positive culture 30 days after finishing treatment (14/50 [28%] with boric acid v 26/52 [50%] with nystatin; OR 0.40, 95% CI 0.18 to 0.89). **Versus intravaginal imidazoles:** See intravaginal imidazoles, p 384.

Harms: One RCT found no reports of adverse effects among 52 women using intravaginal nystatin.[6]

Comment: The *Clinical Evidence* search found no RCTs of nystatin versus placebo; the single RCT cited above[6] is the only published RCT supplied by the Medical Information Department of Bristol Myers Squibb after searching their internal database. We found no RCTs versus other antiseptics, such as gentian violet. The RCT of nystatin versus boric acid found minimal absorption of boric acid, but old case reports have described boron toxicity after intravaginal use.[9]

OPTION **INTRAVAGINAL IMIDAZOLES (CLOTRIMAZOLE, MICONAZOLE, ECONAZOLE, TIOCONAZOLE, BUTOCONAZOLE, TERCONAZOLE, FENTICONAZOLE, AND SERTACONAZOLE)**

Six RCTs have found that intravaginal imidazoles versus placebo reduce persistent symptoms of vulvovaginal candidiasis (NNT 3 after 1 month). Numerous RCTs found no clear evidence that effects differ significantly among the various intravaginal imidazoles. RCTs found no clear evidence of any difference in persistent symptoms between shorter and longer durations of treatment (1–14 days). RCTs have found an increased frequency of mild vulvar irritation with intravaginal imidazoles compared with oral treatments.

Benefits: **Versus placebo:** We found one systematic review (search date 1993[7], 3 RCTs[10–12]) and 3 additional RCTs (see web extra table A at www.clinicalevidence.com).[13–15] Four of the six RCTs found significant reduction of persistent symptoms of vaginal candidiasis 4 weeks after treatment with topical imidazoles versus placebo. One RCT found a non-significant reduction. The sixth RCT (99 women, performed in family practice in Denmark) found no benefit versus placebo, but the follow up rate was low (62/99 [64%]). Overall, we found that intravaginal imidazoles versus placebo significantly reduced persistent symptoms of vaginal candidiasis in the medium term (6 RCTs: 131/392 [33%] with imidazoles v 98/141 [70%] with placebo; OR 0.16, 95% CI 0.04 to 0.60 calculated with a random effects model; see comment below (see web extra figure A at www.clinicalevidence.com). **Versus nystatin:** We found one systematic review (search date 1993, no RCTs)[7] and two additional small RCTs that reported clinical outcomes.[16,17] The first RCT (212 women) compared intravaginal miconazole, clotrimazole, econazole, and nystatin.[16] It found significantly lower symptomatic relapse over 6 months with intravaginal imidazoles versus nystatin (52/167 [31%] with imidazoles v 26/45 [58%] with nystatin; OR 0.32, 95% CI 0.16 to 0.63; NNT 4). The second RCT[17] (70 women) found no significant difference in the proportion of women with persistent symptoms with clotrimazole (100 mg for 14 days) versus high strength nystatin vaginal cream (1 million IU, once daily for 7 days) after 4 weeks (2/33 [6%] with nystatin v 1/37 [3%] with clotrimazole; OR 2.24, 95% CI 0.23 to 22.40). **Versus other imidazoles:** We found one systematic review[7] (search date 1993, 12 RCTs [10,11,18–27]) and 22 additional RCTs (see web extra table B at www.clinicalevidence.com).[17,28-48] Many of the RCTs were too small to exclude clinically important differences. Pooling of the results is difficult because the outcomes vary among the RCTs. The populations selected by each RCTs vary considerably in the prevalence of prognostic risk factors (such as diabetes mellitus or a history of recurrent attacks in the previous year). Together, these RCTs provide no clear evidence of any consistent difference in effectiveness among the different imidazoles. **Duration of treatment:** We found one systematic review (search date 1993, 13 RCTs)[7] and 9 additional RCTs that compared regimens using the same imidazole but for different durations.[11,18,20,24,49-64] These RCTs found no consistent differences in the proportion of women with persistent symptoms, but they were also too small to establish or exclude clinically important differences.

Harms: In the RCTs of intravaginal imidazoles versus placebo, most women did not report any adverse events.[10-15] The commonest adverse event was vulvar irritation. Most RCTs did not report frequencies of specific adverse events with placebo. In one RCT, adverse events were more common in the group of women taking a placebo tablet than among the group using intravaginal imidazole (1 episode of irritation in 23 women using imidazole v 9 adverse events [mainly nausea and headache] in 22 women receiving oral placebo).[12]

Comment: Most RCTs were small and many had weak methods (poorly described randomisation, inadequate concealment and blinding, definitions of cure based on mycology results rather than symptoms). We excluded all RCTs that defined cure only on the basis of mycology results. The RCT that found no benefit with intravaginal clotrimazole versus placebo caused significant heterogeneity of the results (see web extra figure A at www.clinicalevidence.com).

OPTION	ORAL FLUCONAZOLE

We found no RCTs of oral fluconazole versus placebo or no treatment. A systematic review has found no significant difference with oral fluconazole versus intravaginal imidazoles in the symptoms of vulvovaginal candidiasis. RCTs have found that fluconazole is associated with increased frequency of mild nausea, headache, and abdominal pain (NNH 11 after 14 days).

Benefits: **Oral fluconazole versus placebo:** We found no systematic review and no RCTs. **Versus intravaginal nystatin:** We found no RCTs. **Versus intravaginal imidazoles:** We found one systematic review (search date 2000, 6 RCTs, 947 women), which found no significant difference with oral fluconazole versus intravaginal imidazoles (clotrimazole, miconazole, econazole) in persistent symptoms in the short term (124/627 [20%] with oral fluconazole v 121/620 [20%] with intravaginal imidazole; OR 1.00, 95% CI 0.75 to 1.33) or in the medium term (74/432 [17%] v 71/404 [18%]; OR 0.96, 95% CI 0.67 to 1.37).[65] No significant differences were found in any of the subgroup analyses (with different imidazoles, or with single or multiple doses of treatment). For example, three RCTs of oral fluconazole versus intravaginal clotrimazole found no reduction in the persistence of symptoms in the medium term (43/220 [20%] with fluconazole v 40/218 [18%] with topical clotrimazole; OR 1.10, 95% CI 0.68 to 1.79).

Harms: Large RCTs have found that fluconazole is associated with nausea, headache, and abdominal pain.[66–69] In one RCT (429 women) of oral fluconazole versus intravaginal clotrimazole, adverse events were more common with fluconazole (59/217 [27%] with fluconazole v 37/212 [17%]; OR 1.75, 95% CI 1.11 to 2.75; NNH 11 after 14 days).[66] The individual events that were more common with fluconazole were headache (12% v 9%), abdominal pain (7% v 3%), and nausea (4% v 0%). Another RCT (235 women) found that nausea and other gastrointestinal symptoms were significantly more common with fluconazole than with intravaginal econazole (9/121 [7%] v 2/114 [2%]; OR 3.55, 95% CI 1.06 to 11.90) but local vulvar burning and increased vaginal discharge were significantly more common with intravaginal econazole (3/121 [2%] v 25/114 [22%]; OR 0.16, 95% CI 0.07 to 0.35).[67] A third RCT (369 women) found very few adverse events with either fluconazole or clotrimazole (8/188 [4%] v 9/181 [5%]).[68] A fourth RCT (183 women) found that nausea was reported by similar proportions with oral fluconazole versus oral ketoconazole (9/92 [10%] with fluconazole v 13/91 [14%] with ketoconazole).[69]

Comment: We found no evidence of a difference in symptom reduction with oral fluconazole versus intravaginal imidazole, but found evidence that gastrointestinal adverse events are significantly more likely with fluconazole. This is insufficient evidence to conclude that fluconazole is effective compared with placebo. Indirect evidence of the likely effectiveness of oral fluconazole versus placebo can be derived by convoluting the effects for fluconazole versus imidazoles with the effect for imidazoles versus placebo: this gives an indirect estimate, which suggests that fluconazole versus placebo is likely to be effective (calculated OR 0.11, 95% CI 0.03 to 0.41).

OPTION   **ORAL ITRACONAZOLE**

One RCT found that oral itraconazole versus placebo significantly reduced persistent symptoms (NNT 4 after 1 wk). No significant difference in the reduction of persistent symptoms was found between oral itraconazole and intravaginal imidazoles.

Benefits: **Versus oral placebo:** We found one systematic review (search date 2000, 1 RCT[12], 90 women).[65] The RCT found that oral itraconazole (200 mg daily for 3 days) versus placebo significantly reduced the proportion of women with persistent symptoms in the short term (13/48 [27%] with itraconazole v 12/22 [55%] with placebo; ARR 27%, 95% CI 33% to 52%; OR 0.31, 95% CI 0.11 to 0.88; NNT 4). **Versus intravaginal nystatin:** We found no RCTs. **Versus intravaginal imidazoles:** We found one systematic review (search date 2000, 3 RCTs, 300 women), which found no significant difference with oral itraconazole versus intravaginal imidazoles (clotrimazole, econazole) in persistent symptoms in the short term (3 RCTs: 39/162 [24%] with itraconazole v 36/138 [26%] with imidazoles; OR 0.83, 95% CI 0.49 to 1.43) or in the medium term (2 RCTs: 15/74 with itraconazole v 12/54 with imidazoles; OR 0.81, 95% CI 0.34 to 1.94).[65]

Harms: One RCT found that itraconazole versus clotrimazole significantly increased adverse events (17/50 [34%] with itraconazole v 1/23 [4%] with clotrimazole; OR 4.83, 95% CI 1.55 to 15.1); the events with increased frequency were nausea (14%), headache (12%), dizziness (6%), and bloating (6%).[12] However, a second RCT (double blind, 81 women) found similar numbers of adverse events with oral itraconazole versus intravaginal econazole (4/40 [10%] with itraconazole v 8/41 [20%] with econazole; OR 0.48, 95% CI 0.14 to 1.61).[70]

Comment: The evidence suggests that oral itraconazole and intravaginal imidazoles have similar effects on the symptoms of vaginal candidiasis, but itraconazole has more gastrointestinal adverse effects.

| OPTION | ORAL KETOCONAZOLE |

We found no RCT of oral ketoconazole versus placebo or versus no treatment. Four RCTs have found no significant difference with oral ketoconazole versus intravaginal imidazoles in the reduction of persistent symptoms, but found that ketoconazole significantly increased the frequency of minor adverse events (mainly nausea). Case reports have associated ketoconazole with a low risk of serious fulminant hepatitis.

Benefits: **Versus oral placebo:** We found no systematic review or RCT. **Versus intravaginal nystatin:** We found no RCTs. **Versus intravaginal imidazoles:** We found one systematic review (search date 1993, 4 RCTs, 280 women)[7] and three additional RCTs (see web extra table C at www.clinicalevidence.com).[71–73] The systematic review concluded that oral treatment is as effective as topical treatment at eliminating *Candida*, but did not compare clinical outcomes. One additional RCT (140 women) found that oral ketoconazole (400 mg daily for 5 days) versus intravaginal isoconazole (600 mg daily for 5 days) significantly increased persistent symptoms 1 week after treatment (34/64 [53%] with ketoconazole v 11/68 [16%] with isoconazole; ARI 37%, 95% CI 21% to 53%; OR 5.11, 95% CI 2.50 to 10.50) and 1 month after treatment (17/59 [29%] with ketoconazole v 8/61 [13%] with isoconazole; ARI 16%, 95% CI 12% to 30%; OR 2.60, 95% 1.07 to 6.18). Another additional RCT (unblinded, 151 women) recruited women with acute vulvovaginal candidiasis and a history of recurrent attacks (3 or more acute attacks in the previous year).[73] It found that oral ketoconazole (400 mg daily for 14 days) versus intravaginal clotrimazole (100 mg daily for 7 days) had similar rates of recurrent symptomatic relapse after 4 weeks (11/55 [20%] with ketoconazole v 15/57 [26%] with clotrimazole; OR 0.70, 95% CI 0.29 to 1.69). On pooling the results of the 5 RCTs[71–75] that report the number of women with persistent symptoms 1–5 weeks after treatment, we found no significant difference with ketoconazole versus intravaginal imidazole in the proportion of women with persistent symptoms (41/268 [15%] with ketoconazole v 30/211 [14%] with intravaginal imidazoles; OR 1.26, 95% CI 0.52 to 3.05) (see web extra figure B at www.clinicalevidence.com). **Versus oral itraconazole:** We found no systematic review and no RCT. **Versus oral fluconazole:** We found one systematic review (search date 1993[7], 1 RCT[69], 183 women). The RCT found no significant difference with ketoconazole (400 mg daily for 5 days) versus fluconazole (1 dose of 150 mg) in the proportion of women with persistent symptoms after 5–16 days (17/72 [24%] with ketoconazole v 17/80 [21%] with fluconazole; OR 1.15, 95% CI 0.53 to 2.45) or after 27–62 days (14/72 [19%] with ketoconazole v 14/76 [18%] with fluconazole; OR 1.07, 95% CI 0.47 to 2.43).

Harms: In the RCTs, mild adverse effects (nausea, fatigue, headaches, or abdominal pain) were more common with oral ketoconazole than with intravaginal imidazole (3/70 [4%] v 0/70[72]; 0/25 v 0/25[71]; 5/20 [25%] v 1/20 [5%][75]; 3/56 [5%] v 2/47 [4%][76]; overall OR 3.21, 95% CI 1.08 to 9.55) (see web extra figure C at www.clinicalevidence.com). One RCT (151 women) found that ketoconazole versus intravaginal clotrimazole increased rates of headache (23% v 4%), nausea (22% v 1%), abdominal discomfort (14% v 7%), and fatigue (7% v 2%).[73] Minor adverse events were not increased with ketoconazole versus fluconazole (13/91 [14%] v 9/92 [10%]).[69] Observational studies have found that asymptomatic elevation of liver enzymes is common, and fulminant hepatitis was observed in about 1/12 000 courses of treatment with oral ketoconazole.[77]

Comment: In women with uncomplicated vulvovaginal candidiasis, ketoconazole and intravaginal imidazoles have similar effects on persistent symptoms. The possibility of rare but serious hepatitis has led to a consensus that the risks associated with oral ketoconazole may outweigh its benefits in this group of women.

| OPTION | EFFECTS OF TREATING A MALE SEXUAL PARTNER |

Two RCTs found no significant difference with treating versus not treating a woman's male sexual partner in the resolution of the woman's acute vulvovaginal candidiasis symptoms, or in the rate of symptomatic relapse.

Benefits: We found no systematic review but found two RCTs.[78,79] In the first RCT (40 women with acute vulvovaginal candidiasis and their male partners), all the women received itraconazole (100 mg daily for 5 days). Their male partners were randomised to itraconazole (100 mg daily for 5 days) versus placebo. Participants and clinicians were blind to treatment allocation. The RCT found no difference between treating the male partner with itraconazole versus placebo in the number of women with persistent symptoms after 30 days (2/19 [11%] with itraconazole v 4/18 [22%] with placebo; OR 0.43, 95% CI 0.08 to 2.43).[78] The second RCT (117 women with vaginal candidiasis, and their male partners) treated the women with ketoconazole (200–600 mg daily for 3 days) and the male partners were randomised to ketoconazole (400 mg daily) versus placebo for 3 days. The participants and clinicians were blind to treatment allocation. The RCT found no difference in the proportion of women cured 1 week after treatment (48/57 [84%] with partners receiving ketoconazole v 53/60 [88%] with partners receiving placebo; OR 0.71, 0.25 to 2.02; see comment below, or the proportion of initially cured women who relapsed by 4 weeks after treatment (13/48 [27%] with ketoconazole v 19/53 [36%] with placebo; OR 0.67, 95% CI 0.29 to 1.54).[79]

Harms: The RCTs did not report evidence about harms.[78,79]

Comment: The women recruited in the RCTs were not selected because of a history of recurrent vulvovaginal candidiasis. The definition of "cured" and "relapsed" in the second RCT is not clear, but seems to be some combination of improved symptoms and negative cultures. Only a small number of men had any penile symptoms, and these were distributed equally between the ketoconazole and placebo groups. We found no clear evidence that treating male sexual partners influences the recovery of women's vulvovaginal candidiasis. However, the confidence intervals are wide even after pooling the 30 day outcomes from both RCTs (OR 0.85, 95% CI 0.40 to 1.80);[78,79] therefore the evidence is insufficient to establish or to exclude clinically important benefits or harms.

| QUESTION | What are the effects of preventive treatments in non-pregnant women with recurrent vulvovaginal candidiasis |

| OPTION | INTRAVAGINAL IMIDAZOLE |

Two RCTs of regular prophylaxis with intravaginal imidazole versus placebo found inconsistent effects on the proportion of women with symptomatic relapse. Another RCT found that regular prophylactic intravaginal imidazole versus treatment only at the onset of symptoms reduced the frequency of episodes of symptomatic vaginitis, but the difference was not significant. The RCTs were too small to exclude a clinically important reduction.

Benefits: **Versus placebo:** We found one systematic review (search date 1993, 2 RCTs, 89 women with recurrent vulvovaginal candidiasis).[7] The RCTs compared intravaginal clotrimazole (500 mg each month) versus intravaginal placebo (monthly). Both RCTs found that prophylaxis versus placebo reduced the proportion of women with symptomatic relapse, although in one RCT the difference was significant and in the other RCT it was not. On pooling the results, we found no difference with regular prophylaxis versus placebo in the proportion of women with symptomatic relapse (18/48 [38%] with prophylaxis v 31/41 [76%] with placebo; OR [random effects meta-analysis] 0.23, 95% CI 0.05 to 1.12). **Regular prophylactic treatment versus as required treatment:** We found one crossover RCT (unblinded, 23 women with recurrent vaginal candidiasis), which found that regular intravaginal clotrimazole (500 mg each month) versus empirical treatment (clotrimazole 500 mg at the onset of symptoms) reduced the number of symptomatic episodes of vaginitis over 6 months, but the result was not significant (2.2 episodes per person with regular treatment v 3.7 with empirical treatment; P = 0.05).[80] Women used significantly more clotrimazole during the 6 month prophylactic period (7.3 doses of clotrimazole per woman v 3.6 doses of empirical treatment; P < 0.001). In the RCT, significantly more women preferred empirical treatment than prophylactic treatment (74% v 17%).

Harms: See harms of intravaginal imidazoles, p 384.

Comment: One RCT defined recurrent vaginal candidiasis as greater than four proven episodes of candidal vaginitis in the previous year.[80] All three RCTs found that prophylaxis reduces the risk of symptomatic recurrence, but the RCTs were too small to establish or exclude a clinically important reduction.

| OPTION | ORAL FLUCONAZOLE |

We found no evidence about fluconazole and the prevention of recurrent vulvovaginal candidiasis.

Benefits: We found no systematic review and no RCTs.

Harms: We found no evidence.

Comment: None.

| OPTION | ORAL ITRACONAZOLE |

One RCT in women with vulvovaginal candidiasis found that oral itraconazole versus placebo significantly reduced the rate of recurrence (NNT 4 over 6 months). We found no good evidence about oral itraconazole versus intravaginal clotrimazole.

Benefits: We found no systematic review. **Oral itraconazole versus placebo:** One RCT (single blind, 114 women with recurrent vulvovaginal candidiasis)[81] found that oral itraconazole (400 mg monthly) versus placebo significantly reduced recurrence of vulvovaginal candidiasis symptoms (recurrence during 6 months' follow up: 20/55 [36%] with itraconazole v 34/53 [64%] with placebo; ARR 28%, 95% CI 9% to 47%; OR 0.33, 95% CI 0.16 to 0.71; NNT 4). After discontinuation of itraconazole, recurrence rates were similar.[81] **Intermittent oral itraconazole versus intravaginal imidazoles:** We found one RCT (unblinded, 44 women)[82] comparing weekly itraconazole (200 mg twice weekly) versus intravaginal clotrimazole (200 mg twice weekly) for 6 months. One woman withdrew from itraconazole treatment and five withdrew from clotrimazole treatment. It found that oral itraconazole versus intravaginal clotrimazole increased the proportion of women with symptomatic recurrences over 6 months (see comment below); 7/21 [33%] with itraconazole v 0/17 with clotrimazole.[82]

Harms: The first RCT did not report details of any adverse events (see oral itraconazole, p 386).[81]

Comment: The evidence of one RCT suggests that, compared with placebo, oral itraconazole is likely to reduce recurrent symptomatic vaginitis. The results of the comparison between oral itraconazole and intravaginal clotrimazole are difficult to interpret because the study was unblinded, and because the unbalanced withdrawal from the RCT could explain the observed difference between groups.

| OPTION | ORAL KETOCONAZOLE |

One RCT found that oral ketoconazole, given intermittently or continuously at a lower dose versus placebo significantly reduced the rate of symptomatic recurrence (NNT 2–3). This benefit is associated with an increased risk of harms.

Benefits:
Versus placebo or no treatment: We found one systematic review (search date 1993, 1 RCT, 63 women).[7] The RCT (74 women) compared intermittent oral ketoconazole (400 mg daily for 5 days of each menstrual cycle) versus low dose ketoconazole (100 mg daily for 6 months) versus placebo over 6 months.[83] The RCT found that intermittent oral ketoconazole versus placebo reduced symptomatic recurrence of vulvovaginal candidiasis over 6 months (6/21 [29%] with intermittent ketoconazole v 15/21 [71%] with placebo; OR 0.19, 95% CI 0.06 to 0.62; NNT 3) and with continuous ketoconazole versus placebo (1/21 [5%] with continuous ketoconazole; OR 0.06, 95% CI 0.02 to 0.22; NNT 2).
Versus intravaginal imidazoles: We found no systematic review and no RCTs.

Harms:
Ketoconazole is associated with an increased frequency of gastrointestinal adverse effects and case reports of rare fulminant hepatitis (see ketoconazole, p 387).

Comment:
The adverse effects of ketoconazole and no good evidence of increased benefit compared with safer alternatives, has led to a consensus that ketoconazole is likely to be harmful compared with those alternatives.

GLOSSARY

Balanitis Balanitis is inflammation of the glans of the penis. The foreskin is often involved (balanoposthitis).

REFERENCES

1. Sobel JD. Vulvovaginal candidiasis. In: Holmes KK MP-A, Sparling PF, Lemon SM, Stamm WE, Piot P, Wasserheit JN, eds. *Sexually transmitted diseases.* 3rd ed. New York: McGraw-Hill, 1999: 629–639.
2. Sobel JD, Faro S, Force RW, et al. Vulvovaginal candidiasis: epidemiologic, diagnostic, and therapeutic considerations. *Am J Obstet Gynecol* 1998;178:203–211.
3. Foxman B. The epidemiology of vulvovaginal candidiasis: risk factors. *Am J Public Health* 1990; 80:329–331.
4. Geiger AM, Foxman B, Sobel JD. Chronic vulvovaginal candidiasis: characteristics of women with *Candida albicans*, *C glabrata* and no *Candida*. *Genitourin Med* 1995;71:304–307.
5. Geiger AM, Foxman B, Gillespie BW. The epidemiology of vulvovaginal candidiasis among university students. *Am J Public Health* 1995;85: 1146–1148.
6. Isaacs JH. Nystatin vaginal cream in monilial vaginitis. *Illinois Med J* 1973;3:240–241.
7. Reef SE, Levine WC, McNeil MM, et al. Treatment options for vulvovaginal candidiasis, 1993. *Clin Infect Dis* 1995;20:S80–S90. Search date 1993; primary sources Medline and hand search of two textbooks.
8. Van Slyke KK, Michel VP, Rein MF. Treatment of vulvovaginal candidiasis with boric acid powder. *Am J Obstet Gynecol* 1981;141:145–148.
9. Valdes-Dapena MA, Arey JB. Boric acid poisoning: three fatal cases and a review of the literature. *J Paediatr* 1962;61:531.
10. Thomason JL, Gelbart SM, Kellett AV, Scaglione NJ, Gotwalt KT, Broekhuizen FF. Terconazole for the treatment of vulvovaginal candidiasis. *J Reprod Med* 1990;35:992–994.
11. Brown D Jr, Henzl MR, LePage ME, et al. Butoconazole vaginal cream in the treatment of vulvovaginal candidiasis: comparison with miconazole nitrate and placebo. *J Reprod Med* 1986;31:1045–1048.
12. Stein GE, Mummaw N. Placebo-controlled trial of itraconazole for treatment of acute vaginal candidiasis. *Antimicrob Agents Chemother* 1993;37:89–92.
13. Bro F. Single-dose 500-mg clotrimazole vaginal tablets compared with placebo in the treatment of *Candida vaginitis*. *J Fam Pract* 1990;31:148–152.
14. Fleury F, Hodgson C. Single-dose treatment of vulvovaginal candidiasis with a new 500mg clotrimazole vaginal tablet. *Adv Ther* 1984;1: 349–356.
15. Guess EA, Hodgson C. Single-dose topical treatment of vulvovaginal candidiasis with a new 500mg clotrimazole vaginal tablet. *Adv Ther* 1984; 1:137–145.
16. Dennerstein GJ, Langley R. Vulvovaginal candidiasis: treatment and recurrence. *Aust N Z J Obstet Gynaecol* 1982;22:231–233.

Vulvovaginal candidiasis

17. Cassar NL. High-potency nystatin cream in the treatment of vulvovaginal candidiasis. *Curr Ther Res* 1983;34:305–310.

18. Franklin R. Seven-day clotrimazole therapy for vulvovaginal candidiasis. *South Med J* 1978;71:141–143.

19. Corson SL, Kapikian RR, Nehring R. Terconazole and miconazole cream for treating vulvovaginal candidiasis. *J Reprod Med* 1991;36:561–567.

20. Kjaeldgaard A. Comparison of terconazole and clotrimazole vaginal tablets in the treatment of vulvovaginal candidosis. *Pharmatherapeutica* 1986;4:525–531.

21. Stein GE, Gurwith D, Mummaw N, Gurwith M. Single-dose tioconazole compared with 3-day clotrimazole treatment in vulvovaginal candidiasis. *Antimicrob Agents Chemother* 1986;29:969–971.

22. Kaufman RH, Henzl MR, Brown D Jr, et al. Comparison of three-day butoconazole treatment with seven-day miconazole treatment for vulvovaginal candidiasis. *J Reprod Med* 1989;34:479–483.

23. Droegemueller W, Adamson D G, Brown D. Three-day treatment with butoconazole nitrate for vulvovaginal candidiasis. *Obstet Gynecol* 1984;64:530–534.

24. Jacobson JB, Hajman AJ, Wiese J. A new vaginal antifungal agent – butoconazole nitrate. *Acta Obstet Gynecol Scand* 1985;64:241–244.

25. Hajman AJ. Vulvovaginal candidosis: comparison of 3-day treatment with 2% butoconazole nitrate cream and 6-day treatment of 1% clotrimazole cream. *J Int Med Res* 1988;16:367–375.

26. Adamson GD, Brown D Jr, Standard JV, Henzl MR. Three-day treatment with butoconazole vaginal suppositories for vulvovaginal candidiasis. *J Reprod Med Obstet Gynecol* 1986;31:131–132.

27. Bradbeer CS, Mayhew SR, Barlow D. Butaconazole and miconazole in treating vaginal candidiasis. *Genitourin Med* 1985;61:270–272.

28. Glasser A. Single-dose treatment of vaginal mycoses. Effectiveness of clotrimazole and econazole. *Fortschr Med* 1986;104:259–262.

29. Gastaldi A. Treatment of vaginal candidiasis with fenticonazole and miconazole. *Curr Ther Res Clin Exp* 1985;38:489–493.

30. Gabriel G, Thin RN. Clotrimazole and econazole in the treatment of vaginal candidosis. A single-blind comparison. *Br J Ven Dis* 1983;59:56–58.

31. Amrouni B, Pereiro M, Florez A, Pontes C, Izquierdo I, Toribio J. A phase III comparative study of the efficacies of flutrimazole versus clotrimazole for the treatment of vulvovaginal candidiasis. *J Mycol* 2000;10:62–65.

32. Arendt J. Terconazole versus clotrimazole cream in vulvovaginal candidiasis. *Adv Ther* 1989;6:287–294.

33. Gouveia DC, Jones Da Silva C. Oxiconazole in the treatment of vaginal candidiasis: single dose versus 3-day treatment with econazole. *Pharmatherapeutica* 1984;3:682–685.

34. Brewster E, Preti PM, Ruffmann R, Studd J. Effect of fenticonazole in vaginal candidiasis: a double-blind clinical trial versus clotrimazole. *J Int Med Res* 1986;14:306–310.

35. Balsdon M-J. Comparison of miconazole-coated tampons with clotrimazole vaginal tablets in the treatment of vaginal candidosis. *Br J Ven Dis* 1981;57:275–278.

36. Bradbeer CS, Thin RN. Comparison of econazole and isoconazole as single dose treatment for vaginal candidosis. *Genitourin Med* 1985;61:396–398.

37. Brown D Jr, Binder CL, Gardner HL, Wells J. Comparison of econazole and clotrimazole in the treatment of vulvovaginal candidiasis. *Obstet Gynecol* 1980;56:121–123.

38. Brown D, Henzl MR, Kaufman RH, et al. Butoconazole nitrate 2% for vulvovaginal candidiasis. *J Reprod Med* 1999;44:933–938.

39. Cohen L. Single dose treatment of vaginal candidosis: comparison of clotrimazole and isoconazole. *Br J Ven Dis* 1984;60:42–44.

40. Dellenbach P, Thomas J-L, Guerin V, Ochsenbein E, Contet-Audonneau N. Topical treatment of vaginal candidosis with sertaconazole and econazole sustained-release suppositories. *Int J Gynecol Obstet* 2000;71:S47–S42.

41. Wiest W, Azzollini E, Ruffmann R. Comparison of single administration with an ovule of 600 mg fenticonazole versus a 500 mg clotrimazole vaginal pessary in the treatment of vaginal candidiasis. *J Int Med Res* 1989;17:369–372.

42. Palacio-Hernanz A, Sanz-Sanz F, Rodriquez-Noriega A. Double-blind investigation of R-42470 (terconazole cream 0.4%) and clotrimazole (cream 1%) for the topical treatment of mycotic vaginitis. *Chemioterapia* 1984;3:192–195.

43. Lolis D, Kanellopoulos N, Liappas I, Xyngakis A, Zissis NP. Double-blind evaluation of miconazole tampons, compared with clotrimazole vaginal tablets, in vaginal candidiasis. *Clin Ther* 1981;4:212–216.

44. Studd JW, Dooley MM, Welch CC, et al. Comparative clinical trial of fenticonazole ovule (600 mg) versus clotrimazole vaginal tablet (500 mg) in the treatment of symptomatic vaginal candidiasis. *Curr Med Res Opin* 1989;11:477–484.

45. Herbold H. Comparative studies to the clinical efficacy of two 1-dose-therapies of vaginal candidosis. *Med Welt* 1985;36:255–257.

46. Lappin MA, Brooker DC, Francisco CA, Dorfman J. Effect of butoconazole nitrate 2% vaginal cream and miconazole nitrate 2% vaginal cream treatments in patients with vulvovaginal candidiasis. *Infect Dis Obstet Gynecol* 1996;4:323–328

47. Lebherz TB, Goldman L, Wiesmeier E, Mason D, Ford LC. A comparison of the efficacy of two vaginal creams for vulvovaginal candidiasis, and correlations with the presence of *Candida* species in the perianal area and oral contraceptive use. *Clin Ther* 1983;5:409–416.

48. Stettendorf S, Benijts G, Vignali M, Kreysing W. Three-day therapy of vaginal candidiasis with clotrimazole vaginal tablets and econazole ovules: a multicenter comparative study. *Chemotherapy* 1982;28:87–91.

49. Wolfson N, Samuels B, Hodgson C, Graves K. One-day management of vulvovaginal candidiasis. *J La State Med Soc* 1987;139:27–29.

50. Lebherz T, Guess E, Wolfson N. Efficacy of single-versus multiple-dose clotrimazole therapy in the management of vulvovaginal candidiasis. *Am J Obstet Gynecol* 1985;152:965–968.

51. Fleury F, Hughes D, Floyd, R. Therapeutic results obtained in vaginal mycoses after single-dose treatment with 500 mg clotrimazole vaginal tablets. *Am J Obstet Gynecol* 1985;152:968–970.

52. Loendersloot EW, Goormans E, Wiesenhaan PE, Barthel PJ, Branolte JH. Efficacy and tolerability of single-dose versus six-day treatment of candidal vulvovaginitis with vaginal tablets of clotrimazole. *Am J Obstet Gynecol* 1985;152:953–955.

53. Wolfson N, Samuels B, Riley J. A three-day treatment regimen for vulvovaginal candidiasis. *J La State Med Soc* 1982;134:28–31.

54. Oates JK, Davidson F. Treatment of vaginal candidiasis with clotrimazole. *Postgrad Med J* 1974;50:99–102.

55. Lebherz TB, Ford LC, Kleinkopf V. A comparison of a three-day and seven-day clotrimazole regimen for vulvovaginal candidiasis. *Clin Ther* 1981;3: 344–348.

56. Robertson WH. Vulvovaginal candidiasis treated with clotrimazole cream in seven days compared with fourteen day treatment with miconazole cream. *Am J Obstet Gynecol* 1978;132:321–323.

57. Pasquale SA, Lawson J, Sargent EC Jr, Newdeck JP. A dose–response study with Monistat cream. *Obstet Gynecol* 1979;53:250–253.

58. Floyd R, Hodgson C. One-day treatment of vulvovaginal candidiasis with a 500-mg clotrimazole vaginal tablet compared with a three-day regimen of two 100-mg vaginal tablets daily. *Clin Ther* 1986;8:181–186.

59. Hughes D, Kriedman T, Hodgson C. Treatment of vulvovaginal candidiasis with a single 500-mg clotrimazole vaginal tablet compared with two 100-mg tablets daily for three days. *Curr Ther Res Clin Exp* 1986;39:773–777.

60. Mizuno S, Cho N. Clinical evaluation of three-day treatment of vaginal mycosis with clotrimazole vaginal tablets. *J Int Med Res* 1983;11:179–185.

61. Milsom I, Forssman L. Treatment of vaginal candidosis with a single 500-mg clotrimazole pessary. *Br J Ven Dis* 1982;58:124–126.

62. Westphal J. Treatment of *Candida mycoses* of the vulva and vagina with clotrimazole. Comparison of single-dose and six-day therapy. *Fortschr Med* 1988;106:445–448.

63. Upmalis DH, Cone FL, Lamia CA, et al. Single-dose miconazole nitrate vaginal ovule in the treatment of vulvovaginal candidiasis: two single-blind, controlled studies versus miconazole nitrate 100mg cream for 7 days. *J Women's Health Gender-based Medicine.* 2000;9:421–429.

64. Wiest W, Ruffmann R. Short-term treatment of vaginal candidiasis with fenticonazole ovules: a three dose schedule comparative trial. *J Int Med Res* 1987;15:319–325.

65. Watson MC, Grimshaw JM, Bond CM, Mollison J, Ludbrook A. Oral versus intra-vaginal imidazole and triazole anti-fungal treatment of uncomplicated vulvovaginal candidiasis (thrush). In: The Cochrane Library, Issue 4, 2001. Oxford: Update Software. Search date 2000, primary sources Cochrane Library, Medline, Embase, Cochrane Collaboration Sexually Transmitted Disease Group Specialised Register of Controlled Trials, hand search of reference lists, UK manufacturers of anti-fungals.

66. Sobel JD, Brooker D, Stein GE, et al. Single oral dose fluconazole compared with conventional clotrimazole topical therapy of *Candida vaginitis*. *Am J Obstet Gynecol* 1995;172:1263–1268.

67. Osser S, Haglund A, Weström L. Treatment of vaginal candidiasis: a prospective randomized investigator-blind multicenter study comparing topically applied econazole with oral fluconazole. *Acta Obstet Gynecol Scand* 1991;70:73–78.

68. Anon. A comparison of single-dose oral fluconazole with 3-day intravaginal clotrimazole in the treatment of vaginal candidiasis. *Br J Obstet Gynaecol* 1989;96:226–232.

69. Kutzer E, Oittner R, Leodolter S, Brammer KW. A comparison of fluconazole and ketoconazole in the oral treatment of vaginal candidiasis; report of a double-blind multicentre trial. *Eur J Obstet Gynecol Reprod Biol* 1988;29:305–313.

70. Timonen H, Hartikainen-Vahtera P, Kivijarvi A, et al. A double-blind comparison of the effectiveness of itraconazole oral capsules with econazole vaginal capsules in the treatment of vaginal candidosis. *Drug Invest* 1992;4:515–520.

71. Comninos A, Kapellakis I, Pikouli-Giannopoulou P, Manafi Th. Double-blind evaluation of ketoconazole comparatively with clotrimazole in vaginal candidiasis. *Curr Ther Res* 1984;36: 100–104.

72. Farkas B, Simon N. Ergebnisse einer Vergleichsstudie mit einem oral und einem lokal zu applizierenden Antimykotikum bei Vaginalmykosen. *Mykosen* 1984;27:554–561.

73. Sobel JD, Schmitt C, Stein G, Mummaw N, Christensen S, Meriwether C. Initial management of recurrent vulvovaginal candidiasis with oral ketoconazole and topical clotrimazole. *J Reprod Med* 1994;39:517–520.

74. Puolakka J, Tuimala R. Comparison between oral ketoconazole and topical miconazole in the treatment of vaginal candidiasis. *Acta Obstet Gynecol Scand* 1983;62:575–577.

75. Rohde-Werner H. Topical tioconazole versus systemic ketoconazole treatment of vaginal candidiasis. *J Int Med Res* 1984;12:298–302.

76. Bingham JS. Single blind comparison of ketoconazole 200 mg oral tablets and clotrimazole 100 mg vaginal tablets and 1% cream in treating acute vaginal candidosis. *Br J Ven Dis* 1984;60: 175–177.

77. Lake-Bakaar G. Scheuer PJ. Sherlock S. Hepatic reactions associated with ketoconazole in the United Kingdom. *BMJ* 1987;294:419–422.

78. Calderon-Marquez JJ. Itraconazole in the treatment of vaginal candidosis and the effect of treatment of the sexual partner. *Rev Inf Dis* 1987; 9:S143–S145.

79. Bisschop MP, Merkus JM, Scheygrond H, van Cutsem J. Co-treatment of the male partner in vaginal candidosis: a double-blind randomized control study. *Br J Obstet Gynaecol* 1986;93: 79–81.

80. Fong IW. The value of prophylactic (monthly) clotrimazole versus empiric self-treatment in recurrent vaginal candidiasis. *Genitourin Med* 1994;70:124–126.

81. Spinillo A, Colonna L, Piazzi G, Baltaro F, Monaco A, Ferrari A. Managing recurrent vulvovaginal candidiasis. Intermittent prevention with itraconazole. *J Reprod Med* 1997;42:83–87.

82. Fong IW. The value of chronic suppressive therapy with itraconazole versus clotrimazole in women with recurrent vaginal candidiasis. *Genitourin Med* 1992;68:374–377.

83. Sobel JD. Recurrent vulvovaginal candidiasis. A prospective study of the efficacy of maintenance ketoconazole therapy. *N Engl J Med* 1986;315: 1455–1458.

84. Miller PI, Humphries M, Grassick K. A single-blind comparison of oral and intravaginal treatments in acute and recurrent vaginal candidosis in general practice. *Pharmatherapeutica* 1984;3:582–587.

Jeanne Marrazzo

Assistant Professor, Medicine

University of Washington, Seattle, USA

Competing interests: JM has received research funding from Pfizer Pharmaceuticals, the makers of Diflucan.

Note

When looking up a class of drug, the reader is advised to also look up specific examples of that class of drug where additional entries may be found. The reverse situation also applies. Abbreviations used: HIV, human immunodeficiency virus; HSV, herpes simplex virus; NSAIDs, non-steroidal anti-inflammatory drugs.

INDEX

Subject index

The number needed to treat: adjusting for baseline risk

Adapted with permission from Chatellier et al, 1996[1]

BACKGROUND

The number needed to treat (NNT) to avoid a single additional adverse outcome is a meaningful way of expressing the benefit of an active treatment over a control. It can be used both to summarise the results of a therapeutic trial or series of trials and to help medical decision making about an individual patient.

If the absolute risk of adverse outcomes in a therapeutic trial is ARC in the control group and ART in the treatment group, then the absolute risk reduction (ARR) is defined as (ARC − ART). The NNT is defined as the inverse of the ARR:

$$NNT = 1/(ARC - ART)$$

Since the Relative Risk Reduction (RRR) is defined as (ARC − ART)/ARC, it follows that NNT, RRR and ARC are related by their definitions in the following way:

$$NNT \times RRR \times ARC = 1$$

This relationship can be used to estimate the likely benefits of a treatment in populations with different levels of baseline risk (that is different levels of ARC). This allows extrapolation of the results of a trial or meta-analysis to people with different baseline risks. Ideally, there should be experimental evidence of the RRR in each population. However in many trials, subgroup analyses show that the RRR is approximately constant in groups of patients with different characteristics. Cook and Sackett therefore proposed that decisions about individual patients could be made by using the NNT calculated from the RRR measured in trials and the baseline risk in the absence of treatment estimated for the individual patient.[2]

The method may not apply to periods of time different to that studied in the original trials.

USING THE NOMOGRAM

The nomogram shown on the next page allows the NNT to be found directly without any calculation: a straight line should be drawn from the point corresponding to the estimated absolute risk for the patient on the left hand scale to the point corresponding to the relative risk reduction stated in a trial or meta-analysis on the central scale. The intercept of this line with the right hand scale gives the NNT. By taking the upper and lower limits of the confidence interval of the RRR, the upper and lower limits of the NNT can be estimated.

REFERENCES

1. Chatellier G, Zapletal E, Lemaitre D, Menard J, Degoulet P. The number needed to treat: a clinically useful nomogram in its proper context. *BMJ* 1996;321:426–429.
2. Cook RJ, Sackett DL. The number needed to treat: a clinically useful measure of treatment effect. *BMJ* 1995;310:452–454.

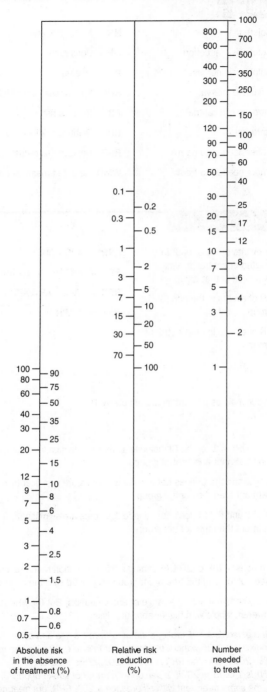

Absolute risk in the absence of treatment (%)	Relative risk reduction (%)	Number needed to treat

Abbreviations

AR	Absolute risk	**NS**	Not significant
ARR	Absolute risk reduction	**OR**	Odds ratio
ARI	Absolute risk increase	**P**	P value
CI	Confidence interval	**RCT**	Randomised controlled trial
CCT	Controlled clinical trial	**RR**	Relative risk
HR	Hazard ratio	**RRI**	Relative risk increase
NNH	Number needed to harm	**RRR**	Relative risk reduction
NNT	Number needed to treat	**WMD**	Weighted mean difference

How to calculate risk

AR = # events (good or bad) in treated or control groups/ # people in that group

ARC = AR of events in the control group

ART = AR of events in the treatment group

ARR = ARC − ART

RR = ART/ARC = 1 − RRR

RRR = (ARC − ART)/ARC = 1 − RR

NNT = 1/ARR

To express decimals as percentages, multiply by 100.

If:

the RR (or OR) = 1, or the CI includes 1, there is no significant difference between treatment and control groups

the RR > 1 and the CI does not include 1, events are significantly more likely in the treatment than the control group

the RR < 1 and the CI does not include 1, events are significantly less likely in the treatment than the control group

RR of 0.8 means a RRR of 20% (meaning a 20% reduction in the relative risk of the specified outcome in the treatment group compared with the control group).

RRR is usually constant across a range of absolute risks. But the ARR is higher and the NNT lower in people with higher absolute risks.

Example: If a person's AR of stroke, estimated from his age and other risk factors (see appendix 1), is 0.25 without treatment but falls to 0.20 with treatment, the ARR is 25% − 20% = 5%; the RRR is (25% − 20%)/25% = 20%; and the NNT is 1/0.05 = 20. In a person with an AR of stroke of only 0.025 without treatment, the same treatment will still produce a 20% RRR, but treatment will reduce her AR of stroke to 0.020, giving a much smaller ARR of 2.5% − 2% = 0.5%, and a NNT of 200.

The American Academy of Pediatrics and the UnitedHealth Foundation are pleased to provide you with this free copy of *Clinical Evidence Pediatrics.* This important resource supports you in your efforts to provide the best health care to your patients. Please take a few moments to answer the following questions to help us better serve you. Just drop the pre-addressed, postage paid card in any mailbox. Your input is valuable to us.

Position *(please mark one in each column)*

Type of Practice	Practice setting
☐ General pediatrics	☐ Pediatrician in practice
☐ Pediatric Subspecialty	☐ Academic medicine
☐ Other.............................	☐ Trainee
☐ Not in direct patient care	

1. How relevant is the content of this book to your practice?

1	2	3	4	5
very relevant				not at all relevant

2. How useful will this book be in your daily practice?

1	2	3	4	5
very useful				not at all useful

3. Comments about the content of the book:

   ....
   ....

4. Suggestions for future topics:

   ....
   ....

5. How likely would you be to purchase this book if that were the only way you could get it?

1	2	3	4	5
very likely				not at all likely

6. How likely are you to use this material on the website or download it to your handheld?

1	2	3	4	5
very likely				not at all likely

Optional:
Name:..
Address: ....
....
Email: ....

Please tear out and return card (no postage necessary) or send us your feedback on the website: www.clinicalevidence.com

For more information on UnitedHealth Foundation, please visit
their website at: **www.unitedhealthfoundation.org**

For more information on American Academy of Pediatrics please visit
their website at: **www.aap.org**